Obstetrics, Gynecology, AND Infertility

Handbook for Clinicians

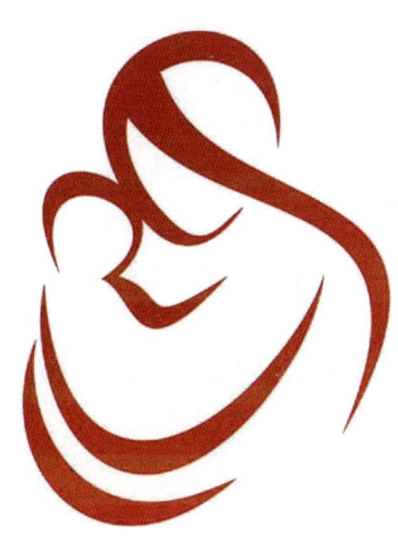

Obstetrics, Gynecology, and Infertility

Handbook for Clinicians
7th Edition

John David Gordon, MD
Co-Director Dominion Fertility Arlington, Virginia
Division Director, Reproductive Endocrinology and Infertility
Inova Fairfax Hospital Falls Church, VA
Clinical Associate Professor VCU School of Medicine

Jan T. Rydfors, MD
Clinical Adjunct Professor
Department of Obstetrics and Gynecology
Stanford University Medical Center
Stanford, California

Maurice L. Druzin, MD
Professor of Gynecology and Obstetrics
Vice Chairman
Department of Obstetrics and Gynecology
Stanford University Medical Center

Yona Tadir, MD
Professor of Obstetrics and Gynecology
Beckman Lase Institute and Medical Clinic
University of California, Irvine
Irvine, California

Yasser El-Sayed, MD
Director Division of Maternal-Fetal Medicine and Obstetrics
Stanford University
Obstetrician-in-Chief
Lucile Packard Children's Hospital Stanford

John Chan, MD
John A. Kerner Distinguished Professor in Gyn-Onc
Director, Division of Gynecologic Oncology
University of California, San Francisco
San Francisco, CA

Dan Israel Lebovic, MD, M.A.
Reproductive Endocrinologist
Center for Reproductive Medicine Minneapolis, MN
Adjunct Professor
University of Minnesota, Department of Obstetrics and Gynecology
Minneapolis, MN

Elizabeth Langen, MD
Clinical Assistant Professor
University of Michigan
Department of Obstetrics and Gynecology
Division of Maternal-Fetal Medicine

Katherine Fuh, MD
Assistant Professor
Division of Gynecologic Oncology
Department of Obstetrics and Gynecology
Washington University
St. Louis, MO

Technical and Computer Support:
Bill Gillespie
Director Emeritus of Computer Operations
Stanford University Medical Center

Scrub Hill Press, Inc.
Arlington, VA 22204
(800) 516-1088
www.scrubhill.com
Copyright © 2017 by Scrub Hill Press, Inc.

ISBN 978-0-9822921-5-0 Pocket Size
ISBN: 978-0-9822921-6-7 Desk Size

Printed in Canada.

All rights reserved. No part of this book may be reproduced, stored in a retrieval system, or transmitted in any form or by any means, electronic, mechanical, photocopying, recording, or otherwise, without written permission from the publisher, except for brief quotations embodied in critical articles and reviews.

The procedures and practices described in this publication should be implemented in a manner consistent with the professional standards set for the circumstances that apply in each specific situation. Every effort has been made to confirm the accuracy of the information presented and to correctly relate generally accepted practices. The authors, editors, and publisher cannot accept responsibility for errors or exclusions or for the outcome of the material presented herein. There is no expressed or implied warranty of this book or information imparted by it. Care has been taken to ensure that drug selection and dosages are in accordance with currently accepted/recommended practice. Off-label uses of drugs may be discussed. Due to continuing research, changes in government policy and regulations, and various effects of drug reactions and interactions, it is recommended that the reader carefully review all materials and literature provided for each drug, especially those that are new or are not frequently used. Some drugs or devices in this publication have clearance for use in a restricted research setting by the Food and Drug and Administration (FDA). Each professional should determine the FDA status of any drug or device prior to use in their practice.

Any review or mention of specific companies or products is not intended as an endorsement by the authors or publisher.

The opinions expressed in this book represent a broad range of opinions, including those of the authors and the volunteer clinical faculty of, but not limited to, the Department of Gynecology and Obstetrics at Stanford University. These opinions are not meant to represent a "standard of care" or a "protocol" but rather a guide to common clinical conditions. Use of these guidelines is obviously influenced by local factors, varying clinical circumstances, and honest differences of opinion.

Publisher: Scrub Hill Press, Inc.
Senior Editor: John David Gordon, MD
Director of Composition: Bill Klump, Scribe Inc. Philadelphia, PA
Cover Design: Rob Johnson

First Edition—1991
Second Edition—1993
Third Edition—1993
Fourth Edition—1995

Revised Fourth Edition—1997
Fifth Edition—2001
Sixth Edition—2007

Publisher's Cataloging-In-Publication Data
(Prepared by The Donohue Group, Inc.)

Names: Gordon, John D. (John David).
Title: Obstetrics, gynecology and infertility : handbook for clinicians / John David Gordon, M.D. [and 9 others].
Description: 7th edition. | Arlington, VA : Scrub Hill Press, Inc., [2016] | Includes bibliographical references and index.
Identifiers: LCCN 2016912399 | ISBN 978-0-9822921-5-0 (pocket size) | ISBN 978-0-9822921-6-7 (desk size)
Subjects: LCSH: Gynecology—Handbooks, manuals, etc. | Obstetrics—Handbooks, manuals, etc. | Infertility—Handbooks, manuals, etc.
Classification: LCC RG110 .O28 2016 | DDC 618—dc23

Library of Congress Control Number: 2016912399

3 4 5 6 7 8 9 10

This book is dedicated to H. Allison Smith, PhD She is my best friend, my loving wife, and the mother of our wonderful children.

JDG

The authors would like to thank all of the publishers and authors for their permission to reproduce various tables and figures in this book.

Advanced Technology Laboratories	Dr. John Bonnar
Advanstar Communications, Inc.	Dr. James Carter
The American College of Obstetricians and Gynecologists	Dr. Frank Chervenak
The American College of Surgeons	Dr. Steven Clark
The American Cancer Society	Dr. Robert Creasy
The American Society of Reproductive Medicine	Dr. Gary Cunningham
The American Heart Association	Dr. Richard Dorr
The American Medical Association	Dr. Arthur Fleischer
The Association of Professors of Gynecology and Obstetrics	Dr. Mark Glezerman
Churchill-Livingston	Dr. Leonard Gomella
Dowden Publishing Company	Dr. Neville Hacker
Elsevier Scientific	Dr. David Halbert
The Female Patient	Dr. Vaclav Insler
Johns Hopkins University Press	Dr. Sidney Joel-Cohen
The Journal of Reproductive Medicine	Dr. Howard Jones, III
Lippincott Williams & Wilkins	Dr. Bruno Lunenfield
The McGraw-Hill Companies	Dr. Fred Miyazaki
The New England Journal of Medicine	Dr. Keith Moore
OBG Management	Dr. John Rock
Oxford University Press	Dr. James Scott
Springer Verlag	Dr. Phillip Sarrel
Thieme Medical Publishers	Dr. Lourdes Scheerer
Wolters-Kluer	Dr. Leonard Speroff
W.B. Saunders	Dr. Richard Sweet
Dr. Emily Baker	Dr. Alan Trounson
Dr. Paul Barash	Dr. Frederick Zuspan
Dr. Arie Bergman	

Dr. Gordon extends his great appreciation to the following physicians for their contributions to this handbook since it was first published:

Dr. John Arpels	Dr. Ian Hardy	Dr. Mary Lake Polan
Dr. Sunil Balgobin	Dr. LeRoy Heinrichs	Dr. Michael Ross
Dr. Susan Ballagh	Dr. Hal Holbrook	Dr. Vicki Seltzer
Dr. Alvaro Cuadros	Dr. Michael Katz	Dr. Dennis Siegler
Dr. Usha Chitkara	Dr. Khoa Lai	Dr. Natalie Sohn
Dr. Babak Edraki	Dr. Emmet Lamb	Dr. Giuliana Songster
Dr. Gretchen Flanagan	Dr. Carl Levinson	Dr. Laurie Swaim
Dr. Linda Giudice	Dr. Jennifer Lublin	Dr. Nelson Teng
Dr. Clifford Goldstein	Dr. Amin Milki	Dr. Shirley Tom
Dr. David Grimes	Dr. Julie Neidich	
Dr. David Halbert	Dr. Katherine O'Hanlan	

Special thanks to the staff of the Inova Fairfax Hospital Medical Library for all of their assistance in retrieving articles.

CONTENTS

Preface to the 7th Edition xiii
Foreword to the 7th Edition xv

Chapter 1: Primary Care 1
Health Screening 1
Colon Cancer Screening 6
Nutrition 10
Body Mass Index 15
Cardiovascular Disease in Women 19
Hypercholesterolemia 21
Lipid Lowering Drugs 29
Hypertension 32
Diabetes Mellitus 38
Tobacco, Alcohol, and Drug Abuse 44
Migraine Headaches 47
Low Back Pain 51
Sinusitis 53
Alternative Medicine/Botanicals 55

Chapter 2: Obstetrics 59
Charting Pearls for Routine Obstetrical Visits 59
Nausea and Vomiting in Pregnancy 61
Nutritional Management during Pregnancy 66
Anemia in Pregnancy 67
Clinical Pelvimetry 69
Assessment of Gestational Age 71
Respiratory Distress Syndrome 72
Normal Labor and Delivery 74
Abnormal Labor and Induction of Labor 76
Shoulder Dystocia 84
Operative Vaginal Delivery 86
Cesarean Delivery 92
Vaginal Birth after Cesarean 100
Care of the Neonate 103
Antepartum Fetal Surveillance 105
Trauma in Pregnancy 112
Guidelines for Diagnostic Imaging in Pregnancy 114
Intrapartum Fetal Evaluation 117
Amnioinfusion 124
Abruptio Placentae 126
Placenta Previa 129
Postpartum Hemorrhage 132
Uterine Inversion 140
Cervical Insufficiency 142

CONTENTS

Preterm Labor 148
Periviable Birth 157
Preterm Premature Rupture of Membranes (PPROM) 159
Multiple Gestation 162
Intrauterine Growth Restriction 167
Asthma in Pregnancy 169
Maternal Heart Disease 172
Diabetes in Pregnancy 178
Hypertensive Disorders of Pregnancy 184
Intrauterine Fetal Demise 201
Nonimmune Hydrops 205
Isoimmunization 209
Systemic Lupus Erythematosus (SLE) and APS in Pregnancy 213
Thromboembolic Disorders 219
Thrombocytopenia in Pregnancy 225
Epilepsy in Pregnancy 227
Thyroid Disease in Pregnancy 230

Chapter 3: Genetics 239

Pan-Ethnic Carrier Screening or Extended Carrier Screening (ECS) 241
Ethnic-Specific Screening 242
Cystic Fibrosis 245
Fragile X 247
Spinal Muscular Atrophy 249
Hemoglobinopathies 251
Chromosome Abnormalities: In the Fetus 254
Genetic Testing 261
Neural Tube Defects 267
Teratogenicity 268

Chapter 4: Ultrasound 273

Transvaginal Sonography 277
Ultrasound Diagnosis of Pregnancy Failure 279
Transvaginal Cervical Length 280

Chapter 5: Contraception 283

Contraceptive Choices 283
Medical Eligibility for Hormonal Contraceptive Use 286
Barrier Contraceptives 291
Oral Contraceptives 292
Metabolic Effects of Oral Contraceptives 294
Oral Contraceptives and Cancer 296
Oral Contraceptives and Reproduction 298
Oral Contraceptive Management Issues 300
Currently Available Oral Contraceptives 302
Oral Contraceptives—Progestin Only 306
Transdermal Contraceptive 307
Injectable Contraceptive 308
Vaginal Contraceptive Ring 310
Progestin Implant (Nexplanon) 311
Emergency PostCoital Oral Contraception 313
Intrauterine Device 316
Female Sterilization 319

CONTENTS

Chapter 6: Gynecology 323
Abnormal Uterine Bleeding 323
Endometrial Ablation 334
Ectopic Pregnancy 336
Pregnancy of Unknown Location 344
False-Positive Beta-hCG 347
Management of First-Trimester Pregnancy Failure 349
Evaluation of the Sexual Assault Patient 352
Pelvic Pain 355
Endometriosis 360
Endometriosis Fertility Index 364
Gonadotropin-Releasing Hormone Analogs 366
Laparoscopy 368
Hysteroscopy 369
Postoperative Management 371
Urogynecology 373
Vulvar Dystrophies 379
Vulvodynia 380
Fibroids 383

Chapter 7: Infectious Diseases 387
Group B *Streptococcus* 387
Intra-Amniotic Infection 394
Febrile Morbidity and Endomyometritis 396
Mastitis and Breast Abscess 397
Hepatitis 399
Hepatitis C 405
Management of Tuberculosis in Pregnancy 407
Human Immunodeficiency Virus 410
Varicella 421
Rubella 422
Toxoplasmosis 424
Cytomegalovirus 427
Zika Virus Infection 428
Immunization during Pregnancy 432
HPV Vaccination 439
Urinary Tract Infections in Pregnancy 440
Vaginitis 444
Sexually Transmitted Infections 446
2015 CDC Guidelines 447
Ulcerative Lesions in STI 449
Herpes Simplex Virus 450
Syphilis 452
Pelvic Inflammatory Disease and Sexually Transmitted Diseases 454
External Genital Warts 457
Tetanus Prophylaxis 459
Antibiotic Prophylaxis 460
MRSA Infections 461
C. Difficile Infections 462

Chapter 8: Infertility 463
Basic Infertility 463
Ovarian Reserve 468
Evaluation of Male Factor Infertility 473
Genetics of Male Subfertility 475

ix

CONTENTS

Basic Fertility Treatment: Ovulation Induction 477
Advanced Fertility Treatment: Superovulation and Intrauterine Insemination (IUI) for Unexplained Infertility 480
Assisted Reproductive Technologies 482
Ovarian Hyperstimulation Syndrome (OHSS) 491
Surgical Treatment of Infertility 495
Recurrent Pregnancy Loss 497
Gamete Preservation 511

Chapter 9: Reproductive Endocrinology 517

Menstrual Cycle 517
Puberty 520
Delayed or Interrupted Puberty 523
Pubertal Variants and Precocious Puberty 526
Amenorrhea 533
Polycystic Ovary Syndrome (PCOS) 537
Congenital Adrenal Hyperplasia 546
Steroid Hormone Biosynthesis 550
Hirsutism 552
Hyperprolactinemia 554
Thyroid Disorders 564

Chapter 10: Menopause 571

Fast Facts 571
Hot Flushes 574
Postmenopausal Osteoporosis 581
Hormone Replacement Therapy 589

Chapter 11: Gyn-Oncology 591

Endometrial Hyperplasia 592
Endometrial Carcinoma 594
Cervical Dysplasia—Cervical Intraepithelial Neoplasia 599
Cervical Cancer 615
Adnexal Masses 620
Epithelial Ovarian Cancer 623
Ovarian Germ Cell Tumors 627
Sex Cord-Stromal Cell Ovarian Tumors 630
Vulvar Intraepithelial Neoplasia (VIN) 631
Vulvar Cancer 632
Gestational Trophoblastic Disease (GTD) and Gestational Trophoblastic Neoplasia (GTN) 635
Dennis Siegler's Top Ten Ways to Survive Gyn-oncology 639
NCCN Guidelines® For Management of Common Problems in Gyn-oncology Patients 640
Other Common Clinical Problems in the Gyn-oncology Patient 657
Helpful Tables 659
Invasive Cardiac Monitoring 660
Coagulation Cascade 665
Thromboembolic Phenomena 666
Sepsis Syndrome 672
Abdominal Dehiscence 673
Hemorrhage 674
Acid/Base Disturbances 675

Chapter 12: Breast Cancer 677

Fast Facts 677
BRCA Screening Tools 684

CONTENTS

Appendix A: Lab Values 689
Stanford University Medical Center Laboratory 689
Endocrine Lab Values 690
English/Metric Weight Conversion 691

Appendix B: Anatomy 693
Location of the Ureter 693
Fetal Circulation 694
Pelvic Blood Supply 695
Bony Pelvis 696

Appendix C: Epidemiology 697
Definition 697
Descriptive Studies 698
Cohort Studies 699
Case Control Studies 700
Randomized Clinical Trials 701

Appendix D: Operative Reports 703
Cesarean Section 703
Tubal Ligation 705
Dilation & Curettage 706
Laparoscopic Tubal Ligation 707
Total Abdominal Hysterectomy 708
Vaginal Hysterectomy 709

Appendix E: Spanish Primer 711
Numbers 711
Years 711
Days of the Week 711
Times 712
Months 712
Anatomy 715
Figures 753

References 719
Illustrations 753
Index 765

PREFACE TO THE 7TH EDITION

Twenty-seven years have passed since I was an anxious PGY-1 at the University of Texas Health Science Center at Houston in July 1989. My transition to Residency was a bit rocky as I followed the advice of my Chairman at Duke (Dr. Charles Hammond) and spent my MS-4 year taking electives that were far-removed from Ob/Gyn. . . . In Houston Dr. Ben Zivney, a calm, cool, and collected PGY-2, took pity on me and did his best to give me guidance and sage advice. One day he confided in me, "All you need is right here in this book." With that comment he handed me his copy of *Obstetrics and Gynecology* by Denise and Elliot Main to inspect. Unfortunately, when I tried to purchase my own copy at the UT Houston Medical Bookstore, I was informed that this title was out of print awaiting a second edition. That second edition was never completed.

Another PGY-2, Dr. Maggie Schleifer-Nachimson, gave us newbies a bunch of helpful papers that included sample operative reports and some other useful guidelines. Tragically, Maggie was killed in a motor vehicle accident just before completing her residency, but I will always remember her kindness. Armed with these papers (and wishing I had a copy of that darn book that Ben had shown me), I muddled through those first few months of internship.

In July 1990, my wife and I moved to Stanford, CA, so she could assume a tenure track position in the School of Engineering. Unfortunately, the lack of PGY-2 positions in the Bay Area led to me repeating my PGY-1 year. Experiencing that second internship year put me in the unique position of having been an Ob/Gyn intern at two very different institutions . . . and seeing firsthand the need for a book like Denise and Elliot had written. Since there was no second edition of Main and Main (as we called it), Jan Rydfors (my chief resident) and I (an intern) resolved to create a similar book to share with the incoming PGY-1 residents at Stanford. So the very first edition of this handbook was created for our new interns (Bertha, Paul, Christie, and Sylvie) that arrived at Stanford in June 1991—just over 25 years ago. . . . and, as they say, the rest is history.

The creation of Scrub Hill Press (named for my parents' summer home in Cape Cod) and the continued success of this book would not have been possible without the support of my late parents, Dr. and Mrs. Edward T. Gordon. I miss them every day.

As always, I again dedicate this book to H. Allison Smith, my loving wife and best friend, for all of her support through medical school, two internships, residency, fellowship training, and beyond. I hope that our next 30 years of marriage will be as wonderful as the first 30 years.

John David Gordon, MD
July 2016
Arlington, VA

FOREWORD TO THE 7TH EDITION

The one book I want with me when I care for obstetrics and gynecology patients on labor and delivery, in my ambulatory practice or the emergency room, is the seventh edition of *Obstetrics, Gynecology, and Infertility*. The book contains all the information you need to care for a broad range of women's health clinical problems that will challenge you in your day-to-day practice.

The book is both comprehensive and concise. Sections of the book focus on primary care, obstetrics, gynecology, gynecologic oncology, reproductive endocrinology, infertility, menopause, breast cancer, ultrasound, genetics, contraception, infectious diseases, anatomy, and epidemiology. The editors have expertly selected the key information necessary to care for patients and presented it in an easy to use manner with many tables, figures, and algorithms. The book is intended for all women's health clinicians, including students, residents, physicians, nurse midwives, nurse practitioners, physician assistants, and nurses. In fact, we give this book to every one of the Harvard medical students who complete their clerkship at Brigham and Women's.

The purpose of a medical textbook is to advance the knowledge and skill of clinicians so that they can continuously improve the health of patients. Most major textbooks languish on the shelf of the busy clinician, accumulating dust. These texts are seldom used to help solve patient problems at the point of care because they cannot be used to quickly provide concise and actionable information about a real patient problem. In contrast, this handbook fits comfortably in your white coat pocket and can be easily accessed every day as you see your patients. This book is the only pocket reference you need to translate knowledge into action while caring for a patient.

With great care and much work, the authors have made a significant contribution to the education of our clinicians. Congratulations on this accomplishment!

Robert Barbieri, MD
Chair, Department of Obstetrics and Gynecology
Brigham and Women's Hospital
Boston, MA

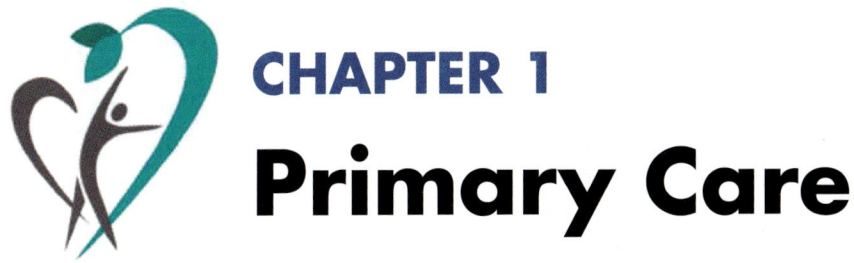

CHAPTER 1
Primary Care

HEALTH SCREENING

Table 1.1. Summary of screening, prevention, and counseling recommendations for adults <65 years

Priority Health Problem	Population	Preventive Intervention(s)*
Cardiovascular disease		
Risk assessment	Patients ≥20 years	CVD risk assessment every 3 to 5 years
Hypertension	All patients	Blood pressure screening/control
Hyperlipidemia	Patients between 17 and 21 years	One-timing screening for dyslipidemia
	Risk factors: women ≥35 years, men ≥25 years	Dyslipidemia screening/control
	Without risk factors: women ≥45 years, men ≥35 years	
Obesity	All patients	Screen with BMI
		Select patients for treatment based on risk factors
Physical activity	All patients	Counseling to exercise
Diabetes mellitus	Adults with hypertension or hyperlipidemia	Screen for diabetes mellitus every 3 years
	Adults with BMI ≥25 kg/m² and additional risk factors	Opportunistic screening

(continued)

PRIMARY CARE — Health Screening

Priority Health Problem	Population	Preventive Intervention(s)*
Cancer		
Breast cancer	Family history	Refer for genetic counseling/testing
	Hereditary breast and ovarian syndrome	Screen per recommendations
	Women 40 to 49 years	Discuss screening with mammography, individual decision
	Women 50 to 70 years	Screen with mammography every 2 years
Cervical cancer	Women 21 to 29 years	Pap smear every 3 years
	Women ≥30 years	Pap smear every 3 years
		Or
		Pap smear + HPV testing every 5 years
Colorectal cancer	Patients with risk factors	Screen per recommendations
	Patients ≥50 years without risk factors	Screening (decide among colonoscopy, flexible sigmoidoscopy, fecal occult blood test)
Lung cancer	Patients 55 to 74 years, ≥30 pack year smoking history and either currently smoking or quit in the past 15 years	Consider screening with low-dose helical CT scan
Prostate cancer	High-risk men 40 to 45 years	Discuss screening, individual decision
	Men ≥50 years without risk factors	Discuss screening, individual decision
Melanoma	High-risk patients	Periodic skin exam
	Average-risk patients	Remain vigilant for suspicious lesions
Immunizations		
Influenza	All patients	Annual influenza vaccination
Tdap/Td	All patients	Tdap at least once
		Td every 10 years
Varicella	Patients without evidence of immunity	Varicella vaccine
HPV	Women until 26 years	HPV vaccine
	Men until 21 years	
	MSM until 26 years	
Zoster	Patients ≥50 years	Zoster vaccine
Pneumococcal disease	Patients with risk factors	Pneumococcal vaccine*
Meningococcal disease	Patients with risk factors	Meningococcal vaccine
Hepatitis B	Patients with risk factors	Hepatitis B vaccine
	All diabetics <60 years, consider in diabetics ≥60 years based on risk factors	
Sexually transmitted infections/blood bourne infections		
Chlamydia	Women <25 years	Screening for chlamydia
	Women at increased risk	
	Men at increased risk	
Gonorrhea	Women at increased risk (including sexually active women <25 years)	Screening for gonorrhea
Hepatitis B	Patients with risk factors	Screening for hepatitis B

(continued)

Health Screening — PRIMARY CARE

Priority Health Problem	Population	Preventive Intervention(s)*
Hepatitis C	Patients born in the US between 1945 and 1965	One-time screening for hepatitis C
	Patients with risk factors	Screening for hepatitis C
HIV	All patients	One-time screening
Syphilis	Patients with risk factors	Screening for syphilis
Psychosocial health concerns		
Depression	All patients	Brief screening
Alcohol	All patients	Screen for alcohol misuse
Tobacco	Smokers and tobacco users	Smoking/tobacco cessation
Other drug use	All patients	Assess for unhealthy drug use
Intimate partner violence	On initial visits or if concerning history or physical exam findings	
Osteoporosis	Postmenopausal women <65 with risk factors	BMD screening
	Men with clinical manifestations of low bone mass	

Refer to individual UpToDate topics for more detailed discussions of screening and preventive counseling.

CVD: cardiovascular disease; BMI: body mass index; Tdap: tetanus, diphtheria, and acellular pertussis vaccination; Td: tetanus, diphtheria vaccine; HPV: human papillomavirus; MSM: men who have sex with men; HIV: human immunodeficiency virus; BMD: bone mineral density.

*The pneumococcal vaccine (23-valent polysaccharide vaccine or 13-valent conjugate vaccine) and schedule varies depending upon the risk factor. Refer to UpToDate topic on pneumococcal vaccination in adults for details.

Source: Reproduced with permission from Park L. Preventive care in adults: recommendations. In: Post, TW, ed. *UpToDate*. Waltham, MA: UpToDate (accessed on February 19, 2016). Copyright © 2016 UpToDate, Inc. For more information, visit www.uptodate.com.

Table 1.2. Summary of screening, prevention, and counseling recommendations for adults ≥65 years

Priority Problem	Brief Recommendation
Historical information and counseling	
Exercise	Moderate to vigorous aerobic activity 3–5 times per week
	Weight training or resistance exercises to maintain strength
	Flexibility activities to maintain range of motion
	Balance training to improve stability and prevent falls
Alcohol use	CAGE questionnaire
	Counseling to stop drinking
Tobacco use	Ongoing regular counseling to stop smoking
	Consideration of pharmacotherapy
Medication use	Regular review of medication list for completeness, accuracy, adherence, and affordability
	Drug-drug, drug-disease interactions
	Careful attention to use of specific drug types/classes, including warfarin, digoxin, antidiabetic, analgesic, antihypertensive, psychotropic, and anticholinergic drugs
Urinary incontinence (UI)	Inquire about presence and severity biannually
	Presence of UI should trigger medication review, GU exam, appropriate blood and urine tests
Driving	Consideration of driving problems in those with problems with vision, mobility, or cognition
	For demented patients, recommend stop driving or refer for detailed driving assessment
Social support	Regular screening for financial and social support
Elder mistreatment	Routine direct questioning about problems with abuse or neglect
Advance directives	Discussion and documentation of preferences with living will and designation of health care power-of-attorney
Physical examination and testing	
Blood pressure	Measure every 1–2 years
	If treatment initiated, monitor orthostatic blood pressure, renal function, and electrolytes
Weight	Weight loss of 10% or more per year triggers assessment of undernutrition, possible medical or medication-related causes, dental status, food security, food-related functional status, appetite and intake, swallow ability, and previous dietary restrictions
Hearing and vision	Annual screening for hearing loss with patient inquiry and exam (Whisper test or handheld audiometry)
	General ophthalmologic examination, including screening for glaucoma, every 1–2 years
Cognition	Targeted screening in patients with memory complaints or new functional impairment with MMSE, Mini-Cog, Clock Drawing Test, or Memory Impairment Screen
Mood	Screen all older adults for depression with two questions:
	1) Feeling depressed or sad?
	2) Loss of interest?
Gait and balance	Get Up and Go Test
Lipids	Screen and treat older adults with CHD risk exceeding 10% over 10 years
Bone density	Screening densitometry for osteoporosis for women beginning at age 65
Abdominal aortic aneurysm	One-time screening ultrasound in men aged 65–75 with any history of smoking or family history of AAA requiring repair

(continued)

Health Screening — PRIMARY CARE

Priority Problem	Brief Recommendation
Cancer screening	
Cancer screening	Key considerations in older adults:
	Life expectancy: will this patient live long enough to benefit?
	Potential harms: procedural complications, anxiety, cost, and overdiagnosis
	Individual patient preference
Breast cancer	Screening mammography every 1–2 years as long as life expectancy at least 5 years
Colorectal cancer	Annual FOBT v.
	Screening colonoscopy every 10 years v.
	Flexible sigmoidoscopy every 5 years as long as life expectancy at least 5 years
Cervical cancer	May safely discontinue Pap smears at or after age 65 after 3 consecutive normals within 10-year period
	May discontinue after hysterectomy for benign indication
Immunization	
Tetanus-diphtheria vaccine	Booster every 10 years in patients who have received primary series (alternative: booster once after age 50)
Influenza vaccine	Annual vaccination
Pneumococcal vaccine (PCV13 and PPSV23)	Give PCV13 followed by PPSV23 6 to 12 months later, once after age 65
	Revaccinate PPSV23 once after age 65 if an initial vaccination was given before age 65 and 5 years have elapsed since the first dose
Herpes zoster vaccine	One-time vaccination after age 60
Other	
Aspirin	Consider daily aspirin in patients with 5-year CHD risk of 3% or greater. Weigh risks of gastrointestinal bleeding
Calcium and vitamin D	1,200 mg of elemental calcium (diet and/or supplement) and at least 800 IU of vitamin D

Source: Reproduced with permission from Park L. Preventive care in adults: recommendations. In: Post TW, ed. *UpToDate*. Waltham, MA. (Accessed on March 18, 2016) Copyright © 2016 UpToDate, Inc. For more information, visit www.uptodate.com.

COLON CANCER SCREENING

Table 1.3. Screening guidelines for the early detection of colorectal cancer and adenomas for average-risk women aged 50 years and older

Test That Detects Adenomatous Polyps and Cancer	Interval	Key Issues for Informed Decisions	Efficacy
Colonoscopy	Every 10 years	• Adenoma removal can possibly prevent colorectal cancer. • Complete bowel preparation is required. • Conscious sedation is used in most centers; patients will miss a day of work and will need a chaperone for transportation from the facility. • Risks include perforation, bleeding, and death, which are rare but potentially serious; most of the risk is associated with polypectomy. • Limitations include significant variability in quality and performance and dependency on the operator's skill.	83% reduction in mortality
Flexible sigmoidoscopy with insertion to 40 cm or to splenic flexure	Every 5 years	• Complete or partial bowel preparation is required. • Sedation usually is not used, so there may be some discomfort during the procedure. • The protective effect of sigmoidoscopy is limited primarily to the portion of the colon examined. • Patients should understand that positive findings on sigmoidoscopy usually result in a referral for colonoscopy. • Complications include colonic perforation, even if no biopsy or polypectomy is performed; this occurs in fewer than 1 in 20,000 examinations.	60–70% reduction in mortality from left colon lesions
CTC[†]	Every 5 years	• Complete bowel preparation is required. • If patients have one or more polyps larger than 6 mm, colonoscopy will be recommended; if same-day colonoscopy is not available, a second complete bowel preparation will be required before colonoscopy. • Risks of CTC are very low; rare cases of perforation have been reported. • Significance of incidental extracolonic findings is not clear. • Increased lifetime cumulative radiation risk needs further evaluation.	Not available
gFOBT with high sensitivity for cancer	Annual	• Depending on manufacturer's recommendations, the test requires two samples from each of three consecutive bowel movements at home; a single sample of stool gathered during a digital examination in the clinical setting is not an acceptable stool test and should not be done.	15–33% reduction in mortality
FIT with high sensitivity for cancer	Annual	• A positive test result is associated with an increased risk of colon cancer and advanced neoplasia; colonoscopy should be recommended if the test result is positive. • If the test result is negative, the test should be repeated annually. • Patients should understand that one-time testing is likely to be ineffective.	74% reduction in mortality

(continued)

Test That Detects Adenomatous Polyps and Cancer	Interval	Key Issues for Informed Decisions	Efficacy
sDNA with high sensitivity	Interval uncertain	• An adequate stool sample must be obtained and packaged with appropriate preservative agents for shipping to the laboratory. • The unit cost of the currently available test is significantly higher than other forms of stool testing. • If the test result is positive, colonoscopy will be recommended. • If the test result is negative, the appropriate interval for a repeat test is uncertain.	Not available

CTC, computed tomography colonography; FIT, fecal immunochemical test; gFOBT, guaiac-based fecal occult blood test; sDNA, stool DNA test.

*These options are acceptable choices for colorectal cancer screening in average-risk adults beginning at age 50 years and at age 45 years for African Americans. Because each of these tests has inherent characteristics related to prevention potential, accuracy, costs, and potential harms, individuals should have an opportunity to make an informed decision when choosing one of these options. In the opinion of the Guidelines Development Committee (of the American Cancer Society, the U.S. Multi-Society Task Force on Colorectal Cancer, and the American College of Radiology), colon cancer prevention should be the primary goal of colorectal cancer screening. Tests that are designed to detect early cancer and adenomatous polyps should be encouraged if resources are available and patients are willing to undergo an invasive test.

†Computed tomography colonography currently is not recommended by the U.S. Preventive Services Task Force, may not be covered by some insurance plans, and currently is not covered under Medicare.

Data from Levin B, Lieberman DA, McFarland B, Andrews KS, Brooks D, Bond J, et al. Screening and surveillance for the early detection of colorectal cancer and adenomatous polyps, 2008: a joint guideline from the American Cancer Society, the U.S. Multi-Society Task Force on Colorectal Cancer, and the American College of Radiology. *Gastroenterology.* 2008;134:1570-95; National Cancer Institute. Colorectal cancer screening (PDQ®). Available at: http://www.cancer.gov/cancertopics/pdq/screening/colorectal/HealthProfessional. Retrieved April 9, 2014; and Telford JJ, Levy AR, Sambrook JC, Zou D, Enns RA. The cost-effectiveness of screening for colorectal cancer. *CMAJ.* 2010;182:1307-13.

Source: Reproduced with permission from American College of Obstetricians and Gynecologists. Committee Opinion No. 609: Colorectal cancer screening strategies. *Obstet Gynecol.* 2014;124:849-55.

Table 1.4. Colorectal cancer screening options based upon risk factors

Individual Risk	Age to Begin Screening, Yr	Interval	Recommended Examination	Alternative Examination	Genetic Testing	Comment
Average risk						
Screening option	50	10 yr	Colonoscopy	FOBT or FIT with FSIG	No	–
Screening option	50	Yearly/5 yr	FOBT or FIT/FSIG	BE every 5 yr or CT colonography every 5 yr	No	Compliance is as important as method
African American screening option	45	10 yr	Colonoscopy	None	No	Higher risk of proximal polyps or cancer at a younger age
Increased risk						
Personal history of polyps						
1–2 small tubular adenomas	–	5–10 yr	Colonoscopy	None	No	–
3–10 adenomas or 1 >1 cm, or high-grade dysplasia without features	–	3 yr	Colonoscopy	None	No	–
>10 adenomas	–	<3 yr	Colonoscopy	None	Possibly	Consider genetic component
Piecemeal excision	–	2–6 mo	Colonoscopy	None	No	–
Personal history of cancer	–	1 yr after operation	Colonoscopy	None	–	If negative, repeat in 3 yr
Family history of cancer (first-degree relatives)	Age 40 or 10 yr before youngest case	5 yr	Colonoscopy	None	Possibly	Look for other cancers linked to genetic transmission
Family history of cancer (second- or third-degree relatives)	50	10 yr	Colonoscopy	None	Possibly	Look for other cancers linked to genetic transmission
IBD	8–10 yr after onset of symptoms	2 yr	Colonoscopy	None	No	–
Hereditary risk						
FAP	10–12	1–2 yr	FSIG	None	Yes	Early screening, early surgery, early genetic testing
HNPCC	Age 20 or 10 yr before youngest family member	1–2 yr	Colonoscopy	None	Yes	Encourage screening of other family members and be vigilant for other associated cancers

BE, barium enema; FAP, familial adenomatous polyposis; FIT, fecal immunohistochemistry testing; FOBT, fecal occult blood testing; FSIG, flexible sigmoidoscopy; HNPCC, hereditary nonpolyposis colorectal cancer; IBD, inflammatory bowel disease.

Source: Reproduced with permission of Springer from Nelson RS, Thorson AG. Colorectal cancer screening. *Curr Oncol Rep.* 2009 Nov;11(6):482-89.

Health Screening
PRIMARY CARE 1

VACCINE ▼ / INDICATION ▶	Pregnancy	Immuno-compromising conditions (excluding HIV infection)[4,6,7,A13]	HIV infection CD4+ count (cells/μL)[4,6,7,A13] < 200	HIV infection CD4+ count (cells/μL)[4,6,7,A13] ≥ 200	Men who have sex with men (MSM)	Kidney failure, end-stage renal disease, on hemodialysis	Heart disease, chronic lung disease, chronic alcoholism	Asplenia and persistent complement component deficiencies[8,11,12]	Chronic liver disease	Diabetes	Healthcare personnel
Influenza*[,2]	1 dose annually										
Tetanus, diphtheria, pertussis (Td/Tdap)*[,3]	1 dose Tdap each pregnancy	Substitute Tdap for Td once, then Td booster every 10 yrs									
Varicella*[,4]	Contraindicated		Contraindicated								
Human papillomavirus (HPV) Female*[,5]		3 doses through age 26 yrs	3 doses through age 26 yrs					2 doses			
Human papillomavirus (HPV) Male*[,5]		3 doses through age 26 yrs			3 doses through age 26 yrs			3 doses through age 21 yrs			
Zoster[6]	Contraindicated	Contraindicated	Contraindicated					1 dose			
Measles, mumps, rubella (MMR)*[,7]	Contraindicated	Contraindicated	Contraindicated					1 or 2 doses depending on indication			
Pneumococcal 13-valent conjugate (PCV13)*[,8]						1 dose					
Pneumococcal polysaccharide (PPSV23)[8]					1, 2, or 3 doses depending on indication						
Hepatitis A*[,9]					2 or 3 doses depending on vaccine						
Hepatitis B*[,10]					3 doses						
Meningococcal 4-valent conjugate (MenACWY) or polysaccharide (MPSV4)*[,11]						1 or more doses depending on indication					
Meningococcal B (MenB)[11]					2 or 3 doses depending on vaccine						
Haemophilus influenzae type b (Hib)*[,12]		3 doses post-HSCT recipients only						1 dose			

*Covered by the Vaccine Injury Compensation Program

Recommended for all persons who meet the age requirement, lack documentation of vaccination, or lack evidence of past infection; zoster vaccine is recommended regardless of past episode of zoster

Recommended for persons with a risk factor (medical, occupational, lifestyle, or other indication)

No recommendation

Contraindicated

These schedules indicate the recommended age groups and medical indications for which administration of currently licensed vaccines is commonly recommended for adults aged ≥19 years, as of February 2016. For all vaccines being recommended on the Adult Immunization Schedule: a vaccine series does not need to be restarted, regardless of the time that has elapsed between doses. Licensed combination vaccines may be used whenever any components of the combination are indicated and when the vaccine's other components are not contraindicated. For detailed recommendations on all vaccines, including those used primarily for travelers or that are issued during the year, consult the manufacturers' package inserts and the complete statements from the Advisory Committee on Immunization Practices (www.cdc.gov/vaccines/hcp/acip-recs/index.html). Use of trade names and commercial sources is for identification only and does not imply endorsement by the U.S. Department of Health and Human Services.

U.S. Department of Health and Human Services
Centers for Disease Control and Prevention

Figure 1.1. Vaccines indicated for various medical conditions
Source: http://www.cdc.gov/vaccines/schedules/downloads/adult/adult-schedule.pdf. Accessed on March 18, 2016.

NUTRITION

Table 1.5. Recommended weekly and occasional food purchases for one person following a healthful diet containing 2100 kcal and 1500 mg of sodium

Type of Food	Servings Per Wk	Serving Size	Total Amount Purchased Per Wk	Recommendations
Weekly purchases				
Market periphery				Do most weekly shopping in this section
Vegetables[†]				
Leafy greens				
Salad greens	4	1 cup	1–2 bags or heads	Lettuce, mixed spring greens, spinach bunch (about 1 lb)
Other greens	4	1/2 cup	1–2 bunches	Kale, collard greens, mustard greens (about 1 lb)
Cruciferous	3	1/2 cup	1–2 heads	Broccoli, cabbage, cauliflower (about 1 lb)
Colorful[‡]	15	1/2 cup	8–12 individual items	Tomatoes, carrots, squash, peppers, sweet potatoes, corn, eggplant, avocados (about 3 lb)
Other	3	1/2 cup	1/2 lb	Celery, green beans, peas, lima beans, sprouts
Fruits				
Fresh	20	1 medium or 1/2 cup chopped	15–20 individual items	Apples, pears, grapes, bananas, peaches, plums, oranges, tangerines, berries, cantaloupe, pineapple
Dried	8	1/4 cup	1 bag	Raisins, apricots, prunes, cherries (about 1/2 lb)
Juice	4	1 glass (8 oz)	1 qt	Orange, grapefruit, unsweetened carrot
Herbs, alliums, and other seasonings	Use freely			Thyme, ginger, garlic, onion, bay leaf, lemon juice
Meat, poultry, and fish				
Fish and shellfish	2	6–8 oz	1 lb	Cod, sea bass, halibut; fresh or canned salmon, tuna, or sardines; mollusks, shrimp, crabmeat
Poultry	2	6–8 oz	1 lb	Turkey, chicken, low-sodium cold cuts
Red meats	1	2–4 oz	1/4 lb	Beef, pork, lamb, low-sodium cold cuts
Dairy products				
Milk	10	1 glass (8 oz)	1/2 gallon	Choose low-fat or nonfat products
Yogurt	3	1 cup	1 container	Choose low-fat or nonfat products (about 32 oz)
Cheese	4	1 slice	1/4 lb	Soft or hard

(continued)

Nutrition

Type of Food	Servings Per Wk	Serving Size	Total Amount Purchased Per Wk	Recommendations
Processed-food aisles				Choose only low-sodium products
Nuts (whole or butter)	10	1 oz	1 bag or jar	Walnuts, almonds, peanuts (about 1/2 lb)
Legumes	3	1 cup	1 can or bag	Chickpeas, lentils, black beans (about 1 lb)
Olives	2	1/2 cup	1 jar	Black, green, stuffed (about 1/4 lb)
Spices	Use freely			Black pepper, cayenne, cinnamon, paprika
Baked goods	20	1 slice	1 bag	Bread, rolls, pancakes, waffles (about 1 1/2 lb); choose wholegrain products
Tomato products	4	2/3 cup	2 jars or cans	Sauce, juice, whole or diced (about 12 oz per jar or can)
Chips and other snacks	3	1/2 cup	3 bags	Tortilla chips, popcorn, pretzels (about 1 1/2 oz per bag)
Chocolate or sweets	1	1 oz	1 bar or similar amount	Granola bars, chocolate bars (about 1 oz)
Other food aisles (sweetened beverages, candy, cookies)				Skip these aisles
Less Frequent Purchases[‖]				
Breakfast cereals	2	1/2 cup	1 1/2 cups	Oats, bran, whole wheat flakes, other whole grains
Pasta, rice, and grains	3	1 cup (cooked)	1/2 cup	Pasta, brown rice, bulgur, quinoa, wheat berries
Cooking oils	12	1 tbs	3/4 cup	Canola, corn, sunflower, olive, soybean
Table fats	16	1 tsp	1/3 cup	Soft, oil-based spreads free of trans fat
Salad dressings and mayonnaise	21	1 tsp	1/2 cup	Choose low-sodium items
Sugars	24	1 tsp	1/2 cup	Table sugar, jelly, honey, maple syrup
Desserts	1	1/2 cup	1/2 cup	Ice cream, sorbet, frozen yogurt, other (4 oz)
Eggs	3	1	3	Large eggs
Salt	7	1/3 tsp	2 1/3 tsp	Salt for cooking or added at the table

[*] Patients should observe the following general recommendations: don't skip meals, and consume one third of daily calorie intake at breakfast; limit eating out to once weekly and choose meals with a low salt content—just one slice of pizza, a turkey sandwich, or a pasta dish can easily contain 2000 mg of sodium. Examples of conversion from standard to metric measures: 1 oz equals 28 g; 1 teaspoon, 5 g; 1 cup leafy greens, about 75 g.

[†] Unsalted frozen or canned vegetables can be substituted for fresh vegetables.

[‡] Choose at least four different types of vegetables from this category.

[§] Also visit the processed-food aisle as needed for other food items in the less frequent purchases category.

[¶] Look for lower-sodium, unsalted, or reduced-salt items. Compare brands and choose those with lower sodium content. The total amount of sodium consumed in a week from processed foods or eating out should not exceed 2000 mg.

[‖] Weekly allowances are provided for items that are generally purchased less than once a week. The amounts for weekly intake should be set aside in individual containers to make it easier to keep track of how much is consumed.

Source: Reproduced with permission from Sacks FM, Campos H. Dietary therapy in hypertension. *N Engl J Med.* 2010 Jun 3;362(22):2102-12. Copyright © 2010 Massachusetts Medical Society. Reprinted with permission from Massachusetts Medical Society.

PRIMARY CARE — Nutrition

Table 1.6. Directory reference intakes (DRIs): recommended dietary allowances and adequate intakes, vitamins

Life Stage Group	Vitamin A (µg/d)[a]	Vitamin C (mg/d)	Vitamin D (µg/d)[b,c]	Vitamin E (mg/d)[d]	Vitamin K (µg/d)	Thiamin (mg/d)	Riboflavin (mg/d)	Niacin (mg/d)E	Vitamin B_6 (mg/d)	Folate (µg/d)F	Vitamin B_{12} (µg/d)	Pantothenic Acid (mg/d)	Biotin (µg/d)	Choline (mg/d)[g]
Infants														
0 to 6 mo	400*	40*	10	4*	2.0*	0.2*	0.3*	2*	0.1*	65*	0.4*	1.7*	5*	125*
6 to 12 mo	500*	50*	10	5*	2.5*	0.3*	0.4*	4*	0.3*	80*	0.5*	1.8*	6*	150*
Children														
1–3 yr	**300**	**15**	**15**	**6**	30*	**0.5**	**0.5**	**6**	**0.5**	**150**	**0.9**	2*	8*	200*
4–8 yr	**400**	**25**	**15**	**7**	55*	**0.6**	**0.6**	**8**	**0.6**	**200**	**1.2**	3*	12*	250*
Males														
9–13 yr	**600**	**45**	**15**	**11**	60*	**0.9**	**0.9**	**12**	**1.0**	**300**	**1.8**	4*	20*	375*
14–18 yr	**900**	**75**	**15**	**15**	75*	**1.2**	**1.3**	**16**	**1.3**	**400**	**2.4**	5*	25*	550*
19–30 yr	**900**	**90**	**15**	**15**	120*	**1.2**	**1.3**	**16**	**1.3**	**400**	**2.4**	5*	30*	550*
31–50 yr	**900**	**90**	**15**	**15**	120*	**1.2**	**1.3**	**16**	**1.3**	**400**	**2.4**	5*	30*	550*
51–70 yr	**900**	**90**	**15**	**15**	120*	**1.2**	**1.3**	**16**	**1.7**	**400**	**2.4**[h]	5*	30*	550*
>70 yr	**900**	**90**	**20**	**15**	120*	**1.2**	**1.3**	**16**	**1.7**	**400**	**2.4**[h]	5*	30*	550*
Females														
9–13 yr	**600**	**45**	**15**	**11**	60*	**0.9**	**0.9**	**12**	**1.0**	**300**	**1.8**	4*	20*	375*
14–18 yr	**700**	**65**	**15**	**15**	75*	**1.0**	**1.0**	**14**	**1.2**	**400**[i]	**2.4**	5*	25*	400*
19–30 yr	**700**	**75**	**15**	**15**	90*	**1.1**	**1.1**	**14**	**1.3**	**400**[i]	**2.4**	5*	30*	425*
31–50 yr	**700**	**75**	**15**	**15**	90*	**1.1**	**1.1**	**14**	**1.3**	**400**[i]	**2.4**	5*	30*	425*
51–70 yr	**700**	**75**	**15**	**15**	90*	**1.1**	**1.1**	**14**	**1.5**	**400**	**2.4**[h]	5*	30*	425*
>70 yr	**700**	**75**	**20**	**15**	90*	**1.1**	**1.1**	**14**	**1.5**	**400**	**2.4**[h]	5*	30*	425*
Pregnancy														
14–18 yr	**750**	**80**	**15**	**15**	75*	**1.4**	**1.4**	**18**	**1.9**	**600**[i]	**2.6**	6*	30*	450*
19–30 yr	**770**	**85**	**15**	**15**	90*	**1.4**	**1.4**	**18**	**1.9**	**600**[i]	**2.6**	6*	30*	450*
31–50 yr	**770**	**85**	**15**	**15**	90*	**1.4**	**1.4**	**18**	**1.9**	**600**[i]	**2.6**	6*	30*	450*
Lactation														
14–18 yr	**1,200**	**115**	**15**	**19**	75*	**1.4**	**1.6**	**17**	**2.0**	**500**	**2.8**	7*	35*	550*
19–30 yr	**1,300**	**120**	**15**	**19**	90*	**1.4**	**1.6**	**17**	**2.0**	**500**	**2.8**	7*	35*	550*
31–50 yr	**1,300**	**120**	**15**	**19**	90*	**1.4**	**1.6**	**17**	**2.0**	**500**	**2.8**	7*	35*	550*

NOTE: This table (taken from the DRI reports, see www.nap.edu) presents Recommended Dietary Allowances (RDAs) in **bold type** and Adequate Intakes (AIs) in ordinary type followed by an asterisk (*). An RDA is the average daily dietary intake level, sufficient to meet the nutrient requirements of nearly all (97-98%) healthy individuals in a group. It is calculated from an Estimated Average Requirement (EAR). If sufficient scientific evidence is not available to establish an EAR, and thus calculate an RDA, an AI is usually developed. For healthy breastfed infants, an AI is the mean intake. The AI for other life stage and gender groups is believed to cover the needs of all healthy individuals in the groups, but lack of data or uncertainty in the data prevent being able to specify with confidence the percentage of individuals covered by this intake.

^{a}As retinol activity equivalents (RAEs). 1 RAE = 1 μg retinol, 12 μg β-carotene, 24 μg α-carotene, or 24 μg β-cryptoxanthin. The RAE for dietary provitamin A carotenoids is two-fold greater than retinol equivalents (RE), whereas the RAE for preformed vitamin A is the same as RE.

^{b}As cholecalciferol. 1 μg cholecalciferol = 40 IU vitamin D.

^{c}Under the assumption of minimal sunlight.

^{d}As α-tocopherol. α-Tocopherol includes *RRR*-α-tocopherol, the only form of α-tocopherol that occurs naturally in foods, and the 2*R*-stereoisomeric forms of α-tocopherol (*RRR*-, *RSR*-, *RRS*-, and *RSS*-α-tocopherol) that occur in fortified foods and supplements. It does not include the 2*S*-stereoisomeric forms of α-tocopherol (*SRR*-, *SSR*-, *SRS*-, and *SSS*-α-tocopherol), also found in fortified foods and supplements.

^{e}As niacin equivalents (NE). 1 mg of niacin = 60 mg of tryptophan; 0–6 months = preformed niacin (not NE).

^{f}As dietary folate equivalents (DFE). 1 DFE = 1 μg food folate = 0.6 μg of folic acid from fortified food or as a supplement consumed with food = 0.5 μg of a supplement taken on an empty stomach.

^{g}Although AIs have been set for choline, there are few data to assess whether a dietary supply of choline is needed at all stages of the life cycle, and it may be that the choline requirement can be met by endogenous synthesis at some of these stages.

^{h}Because 10 to 30% of older people may malabsorb food-bound B12, it is advisable for those older than 50 years to meet their RDA mainly by consuming foods fortified with B12 or a supplement containing B12.

^{i}In view of evidence linking folate intake with neural tube defects in the fetus, it is recommended that all women capable of becoming pregnant consume 400 μg from supplements or fortified foods in addition to intake of food folate from a varied diet.

^{j}It is assumed that women will continue consuming 400 μg from supplements or fortified food until their pregnancy is confirmed and they enter prenatal care, which ordinarily occurs after the end of the periconceptional period—the critical time for formation of the neural tube.

Source: Reproduced with permission from Otten JJ, Hellwig JP, Meyers LD. *DRI, Dietary Reference Intakes: The Essential Guide to Nutrient Requirements*. Washington, DC: National Academies Press; 2006. Reprinted with permission from the National Academies Press, Copyright © 2006, National Academy of Sciences. These reports may be accessed via www.nap.edu.

Table 1.7. Directory reference intakes (DRIs): recommended dietary allowances and adequate intakes, elements

Life Stage Group	Calcium (mg/d)	Chromium (µg/d)	Copper (µg/d)	Fluoride (mg/d)	Iodine (µg/d)	Iron (mg/d)	Magnesium (mg/d)	Manganese (mg/d)	Molybdenum (µg/d)	Phosphorus (mg/d)	Selenium (µg/d)	Zinc (mg/d)	Potassium (g/d)	Sodium (g/d)	Chloride (g/d)
Infants															
0 to 6 mo	200*	0.2*	200*	0.01*	110*	0.27*	30*	0.003*	2*	100*	15*	2*	0.4*	0.12*	0.18*
6 to 12 mo	260*	5.5*	220*	0.5*	130*	**11**	75*	0.6*	3*	275*	20*	**3**	0.7*	0.37*	0.57*
Children															
1–3 yr	**700**	11*	**340**	0.7*	**90**	**7**	**80**	1.2*	**17**	**460**	**20**	**3**	3.0*	1.0*	1.5*
4–8 yr	**1,000**	15*	**440**	1*	**90**	**10**	**130**	1.5*	**22**	**500**	**30**	**5**	3.8*	1.2*	1.9*
Males															
9–13 yr	**1,300**	25*	**700**	2*	**120**	**8**	**240**	1.9*	**34**	**1,250**	**40**	**8**	4.5*	1.5*	2.3*
14–18 yr	**1,300**	35*	**890**	3*	**150**	**11**	**410**	2.2*	**43**	**1,250**	**55**	**11**	4.7*	1.5*	2.3*
19–30 yr	**1,000**	35*	**900**	4*	**150**	**8**	**400**	2.3*	**45**	**700**	**55**	**11**	4.7*	1.5*	2.3*
31–50 yr	**1,000**	35*	**900**	4*	**150**	**8**	**420**	2.3*	**45**	**700**	**55**	**11**	4.7*	1.5*	2.3*
51–70 yr	**1,000**	30*	**900**	4*	**150**	**8**	**420**	2.3*	**45**	**700**	**55**	**11**	4.7*	1.3*	2.0*
>70 yr	**1,200**	30*	**900**	4*	**150**	**8**	**420**	2.3*	**45**	**700**	**55**	**11**	4.7*	1.2*	1.8*
Females															
9–13 yr	**1,300**	21*	**700**	2*	**120**	**8**	**240**	1.6*	**34**	**1,250**	**40**	**8**	4.5*	1.5*	2.3*
14–18 yr	**1,300**	24*	**890**	3*	**150**	**15**	**360**	1.6*	**43**	**1,250**	**55**	**9**	4.7*	1.5*	2.3*
19–30 yr	**1,000**	25*	**900**	3*	**150**	**18**	**310**	1.8*	**45**	**700**	**55**	**8**	4.7*	1.5*	2.3*
31–50 yr	**1,000**	25*	**900**	3*	**150**	**18**	**320**	1.8*	**45**	**700**	**55**	**8**	4.7*	1.5*	2.3*
51–70 yr	**1,200**	20*	**900**	3*	**150**	**8**	**320**	1.8*	**45**	**700**	**55**	**8**	4.7*	1.3*	2.0*
>70 yr	**1,200**	20*	**900**	3*	**150**	**8**	**320**	1.8*	**45**	**700**	**55**	**8**	4.7*	1.2*	1.8*
Pregnancy															
14–18 yr	**1,300**	29*	**1,000**	3*	**220**	**27**	**400**	2.0*	**50**	**1,250**	**60**	**12**	4.7*	1.5*	2.3*
19–30 yr	**1,000**	30*	**1,000**	3*	**220**	**27**	**350**	2.0*	**50**	**700**	**60**	**11**	4.7*	1.5*	2.3*
31–50 yr	**1,000**	30*	**1,000**	3*	**220**	**27**	**360**	2.0*	**50**	**700**	**60**	**11**	4.7*	1.5*	2.3*
Lactation															
14–18 yr	**1,300**	44*	**1,300**	3*	**290**	**10**	**360**	2.6*	**50**	**1,250**	**70**	**13**	5.1*	1.5*	2.3*
19–30 yr	**1,000**	45*	**1,300**	3*	**290**	**9**	**310**	2.6*	**50**	**700**	**70**	**12**	5.1*	1.5*	2.3*
31–50 yr	**1,000**	45*	**1,300**	3*	**290**	**9**	**320**	2.6*	**50**	**700**	**70**	**12**	5.1*	1.5*	2.3*

NOTE: This table (taken from the DRI reports, see www.nap.edu) presents Recommended Dietary Allowances (RDAs) in **bold type** and Adequate Intakes (AIs) in ordinary type followed by an asterisk (*). An RDA is the average daily dietary intake level, sufficient to meet the nutrient requirements of nearly all (97-98%) healthy individuals in a group. It is calculated from an Estimated Average Requirement (EAR). If sufficient scientific evidence is not available to establish an EAR, and thus calculate an RDA, an AI is usually developed. For healthy breastfed infants, an AI is the mean intake. The AI for other life stage and gender groups is believed to cover the needs of all healthy individuals in the groups, but lack of data or uncertainty in the data prevent being able to specify with confidence the percentage of individuals covered by this intake.

Source: See reference on previous page. Copyright © 2006 National Academy of Sciences.

Nutrition — PRIMARY CARE

BODY MASS INDEX
Nomogram

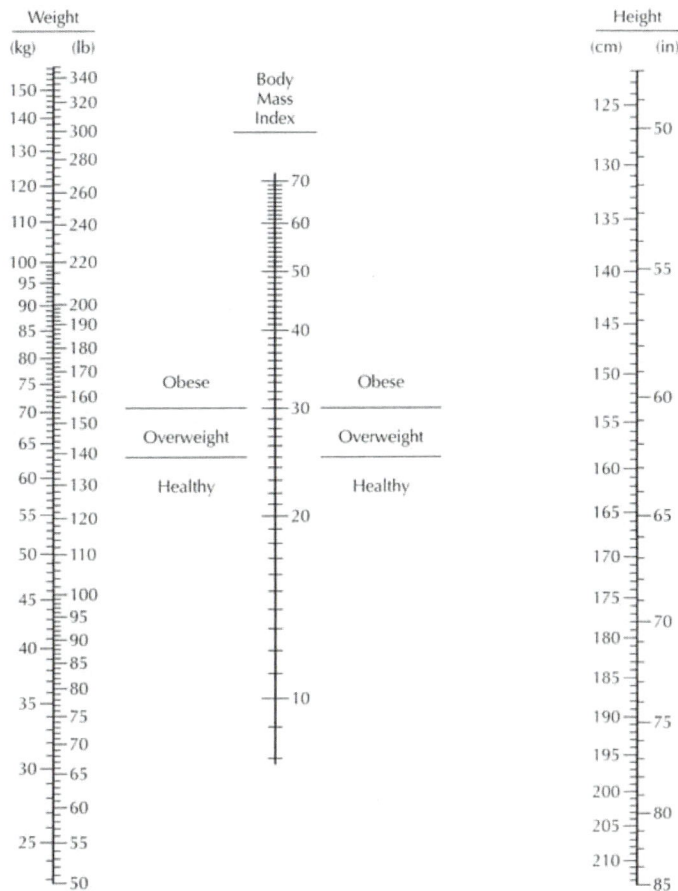

Figure 1.2. Body mass index (BMI) nomogram
Source: Reprinted by permission from Macmillan Publishers Ltd: Bray GA. Definition, measurement, and classification of the syndromes of obesity. *Int J Obes.* 1978;2(2):99-112. Copyright © 1978.

Table 1.8. Body mass index nomogram

BMI	Normal						Overweight					Obese						
Height (in)	19	20	21	22	23	24	25	26	27	28	29	30	31	32	33	34	35	36
							Body Weight (lb)											
58	91	96	100	105	110	115	119	124	129	134	138	143	148	153	158	162	167	172
59	94	99	104	109	114	119	124	128	133	138	143	148	153	158	163	168	173	178
60	97	102	107	112	118	123	128	133	138	143	148	153	158	163	168	174	179	184
61	100	106	111	116	122	127	132	137	143	148	153	158	164	169	174	180	185	190
62	104	109	115	120	126	131	136	142	147	153	158	164	169	175	180	186	191	196
63	107	113	118	124	130	135	141	146	152	158	163	169	175	180	186	191	197	203
64	110	116	122	128	134	140	145	151	157	163	169	174	180	186	192	197	204	209
65	114	120	126	132	138	144	150	156	162	168	174	180	186	192	198	204	210	216
66	118	124	130	136	142	148	155	161	167	173	179	186	192	198	204	210	216	223
67	121	127	134	140	146	153	159	166	172	178	185	191	198	204	211	217	223	230
68	125	131	138	144	151	158	164	171	177	184	190	197	203	210	216	223	230	236
69	128	135	142	149	155	162	169	176	182	189	196	203	209	216	223	230	236	243
70	132	139	146	153	160	167	174	181	188	195	202	209	216	222	229	236	243	250
71	136	143	150	157	165	172	179	186	193	200	208	215	222	229	236	243	250	257
72	140	147	154	162	169	177	184	191	199	206	213	221	228	235	242	250	258	265
73	144	151	159	166	174	182	189	197	204	212	219	227	235	242	250	257	265	272
74	148	155	163	171	179	186	194	202	210	218	225	233	241	249	256	264	272	280
75	152	160	168	176	184	192	200	208	216	224	232	240	248	256	264	272	279	287
76	156	164	172	180	189	197	205	213	221	230	238	246	254	263	271	279	287	295

Nutrition

PRIMARY CARE

BMI	Obese			Extreme Obesity														
Height (in)	37	38	39	40	41	42	43	44	45	46	47	48	49	50	51	52	53	54
								Body Weight (lb)										
58	177	181	186	191	196	201	205	210	215	220	224	229	234	239	244	248	253	258
59	183	188	193	198	203	208	212	217	222	227	232	237	242	247	252	257	262	267
60	189	194	199	204	209	215	220	225	230	235	240	245	250	255	261	266	271	276
61	195	201	206	211	217	222	227	232	238	243	248	254	259	264	269	275	280	285
62	202	207	213	218	224	229	235	240	246	251	256	262	267	273	278	284	289	295
63	208	214	220	225	231	237	242	248	254	259	265	270	278	282	287	293	299	304
64	215	221	227	232	238	244	250	256	262	267	273	279	285	291	296	302	308	314
65	222	228	234	240	246	252	258	264	270	276	282	288	294	300	306	312	318	324
66	229	235	241	247	253	260	266	272	278	284	291	297	303	309	315	322	328	334
67	236	242	249	255	261	268	274	280	287	293	299	306	312	319	325	331	338	344
68	243	249	256	262	269	276	282	289	295	302	308	315	322	328	335	341	348	354
69	250	257	263	270	277	284	291	297	304	311	318	324	331	338	345	351	358	365
70	257	264	271	278	285	292	299	306	313	320	327	334	341	348	355	362	369	376
71	265	272	279	286	293	301	308	315	322	329	338	343	351	358	365	372	379	386
72	272	279	287	294	302	309	316	324	331	338	346	353	361	368	375	383	390	397
73	280	288	295	302	310	318	325	333	340	348	355	363	371	378	386	393	401	408
74	287	295	303	311	319	326	334	342	350	358	365	373	381	389	396	404	412	420
75	295	303	311	319	327	335	343	351	359	367	375	383	391	399	407	415	423	431
76	304	312	320	328	336	344	353	361	369	377	385	394	402	410	418	426	435	443

Source: NHLBI Obesity Education Initiative Expert Panel on the Identification, Evaluation, and Treatment of Obesity in Adults (US). *Clinical Guidelines on the Identification, Evaluation, and Treatment of Overweight and Obesity in Adults: The Evidence Report.* Bethesda, MD: National Heart, Lung, and Blood Institute; 1998. Available from: http://www.ncbi.nlm.nih.gov/books/NBK2003/.

Table 1.9. Body mass index table

Weight Category	BMI
Underweight	<18.5
Normal weight	18.5–24.9
Overweight	25–29.9
Obesity (Class I)	30–34.9
Obesity (Class II)	35–39.9
Extreme Obesity (Class III)	<40

Source: NHLBI Obesity Education Initiative Expert Panel on the Identification, Evaluation, and Treatment of Obesity in Adults (US). *Clinical Guidelines on the Identification, Evaluation, and Treatment of Overweight and Obesity in Adults: The Evidence Report.* Bethesda, MD: National Heart, Lung, and Blood Institute; 1998. Available from: http://www.ncbi.nlm.nih.gov/books/NBK2003/.

Cardiovascular Disease and Hypercholesterolemia **PRIMARY CARE**

CARDIOVASCULAR DISEASE IN WOMEN

Table 1.10. Classification of CVD risk in women

Risk Status	Criteria
High risk (≥1 high-risk states)	Clinically manifest CHD
	Clinically manifest cerebrovascular disease
	Clinically manifest peripheral arterial disease
	Abdominal aortic aneurysm
	End-stage or chronic kidney disease
	Diabetes mellitus
	10-yr Predicted CVD risk ≥10%
At risk (≥1 major risk factor[s])	Cigarette smoking
	SBP ≥120 mm Hg, DBP ≥80 mm Hg, or treated hypertension
	Total cholesterol ≥200 mg/dL, HDL-C <50 mg/dL, or treated for dyslipidemia
	Obesity, particularly central adiposity
	Poor diet
	Physical inactivity
	Family history of premature CVD occurring in first-degree relatives in men <55 yr of age or in women <65 yr of age
	Metabolic syndrome
	Evidence of advanced subclinical atherosclerosis (e.g., coronary calcification, carotid plaque, or thickened IMT)
	Poor exercise capacity on treadmill test and/or abnormal heart rate recovery after stopping exercise
	Systemic autoimmune collagen-vascular disease (e.g., lupus or rheumatoid arthritis)
	History of preeclampsia, Gestational diabetes, or pregnancy-induced hypertension
Ideal cardiovascular health (all of these)	Total cholesterol <200 mg/dL (untreated)
	BP <120/<80 mm Hg (untreated)
	Fasting blood glucose <100 mg/dL (untreated)
	Body mass index <25 kg/m^2
	Abstinence from smoking
	Physical activity at goal for adults >20 yr of age: ≥150 min/wk moderate intensity, ≥75 min/wk vigorous intensity, or combination
	Healthy (DASH-like) diet (see Appendix)

CVD indicates cardiovascular disease; CHD, coronary heart disease; SBP, systolic blood pressure; DBP, diastolic blood pressure; HDL-C, high-density lipoprotein cholesterol; IMT, intima-media thickness; BP, blood pressure; and DASH, Dietary Approaches to Stop Hypertension.

Source: Reproduced with permission from Mosca L, Benjamin EJ, Berra K, et al. Effectiveness-based guidelines for the prevention of cardiovascular disease in women—2011 update: a guideline from the American Heart Association. *J Am Coll Cardiol.* 2011;57:1404-23. © 2011 American Heart Association, Inc

PRIMARY CARE — Cardiovascular Disease and Hypercholesterolemia

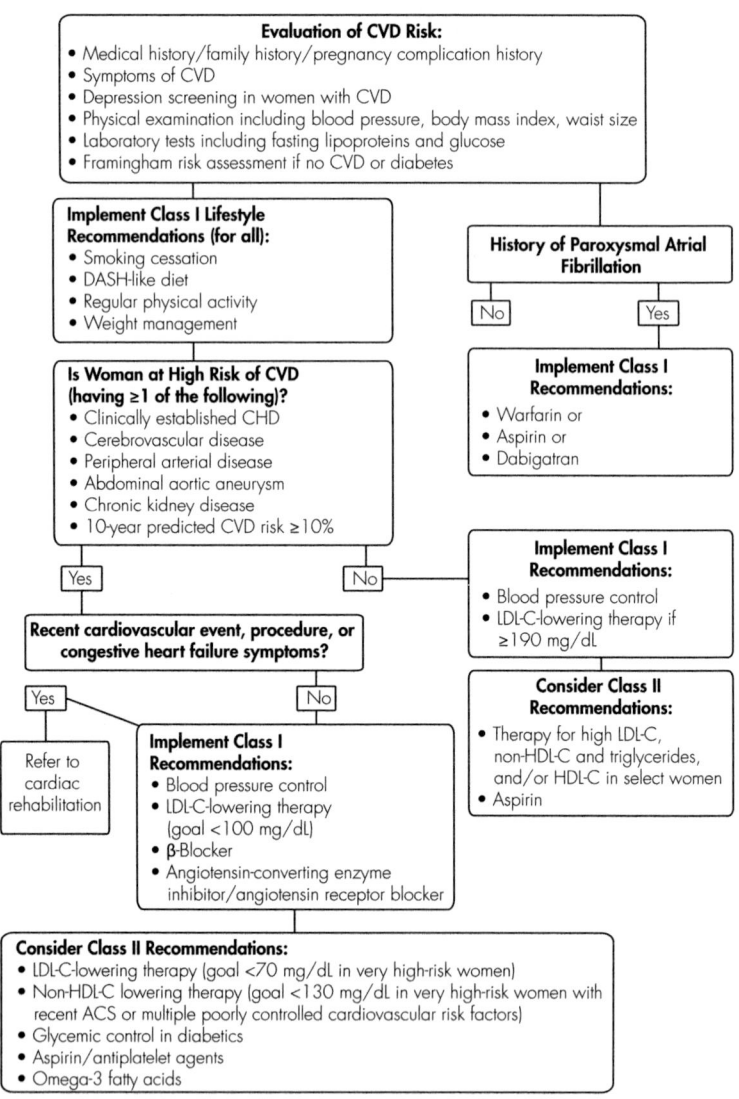

Figure 1.3. Flow diagram for CVD preventative care in women
CVD indicates cardiovascular disease; DASH, Dietary Approaches to Stop Hypertension; CHD, coronary heart disease; LDL-C, low-density lipoprotein cholesterol; HDL-C, high-density lipoprotein cholesterol; and ACS, acute coronary syndrome.
Source: Reproduced with permission from Mosca L, Benjamin EJ, Berra K, et al. Effectiveness-based guidelines for the prevention of cardiovascular disease in women—2011 update: a guideline from the American Heart Association. J Am Coll Cardiol. 2011;57:1404-23. © 2011 American Heart Association, Inc.

Cardiovascular Disease and Hypercholesterolemia — PRIMARY CARE

HYPERCHOLESTEROLEMIA
Fast Facts
- Cholesterol is an essential component of human cell membranes and also act as a precursor to all steroid hormones.
- High levels of cholesterol, however, are associated with cardiovascular disease, since they promote plaque development in arteries, which leads to myocardial infarction, stroke and peripheral vascular disease also known as Arteriosclerotic cardiovascular diseases (ASCVD).
- The 10-year risk for ASCVD is currently used as the main method to determine when to initiate statin treatment. The 10-year risk for ASCVD can be determined by the calculator at this link: http://reference.medscape.com/calculator/framingham-cardiovascular-disease-risk.
- Statins are HMG CoA reductase inhibitors and result in:
  - 30–50% decrease in LDL
  - 5% increase in HDL
  - 20–30% decrease in triglycerides
- All patients, including those with hypercholesterolemia, should be counseled to exercise, eat a prudent diet, and lose weight even if statins are initiated.
- Measuring LDL-C response at 6 weeks after initiating therapy and every 6 to 12 months thereafter may be helpful in assessing medication adherence but is NOT necessary, since intensifying the regiment based upon a particular level of LDL-C response is not recommended anymore.
- In primary prevention, in patients who do not tolerate statins, a nonstatin lipid-lowering medication is recommended. Potential interventions include lifestyle modification and, in higher-risk patients, antiplatelet therapy.
- Statin hepatotoxicity occurs in 0.5–3% of users. Per FDA recommendations (2012), check ALT before start of Rx is recommended, but repeat only if clinically indicated. If ALT is ≥3x, consider changing the statin.
- Severe statin muscle toxicity occurs in 0.5% of users. It is often associated with low CoQ10, low vitamin D, and being hypothyroid. Check Creatinine Kinase (CK) levels at start of treatment, but only repeat the CK level if clinically indicated. If CK is ≥10 × the upper limits normal level, the statin should be discontinued. Do note that pravastatin and fluvastatin have less muscle toxicity than the others.
- Statins may result in a minor increase risk for diabetes mellitus.
- Cholesterol levels will usually increase in pregnancy but do note that statins are contraindicated in pregnant women.

When to Initiate Statins:
New guidelines for treatment of high cholesterol were released in 2013 by the American College of Cardiology and the American Heart Association. These new recommendation suggest that if you are in one of the following 4 groups, treatment with statins will reduce your risk of Arteriosclerotic cardiovascular diseases (ASCVD) and should be recommended.

1. Individuals with existing clinical ASCVD.
2. Individuals with primary elevations of LDL-C ≥190 mg/dL.
3. Individuals 40 to 75 years of age with diabetes and LDL-C 70 to 189 mg/dL without clinical ASCVD.

4. Individuals without clinical ASCVD or diabetes who are 40 to 75 years of age and have LDL-C 70 to 189 mg/dL and an estimated 10-year ASCVD risk of ≥7.5%.

In addition to the 4 groups above, there is also moderate support to treat patients with 10-year ASCVD risk of 5–7.5%.
Link to the 10-year ASCVD calculator: http://reference.medscape.com/calculator/framingham-cardiovascular-disease-risk.

Intensity Level of Treatment

Along with lifestyle counseling, there are 3 levels of intensity statin treatment that can be initiated. Low, moderate and high intensity levels (see table).

Table 1.11. High-, moderate-, and low-intensity statin therapy

High-intensity Statin Therapy	Moderate-intensity Statin Therapy	Low-intensity Statin Therapy
Daily dose lowers LDL-C, on average, by approximately 50%	Daily dose lowers LDL-C, on average, by approximately 30% to <50%	Daily dose lowers LDL-C, on average, by <30%
Atorvastatin (40^y)–80 mg	**Atorvastatin 10 (20) mg**	Simvastatin 10 mg
Rosuvastatin 20 (40) mg	**Rosuvastatin (5) 10 mg**	**Pravastatin 10–20 mg**
	Simvastatin 20–40 mg^z	**Lovastatin 20 mg**
	Pravastatin 40 (80) mg	Fluvastatin 20–40 mg
	Lovastatin 40 mg	Pitavastatin 1 mg
	Fluvastatin XL 80 mg	
	Fluvastatin 40 mg BID	
	Pitavastatin 2–4 mg	

Boldface type indicates specific statins and doses that were evaluated in RCTs included in CQ1, CQ2, and the Cholesterol Treatment Trialists 2010 meta-analysis included in CQ3. All of these RCTs demonstrated a reduction in major cardiovascular events. *Italic type* indicates statins and doses that have been approved by the FDA but were not tested in the RCTs reviewed.

*Individual responses to statin therapy varied in the RCTs and should be expected to vary in clinical practice. There might be a biological basis for a less-than-average response.

^{y}Evidence from 1 RCT only: down-titration if unable to tolerate atorvastatin 80 mg in the IDEAL (Incremental Decrease through Aggressive Lipid Lowering) study (47).

^{z}Although simvastatin 80 mg was evaluated in RCTs, initiation of simvastatin 80 mg or titration to 80 mg is not recommended by the FDA because of the increased risk of myopathy, including rhabdomyolysis.

BID indicates twice daily; CQ, critical question; FDA, Food and Drug Administration; LDL-C, low-density lipoprotein cholesterol; and RCTs, randomized controlled trials.

Source: Reproduced with permission from Stone NJ, Robinson JG, Lichtenstein AH, et al. American College of Cardiology/American Heart Association Task Force on Practice Guidelines. 2013 ACC/AHA guideline on the treatment of blood cholesterol to reduce atherosclerotic cardiovascular risk in adults: a report of the American College of Cardiology/American Heart Association Task Force on Practice Guidelines. *Circulation.* 2014;129:S1-S45. © 2014 American Heart Association, Inc.

Cardiovascular Disease and Hypercholesterolemia — PRIMARY CARE

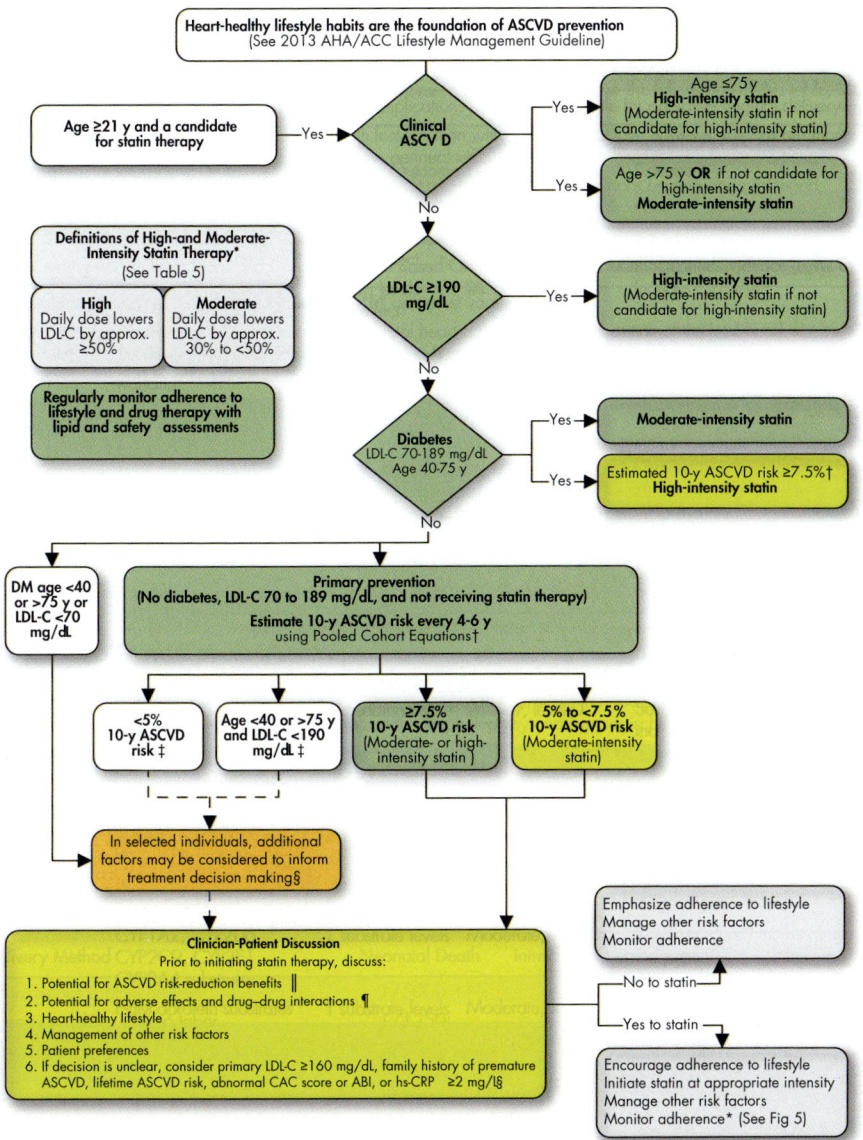

Figure 1.4. Algorithm summarizing the initiation of statin therapy
See source document for color definitions. Assessment of the potential for benefit and risk from statin therapy for ASCVD prevention provides the framework for clinical decision making incorporating patient preferences.

*Percent reduction in LDL-C can be used as an indication of response and adherence to therapy, but is not in itself a treatment goal.

^{y}The Pooled Cohort Equations can be used to estimate 10-year ASCVD risk in individuals with and without diabetes. The estimator within this application should be used to inform decision making in primary prevention patients not on a statin.

^{z}Consider moderate-intensity statin as more appropriate in low-risk individuals.

^{x}For those in whom a risk assessment is uncertain, consider factors such as primary LDL-C ≥160 mg/dL or other evidence of genetic hyperlipidemias, family history of premature ASCVD with onset <55 years of age in a first-degree male relative or <65 years of age in a first-degree female relative, hs-CRP ≥2 mg/L, CAC score ≥300 Agatston units, or ≥75th percentile for age, sex, and ethnicity (for additional information, see http://www.mesa-nhlbi.org/CACReference.aspx), ABI <0.9, or lifetime risk of ASCVD. Additional factors that may aid in individual risk assessment may be identified in the future.

^{k}Potential ASCVD risk-reduction benefits. The absolute reduction in ASCVD events from moderate- or high-intensity statin therapy can be approximated by multiplying the estimated 10-year ASCVD risk by the anticipated relative-risk reduction from the intensity of statin initiated (w30% for moderate-intensity statin or w45% for high-intensity statin therapy). The net ASCVD risk-reduction benefit is estimated from the number of potential ASCVD events prevented with a statin, compared to the number of potential excess adverse effects. The excess risk of diabetes is the main consideration in w0.1 excess cases per 100 individuals treated with a moderate-intensity statin for 1 year and w0.3 excess cases per 100 individuals treated with a high-intensity statin for 1 year. In RCTs, both statin-treated and placebo-treated participants experienced the same rate of muscle symptoms. The actual rate of statin-related muscle symptoms in the clinical population is unclear. Muscle symptoms attributed to statin therapy should be evaluated (see Table 8, Safety Recommendation 8 in Stone (2014)).

ABI indicates ankle-brachial index; ASCVD, atherosclerotic cardiovascular disease; CAC, coronary artery calcium; hs-CRP, high-sensitivity C-reactive protein; LDL-C, low-density lipoprotein cholesterol; MI, myocardial infarction; and RCT, randomized controlled trial.

Source: Reproduced with permission from Stone NJ, Robinson JG, Lichtenstein AH, et al. American College of Cardiology/American Heart Association Task Force on Practice Guidelines. 2013 ACC/AHA guideline on the treatment of blood cholesterol to reduce atherosclerotic cardiovascular risk in adults: a report of the American College of Cardiology/American Heart Association Task Force on Practice Guidelines. *Circulation.* 2014;129:S1-S45. © 2014 American Heart Association, Inc.

Cardiovascular Disease and Hypercholesterolemia **PRIMARY CARE**

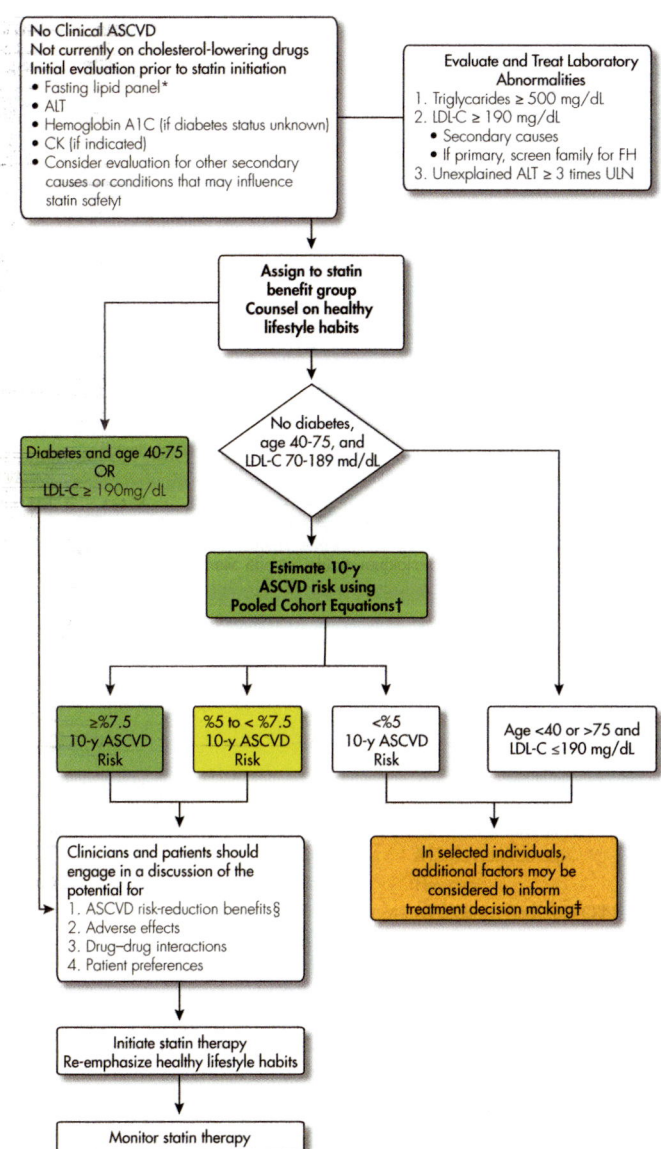

Figure 1.5. Algorithm for the initiation of statin therapy in individuals without ASCVD
See source document for color definitions.
*Fasting lipid panel preferred. In a nonfasting individual, a non-HDL-C level ≥220 mg/dL could indicate genetic hypercholesterolemia that requires further evaluation or a secondary etiology. If nonfasting triglycerides are ≥500 mg/dL, a fasting lipid panel is required.

ʸThe Pooled Cohort Equations can be used to estimate 10-year ASCVD risk in individuals with and without diabetes.

A downloadable spreadsheet enabling estimation of 10-year and lifetime risk for ASCVD and a web-based calculator are available at http://my.americanheart.org/cvriskcalculator and http://www.cardiosource.org/en/Science-And-Quality/Practice-Guidelines-and-Quality-Standards/2013-Prevention-Guideline-Tools.aspx.

ᶻFor those in whom a risk assessment is uncertain, consider factors such as primary LDL-C ≥160 mg/dL or other evidence of genetic hyperlipidemias; family history of premature ASCVD with onset <55 years of age in a first-degree male relative or <65 years of age in a first-degree female relative, high-sensitivity C-reactive protein ≥2 mg/L; CAC ≥300 Agatston units or ≥75th percentile for age, sex, and ethnicity (for additional information, see http://www.mesa-nhlbi.org/CACReference.aspx); ABI <0.9; or lifetime risk of ASCVD. Additional factors that may aid in individual risk assessment could be identified in the future.

ˣ(1) Potential ASCVD risk-reduction benefits. The absolute reduction in ASCVD events from moderate- or high-intensity statin therapy can be approximated by multiplying the estimated 10-year ASCVD risk by the anticipated relative-risk reduction from the intensity of statin initiated (w30% for moderate-intensity statin or w45% for high-intensity statin therapy). The net ASCVD risk-reduction benefit is estimated from the number of potential ASCVD events prevented with a statin, compared to the number of potential excess adverse effects. (2) Potential adverse effects. The excess risk of diabetes is the main consideration in w0.1 excess cases per 100 individuals treated with a 1 year and 1 year and w0.3 excess cases per 100 individuals treated with a high-intensity statin for 1 year. In RCTs, both statin-treated and placebo-treated participants experienced the same rate of muscle symptoms. The actual rate of statin-related muscle symptoms in the clinical population is unclear. Muscle symptoms attributed to statin therapy should be evaluated (see Table 8, Safety Recommendation 8 in Stone (2014)).

ABI indicates ankle-brachial index; ALT, alanine transaminase; ASCVD, atherosclerotic cardiovascular disease; CAC, coronary artery calcium; CK, creatine kinase; FH, familial hypercholesterolemia; LDL-C, low-density lipoprotein cholesterol; MI, myocardial infarction; RCT, randomized controlled trial; and ULN, upper limit of normal.

Source: Reproduced with permission from Stone NJ, Robinson JG, Lichtenstein AH, et al. American College of Cardiology/American Heart Association Task Force on Practice Guidelines. 2013 ACC/AHA guideline on the treatment of blood cholesterol to reduce atherosclerotic cardiovascular risk in adults: a report of the American College of Cardiology/American Heart Association Task Force on Practice Guidelines. *Circulation.* 2014;129:S1-S45. © 2014 American Heart Association, Inc.

Cardiovascular Disease and Hypercholesterolemia — PRIMARY CARE

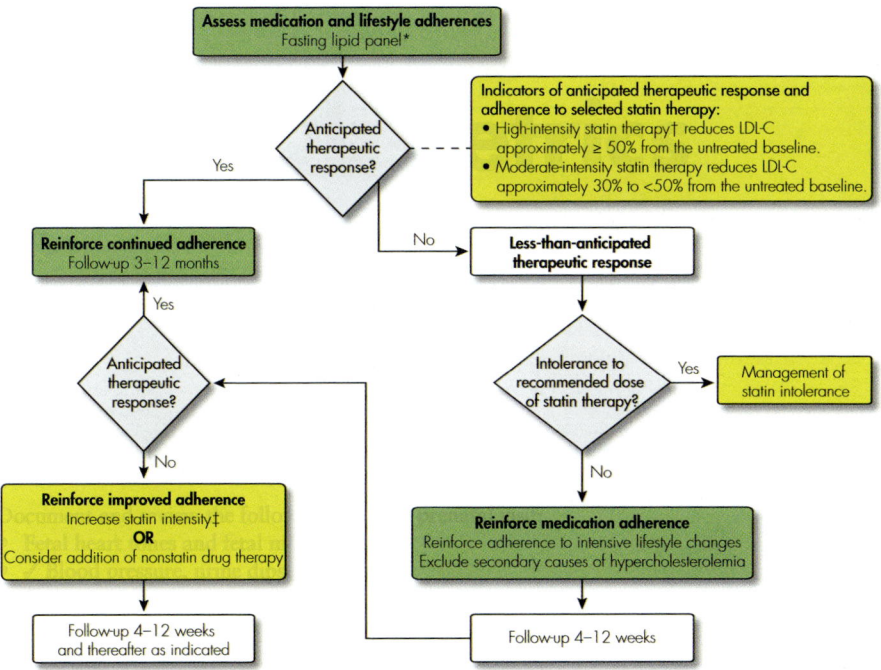

Figure 1.6. Statin therapy: monitoring therapeutic response and adherence

See source document for color definitions.

*Fasting lipid panel preferred. In a nonfasting individual, a non-HDL-C level ≥220 mg/dL may indicate genetic hypercholesterolemia that requires further evaluation or a secondary etiology. If nonfasting triglycerides are ≥500 mg/dL, a fasting lipid panel is required.

†In those already on a statin, in whom baseline LDL-C is unknown, an LDL-C <100 mg/dL was observed in most individuals receiving high-intensity statin therapy in RCTs (See Section 6.3.1 in Stone (2014)).

HDL-C indicates high-density lipoprotein cholesterol; LDL-C, low-density lipoprotein cholesterol; and RCTs, randomized clinical trials.

Source: Reproduced with permission from Stone NJ, Robinson JG, Lichtenstein AH, et al. American College of Cardiology/American Heart Association Task Force on Practice Guidelines. 2013 ACC/AHA guideline on the treatment of blood cholesterol to reduce atherosclerotic cardiovascular risk in adults: a report of the American College of Cardiology/American Heart Association Task Force on Practice Guidelines. *Circulation.* 2014;129:S1-S45. © 2014 American Heart Association, Inc.

Table 1.12. Secondary causes of hyperlipidemia most commonly encountered in clinical practice

Secondary Cause	Elevated LDL-C	Elevated Triglycerides
Diet	Saturated or trans fats, weight gain, anorexia nervosa	Weight gain, very low-fat diets, high intake of refined carbohydrates, excessive alcohol intake
Drugs	Diuretics, cyclosporine, glucocorticoids, amiodarone	Nephrotic syndrome, chronic renal failure, lipodystrophies
Disorders and altered states of metabolism	Hyperthyroidism, obesity, pregnancy*	Diabetes (poorly controlled), hypothyroidism, obesity, pregnancy*

*Cholesterol and triglycerides rise progressively throughout pregnancy (80); treatment with statins, niacin, and ezetimibe are contraindicated during pregnancy and lactation.

LDL-C indicates low-density lipoprotein cholesterol.

Source: Reproduced with permission from Stone NJ, Robinson JG, Lichtenstein AH, et al. American College of Cardiology/American Heart Association Task Force on Practice Guidelines. 2013 ACC/AHA guideline on the treatment of blood cholesterol to reduce atherosclerotic cardiovascular risk in adults: a report of the American College of Cardiology/American Heart Association Task Force on Practice Guidelines. *Circulation.* 2014;129:S1-S45. © 2014 American Heart Association, Inc.

Cardiovascular Disease and Hypercholesterolemia **PRIMARY CARE**

LIPID LOWERING DRUGS

Table 1.13. Adult dosing, side effects, and drug interactions of lipid-lowering drugs

Drug Class	Dose	Dosing	Major Side Effects and Drug Interactions
Statins (HMG coa reductase inhibitors)			
Lovastatin	20–80 mg/day	IR take with evening meal. BID with meals if dose >20 mg/day. XR take any time.	Headache; nausea; sleep disturbance; elevations in hepatocellular enzymes and alkaline phosphatase. Myositis and rhabdomyolysis, primarily when given with gemfibrozil or cyclosporine; myositis is also seen with severe renal insufficiency (CrCl <30 mL/min). Lovastatin, atorvastatin, rosuvastatin, and simvastatin potentiate effect of warfarin; this interaction is not seen with pravastatin, fluvastatin, or pitavastatin. Most statins can also affect digoxin metabolism and levels.
Pravastatin	10–80 mg/day		
Simvastatin	5–40 mg/day	Take in the evening	
Fluvastatin	20–80 mg/day	IR take in the evening; if dose >40 mg/day take morning and evening. XR take any time.	
	80 mg XR/day		
Atorvastatin	10–80 mg/day		
Rosuvastatin	5–50 mg/day		
Pitavastatin	1–4 mg/day		
Gemfibrozil	600 mg BID	30 to 60 min before meals	Potentiates warfarin action. Absorption of gemfibrozil diminished by bile acid sequestrants.
Fenofibrate	Nanocrystal 145 mg/day	Micronized taken with meals. Use lower doses with renal insufficiency. Skin rash, gastrointestinal (nausea, bloating, cramping), myalgia; lowers blood cyclosporine levels; potentially nephrotoxic in cyclosporine-treated patients. Avoid in patients with CrCl <30 mL/min.	
	Micronized 160–200 mg/day		
Nicotinic acid	1–12 g/day	Given with meals. Start with 100 mg BID and titrate to 500 mg TID. After 6 weeks, check lipids, glucose, liver function, and Uric acid. Increase dose as needed.	Prostaglandin-mediated cutaneous flushing, headache, warm sensation, and pruritus; hyperpigmentation (particularly in intertriginous regions); acanthosis nigricans; dry skin; nausea; vomiting; diarrhea; and myositis.

(continued)

PRIMARY CARE — Cardiovascular Disease and Hypercholesterolemia

Drug Class	Dose	Dosing	Major Side Effects and Drug Interactions
Bile acid sequestrants			
Cholestyramine	4–24 g/day	Take within 30 min of a meal. A double dose with dinner produces the same lipid-lowering effect as BID dosing.	Nausea, bloating, cramping, and constipation; elevations in hepatic transaminases and alkaline phosphatase. Impaired absorption of fat soluble vitamins, digoxin, warfarin, thiazides, β-blockers, thyroxine, and phenobarbital.
Colesevelam	3.75 g/day	Taken with meals QD or divided BID	Similar
Cholesterol absorption inhibitors			
Ezetimibe	10 mg/day		Increased transaminases in combination with statins
Neomycin	1 g BID		Ototoxicity; nephrotoxicity
Probucol	500 mg BID		Loose stools; eosinophilia; QT prolongation; angioneurotic edema

BID: twice daily; QD: daily; TID: three times daily; IR: immediate release; XR: extended release; CrCl: creatinine clearance.

Source: Reproduced with permission from Rosenson RS. Lipid lowering with drugs other than statins and fibrates. In: UpToDate, Post TW (Ed), UpToDate, Waltham, MA. (Accessed on March 18, 2016) Copyright © 2016 UpToDate, Inc. For more information, visit www.uptodate.com.

Table 1.14. Properties of statins

Variable	Atorvastatin	Fluvastatin	Lovastatin	Pitavastatin	Pravastatin	Rosuvastatin	Simvastatin
LDL cholesterol reductions (dose range, mg)	38 to 54% (10 to 80)	17 to 33% (20 to 80)	29 to 48% (20 to 80)	31 to 41% (1 to 4)	19 to 40% (10 to 40)	52 to 63% (10 to 40)	28 to 41% (10 to 40)
Elimination half-life, hours	15 to 30	0.5 to 2.3	2.9	12	1.3 to 2.8	19	2 to 3
Bioavailability, percent	12	19 to 29	5	51	18	20	5
Protein binding, percent	80 to 90	>99	>95	99	43 to 55	88	94 to 98
Solubility	Lipophilic	Lipophilic	Lipophilic	Lipophilic	Hydrophilic	Hydrophilic	Lipophilic
Cytochrome 450 metabolism and isozyme	3A4	2C9	3A4	Limited 2C9, 2C8	-	Limited 2C9	3A4, 3A5
Active metabolites	Yes	No	Yes	Yes	No	No	Yes
Effect of food absorption on drug	None	Negligible	Increased absorption	Decreases	Decreased absorption	None	None
Optimal time of administration	Anytime	IR: evening (or morning and evening if taken twice daily)	IR: with evening meal (or with morning and evening meal if taken twice daily)	Anytime	Anytime	Anytime	Evening
		XR: anytime	XR: anytime				
Renal excretion of absorbed dose, percent	2	<6	10	15	20	10	13

IR: immediate release; XR: extended release.

Source: Reproduced with permission from Rosenson RS. Statins: actions, side effects, and administration. In: UpToDate, Post TW (Ed), UpToDate, Waltham, MA. (Accessed on March 18, 2016) Copyright © 2016 UpToDate, Inc. For more information, visit www.uptodate.com.

HYPERTENSION

Fast Facts
- Hypertension (HTN) is the most common condition seen in primary care.
- HTN may lead to myocardial infarction, stroke, renal failure, and death if not treated appropriately.
- Reverse risk factors include:
  - BMI of 25 kg/m^2 or less
  - daily 30 min exercise
  - following a Dietary Approaches to Stop Hypertension (DASH) diet, which is composed of four to five servings of fruit, four to five servings of vegetables, two to three servings of low-fat dairy per day, and <25% dietary fat
  - low alcohol intake
  - infrequent use of non narcotic analgesics
  - folate intake of ≥400mcg
- Normal BP is systolic <120 mm Hg and diastolic <80 mm Hg.
- Prehypertension is systolic 120 to 139 mm Hg or diastolic 80 to 89 mm Hg.
  Patients with prehypertension, but without diabetes, chronic kidney disease, or cardiovascular disease, are treated with nonpharmacologic therapies such as weight reduction, sodium restriction, and avoidance of excess alcohol. They should also have their blood pressure measured at least annually, or more frequently if home monitoring is available, since they are at significant risk of developing hypertension over time
- Isolated systolic hypertension is considered to be present when the blood pressure is ≥140/<90 mm Hg.
- Hypertension:
  - Stage 1: systolic 140 to 159 mm Hg or diastolic 90 to 99 mm Hg
  - Stage 2: systolic ≥160 mm Hg or diastolic ≥100 mm Hg
- Patients with office hypertension, normal values at home, and no evidence of end-organ damage should undergo ambulatory blood pressure monitoring to see whether they are truly hypertensive.
- In the absence of end-organ damage, a patient should not be labeled as having hypertension unless the blood pressure is persistently elevated after three to six visits over a several-month period.
- Systolic and diastolic hypertension, isolated systolic hypertension, and isolated diastolic hypertension all should be treated. Isolated diastolic hypertension is associated with increased cardiovascular risk, but there are no treatment trials to prove benefit from antihypertensive therapy.
- In summary, antihypertensive medications should generally be begun if the systolic pressure is persistently ≥140 mm Hg (in patients younger than 60 years) and/or the diastolic pressure is persistently ≥90 mm Hg in the office and at home, despite attempted nonpharmacologic therapy. See below for more detail regarding latest recommendations.

Latest Recommendations regarding When to Start Treatment

ALL patients should undergo appropriate lifestyle (nonpharmacologic) modification before treatment starts.

1. In patients aged **≥60 years**, initiate pharmacologic treatment at:
   - systolic BP ≥150 mm Hg or diastolic BP ≥90 mm Hg
   - treat to a goal systolic BP <150 mm Hg and goal diastolic BP <90 mm Hg
2. In patients aged **<60 years**, initiate pharmacologic treatment at:
   - diastolic BP ≥90 mm Hg
   - treat to a goal <90 mm Hg

Hypertension

3. In patients aged **<60 years**, initiate pharmacologic treatment at:
   o systolic BP ≥140 mm Hg
   o treat to a goal <140 mm Hg
4. In patients aged **≥18 years** with chronic kidney disease, initiate pharmacologic treatment at:
   o systolic BP ≥140 mm Hg or diastolic BP ≥90 mm Hg
   o treat to goal systolic BP <140 mm Hg and goal diastolic BP <90 mm Hg
5. In patients aged **≥18** years with diabetes, initiate pharmacologic treatment at:
   o systolic BP ≥140 mm Hg or diastolic BP ≥90 mm Hg
   o treat to a goal systolic BP <140 mm Hg and goal diastolic BP <90 mm Hg
6. In the general nonblack population, including those with diabetes, initial antihypertensive treatment should include either one of the listed:
   o Calcium channel blocker (CCB)
   o Angiotensin converting enzyme (ACE) inhibitor
   o Angiotensin receptor blocker (ARB)
7. In the general black population, including those with diabetes, initial antihypertensive treatment should include either one of the listed:
   o thiazide-type diuretic
   o CCB
8. In the population aged ≥18 years with chronic kidney disease, initial (or add-on) antihypertensive treatment should include an ACE inhibitor or ARB to improve kidney outcomes.
9. If goal BP is not reached within a month of treatment, increase the dose of the initial drug or add a second drug from one of the classes in Recommendation 6. If goal BP cannot be reached with two drugs, add and titrate a third drug from the list provided. Do not use an ACEI and an ARB together in the same patient. If goal BP cannot be reached using only the drugs in Recommendation 6 because of a contraindication or the need to use more than 3 drugs to reach goal BP, antihypertensive drugs from other classes can be used.

Principles of Lifestyle Modifications

- Encourage healthy lifestyles for all individuals.
- Prescribe lifestyle modifications for all patients with prehypertension and hypertension.
- Components of lifestyle modifications include weight reduction, DASH eating plan, dietary sodium reduction, aerobic physical activity, and moderation of alcohol consumption.

Table 1.15. Lifestyle modification recommendations

Modification	Recommendation	Avg. SBP Reduction Range[a]
Weight reduction	Maintain normal body weight (body mass index 18.5–24.9 kg/m^2).	5–20 mm Hg/10 kg
DASH eating plan	Adopt a diet rich in fruits, vegetables, and low-fat dairy products with reduced content of saturated and total fat.	8–14 mm Hg
Dietary sodium reduction	Reduce dietary sodium intake to ≤100 mmol per day (2.4 g sodium or 6 g sodium chloride).	2–8 mm Hg
Aerobic physical activity	Regular aerobic physical activity (e.g., brisk walking) at least 30 mins per day, most days of the week.	4–9 mm Hg
Moderation of alcohol consumption	Men: limit to ≤2 drinks[b] per day. Women and lighter weight persons: limit to ≤1 drink[b] per day.	2–4 mm Hg

[a] Effects are dose and time dependent.
[b] 1 drink = 1/2 oz or 15 mL ethanol (e.g., 12 oz beer, 5 oz wine, 1.5 oz 80 proof whiskey).

Source: Reproduced from Seventh Report of the Joint National Committee on Prevention, Detection, Evaluation, and Treatment of High Blood Pressure (JNC 7 Express). U.S. Department of Health and Human Services. NIH Publication No. 03-5233, December 2003.

Table 1.16. Evidence-based dosing for antihypertensive drugs

Antihypertensive Medication	Initial Daily Dose, mg	Target Dose in RCTs Reviewed, mg	No. of Doses Per Day
ACE inhibitors			
Captopril	50	150–200	2
Enalapril	5	20	1–2
Lisinopril	10	40	1
Angiotensin receptor blockers			
Eprosartan	400	600–800	1–2
Candesartan	4	12–32	1
Losartan	50	100	1–2
Valsartan	40–80	160–320	1
Irbesartan	75	300	1
β-blockers			
Atenolol	25–50	100	1
Metoprolol	50	100–200	1–2
Calcium channel blockers			
Amlodipine	2.5	10	1
Diltiazem extended release	120–180	360	1
Nitrendipine	10	20	1–2
Thiazide-type diuretics			
Bendroflumethiazide	5	10	1
Chlorthalidone	12.5	12.5–25	1
Hydrochlorothiazide	12.5–25	25–100[a]	1–2
Indapamide	1.25	1.25–2.5	1

ACE, angiotensin-converting enzyme; RCT, randomized controlled trial.

[a]Current recommended evidence-based dose that balances efficacy and safety is 25–50 mg daily.

Reproduced with permission from James PA, Oparil S, Carter BL, et al. 2014 evidence-based guideline for the management of high blood pressure in adults: report from the panel members appointed to the Eighth Joint National Committee (JNC 8). *JAMA.* 2014 Feb 5;311(5):507-520. Copyright © 2014 American Medical Association. All rights reserved.

Table 1.17. Strategies to dose antihypertensive drugs

Strategy	Description	Details
A	Start one drug, titrate to maximum dose, and then add a second drug	If goal BP is not achieved with the initial drug, titrate the dose of the initial drug up to the maximum recommended dose to achieve goal BP
		If goal BP is not achieved with the use of one drug despite titration to the maximum recommended dose, add a second drug from the list (thiazide-type diuretic, CCB, ACEI, or ARB) and titrate up to the maximum recommended dose of the second drug to achieve goal BP
		If goal BP is not achieved with 2 drugs, select a third drug from the list (thiazide-type diuretic, CCB, ACEI, or ARB), avoiding the combined use of ACEI and ARB. Titrate the third drug up to the maximum recommended dose to achieve goal BP
B	Start one drug and then add a second drug before achieving maximum dose of the initial drug	Start with one drug then add a second drug before achieving the maximum recommended dose of the initial drug, then titrate both drugs up to the maximum recommended doses of both to achieve goal BP
		If goal BP is not achieved with 2 drugs, select a third drug from the list (thiazide-type diuretic, CCB, ACEI, or ARB), avoiding the combined use of ACEI and ARB. Titrate the third drug up to the maximum recommended dose to achieve goal BP
C	Begin with 2 drugs at the same time, either as 2 separate pills or as a single pill combination	Initiate therapy with 2 drugs simultaneously, either as 2 separate drugs or as a single pill combination. Some committee members recommend starting therapy with ≥2 drugs when SBP is >160 mm Hg and/or DBP is >100 mm Hg, or if SBP is >20 mm Hg above goal and/or DBP is >10 mm Hg above goal. If goal BP is not achieved with 2 drugs, select a third drug from the list (thiazide-type diuretic, CCB, ACEI, or ARB), avoiding the combined use of ACEI and ARB. Titrate the third drug up to the maximum recommended dose.

ACEI, angiotensin-converting enzyme; ARB, angiotensin receptor blocker; BP, blood pressure; CCB, calcium channel blocker; DBP, diastolic blood pressure; SBP, systolic blood pressure.

[a]This table is not meant to exclude other agents within the classes of antihypertensive medications that have been recommended but reflects those agents and dosing used in randomized controlled trials that demonstrated improved outcomes.

Reproduced with permission from James PA, Oparil S, Carter BL, et al. 2014 evidence-based guideline for the management of high blood pressure in adults: report from the panel members appointed to the Eighth Joint National Committee (JNC 8). *JAMA.* 2014 Feb 5;311(5):507-520. Copyright © 2014 American Medical Association. All rights reserved.

Table 1.18. Guideline comparisons of goal BP and initial drug therapy for adults with hypertension

Guideline	Population	Goal BP, mm Hg	Initial Drug Treatment Options
2014 hypertension guideline	General ≥60 yr	<150/90	Nonblack: thiazide-type diuretic, ACEI, ARB, or CCB; black: thiazide-type diuretic or CCB
	General <60 yr	<140/90	
	Diabetes	<140/90	Thiazide-type diuretic, ACEI, ARB, or CCB
	CKD	<140/90	ACEI or ARB
ESH/ESC 2013	General nonelderly	<140/90	Diuretic, β-blocker, CCB, ACEI, or ARB
	General elderly <80 yr	<150/90	
	General ≥80 yr	<150/90	
	Diabetes	<140/85	ACEI or ARB
	CKD no proteinuria	<140/90	ACEI or ARB
	CKD + proteinuria	<130/90	
CHEP 2013	General <80 yr	<140/90	Thiazide, β-blocker (age <60 yr), ACEI (nonblack), or ARB
	General ≥80 yr	<150/90	
	Diabetes	<130/80	ACEI or ARB with additional CVD risk
			ACEI, ARB, thiazide, or DHPCCB without additional CVD risk
	CKD	<140/90	ACEI or ARB
ADA 2013	Diabetes	<140/80	ACEI or ARB
KDIGO 2012	CKD no proteinuria	≤140/90	ACEI or ARB
	CKD + proteinuria	≤130/80	
NICE 2011	General <80 yr	<140/90	<55 yr: ACEI or ARB
	General ≥80 yr	<150/90	≥55 yr or black: CCB
ISHIB 2010	Black, lower risk	<135/85	Diuretic or CCB
	Target organ damage or CVD risk	<130/80	

ADA, American Diabetes Association; ACEI, angiotensin-converting enzyme inhibitor; ARB, angiotensin receptor blocker; CCB, calcium channel blocker; CHEP, Canadian Hypertension Education Program; CKD, chronic kidney disease; CVD, cardiovascular disease; DHPCCB, dihydropyridine calcium channel blocker; ESC, European Society of Cardiology; ESH, European Society of Hypertension; ISHIB, International Society for Hypertension in Blacks; JNC, Joint National Committee; KDIGO, Kidney Disease: Improving Global Outcome; NICE, National Institute for Health and Clinical Excellence.

Reproduced with permission from James PA, Oparil S, Carter BL, et al. 2014 evidence-based guideline for the management of high blood pressure in adults: report from the panel members appointed to the Eighth Joint National Committee (JNC 8). *JAMA*. 2014 Feb 5;311(5):507-520. Copyright © 2014 American Medical Association. All rights reserved.

Hypertension

PRIMARY CARE

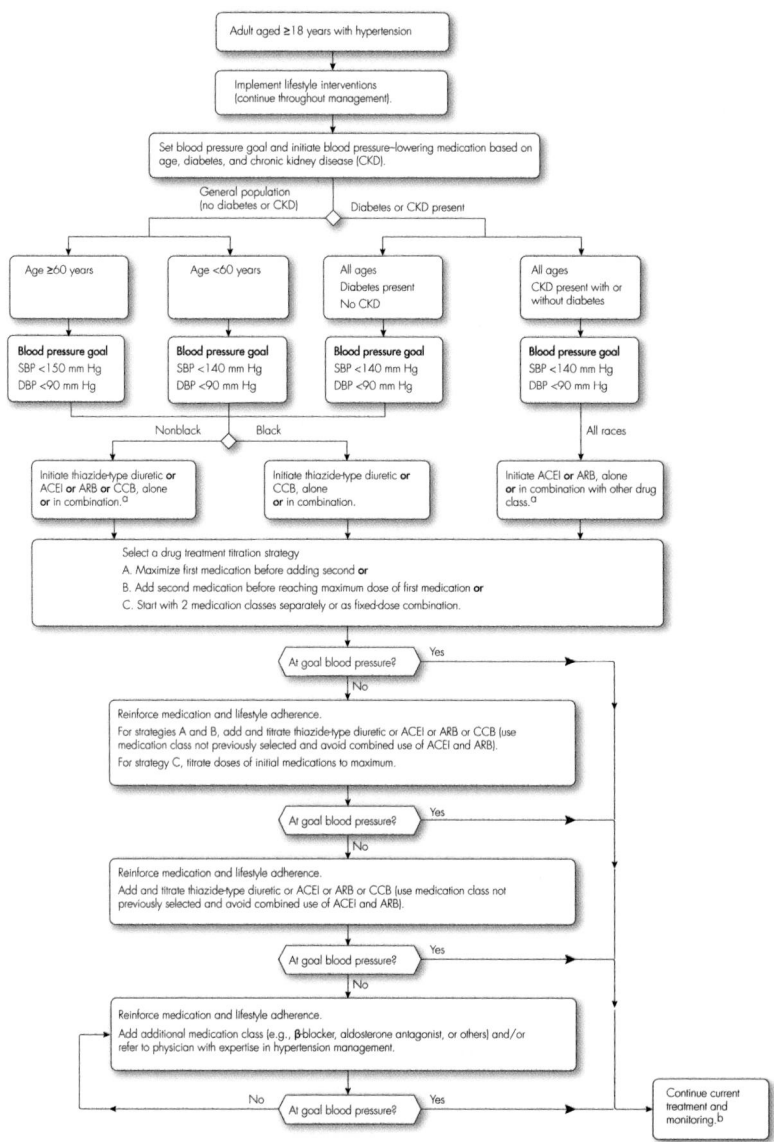

Figure 1.7. Algorithm for the management of high blood pressure in adults
Source: Reproduced with permission from James PA, Oparil S, Carter BL, et al. 2014 evidence-based guideline for the management of high blood pressure in adults: report from the panel members appointed to the Eighth Joint National Committee (JNC 8). *JAMA.* 2014 Feb 5;311(5):507-520. Copyright © 2014 American Medical Association. All rights reserved.

DIABETES MELLITUS

Fast Facts
- Type 2 diabetes results in enormous human suffering and economic cost.
- Complications can be reduced by achieving nondiabetic glucose levels.
- First line of treatment is lifestyle modification and metformin.
- Early addition of insulin is recommended if goals not achieved.

Table 1.19. Initial evaluation of type 2 diabetes

Medical History
- Age and characteristics of onset of diabetes (e.g., DKA, asymptomatic laboratory finding)
- Eating patterns, nutritional status, and weight history; growth and development in children and adolescentss
- Diabetes education history
- Review of previous treatment regimens and response to therapy (A1C records)
- Current treatment of diabetes, including medications, meal plan, physical activity patterns, and results of glucose monitoring
- patterns, and results of glucose monitoring and patient's use of data
- DKA frequency, severity, and cause
- Hypoglycemic episodes
  - Hypoglycemia awareness
  - Any severe hypoglycemia: frequency and cause
- History of diabetes-related complications
  - Microvascular: retinopathy, nephropathy, neuropathy (sensory, including history of foot lesions; autonomic including sexual dysfunction and gastroparesis)
  - Macrovascular: CHD, cerebrovascular disease, PAD
  - Other: psychosocial problems,* dental disease*

Physical Examination
- Height, weight, BMI
- Blood pressure determination, including orthostatic measurements when indicated
- Fundoscopic examination*
- Thyroid palpation
- Skin examination (for acanthosis nigracans and insulin injection sites)
- Comprehensive foot examination:
  - Inspection
  - Palpation of dorsalis pedis and posterior tibial pulses
  - Presence/absence of patellar and Achilles reflexes
  - Determination of proprioception, vibration, and monofilament sensation

Laboratory Evaluation
- A1C, if results not available within past 2–3 months

If Not Performed/Available Within Past Year:
- Fasting lipid profile, including total, LDL, and HDL cholesterol and triglycerides
- Liver function tests
- Test for urine albumin excretion with spot urine albumin-to-creatinine ratio
- Serum creatinine and calculated GFR
- Thyroid-stimulating hormone in type 1 diabetes, dyslipidemia or women over age 50

(continued)

Diabetes Mellitus **PRIMARY CARE**

Referrals

- Annual dilated eye exam
- Family planning for women of reproductive age
- Registered dietitian for MNT
- Diabetes self-management education
- Dental examination
- Mental health professional, if needed

*See appropriate referrals for these categories.

Source: Reproduced with permission from American Diabetes Association. Standards of medical care in diabetes—2008. *Diabetes Care.* 2008 Jan;31 Suppl 1:S12-54. Copyright © 2008, American Diabetes Association.

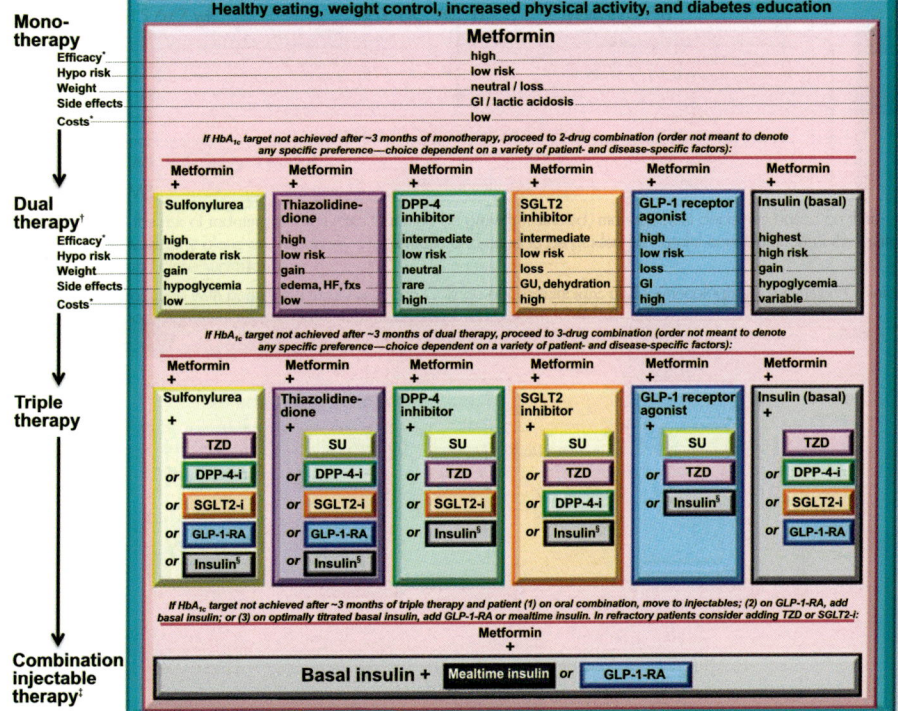

Figure 1.8. Antihyperglycemic therapy in type 2 diabetes: general recommendations

Source: Reproduced with permission from Inzucchi SE, Bergenstal RM, Buse JB, et al. Management of hyperglycemia in type 2 diabetes, 2015: a patient-centered approach: update to a position statement of the American Diabetes Association and the European Association for the Study of Diabetes. *Diabetes Care.* 2015 Jan;38(1):140-149 Copyright © 2015, American Diabetes Association.

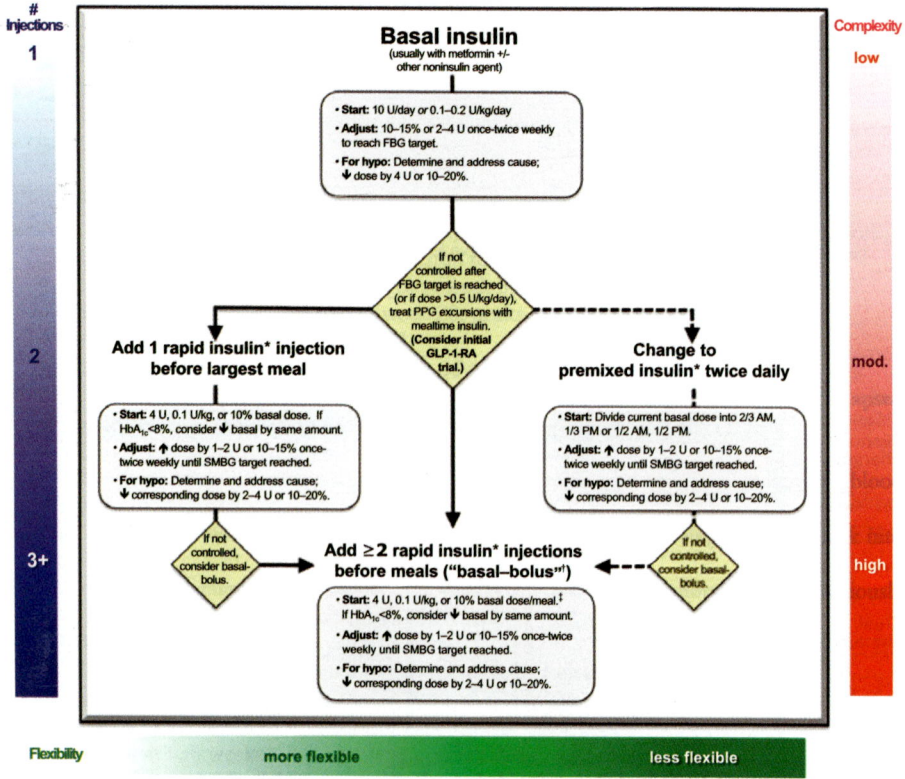

Figure 1.9. Approach to starting and adjusting insulin in type 2 diabetes
Source: Reproduced with permission from Inzucchi SE, Bergenstal RM, Buse JB, et al. Management of hyperglycemia in type 2 diabetes, 2015: a patient-centered approach: update to a position statement of the American Diabetes Association and the European Association for the Study of Diabetes. *Diabetes Care*. 2015 Jan;38(1):140-149 Copyright © 2015, American Diabetes Association.

Diabetes Mellitus **PRIMARY CARE**

Table 1.20. Properties of available glucose-lowering agents in the U.S. and Europe that may guide individualized treatment choices in patients with type 2 diabetes

Class	Compound(s)	Cellular Mechanism(s)	Primary Physiological Action(s)	Advantages	Disadvantages	Cost*
Biguanides	• Metformin	Activates AMP-kinase (? other)	• ↓ Hepatic glucose production	• Extensive experience • No hypoglycemia • ↓ CVD events (UKPDS)	• Gastrointestinal side effects (diarrhea, abdominal cramping) • Lactic acidosis risk (rare) • Vitamin B12 deficiency • Multiple contraindications: CKD, acidosis, hypoxia, dehydration, etc.	Low
Sulfonylureas	Second Generation • Glyburide/ glibenclamide • Glipizide • Gliclazide[†] • Glimepiride	Closes K_{ATP} channels on β-cell plasma membranes	• ↑ Insulin secretion	• Extensive experience • ↓ Microvascular risk (UKPDS)	• Hypoglycemia • ↑ Weight • ? Blunts myocardial ischemic preconditioning • Low durability	Low
Meglitinides (glinides)	• Repaglinide • Nateglinide	Closes K_{ATP} channels on β-cell plasma membranes	• ↑ Insulin secretion	• ↓ Postprandial glucose excursions • Dosing flexibility	• Hypoglycemia • ↑ Weight • ? Blunts myocardial ischemic preconditioning • Frequent dosing schedule	Moderate
TZDs	• Pioglitazone[‡] • Rosiglitazone[§]	Activates the nuclear transcription factor PPAR-γ	• ↑ Insulin sensitivity	• No hypoglycemia • Durability • ↑ HDL-C • ↓ Triglycerides (pioglitazone) • ? ↓ CVD events (PROactive, pioglitazone)	• ↑ Weight • Edema/heart failure • Bone fractures • ↑ LDL-C (rosiglitazone) • ? ↑ MI (meta-analyses, rosiglitazone)	Low
α-glucosidase inhibitors	• Acarbose • Miglitol	Inhibits intestinal α-glucosidase	• Slows intestinal carbohydrate digestion/absorption	• No hypoglycemia • ↓ Postprandial glucose excursions • ? ↓ CVD events (STOP-NIDDM) • Nonsystemic	• Generally modest HbA1C efficacy • Gastrointestinal side effects (flatulence, diarrhea) • Frequent dosing schedule	Moderate

(continued)

Class	Compound(s)	Cellular Mechanism(s)	Primary Physiological Action(s)	Advantages	Disadvantages	Cost*
DPP-4 inhibitors	• Sitagliptin • Vildagliptin† • Saxagliptin • Linagliptin • Alogliptin	Inhibits DPP-4 activity, increasing postprandial active incretin (GLP-1, GIP) concentrations	• ↑ Insulin secretion (glucose-dedependent) • ↓ Glucagon secretion (glucose-dependent)	• No hypoglycemia • Well tolerated	• Angioedema/ urticaria and other immune-mediated dermatological effects • ? Acute pancreatitis • ? ↑ Heart failure hospitalizations	High
Bile acid sequestrants	• Colesevelam	Binds bile acids in intestinal tract, increasing hepatic bile acid production	• ? ↓ Hepatic glucose production • ? ↑ Incretin levels	• No hypoglycemia • ↓ LDL-C	• Generally modest HbA1C efficacy • Constipation • ↑ Triglycerides • May ↓ absorption of other medications	High
Dopamine-2 agonists	• Bromocriptine (quick release)§	Activates dopaminergic receptors	• Modulates hypothalamic regulation of metabolism • ↑ Insulin sensitivity	• No hypoglycemia • ? ↓ CVD events (Cycloset Safety Trial)	• Generally modest HbA1C efficacy • Dizziness/ syncope • Nausea • Fatigue • Rhinitis	High
SGLT2 inhibitors	• Canagliflozin • Dapagliflozin‡ • Empagliflozin	Inhibits SGLT2 in the proximal nephron	• Blocks glucose reabsorption by the kidney, increasing glucosuria	• No hypoglycemia • ↓ Weight • ↓ Blood pressure • Effective at all stages of T2DM	• Genitourinary infections • Polyuria • Volume depletion/ hypotension/ dizziness • ↑ LDL-C • ↑ Creatinine (transient)	High
GLP-1 receptor agonists	• Exenatide • Exenatide extended release • Liraglutide • Albiglutide • Lixisenatide† • Dulaglutide	Activates GLP-1 receptors	• ↑ Insulin secretion (glucose-dependent) • ↓ Glucagon secretion (glucose-dependent) • Slows gastric emptying • ↑ Satiety	• No hypoglycemia • ↓ Weight • ↓ Postprandial glucose excursions • ↓ Some cardiovascular risk factors	• Gastrointestinal side effects (nausea/vomiting/ diarrhea) • ↑ Heart rate • ? Acute pancreatitis • C-cell hyperplasia/medullary thyroid tumors in animals • Injectable • Training requirements	High

(continued)

Diabetes Mellitus

Class	Compound(s)	Cellular Mechanism(s)	Primary Physiological Action(s)	Advantages	Disadvantages	Cost*
Amylin mimetics	• Pramlintide§	Activates amylin receptors	• ↓ Glucagon secretion • Slows gastric emptying • ↑ Satiety	• ↓ Postprandial glucose excursions • ↓ Weight	• Generally modest HbA1C efficacy • Gastrointestinal side effects (nausea/vomiting) • Hypoglycemia unless insulin dose is simultaneously reduced • Injectable • Frequent dosing schedule • Training requirements	High

Insulins	• Rapid-acting analogs
	  ○ Lispro
	  ○ Aspart
	  ○ Glulisine
	• Short-acting
	  ○ Human Regular
	• Intermediate-acting
	  ○ Human NPH
	• Basal insulin analogs
	  ○ Glargine
	  ○ Detemir
	  ○ Degludec†
	• Premixed (several types)
		Activates insulin receptors	• ↑ Glucose disposal
			• ↓ Hepatic glucose production
			• Other
				• Nearly universal response
				• Theoretically unlimited efficacy
				• ↓ Microvascular risk (UKPDS)
					• Hypoglycemia
					• Weight gain
					• ? Mitogenic effects
					• Injectable
					• Patient reluctance
					• Training requirements
						Variable#

CVD, cardiovascular disease; GIP, glucose-dependent insulinotropic peptide; HDL-C, HDL cholesterol; LDL-C, LDL cholesterol; MI, myocardial infarction; PPAR-γ, peroxisome proliferator-activated receptor γ; PROactive, Prospective Pioglitazone Clinical Trial in Macrovascular Events (26); STOP-NIDDM, Study to Prevent Non-Insulin-Dependent Diabetes Mellitus (60); T2DM, type 2 diabetes mellitus; UKPDS, UK Prospective Diabetes Study (4,61). Cycloset trial of quick-release bromocriptine (62).

*Cost is based on lowest-priced member of the class.
†Not licensed in the U.S.
‡Initial concerns regarding bladder cancer risk are decreasing after subsequent study.
§Not licensed in Europe for type 2 diabetes.
#Cost is highly dependent on type/brand (analogs > human insulins) and dosage.

Source: Reproduced with permission from Inzucchi SE, Bergenstal RM, Buse JB, et al. Management of hyperglycemia in type 2 diabetes, 2015: a patient-centered approach: update to a position statement of the American Diabetes Association and the European Association for the Study of Diabetes. *Diabetes Care.* 2015 Jan;38(1):140-49. Copyright © 2015, American Diabetes Association.

TOBACCO, ALCOHOL, AND DRUG ABUSE

Table 1.21. Agents to help smokers quit

Factor	Bupropion Hydrochloride SR (Zyban®, Wellbutrin®)	Patch (Various)	Gum (Nicorette®)
Treatment Period	7–12 wk Take for 1–2 wk before quitting smoking May use for maintenance for up to 6 mo	6–8 wk	Up to 12 wk May use for longer time as needed
Dosage	Days 1–3: 150-mg tablet each morning Days 4–end: 150-mg tablet in morning and evening 14 mg for 2 wk 7 mg for 2 wk No taper if using 15 mg for 8 wk Light smokers (≤10 cigarettes/day) can start with lower dose	One patch each day Taper dose if using 21 mg for 4 wk Many people do not use enough gum—chew gum whenever you need it!	2 mg 4 mg (heavy smokers) Chew one piece every 1–2 hr (10–15 pieces/day)
Pros	Easy to use Reduces urges to smoke	Easy to use Steady dose of nicotine	Can control your own dose Helps with predictable urges (e.g., after meals) Keeps mouth busy
Cons	May disturb sleep May cause dry mouth	May irritate skin May disturb sleep Cannot adjust amount of nicotine in response to urges	Need to chew correctly—"chew and park" May stick to dentures Should not drink acidic beverages while chewing gum
Availability	Prescription only	Over the counter	Over the counter
Factor	Inhaler (Nicotrol®)	Nasal Spray (Nicotrol®)	Lozenge (Commit™)
Treatment Period	3–6 mo Taper use over last few wk	3–6 mo Taper use over last few wk	12 wk
Dosage	6–16 cartridges/day Need to inhale about 80 times to use up cartridge Can use part of cartridge, save rest for later that day	One dose equals one squirt to each nostril Dose 1–2 times/hr as needed Minimum = 8 doses/day Maximum = 40 doses/day	Take one 2-mg lozenge (if you smoke first cigarette more than 30 mins after waking up) or one 4-mg lozenge (if you smoke first cigarette within 30 mins of waking up) every 1–2 hr/day (wk 1–6); every 2–4 hr (wk 7–9); every 4–8 hr (wk 10–12)
Pros	Can control your own dose Helps with predictable urges Keeps hands and mouth busy	Can control your own dose Fastest acting for relief of urges	Easy to use Takes about 20–30 mins to dissolve completely

(continued)

Factor	Inhaler (Nicotrol®)	Nasal Spray (Nicotrol®)	Lozenge (Commit™)
Cons	May irritate mouth and throat (improves with use)	Need to use correctly (do not inhale it)	May cause hiccups, heartburn, nausea, or other side effects if used continuously
	Does not work well <40°F	May irritate nose (improves with use)	Do not chew or swallow lozenge
	Should not drink acidic beverages while using inhaler	May cause dependence	Cannot eat or drink 15 mins before using or while lozenge is in mouth
Availability	Prescription only	Prescription only	Over the counter

Source: Reproduced with permission from Anderson JE, Jorenby DE, Scott WJ, Fiore MC. Treating tobacco use and dependence: an evidence-based clinical practice guideline for tobacco cessation. *Chest.* 2002 Mar;121(3):932-34. Copyright © 2002 Elsevier.

Table 1.22. Limits of drug detection in urine and blood samples according to length of time from last use

Substance	Urine	Blood
Alcohol	12 hours	12 hours
Amphetamine (except methamphetamine)	1–2 days	12 hours
Methamphetamine	1–2 days	1–3 days
MDMA (Ecstasy)	1–2 days	25 hours
Barbiturates (except phenobarbital)	Short acting: 2 days	1–2 days
	Long acting: 1–3 weeks	2–3 weeks
Phenobarbital		4–7 days
Benzodiazepines	Therapeutic use: 3 days	6–48 hours
	Chronic use: 4–6 weeks	
Cannabis	Single use: 2–7 days	Infrequent use: 2–3 days
	Prolonged use: 1–2 months	Frequent use: up to 2 weeks
Cocaine	2–4 days	24 hours
Codeine	2 days	12 hours
Cotinine (metabolite of cigarettes)	2–4 days	2–4 days
Morphine	2 days	6 hours
Heroin	2 days	6 hours
LSD	1–3 days	0–3 hours
Methadone	3 days	24 hours
PCP	Single use: 14 days	1–3 days
	Chronic use: up to 30 days	

LSD indicates lysergic acid diethylamide; MDMA, 3,4-methylenedioxymethamphetamine; PCP, phencyclidine

Source: Reproduced with permission from Wenstrom KD. Substance abuse. In *Precis: an update in obstetrics and gynecology. Obstetrics, 4th ed.* Washington, DC: American College of Obstetricians and Gynecologists; 2010. Copyright © 2010 The American College of Obstetricians and Gynecologists.

PRIMARY CARE Tobacco, Alcohol, and Drug Abuse

Table 1.23. The TWEAK screening test for alcohol abuse

The TWEAK test, which screens for alcohol abuse, is a self-administered test that includes five questions:

T	**T**olerance—How many drinks can you hold? *(If 5 or more drinks, score 2 points.)*
W	Have close friends or relatives **W**orried or complained about your drinking in the past year? *(If "Yes," score 2 points.)*
E	**E**ye Opener—Do you sometimes take a drink in the morning when you get up? *(If "Yes," score 1 point.)*
A	**A**mnesia—Has a friend or family member ever told you about things you said or did while *you were* drinking that *you could* not remember? *(If "Yes," score 1 point.)*
K(C)	Do you sometimes feel the need to **C**ut down on your drinking? *(If "Yes," score 1 point.)*

The TWEAK test is used to screen for pregnant at-risk drinking, defined here as the consumption of 1 oz or more of alcohol per day while pregnant. A total score of 2 points or more indicates a positive result for pregnancy risk drinking.

Source: Modified from Chan AW, Pristach EA, Welte JW, Russell M. Use of the TWEAK test in screening for alcoholism/heavy drinking in three populations. *Alcohol Clin Exp Res.* 1993 Dec;17(6):1188-92.

Table 1.24. The CAGE screening test for alcohol abuse

The CAGE test, another simple test that can be used for either alcohol or illicit drug screening, is based on four questions:

1. Do you feel that you should **C**ut down on your narcotic or alcohol use?

2. Have you been **A**nnoyed by people criticizing your narcotic or alcohol use?

3. Do you ever feel **G**uilty about narcotic or alcohol use?

4. Do you feel **E**dgy if you do not use narcotics or alcohol? or Do you ever need an **E**ye opener to get going in the morning?

Two affirmative answers to the CAGE test indicate problems with narcotics or alcohol.

Source: Modified from Ewing JA. Detecting alcoholism: the CAGE questionnaire. *JAMA.* 1984;252(14):1905-07.

MIGRAINE HEADACHES

Fast Facts
- A migraine is a common disabling headache often associated with nausea as well as light and sound sensitivity.
- Lifestyle optimization is important (sleep hygiene, routine meals and exercise, avoidance of oral migraine triggers).

Treatment of Acute Migraines
- Acute abortive therapy for migraine should be migraine specific and should be used early in the course of the migraine for best results.
- Mild to moderate attacks are best treated with NSAID (e.g., naproxen 500 mg)/acetaminophen (1000 mg) and if needed, an antiemetic (metoclopramide 10 mg PO/IV, prochloperazine 10 mg PO/IV/IM).
- Moderate to severe attacks are best treated with a triptan is the first line of treatment—if severe nausea, nonoral triptan is used.
- Triptans are serotonin agonists and are effective to treat migraines. There are 7 available. They often equally effective and the choice of agent should be individualized.
- Sumatriptan has the most options for route of delivery and is available as PO/IM/Nasal spray. Zolmitriptan is available as PO/Nasal spray. All others are PO only.
- Synergy is seen if a NSAID is added to the triptan (e.g., Naproxen 500 mg).
- Opiates and barbiturate should NOT be used as a first-line treatment of migraines.

Table 1.25. Characteristics of migraine, cluster, and tension-type headaches

Characteristic	Migraine	Cluster	Tension-type
Onset	Peak incidence in adolescence	30s or 40s	Variable, generally problematic in the 20s or beyond
Frequency	1 or 2 attacks per mo, often with menses	1 or more attacks per day for 6 to 8 wk	*Episodic*—less than 15 days per mo *Chronic*—more than 15 days per mo
Location	Unilateral > bilateral Fronto-temporal or orbital	100% unilateral; generally orbito-temporal	Bifrontal, biocciptal, neck
Description	Throbbing or intense pressure	Nonthrobbing, excruciating, boring, penetrating	Squeezing, pressing, aching
Duration	4–72 hr, usually 12–24 hr	30 mins to 2 hr, usually 45–90 mins	*Episodic*—several hr *Chronic*—all day
Prodrome	Changes in mood, energy, appetite	May include brief mild burning in the ipsilateral inner canthus or internal nares	None
Aura	Up to 60 mins, usually 20 mins, often visual	None	None
Associated symptoms	Nausea, vomiting, sonophobia and photophobia, sensitivity, occasional ptosis	Ipsilateral ptosis–miosis, conjunctival injection, lacrimation; ipsilateral stuffed and running nostril	*Episodic*—loss of appetite, either light or sound sensitivity *Chronic*—light or sound sensitivity or presence of nausea
Behavior	Retreat to a dark, quiet room (hibernate)	Frenetic pacing, rocking	Generally not affected; may have mild reduction in functional capacity

Source: Reproduced with permission from Marks DR, Rapoport AM. Practical evaluation and diagnosis of headache. *Semin Neurol.* 1997;17:309. Copyright © 1997 Georg Thieme Verlag KG.

PRIMARY CARE — Migraine Headaches

Table 1.26. Available triptans and their doses

Drug	Available Formulations and Recommended Doses	Commonly Prescribed Initial Dose	Half-life hr	Selected Drug Interactions	Minimum Interval Before Repeating Dose hr	Highest Approved Dose Per 24 hr
Almotriptan (Axert)	Tablet: 6.25 and 12.5 mg	12.5 mg	3–4	Contains a sulfa group—contraindicated in patients with sulfonamide allergies; dose reduction to 6.25 mg suggested when used with potent CYP3A4 inhibitor, such as ketoconazole, itraconazole, nefazodone, troleandomycin, clarithromycin, ritonavir, or nelfinavir	2	25 mg
Eletriptan (Relpax)	Tablet: 20 and 40 mg	40 mg	4	Metabolized by CYP3A4 enzyme—should not be used within 3 days after potent CYP3A4 inhibitor, such as ketoconazole, itraconazole, nefazodone, troleandomycin, clarithromycin, ritonavir, or nelfinavir	2	80 mg
Frovatriptan (Frova)	Tablet: 2.5 mg	2.5 mg	26		2	7.5 mg
Naratriptan (Amarge)	Tablet: 1 and 2.5 mg	2.5 mg	6		4	5 mg
Rizatriptan (Maxalt)	Tablet: 5 and 10 mg Orally dissolving wafer: 5 and 10 mg	Tablet: 10 mg Wafer: 10 mg	2–3	Dose reduction to 5 mg recommended in patients taking propranolol; should not be used within 2 wk after monoamine oxidase inhibitor	Tablet: 2	30 mg (15 mg for cases in which initial dose must be reduced to 5 mg)
Sumatriptan (Imitrex)	Tablet: 25, 50, and 100 mg Nasal spray: 5 and 20 mg Single-dose vial: 6 mg/0.5 mL of solution for subcutaneous injection Cartridges used in reusable autoinjector device: 4 and 6 mg Needle-free, single-use device for subcutaneous administration: 6 mg Fixed-dose combination tablet: 85 mg of sumatriptan with 500 mg of naproxen sodium	Tablet: 50 or 100 mg Nasal spray: 20 mg Subcutaneous injection cartridge: 6 mg	2.5	Should not be used within 2 wk after monoamine oxidase inhibitor	Tablet: 2 Nasal spray: 2 Subcutaneous injection: 1 Sumatriptan-naproxen tablet: 2	200 mg 40 mg 12 mg 2 tablets

(continued)

Drug	Available Formulations and Recommended Doses	Commonly Prescribed Initial Dose	Half-life hr	Selected Drug Interactions	Minimum Interval Before Repeating Dose hr	Highest Approved Dose Per 24 hr
Zolmitriptan (Zomig)	Tablet: 2.5 and 5 mg Orally dissolving wafer: 2.5 and 5 mg Nasal spray: 5 mg	Tablet: 5 mg Wafer: 5 mg Nasal spray: 5 mg	3	Should not be used within 2 wk after monoamine oxidase inhibitor	Tablet or wafer: 2 Nasal spray: 2	10 mg 10 mg

*Information on dosing is from package inserts.

Source: Reproduced from Loder E. Triptan therapy in migraine. *N Engl J Med*. 2010 Jul 1;363(1):63-70. Copyright © 2010 Massachusetts Medical Society. Reprinted with permission from Massachusetts Medical Society.

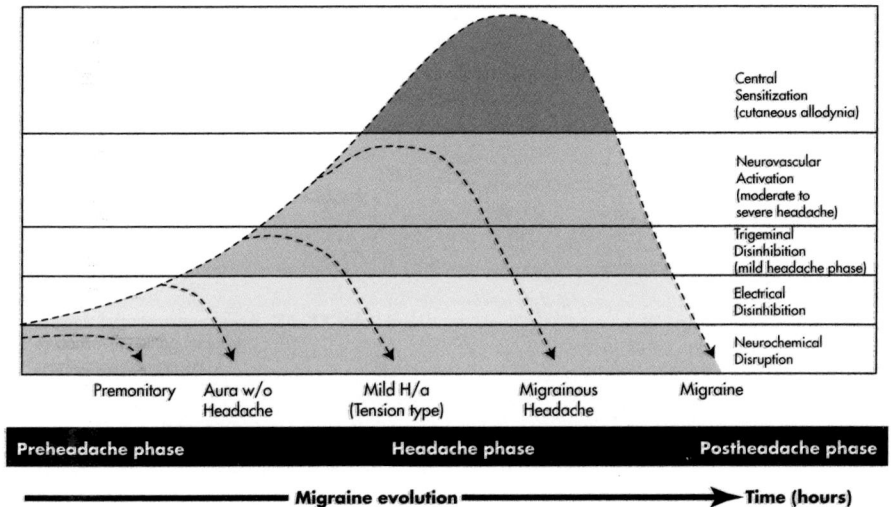

Figure 1.10. Typical migraine evolution over time
Source: Reproduced with permission from Schreiber CP. The pathophysiology of primary headache. *Prim Care*. 2004 Jun;31(2):261-76, v-vi. Copyright © 2004 Elsevier.

Preventative Treatment of Migraines

- Preventive treatment is recommended if ≤14 days of headaches are noted per month.
- Treatment will results in 50% to 75% of patients having a 50% reduction of headaches.
- Relief is usually noted first after 4 weeks of Rx.

Table 1.27. Classification of migraine preventive therapies (available in the United States)

Level A: Medications with Established Efficacy (≥2 Class I Trials)	Level B: Medications Are Probably Effective (1 Class I or 2 Class II Studies)	Level C: Medications Are Possibly Effective (1 Class II Study)	Level U: Inadequate or Conflicting Data to Support Or Refute Medication Use	Other: Medications That Are Established As Ineffective, Probably Ineffective, Or Possibly Ineffective
Antiepileptic drugs	Antidepressants/ SSRI/SSNRI/TCA	ACE inhibitors	α-Agonists	Established as ineffective
Divalproex sodium	Amitriptyline	Lisinopril	Clonidine[a]	Lamotrigine
Sodium valproate	Venlafaxine	α-Agonists	Antidepressants/SSRI/SSNRI	Probably ineffective
Topiramate	β-Blockers	Guanfacine[a]	Fluoxetine	Clomipramine[a]
β-Blockers	Atenolol[a]	Angiotensin receptor blockers	Fluvoxamine[a]	Possibly ineffective
Metoprolol	Nadolol[a]	Candesartan	Antiepileptic drugs	Acebutolol[a]
Propranolol	Triptans (MRM[b])	Antiepileptic drugs	Gabapentin	Clonazepam[a]
Timolol[a]	Naratriptan[b]	Carbamazepine[a]	Antithrombotics	Nabumetone[a]
Triptans (MRM[b])	Zolmitriptan[b]	Antihistamines	Acenocoumarol	Oxcarbazepine
Frovatriptan[b]		Cyproheptadine	Coumadin	Telmisartan
		β-Blockers	Picotamide	
		Nebivolol	β-Blockers	
		Ca++ blockers	Bisoprolol[a]	
		Nicardipine[a]	Pindolol[a]	
			Ca++ blockers	
			Nifedipine[a]	
			Nimodipine	
			Verapamil	
			Carbonic anhydrase inhibitor	
			Acetazolamide	
			Direct vascular smooth muscle relaxants	
			Cyclandelate	
			TCAs	
			Protriptyline[a]	

ACE, angiotensin-converting-enzyme; Ca++ blockers, calcium channel blockers; MRM, menstrually related migraine; SSNRI, selective serotonin-norepinephrine reuptake inhibitor; SSRI, selective serotonin reuptake inhibitor; TCA, tricyclic antidepressant.

[a]Classification based on original guideline and new evidence not found for this report.
[b]For short-term prophylaxis of MRM.

Source: Reproduced with permission from Silberstein SD, Holland S, Freitag F, et al. Evidence-based guideline update: pharmacologic treatment for episodic migraine prevention in adults: report of the Quality Standards Subcommittee of the American Academy of Neurology and the American Headache Society. *Neurology*. 2013 Feb 26; 80(9):871. Copyright © 2013 American Academy of Neurology (AAN Enterprises).

LOW BACK PAIN

Fast Facts

- One of the leading causes of MD clinic visits.
- Most of the time, it is self-limiting.
- 90% are pain free within 3 months and, of those, 90% are pain free in 4 weeks.
- Important to rule out serious causes such as malignancy, infection, trauma, or significant neurological compromise.
- Positive straight leg test (SLT) often indicates disc herniation.
- Location on pain with SLT will often indicate the anatomical location of the lesion.
- Laboratory tests are rarely needed.
- Activity, NSAIDs, Ultram, and physical therapy are useful for uncomplicated low back pain.

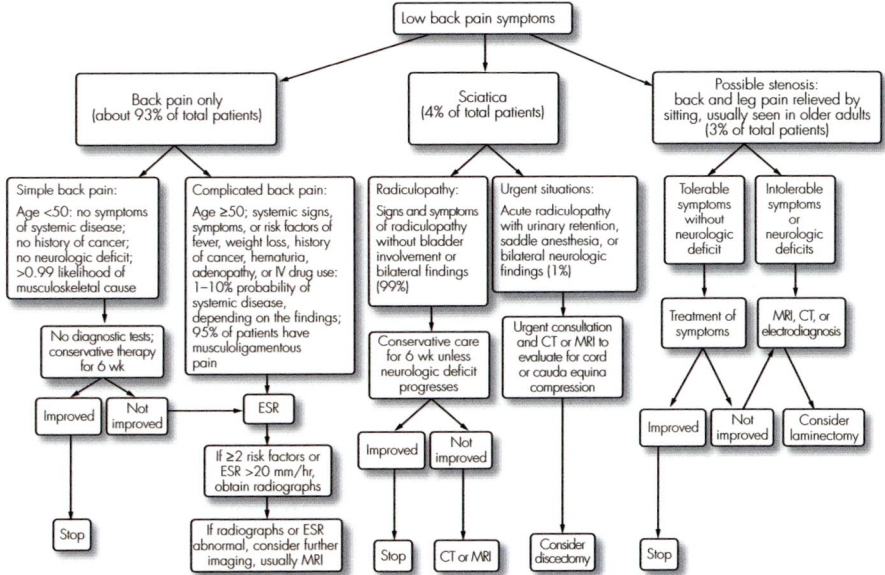

Figure 1.11. Algorithm for the diagnostic evaluation of back pain
CT, computed tomography; ESR, erythrocyte sedimentation rate; MRI, magnetic resonance imaging.
Source: Reproduced with permission from Jarvik J, Deyo R. Diagnostic evaluation of low back pain with emphasis on imaging. *Ann Intern Med.* 2002;137:586-95.

Table 1.28. Summary of the nonsurgical treatment options for low back pain

Treatment Modality	Recommendation	Grade	Comment
Bed rest	To be avoided	A	Bed rest should be avoided; patients should be instructed to remain as active as possible within the limits of their pain.
Lifestyle modification: weight loss, tobacco cessation, exercise program	Recommended	C	Limited evidence as these nonmedical therapies do not lend themselves to easy comparison and analysis via RCT.
Physical therapy	Recommended	D	Limited evidence to document efficacy, but most clinicians agree that PT should be routinely recommended.
NSAIDs	Recommended	A	Drugs of choice for management of acute LBP.
Acetaminophen	Not routinely recommended	B	Inconsistent evidence suggests that NSAIDs may be superior to acetaminophen.
COX-2 inhibitors	Not recommended	B	No more efficacious than traditional NSAIDs. Have been touted for their beneficial GI side effect profile; however, new data regarding prothrombotic risk is concerning.
Muscle relaxants	May be helpful for bothersome night symptoms	B	Can be helpful for short courses, but the benefit arises with significant side effects, particularly sedation.
Narcotic analgesics	Recommended only for severe LBP	C	Studies comparing narcotics to NSAIDs and acetaminophen are of low quality. Narcotic analgesics may be helpful for severe cases of LBP with marked functional limitations.
Tramadol	Recommended for moderate to severe pain	A	Tramadol can be used as an adjunct to NSAIDs.
Epidural steroid injections	Recommended in carefully selected patients	D	Limited evidence for utility, but low methodologic quality of studies.
Spinal manipulation	Not routinely recommended	C	No documented benefit, but a generally safe modality.
Chiropractic manipulation	Not routinely recommended	D	Not more effective than other treatment modalities, but patient satisfaction is high with chiropractic treatment.
TENS	Not routinely recommended	B	Limited evidence to support its use, but a safe modality.
Prolotherapy	Not recommended	D	Evidence is lacking, and there are limited long-term data to document safety.
Acupuncture/massage	Not routinely recommended	B	No high-quality evidence available to support its use, but a generally safe modality.
Back school	Reserved for patients with chronic LBP with marked functional impairment	B	Cost-effectiveness data unavailable.
Heat or cryotherapy	Recommended	C	No high-quality evidence to support its use. Safe, minimally invasive modality.

LBP, low back pain; NSAID, nonsteroidal antiinflammatory drug; PT, physical therapy; RCT, randomized control trial.

Source: Reproduced with permission from Harwood MI, Smith BJ. Low back pain: a primary care approach. *Clinics in Family Practice.* 2005; 7(2):279-303. Copyright © 2005 W. B. Saunders Company.

SINUSITIS
Fast Facts
Four Types of Bacterial Sinusitis
Acute Bacterial Sinusitis
- Symptoms of purulent rhinorrhea, postnasal drainage, pain over sinuses.
- Often proceeded by viral infection.
- Mostly caused by *S. pneumoniae*, *H. influenzae*, and *M. catarrhalis*.
- Due to a high percentage of viral sinusitis, wait to treat for full 10 days unless severe symptoms such as temp >39°C (102°F) or ≥3 days of facial pain/purulent nasal discharge.
- Treatment consists of 5–7 days of antibiotics.
- First-line treatment is amoxicillin-clavulanate 500 mg/125 mg orally three times daily or 875 mg/125 mg orally twice daily.
- If penicillin allergic, doxycycline or a fluoroquinolone (levofloxacin or moxifloxacin) for 5–7 days are alternative first-line treatment.
- Nasal corticosteroids and saline nasal sprays/lavage might be helpful.
- Topical and oral decongestants are not helpful.

Acute Sinusitis with Treatment Failure
- If no improvement in 3–5 days or if symptoms worsen after ≥2 days, the following should be given for 7–10 days: amoxicillin-clavulanate 2000 mg/125 mg orally twice daily or Levofloxacin 500 mg orally once daily or moxifloxacin 400 mg orally once daily.
- If still not improved, consider CT scan/MRI and meatal/sinus cultures along with referral to allergist and/or ENT.

Chronic Sinusitis
- Symptoms similar to acute sinusitis but more subtle.
- Often caused by noninfectious reasons.
- If infectious component, mostly caused by *S. aureus*, gram-negative enteric bacteria, anaerobes.
- Consider referral to allergist and/or ENT.

Recurrent Sinusitis
- Consider referral to allergist and/or ENT.

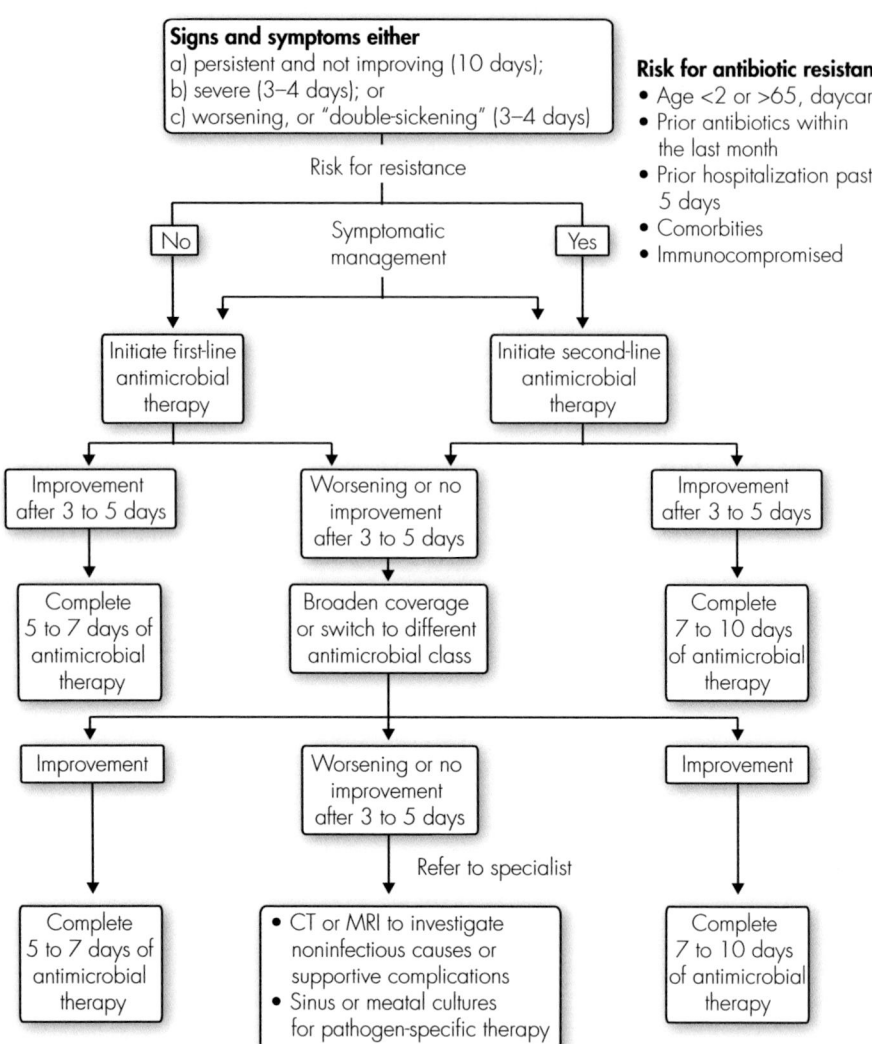

Figure 1.12. Algorithm for the management of acute bacterial rhinosinusitis
Source: Reproduced from Chow AW, Benninger MS, Brook I, et al. IDSA clinical practice guideline for acute bacterial rhinosinusitis in children and adults. *Clin Infect Dis*. 2012; 54:e72. By permission of the Infectious Diseases Society of America and Oxford University Press.

ALTERNATIVE MEDICINE/BOTANICALS

Table 1.29. Drug interactions with complementary medicines

This table shows complementary medicines with at least one "major" interaction. For the full version of this table, see this article online at www.australianprescriber.com

Complementary Medicine	Interacting Drug	Possible Outcome	Severity and Level of Evidence*	Proposed Mechanisms/ Comment
Evening primrose oil	Antiplatelet drugs, warfarin	↑ drug effect	**Major**, level B	Contains gamma-linolenic acid, probable anticoagulant
Garlic	Contraceptives, oral	↓ drug effect	Moderate, level D	Induces CYP3A4
	Saquinavir/nonnucleoside reverse transcriptase inhibitors	↓ drug levels and effect	**Major**, level B	Induces CYP3A4
	Antiplatelet drugs, warfarin	↑ bleeding risk	Moderate, level D	Theoretical antiplatelet activity
Ginkgo	Anticonvulsants	↑ seizure risk	Moderate, level D	Large amounts of ginkgotoxin can cause neurotoxicity
	Warfarin, antiplatelet drugs	↑ bleeding risk	**Major**, level D	Antiplatelet activity after several weeks
	CYP2C9 substrates (e.g., glipizide, warfarin, celecoxib)	↑ substrate levels	Moderate, level D	Inhibits CYP2C9 activity
	CYP1A2, CYP2C19, CYP2D6 and CYP3A4 substrates	↑ substrate levels	Moderate, level B	Potentially inhibits these enzymes
	Hypoglycaemic drugs	↑↓ drug effect	Moderate, level B	Variably affects blood glucose concentrations
Glucosamine	Warfarin	↑ bleeding risk	**Major**, level D	Several case reports of increased INR
Hawthorn	Calcium channel blockers, nitrates, phosphodiesterase inhibitors	↑ drug effect	**Major**, level D	Additive vasodilator effects
	Digoxin, beta blockers	↑ drug effect	**Major**, level D	Additive effects on heart rate and/or blood pressure. Hawthorn has cardiotonic effects.
Kava	CNS depressants	↑ drug effect	**Major**, level A	Additive somnolence
	CYP1A2, CYP2D6, CYP2C9, CYP2E1, CYP3A4 substrates	↑ substrate levels	Moderate, level B	Kava potentially inhibits these enzymes
	P-glycoprotein substrates	↑ substrate levels	Moderate, level D	
St. John's wort	Alprazolam	↓ drug levels and effect	**Major**, level B	Increased clearance; half-life reduced by 50%
	Amitriptyline	↑ drug effect	**Major**, level B	Increased risk of serotonin syndrome
	Antidepressants, tramadol	↑ drug effect	**Major**, level D	
	Pethidine	↑ drug effect	**Major**, level D	
	Triptans	↑ drug effect	Moderate, level D	
	Clopidogrel	↑ bleeding risk	Moderate, level B	Increased conversion to active metabolite

(continued)

PRIMARY CARE — Alternative Medicine/Botanicals

This table shows complementary medicines with at least one "major" interaction. For the full version of this table, see this article online at www.australianprescriber.com

Complementary Medicine	Interacting Drug	Possible Outcome	Severity and Level of Evidence*	Proposed Mechanisms/Comment
St. John's wort	CYP1A2, CYP2C9, CYP3A4 substrates (e.g., imatinib, indinavir, tacrolimus, carbamazepine, phenytoin)	↓ drug levels and effect	CYP3A4 = **Major**, level B CYP1A2, CYP2C9 = Moderate, level B	Induces CYP enzymes
	Non-nucleoside reverse transcriptase inhibitors, protease inhibitors	↓ drug levels and effect	**Major**, level B	Induces CYP3A4
	Oral contraceptives	↓ drug levels	**Major**, level B	Risk of breakthrough bleeding/contraceptive failure
	P-glycoprotein substrates (e.g., digoxin, fexofenadine, irinotecan)	↓ drug levels and effect	**Major**, level B	Induces intestinal P-glycoprotein
	Simvastatin	↓ drug levels	Moderate, level B	Statin levels reduced by up to 28%
	Warfarin	↓ drug effect	**Major**, level B	Induces CYP1A2, CYP2C9, and CYP3A4
Valerian	Alprazolam	↑ drug levels	**Major**, level B	CYP3A4 inhibitor. Alprazolam increased by 19% in one study
	CNS depressants	↑ drug effect	**Major**, level D	Pharmacodynamic effect
	CYP3A4 substrates	↑ substrate effect	Moderate, level D	

CYP, cytochrome P450; INR, international normalised ratio; CNS, central nervous system

*Interaction rating adapted from Natural Medicines Comprehensive Database.[11] The level of severity (major, moderate, minor) has been calculated using the evidence and probability of harm. This rating is linked with a generic recommendation for management.

Major Strongly discourage patients from using this combination, as a serious adverse outcome could occur. If used, patient should be monitored closely for potential adverse outcomes.

Moderate Use cautiously or avoid combination, as a significant adverse outcome could occur. If used, monitor for potential adverse outcomes.

Minor Be aware that there is a chance of an interaction. Advise patients of symptoms that may occur and an action plan to follow.

Level of evidence ratings:

A High-quality randomised controlled trial or meta-analysis

B Non-randomised clinical trial, literature review, clinical cohort or case-control study, historical control, or epidemiologic study

C Consensus or expert opinion

D Anecdotal evidence; in vitro or animal study or theoretical based on pharmacology

Reproduced with permission from Moses, GM and McGuire TM. Drug interactions with complementary medicines. Aust Prescr. 2010; 33:177-80. Copyright © 2010 NPS MedicineWise.

Alternative Medicine/Botanicals **PRIMARY CARE**

Table 1.30. Commonly used botanicals and vitamins and their possible effects in the surgical patient

Substance	Potential Negative Effect
Chaparral	Hepatotoxicity
Chondroitin	Anticoagulative properties
Chromium	Hypoglycemia
Dong quai	Anticoagulative properties
Echinacea	Hepatotoxicity
Feverfew	Anticoagulative properties
Garlic	Anticoagulative properties
Ginger	Anticoagulative properties
Ginkgo	Anticoagulative properties
Ginseng	Anticoagulative properties; hypertension; hypoglycemia
Goldenseal	Can reduce effect of antihypertensives
Kava	Potentiates the sedative effects of anesthetics; hepatotoxicity
Licorice root	Hypertension; hyperkalemia; hypokalemia; hypernatremia; edema
Ma huang (ephedra)	Arrhythmias; hypertension
Red yeast rice	Hepatotoxicity
St. John's wort	Prolongs anesthetic effects; inhibits reuptake of serotonin, dopamine, and noradrenaline
Valerian	Prolongs anesthetic effects; hepatotoxicity
Vitamin E	Anticoagulative properties

Reproduced with permission from Gaudet T. Complementary and Alternative Medicine. *Clin Update Womens Health Care.* 2011; X(4):66. Copyright © 2011 The American College of Obstetricians and Gynecologists.

CHAPTER 2
Obstetrics

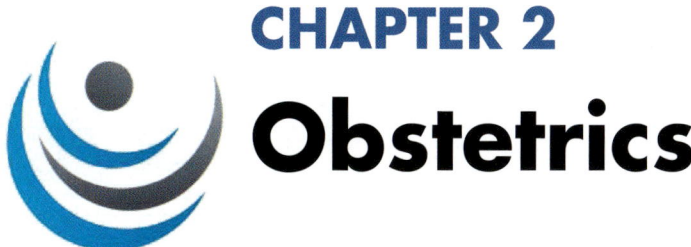

CHARTING PEARLS FOR ROUTINE OBSTETRICAL VISITS

Document and review the following for each prenatal visit:
- Fetal heart tones and fetal movement.
- ✓ Blood pressure, urine dipstick protein.
- Outstanding lab results.
- Presentation and assessment of fetal growth.
- Estimated gestational age and method by which this was assigned.
- Date of return visit.
- Confirm and note type of uterine incision if previous cesarean delivery (C/D).
- Confirm and note discussion regarding postpartum contraception.
- Confirm and note discussion of trial of labor after cesarean delivery (TOLAC) if previous Low transverse C/S.
  - Consider TOLAC consent form.
- Presence or absence of preterm labor symptoms, bleeding, vaginal discharge, or spontaneous rupture of membranes.
- Presence or absence of symptoms of preeclampsia.
  - Blurred vision
  - Scotoma
  - Headache
  - Rapid weight gain and edema

Table 2.1. Routine prenatal laboratories

First Visit	Comments
Type and screen	
Varicella immunity	Document by patient history or antibody status
Rubella immunity	Administer vaccine postpartum
VDRL	Syphilis testing; same as RPR
HBsAg	
HIV	
Pap smear	As indicted by ASCCP guidelines
Cervical cultures for GC and chlamydia	Include group B strep depending on clinic protocol
Complete blood count (CBC)	
Hemoglobin electrophoresis	When indicated
PPD	When indicated
Discuss genetic screening and diagnostic testing	e.g., Tay-Sachs, Canavan's, cystic fibrosis, risk for aneuploidy and/or CVS vs. amniocentesis
9–14 Wk Gestation	
Offer first trimester genetic screening	PAPP-A, free β-hCG and nuchal translucency screening (see page 263) or cell free fetal DNA (see page 264)
15–20 wk gestation	
Offer "quad screen" genetic screening	β-hCG, estrogen, AFP, inhibin (see page 263)
Discuss weekly 17 hydroxy progesterone caproate injections (16–36 weeks)	If at risk for recurrent preterm delivery
18–22 wk gestation	
Ultrasound examination	Anatomic survey with fetal cardiac echo at 20–22 weeks as indicated
24–28 wk gestation	
Gestational diabetes screening	See comments on page 178
Repeat CBC	As indicated
28–30 wk gestation	
RhoGAM administration	Must have negative antibody screen prior to RhoGAM
35–37 wk gestation	
Group B strep culture	
34–40 wk gestation	
Repeat STI screening with HIV	In high-risk patients
Discuss HSV suppressive therapy with acyclovir or valacyclovir	In patient with history of genital HSV

AFP, alpha-fetoprotein; β-hCG, β human chorionic gonadotrophin; GC, neisseria gonorrhoeae; HIV, human immunodeficiency virus; MSAFP, maternal serum alpha-fetal protein; RPR, rapid plasma reagent; VDRL, Venereal Disease Research Laboratory test of syphilis; HSV, herpes simplex virus.

NAUSEA AND VOMITING IN PREGNANCY
Fast Facts
- A very common condition with 50–80% of pregnant women reporting nausea and 50% with nausea and vomiting.
- Hyperemesis gravidarum is extreme example affecting 03–3% of pregnancies.
- Typically, nausea and vomiting almost always presents before 9 weeks of pregnancy, so symptoms that first manifest after 9 weeks warrant further evaluation.

Nonpharmacologic Treatment
- Rest and avoidance of stimuli that trigger symptoms.
- Small, frequent meals with bland foods and high protein content may be helpful.
- Several studies demonstrate efficacy of ginger.
- Acupressure, acupuncture, or electric nerve stimulation (acustimulation) at the P6 (or Neiguan) point on the inside of the wrist has been recommended but may not be better than placebo.

Pharmacologic Treatment
- Vitamin B6 or vitamin B6 plus doxylamine (McKeigue 1994; Neutel 1995).
  - Safe and effective
  - FDA-approved formulation available (Diclegis)
- Phenothiazines probably safe, but one study suggested a possible association with fetal malformations.
- Corticosteroids may be of benefit, but three studies have confirmed an association between oral clefts and methylprednisolone use in the first trimester (Carmichael 1999; Park-Wyllie 2000; Rodriguez-Pinilla 1998).
  - The teratogenic effect is weak, probably accounting for no more than one or two cases per 1,000 treated women (Shepard 2002).
  - Corticosteroid use for hyperemesis gravidarum should be used with caution and avoided as a first-line agent before 10 weeks of gestation.
- Metoclopramide: some safety data available but limited studies on efficacy.

Odansteron (Zofran) as a Treatment
- Possibly more effective than vitamin B6 and doxylamine (Oliveira 2014).
- High doses of IV odansteron carry potential cardiac risk of QT interval prolongation leading to torsades de pointes, a potentially fatal heart rhythm.
- Some studies have shown an increased rate of birth defects with early odansteron use. The potential risks and benefits need to be weighed in each case.

Source: American College of Obstetricians and Gynecologists. Practice Bulletin No. 153: Nausea and Vomiting of Pregnancy. *Obstet Gynecol*. 2015 Sep;126(3):e12-24.

OBSTETRICS

Table 2.2. Contraindicated medications for patients receiving odansetron

Examples of medications to be avoided by patients receiving ondansetron include, but are not limited to, the following:
- Antihistamines (hydroxyzine)
- Analgesics and sedatives (methadone, oxycodone, and chloral hydrate)
- Diuretics
- Anticholinergics
- Antiarrhythmics (amiodarone, sotalol, quinidine, procainamide, and flecainide)
- Antipsychotics (thioridazine, haloperidol, chlorpromazine, and clozapine)
- Tricyclic and tetracyclic antidepressants (amitriptyline, imipramine, and clomipramine)
- Macrolide antibiotics (erythromycin and azithromycin)
- Trazodone
- Fluoxetine
- Antimalarials (chloroquine, mefloquine, and quinine)
- Metronidazole
- Human immunodeficiency virus (HIV) protease inhibitors

Source: Reproduced with permission from American College of Obstetricians and Gynecologists. Practice Bulletin No. 153: Nausea and Vomiting of Pregnancy. *Obstet Gynecol.* 2015 Sep;126(3):e12-24. Copyright © 2015 The American College of Obstetricians and Gynecologists.

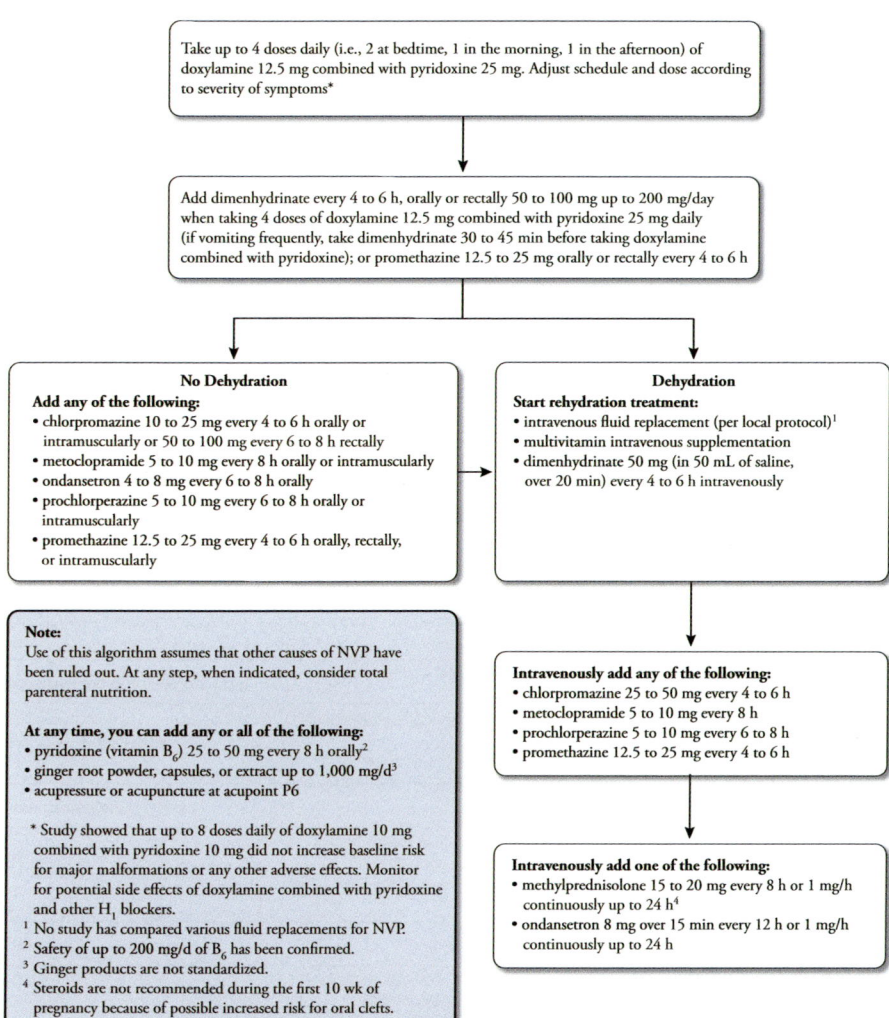

Figure 2.1. Management algorithm for prevention and treatment of nausea and vomiting of pregnancy

Source: Reproduced with permission from Einarson A, Maltepe C, Boskovic R, et al. Treatment of nausea and vomiting in pregnancy: an updated algorithm. *Can Fam Physician.* 2007 Dec;53(12):2109-11. Copyright © The College of Family Physicians of Canada.

Table 2.3. Pharmacologic treatment of nausea and vomiting in pregnancy

Agent	Oral Dose	Side Effects	FDA Category[†]	Comments
Vitamin B6 (pyridoxine)	10–25 mg every 8 hr		A	Vitamin B6 or vitamin B6-antihistamine combination recommended as first-line treatment
Vitamin B6-doxylamine combination	Pyridoxine, 10–25 mg every 8 hr; doxylamine, 25 mg at bedtime, 12.5 mg in the morning as needed, plus 12.5 in the afternoon as needed	Sedation	A	
Vitamin B6-doxylamine combination, delayed-release formulation (Diclectin, Canada)	10 mg pyridoxine and 10 mg doxylamine, extended release; 2 tablets at bedtime, 1 tablet in the morning as needed, plus 1 tablet in the afternoon as needed			
Antihistamines		Sedation		
Doxylamine (Unisom SleepTabs)	12.5–25 mg every 8 hr		A	
Diphenhydramine (Benadryl)	25–50 mg every 8 hr		B	
Meclizine (Bonine)	25 mg every 6 hr		B	
Hydroxyzine (Atarax, Vistaril)	50 mg every 4–6 hr		C	
Dimenhydrinate (Dramamine)	50–100 mg every 4–6 hr		B	
Phenothiazines		Extrapyramidal symptoms, sedation		
Promethazine (Phenergan)	25 mg every 4–6 hr		C	Severe tissue injuries with intravenous use (black-box warning); oral, rectal, or intramuscular administration preferred
Prochlorperazine (Compazine)	5–10 mg every 6 hr		C	Also available as buccal tablet
Dopamine antagonists		Sedation, anticholinergic effects		
Trimethobenzamide (Tigan)	300 mg every 6–8 hr		C	
Metoclopramide (Reglan)	10 mg every 6 hr	Tardive dyskinesia (black-box warning)	B	Treatment for more than 12 wk increases risk of tardive dyskinesia
Droperidol (Inapsine)	1.25–2.5 mg intramuscularly or intravenously only		C	Black-box warning regarding torsades de pointes

(continued)

Agent	Oral Dose	Side Effects	FDA Category[†]	Comments
5-hydroxytryptamine$_3$-receptor antagonist		Constipation, diarrhea, headache, fatigue		
Ondansetron (Zofran)	4–8 mg every 6 hr	See page 61	B	Also available as oral disintegrating tablet; more costly than oral ondansetron tablets
Glucocorticoid				
Methylprednisolone (Medrol)	16 mg every 8 hr for 3 days, then taper over 2 wk	Small increased risk of cleft lip if used before 10 wk of gestation	C	Avoid use before 10 wk of gestation; maximum duration of therapy 6 wk to limit serious maternal side effects
Ginger extract	125–250 mg every 6 hr	Reflux, heartburn	C	Available over the counter as a food supplement

[*] This list of agents is not exhaustive. FDA denotes Food and Drug Administration.

[†] FDA categories are as follows: A, controlled studies show no risk; B, no evidence of risk in humans; C, risk cannot be ruled out; D, positive evidence of risk; and X, contraindicated in pregnancy.

Source: Reproduced with permission from Niebyl JR. Clinical practice. Nausea and vomiting in pregnancy. *N Engl J Med*. 2010 Oct 14;363(16):1544-50. Copyright © 2010 Massachusetts Medical Society. Reprinted with permission from Massachusetts Medical Society.

NUTRITIONAL MANAGEMENT DURING PREGNANCY
Weight Gain
- Recommendations based on body mass index (BMI) or IBW.
- Adolescents should strive for gains at the upper end of the range.
- Short women (<157 cm or 62 in) should aim for the lower end of the range.
- Obese women should gain at least 6 kg.

Table 2.4. New recommendations for total and rate of weight gain during pregnancy

Prepregnancy BMI	BMI+ (kg/m^2) (WHO)	Total Weight Gain Range (lbs)	Rates of Weight Gain* Second and Third Trimester (Mean Range in lbs/wk)
Underweight	<18.5	28–40	1 (1–1.3)
Normal weight	(18.5–24.9)	25–35	1 (0.8–1)
Overweight	25.0–29.9	15–25	0.6 (0.5–0.7)
Obese (includes all classes)	≥30.0	11–20	0.5 (0.4–0.6)

+To calculate BMI, go to www.nhlbisupport.com/bmi/.

*Calculations assume a 0.5–2 kg (1.1–4.4 lbs) weight gain in the first trimester (based on Siega-Riz, et al. 1994; Abrams, et al. 1995; Carmichael, et al. 1997).

Source: Reproduced from http://www.iom.edu/en/Reports/2009/Weight-Gain-During-Pregnancy-Reexamining-the-Guidelines.aspx. Accessed on May 24, 2015.

Caloric Requirements
- First and early second trimester: 25–30 kcal/kg IBW.
- Late second and early third trimester: 25–35 kcal/kg IBW.

Iron Supplementation
- Total iron requirement during pregnancy: 1000 mg.
- 27 mg/day of elemental iron/day recommended (U.S. Centers for Disease Control and Prevention recommends starting at the first prenatal visit).
  - 150 mg ferrous sulfate or
  - 300 mg ferrous gluconate or
  - 100 mg ferrous fumarate

Folate Supplementation
- Routine supplementation is now recommended for all women of reproductive age (0.4 mg/day = amount in most prenatal vitamins) at least 1 month before conception.
- For women with a history of neural tube defects, many experts recommend 4 mg of folic acid daily.
- All women should begin supplementation prepregnancy (*MMWR* 40: 513–16, 1991).

Special Needs (See Tables 1.6 and 1.7)
- Vitamin D: 51 mcg (600 IU) daily for complete vegetarians.
- Vitamin B12: 2.6 mcg daily for all women.
- Calcium: 1300 mg daily for women <19 years old, 1000 mg daily for women 19–50 years old.

ANEMIA IN PREGNANCY

Table 2.5. Classifications of anemia in pregnancy

Anemia Classification

Acquired

- Deficiency anemia (e.g., iron, vitamin B12, folate)
- Hemorrhagic anemia
- Anemia of chronic disease
- Acquired hemolytic anemia
- Aplastic anemia

Inherited

- Thalassemias
- Sickle cell anemia
- Hemoglobinopathies (other than sickle cell anemia)
- Inherited hemolytic anemias

Anemias Characterized by Mechanism

Decreased red blood cell production

- Iron deficiency anemia
- Anemia associated with vitamin B12 deficiency
- Folic acid deficiency anemia
- Anemia associated with bone marrow disorders
- Anemia associated with bone marrow suppression
- Anemia associated with low levels of erythropoietin
- Anemia associated with hypothyroidism

Increased red blood cell destruction

- Inherited hemolytic anemias
    - Sickle cell anemia
    - Thalassemia major
    - Hereditary spherocytosis
- Acquired hemolytic anemias
    - Autoimmune hemolytic anemia
    - Hemolytic anemia associated with thrombotic thrombocytopenic purpura
    - Hemolytic anemia associated with hemolytic uremic syndrome
    - Hemolytic anemia associated with malaria
- Hemorrhagic anemia

(continued)

Anemias Classified by Mean Corpuscular Volume

Microcytic (MCV less than 80 fl)
- Iron deficiency anemia
- Thalassemias
- Anemia of chronic disease
- Sideroblastic anemia
- Anemia associated with copper deficiency
- Anemia associated with lead poisoning

Normocytic (MCV 80–100 fl)
- Hemorrhagic anemia
- Early iron deficiency anemia
- Anemia of chronic disease
- Anemia associated with bone marrow suppression
- Anemia associated with chronic renal insufficiency
- Anemia associated with endocrine dysfunction
- Autoimmune hemolytic anemia
- Anemia associated with hypothyroidism or hypopituitarism
- Hereditary spherocytosis
- Hemolytic anemia associated with paroxysmal nocturnal hemoglobinuria

Macrocytic (MCV greater than 100 fl)
- Folic acid deficiency anemia
- Anemia associated with vitamin B12 deficiency
- Drug-induced hemolytic anemia (e.g., zidovudine)
- Anemia associated with reticulocytosis
- Anemia associated with liver disease
- Anemia associated with ethanol abuse
- Anemia associated with acute myelodysplastic syndrome

MCV, mean corpuscular volume.

Source: Reproduced with permission from American College of Obstetricians and Gynecologists. ACOG Practice Bulletin No. 95: Anemia in pregnancy. *Obstet Gynecol.* 2008 Jul;112(1):201-207. Copyright © 2008 The American College of Obstetricians and Gynecologists.

CLINICAL PELVIMETRY

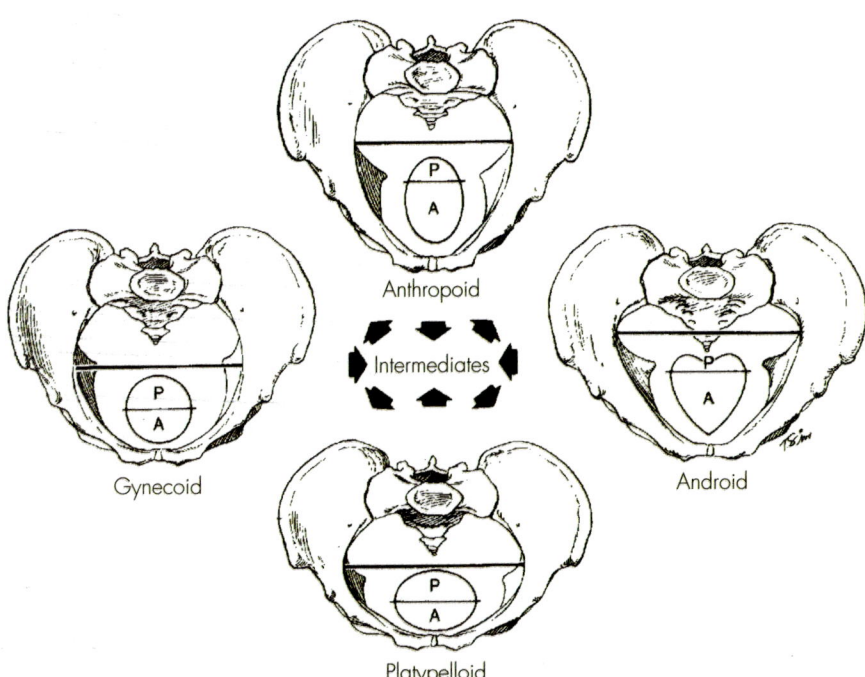

Figure 2.2. Caldwell-Moloy classification of the female pelvis
Source: Reproduced with permission from Cunningham FG, MacDonald PC, Gant NF, et al. Anatomy of the female reproductive tract. In: *Williams Obstetrics*. 20th Ed. Norwalk, CT: Appleton-Lange, 1997. Copyright © McGraw-Hill Education.

Table 2.6. Classification of the bony pelvis

Classification	Forepelvis	Sidewalk	Sacrum Inclination	Sacrosciatic Notch	Ischial Spines	Arch
Gynecoid	wide	straight	medium	medium	not prominent	wide
Android	narrow	convergent	forward	narrow	prominent	narrow
Anthropoid	narrow	divergent	backward	wide	not prominent	medium
Platypelloid	wide	straight	forward	narrow	not prominent	medium

Source: Bochner C. Anatomic characteristics of the fetal head and maternal pelvis. In: Hacker NF, Moore JG, ed. *Essentials of Obstetrics and Gynecology, 2nd Ed.* Philadelphia: Saunders; 1992. Copyright © Elsevier.

OBSTETRICS Clinical Pelvimetry

Table 2.7. Average measurements of the female pelvis

Pelvic Plane	Diameter	Average Length (cm)
Inlet	True conjugate	11.5
	Obstetric conjugate	11
	Transverse	13.5
	Oblique	12.5
	Posterior sagittal	4.5
Greatest diameter	A-P	12.75
	Transverse	12.5
Mid-plane	A-P	12
	Bispinous	10
	Posterior sagittal	4.5–5
Outlet	Anatomic A-P	9.5
	Obstetric A-P	11.5
	Bituberous	11
	Posterior sagittal	7.5

Source: Bochner C. Anatomic characteristics of the fetal head and maternal pelvis. In: Hacker NF, Moore JG, ed. *Essentials of Obstetrics and Gynecology, 2nd Ed.* Philadelphia: Saunders; 1992. Copyright © Elsevier.

ASSESSMENT OF GESTATIONAL AGE
Fast Facts
- First trimester ultrasound is the most accurate method to establish dating.
- If pregnancy was conceived by assisted reproductive technology, this should be used to date the pregnancy.
- Up to 40% of first trimester pregnancies will have their EDC based on LMP adjusted if an early ultrasound is preformed.

Table 2.8. Guidelines for redating gestational age based upon ultrasonography

Gestational Age Range*	Method of Measurement	Discrepancy Between Ultrasound Dating and LMP Dating that Supports Redating
≤13 6/7 wk	CRL	
∘ ≤ 8 6/7 wk		More than 5 d
∘ 9 0/7 wk to 13 6/7 wk		More than 7 d
14 0/7 wk to 15 6/7 wk	BPD, HC, AC, FL	More than 7 d
16 0/7 wk to 21 6/7 wk	BPD, HC, AC, FL	More than 10 d
22 0/7 wk to 27 6/7 wk	BPD, HC, AC, FL	More than 14 d
†28 0/7 wk and beyond	BPD, HC, AC, FL	More than 21 d

AC, abdominal circumference; BPD, biparietal diameter; CRL, crown-rump length; FL, femur length; HC, head circumference; LMP, last menstrual period.

*Based on LMP.

†Because of the risk of redating a small fetus that may be growth restricted, management decisions based on third-trimester ultrasonography alone are especially problematic and need to be guided by careful consideration of the entire clinical picture and close surveillance.

Source: Reproduced with permission from American College of Obstetricians and Gynecologists. Committee Opinion No. 611: Method for estimating due date. *Obstet Gynecol.* 2014 Oct;124(4):863-66.

RESPIRATORY DISTRESS SYNDROME
Epidemiology
- Incidence—20/100,000 infant deaths due to RDS
- Age—more common the younger the gestational age
- Sex—M>F (minimal)

Pathophysiology
- Pulmonary surfactants are synthesized by type II pneumocytes and packaged into storage granules called lamellar bodies; these function to decrease alveolar surface tension.
  - Lecithin—detected at week 28; surges at week 36
  - Phosphatidylinositol—detected at week 28; peaks at week 35
  - Sphingomyelin—detected at week 28
  - Phosphatidylglycerol—detected at week 36 with increases until delivery
- RDS is caused by insufficient concentrations of pulmonary surfactants, resulting in collapsed alveoli (alveoli are perfused but hypoventilated).
  - Leads to hypoxia, hypercapnia, and respiratory acidosis
  - Conditions cause vasoconstriction of pulmonary arteries and decreased pulmonary blood flow
    - Pulmonary vasoconstriction causes epithelial cell damage, allowing plasma to leak into alveoli.
      - Fibrin accumulation and necrotic cells create a hyaline membrane (RDS previously called hyaline membrane disease).
- Nearly always associated with preterm birth.
  - Risk of RDS is inversely related to gestational age at birth:
    - >60% at <30 weeks
    - 20% at 34 weeks
    - <5% at >36 weeks
  - Measurement of fetal lung maturity through biochemical testing of amniotic fluid helps predict risk of RDS

Recent Changes in Clinical Practice
- Fetal lung maturity (FLM) tests have historically been performed to predict whether a fetus's lungs are developed enough for delivery. However, FLM testing has limited value in light of the most recent ACOG guidelines (2013), which advise against delivery <39 weeks unless medically mandated due to potential serious morbidity when compared to those delivered ≥39 weeks in spite of mature FLM tests.
- FLM testing may have value in the following clinical situations:
  - Premature rupture of membranes (≥32 weeks)—if FLM test is mature, delivery is likely safer than "wait and see" approach.
  - Assessment of need for NICU—possible only if early delivery has medical mandate and time allows for FLM testing.
  - Other selected late preterm and early preterm pregnancy issues where FLM may guide management of at-risk pregnancy.

Table 2.9. Comparison of FLM laboratory testing options (all testing requires amniotic fluid)

Lamellar Body Count (LBC)	Phosphatidylglycerol (PG)	Lecithin-Sphingomyelin Ratio (L/S)

• Initial FLM of choice
• Rapid, sensitive
• New data indicates that one can estimate risk of respiratory distress syndrome (RDS) as a function of gestational age and LBC
• Unclear whether *ACOG cascade should be followed if LBC is immature
	• Not useful unless gestational age ≥35 weeks
	• Limited availability
	• Sensitive
	• Unclear whether *ACOG cascade should be followed if PG is immature
		• Main role is in adjudication of immature LBC or PG
		• Last test of choice
		  ◦ Labor intensive, imprecise
		  ◦ Limited availability
		  ◦ Results take >24 hr unless performed at a local laboratory

*Refer to Diagnosis section for ACOG cascade, which is from ACOG Practice Bulletin 97 (which has been withdrawn). See above website to access this cascade.

Note: in general, mature results suggest RDS unlikely.

Source: Courtesy of David G. Grenache, PhD Adapted from Fetal Lung Maturity—Neonatal Respiratory Distress Syndrome. AARUP Consult (https://www.arupconsult.com), an ARUP Laboratories test selection tool for healthcare professionals. Copyright © 2016. All rights reserved.

NORMAL LABOR AND DELIVERY
Labor—Normal
- Ideally each patient should be evaluated at least q2 hr (with or without an exam).
- Labor is a physiologic, not pathologic, process.
- Contemporary labor curves suggest that active labor starts at 6 cm dilation.

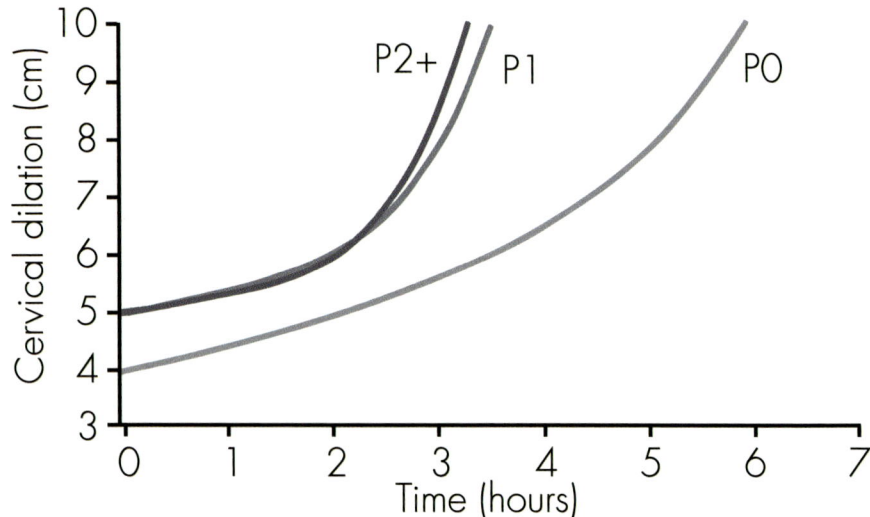

Figure 2.3. Average labor curves by parity in singleton, term pregnancies
Source: Reproduced with permission from Zhang J, Landy HJ, Branch DW, et al. Contemporary patterns of spontaneous labor with normal neonatal outcomes. *Obstet Gynecol.* 2010;116(6):1281-87. Copyright © 2010 The American College of Obstetricians and Gynecologists.

Table 2.10. Spontaneous labor progress stratified by cervical dilation and parity

	Median Elapsed Time (Hr)		
Cervical Dilation (cm)	Parity 0 (95th percentile)	Parity 1 (95th percentile)	Parity 2 or greater (95th percentile)
3–4	1.8 (8.1)	—	—
4–5	1.3 (6.4)	1.4 (7.3)	1.4 (7.0)
5–6	0.8 (3.2)	0.8 (3.4)	0.8 (3.4)
6–7	0.6 (2.2)	0.5 (1.9)	0.5 (1.8)
7–8	0.5 (1.6)	0.4 (1.3)	0.4 (1.2)
8–9	0.5 (1.4)	0.3 (1.0)	0.3 (0.9)
9–10	0.5 (1.8)	0.3 (0.9)	0.3 (0.8)

Source: Reproduced with permission from Zhang J, Landy HJ, Branch DW, et al. Contemporary patterns of spontaneous labor with normal neonatal outcomes. *Obstet Gynecol.* 2010;116(6):1281-87. Copyright © 2010 The American College of Obstetricians and Gynecologists.

Labor—Normal **OBSTETRICS** 2

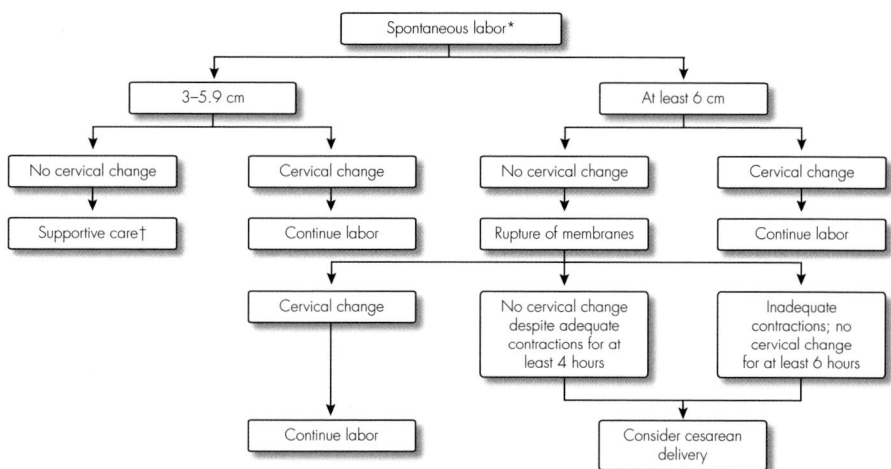

Figure 2.4. Algorithm for spontaneous labor
Reproduced with permission from Spong CY, Berghella V, Wenstrom KD, et al. Preventing the first cesarean delivery: summary of a joint Eunice Kennedy Shriver National Institute of Child Health and Human Development, Society for Maternal-Fetal Medicine, and American College of Obstetricians and Gynecologists Workshop. *Obstet Gynecol.* 2012 Nov;120(5):1181-93. Copyright © 2012 The American College of Obstetricians and Gynecologists.

ABNORMAL LABOR AND INDUCTION OF LABOR
Induction of Labor
Fast Facts
- Elective induction of labor should not occur prior to 39 weeks gestation.
- Bishop score >6 is one favorable for success (see table below).
- Misoprostol (prostaglandin E1) should be discouraged in women with a history of prior C/D, but pitocin and/or foley bulb can be considered. Data on the use of prostaglandin E2 in women with a prior cesarean delivery is limited. (See ACOG Practice Bulletin No. 115: Vaginal birth after previous cesarean delivery, 2010 Aug.)

Table 2.11. Bishop scoring for cervical ripening

Factor	0	1	2	3
Cervical dilation (cm)	closed	1–2	3–4	5+
Cervical effacement (%)	0–30	40–50	60–70	80+
Fetal station	−3	−2	−1	+1, +2
Cervical consistency	firm	medium	soft	•
Cervical position	posterior	mid	anterior	•

Add 1 point for preeclampsia and each prior vaginal delivery.

Deduct 1 point for postdates, nulliparity, preterm or prolonged PROM. Predicted values for success: Score 0–4 (45–50% failure); score 5–9 (10% failure), score 10–13 (0% failure).

Source: Reproduced from Bishop EH Pelvic scoring for elective induction. *Obstet Gynecol.* 1964 Aug;24:266-68; and Xenakis EM, Piper JM, Conway DL, Langer O. Induction of labor in the nineties: conquering the unfavorable cervix. *Obstet Gynecol.* 1997 Aug;90(2):235-39. Copyright © 1964 The American College of Obstetricians and Gynecologists.

Table 2.12. Attributes of commercially available prostaglandin analogues

	Dinoprostone (GE2 Cervical Gel)	Dinoprostone (PGE2 Vaginal Insert)	Misoprostol (PGE1 Analogue)
Description	Sterile, semitranslucent viscous preparation for endocervical application of 0.5 mg PGE2 per 3.0 g, in syringe	Thin, flat polymeric slab of 10 mg dinoprostone pessary contained within knitted polyester retrieval system	100 or 200 mcg oral tablets, divided in the pharmacy into 25- and 50-mcg doses; intravaginal use more preferable than oral
FDA status	FDA approved for cervical ripening	FDA approved for cervical ripening	FDA approved as an ulcer medication; Class X drug with black box warning contraindicating use by pregnant women; documented abortifacient properties
Pharmacokinetics	Half-life <5 mins; extensively metabolized in the lungs; rapidly absorbed; T_{max} of 0.5–0.75 hr	2.5–5-min half-life; 95% is cleared on first pass through pulmonary circulation; controlled release of approximately 0.3 mg/hr in vivo	20–40-min half-life; no industry standard dosing schedule
Initial dose	0.5 mg	10 mg	25–50 mcg
Route	Intracervical	Intravaginal	Intravaginal
Maximum number of doses	3 doses per 24 hr	1 dose	6 doses per 24 hr
Mechanisms of action	Softens the cervix; relaxes cervical smooth muscle; causes uterine contractions	Softens the cervix; relaxes cervical smooth muscle; causes uterine contractions	Causes uterine contractions
Use in VBAC	Implicated in the literature for increased risk of uterine rupture	Implicated in the literature for increased risk of uterine rupture	Specifically contraindicated by ACOG due to risk of uterine rupture
Price per dose	Approximately $150; usually requires more than 1 dose	Approximately $175; only 1 dose needed	Approximately $1.00
Refrigeration	Required	Required	Not required
Uterine hyperstimulation	Tocolytic agents must be administered	Resolves immediately upon removal of vaginal pessary	Tocolytic agents must be administered
Oxytocin administration	6–12 hr after administration of the last dose of the gel	30–60 mins after removal of pessary	Minimum of 3 hr after administration of the last dose of PGE1
Efficacy as cervical ripener	Comparable	Comparable	Comparable
Medicolegal	Labeled use precludes additional action	Labeled use precludes additional action	Off-label use requires informed consent
Cesarean delivery rate	No diminishment	No diminishment	No diminishment

ACOG, American College of Obstetricians and Gynecologists; FDA, Food and Drug Administration; PGE1, prostaglandin E1; PGE2, prostaglandin E2; VBAC, vaginal birth after cesarean delivery.

Source: Reproduced with permission from Witter F, Devoe L. Update on successful induction of labor. *Adv Stud Med.* 2005;5(9D):s888-s892.

Foley Catheter
- Comparable success to medical methods.
- Insert sterile speculum and clean cervix with Betadine or other antiseptic.
- Use ring forceps to insert tip of Foley catheter just beyond internal cervical os (may need to use a stylet).
- Use a 26 french catheter with 30 cc balloon.
- Fill balloon with 30–60 cc of normal saline over 1 minute.
- Retract the balloon so that it rests at the internal cervical os.
- Tape to patient's thigh with the traction in place.
- Foley will fall out when cervix has dilated to 3–4 cm in response to the pressure applied.
- May attach a 1 liter IV fluid bag to end of catheter and let hang out of the bed.
- Remove 6 hours later or at time of the rupture of membranes or spontaneous expulsion.
- May be combined with Pitocin administration.

    Source: Culver J, et al. A randomized trial comparing vaginal misoprostol versus Foley catheter with concurrent oxytocin for labor induction in nulliparous women. *Am J Perinatol.* 2004;21(3);139–146.

Cook® Cervical Ripening Balloon
- 2 separate balloons, one is placed against the internal cervical os and the second one is placed outside the external cervical os.
- 40 to 80 cc of saline is inflated into both balloons.
- The cervix is then squeezed open by the two balloons.
- The end of the catheter may be taped to the patient's thigh, but this is not necessary.

Pitocin
- Multiple protocols with either low- or high-dose Pitocin have been studied.
- Most institutions will have standard protocols for Pitocin augmentation.
- There is conflicting evidence regarding the use of Pitocin in women with a history of a prior C/D. Studies that show an increase in rate of uterine rupture with use of Pitocin for induction still report a rupture rate of less than 1% (see page 102).

Induction of Labor

Precautions
- Document indication, estimated fetal weight, and presentation (by ultrasound) clearly in chart.
- No elective inductions should be scheduled prior to 39 weeks and zero days.
- Document normal fetal heart rate (FHR) and less than 3 contractions per 10 minutes prior to placement of prostaglandins.
- Monitor FHR and uterine activity for at least 30 minutes to 2 hours after administration of gel or continuously with misoprostol.
- Use caution in patients with asthma, glaucoma, or renal, pulmonary, and hepatic disease.

Table 2.13. Neonatal and infant mortality rates associated with late-preterm and early-term deliveries

Gestational Age (Wk)	Neonatal Mortality Rate (Per 1,000 Live Births)	Relative Risk (95% CI)	Infant Mortality Rate (Per 1,000 Live Births)	Relative Risk (95% CI)
34*	7.1	9.5 (8.4–10.8)	11.8	5.4 (4.9–5.9)
35*	4.8	6.4 (5.6–7.2)	8.6	3.9 (3.6–4.3)
36*	2.8	3.7 (3.3–4.2)	5.7	2.6 (2.4–2.8)
37*	1.7	2.3 (2.1–2.6)	4.1	1.9 (1.8–2.0)
38*	1.0	1.4 (1.3–1.5)	2.7	1.2 (1.2–1.3)
39	0.8	1.00†	2.2	1.00†
40	0.8	1.0 (0.9–1.1)	2.1	0.9 (0.9–1.0)

CI, confidence interval.
*P<.001.
†Reference group.

Source: American College of Obstetricians and Gynecologists. ACOG Committee Opinion No. 561: Nonmedically indicated early-term deliveries. *Obstet Gynecol.* 2013 Apr;121(4):911-15. Copyright © 2013 The American College of Obstetricians and Gynecologists.

Table 2.14. Recommendations for timing of delivery when conditions complicate pregnancy at or after 34 weeks of gestation

Condition	Gestational Age* at Delivery	Grade of Recommendation†
Placental and uterine issues		
Placenta previa‡	**36–37 wk**	B
Suspected placenta accreta, increta, or percreta with placenta previa‡	**34–35 wk**	B
Prior classical cesarean (upper segment uterine incision)‡	**36–37 wk**	B
Prior myomectomy necessitating cesarean delivery‡	37–38 wk (may require earlier delivery, similar to prior classical cesarean, in situations with more extensive or complicated myomectomy)	B
Fetal issues		
Fetal growth restriction-singleton	**38–39 wk:**	
	• Otherwise uncomplicated, no concurrent findings	B
	34–37 wk:	
	• Concurrent conditions (oligohydramnios, abnormal Doppler studies, maternal risk factors, comorbidity)	B
	Expeditious delivery regardless of gestational age:	
	• Persistent abnormal fetal surveillance suggesting imminent fetal jeopardy	
Fetal growth restriction-twin gestation	**36–37 wk:**	
	• Dichorionic-diamniotic twins with isolated fetal growth restriction	B
	32–34 wk:	
	• Monochorionic-diamniotic twins with isolated fetal growth restriction	B
	• Concurrent conditions (oligohydramnios, abnormal Doppler studies, maternal risk factors, comorbidity)	B
	Expeditious delivery regardless of gestational age:	
	• Persistent abnormal fetal surveillance suggesting imminent fetal jeopardy	B
Fetal congenital malformations‡	**34–39 wk:**	B
	• Suspected worsening of fetal organ damage	
	• Potential for fetal intracranial hemorrhage (e.g., vein of Galen aneurysm, neonatal alloimmune thrombocytopenia)	
	• When delivery prior to labor is preferred (e.g., EXIT procedure)	
	• Previous fetal intervention	
	• Concurrent maternal disease (e.g., preeclampsia, chronic hypertension)	
	• Potential for adverse maternal effect from fetal condition	

(continued)

Induction of Labor — OBSTETRICS

Condition	Gestational Age* at Delivery	Grade of Recommendation†
	Expeditious delivery regardless of gestational age:	B
	• When intervention is expected to be beneficial	
	• Fetal complications develop (abnormal fetal surveillance, new-onset hydrops fetalis, progressive or new-onset organ injury)	
	• Maternal complications develop (mirror syndrome)	
Multiple gestations: dichorionic-diamniotic‡	**38 wk**	B
Multiple gestations: monochorionic-diamniotic‡	**34–37 wk**	B
Multiple gestations: dichorionic-diamniotic or monochorionic-diamniotic with single fetal death‡	If occurs at or after 34 wk, consider delivery (recommendation limited to pregnancies at or after 34 wk; if occurs before 34 wk, individualize based on concurrent maternal or fetal conditions)	B
Multiple gestations: monochorionic-monoamniotic‡	**32–34 wk**	B
Multiple gestations: Monochorionic-monoamniotic with single fetal death‡	Consider delivery; individualized according to gestational age and concurrent complications	B
Oligohydramnios—isolated and persistent‡	**36–37 wk**	B
Maternal issues	**38–39 wk**	B
Chronic hypertension—no medications‡ Chronic hypertension—controlled on medication‡	**37–39 wk**	B
Chronic hypertension—difficult to control (requiring frequent medication adjustments) ‡	**36–37 wk**	B
Gestational hypertension§	**37–38 wk**	B
Preeclampsia—severe‡	At diagnosis (recommendation limited to pregnancies at or after 34 wk)	C
Preeclampsia—mild‡	**37 wk**	B
Diabetes—pregestational well controlled‡	LPTB or ETB not recommended	B
Diabetes—pregestational with vascular disease‡	**37–39 wk**	B
Diabetes—pregestational, poorly controlled‡	**34–39 wk** (individualized to situation)	B
Diabetes—gestational well controlled on diet‡	LPTB or ETB not recommended	B
Diabetes—gestational well controlled on medication‡	LPTB or ETB not recommended	B
Diabetes—gestational poorly controlled on medication‡	**34–39 wk** (individualized to situation)	B
Obstetric issues		

(continued)

OBSTETRICS — Induction of Labor

Condition	Gestational Age* at Delivery	Grade of Recommendation†
Prior stillbirth-unexplained‡	LPTB or ETB not recommended	B
	Consider amniocentesis for fetal pulmonary maturity if delivery planned at less than 39 wk	C
Spontaneous preterm birth: preterm premature rupture of membranes‡	**34 wk** (recommendation limited to pregnancies at or after 34 wk)	B
Spontaneous preterm birth: active preterm labor‡	Delivery if progressive labor or additional maternal or fetal indication	B

LPTB, late-preterm birth at 34 0/7 weeks through 36 6/7 weeks; ETB, early-term birth at 37 0/7 weeks through 38 6/7 weeks.

*Gestational age is in completed weeks; thus, 34 weeks includes 34 0/7 weeks through 34 6/7 weeks.

† Grade of recommendations are based on the following: recommendations or conclusions or both are based on good and consistent scientific evidence (A); limited or inconsistent scientific evidence (B); primarily consensus and expert opinion (C). The recommendations regarding expeditious delivery for imminent fetal jeopardy were not given a grade. The recommendation regarding severe preeclampsia is based largely on expert opinion; however, higher-level evidence is not likely to be forthcoming because this condition is believed to carry significant maternal risk with limited potential fetal benefit from expectant management after 34 weeks.

‡ Uncomplicated, thus no fetal growth restriction, superimposed preeclampsia, etc. If these are present, then the complicating conditions take precedence and earlier delivery may be indicated.

§ Maintenance antihypertensive therapy should not be used to treat gestational hypertension.

Source: Modified from Spong CY, Mercer BM, D'Alton M, Kilpatrick S, Blackwell S, Saade G. Timing of Indicated Late-Preterm and Early-Term Birth. *Obstet Gynecol.* 2011;118(2 Pt 1):323-33. Reproduced with permission from American College of Obstetricians and Gynecologists. ACOG Committee Opinion No. 561: Nonmedically indicated early-term deliveries. *Obstet Gynecol.* 2013 Apr;121(4):911-15. Copyright © 2013 The American College of Obstetricians and Gynecologists.

Algorithm for Induction of Labor

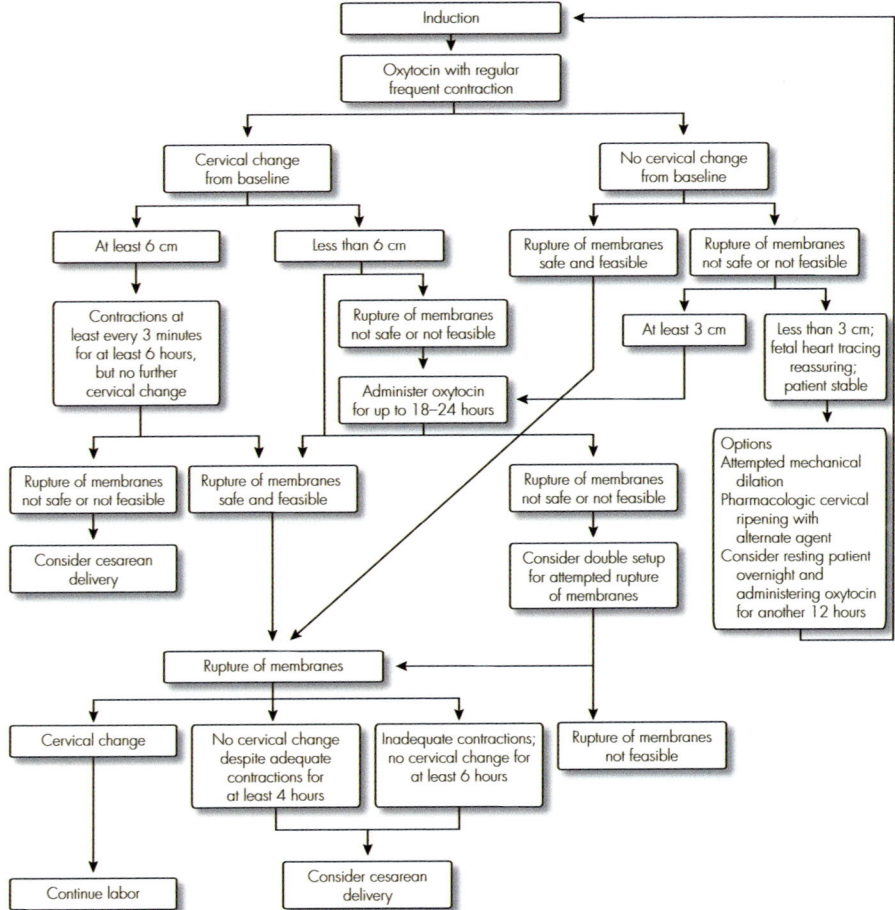

Figure 2.5. Algorithm for induction of labor
Reproduced with permission from Spong CY, Berghella V, Wenstrom KD, et al. Preventing the first cesarean delivery: summary of a joint Eunice Kennedy Shriver National Institute of Child Health and Human Development, Society for Maternal-Fetal Medicine, and American College of Obstetricians and Gynecologists Workshop. *Obstet Gynecol.* 2012 Nov;120(5):1181-93. Copyright © 2012 The American College of Obstetricians and Gynecologists.

SHOULDER DYSTOCIA

Definition
"Delivery that requires additional maneuvers following failure of gentle downward traction on the fetal head to effect delivery of the shoulders." (Source: ACOG Practice Bulletin No. 40: Shoulder dystocia, 2002 Nov.)

Incidence
- 0.6–1.4% of all deliveries.

Risk Factors
- Maternal obesity, diabetes, history of macrosomic infant, current macrosomia, history of prior shoulder dystocia.

Table 2.15. Risk of shoulder dystocia (%) as a function of birthweight

Reference	2500–2999 G	3000–3499 G	3500–3999 G	4000–4499 G	4500–5000 G	>5000 G
Acker 1985	0.2	0.6	2.3	10.3	23.9	
Spellacy 1985	0.3		N/A		7.3	14.6
Benedetti 1978	1.5		3.0			

- 2/3 occur with birthweight <4000 g.
- Diabetic pregnancies are at higher risk.
- Consideration of cesarean delivery to avoid should dystocia is reasonable if the estimated fetal weight is >5,000 gm in a nondiabetic mother or 4,500 gm in a pregnancy complicated by diabetes.
- The recurrence of shoulder dystocia in a subsequent pregnancy is between 1–16.7%. Cesarean delivery may be offered after considering the patient's history and current pregnancy. (Source: ACOG Practice Bulletin No. 40: Shoulder dystocia. *Int J Gynaecol Obstet*. 2003;80:87.)

Warning Signs
- Anticipation is key!
- Prolonged second stage of labor
- Recoil of head on perineum (turtle sign)
- Lack of spontaneous restitution

Treatment
- Alert all members of the delivery team.
- Call for additional obstetrical and neonatal help.
- McRobert's Maneuver: dorsiflexion of hips against abdomen and abduction.
- Suprapubic pressure (NOT fundal pressure).
- Constant moderate DOWNWARD pressure.
- Cut episiotomy if needed to perform other maneuvers.
- Rubin's Screw Maneuver: push the most accessible shoulder to the fetal chest.
- Attempt Wood's Screw: place your hand behind the posterior shoulder and rotate the fetus 180 degrees to disimpact the anterior shoulder.

- Attempt delivery of posterior arm by flexing the arm over the fetal chest with 2 fingers to allow for delivery (may fracture humerus).
- Gaskin Maneuver: position the patient on hands and knees.
- Fracture the fetal clavicle.
- Zavenelli Maneuver: cephalic replacement/abdominal rescue (high rates of fetal injury/death and uterine rupture).

Fetal Complications
- Brachial plexus injuries occur in 4–40% of deliveries complicated by shoulder dystocia. Fewer than 10% of brachial plexus injuries are permanent.
- Common injuries include brachial plexus injury, clavicle fracture, and humerus fracture.
- <10% have permanent injuries.
- Increased risk of hypoxic-ischemic encephalopathy and death.

Maternal Complications
- 11% risk of postpartum hemorrhage
- 3.8% risk of fourth-degree laceration

OPERATIVE VAGINAL DELIVERY
Fast Facts
- Have a clear indication for the operative vaginal delivery.
- Obtain consent from the patient.
- Know the fetal position.
- Assure adequate anesthesia.
- Empty the maternal bladder.
- Have pediatrics available to assess the infant after delivery.

Source: Personal communication, Dr. Shirley Tom, FACOG.

Table 2.16. Criteria for types of forceps delivery

Outlet Forceps
Scalp is visible at the introitus without separating the labia.
Fetal skull has reached the pelvic floor.
Fetal head is at or on perineum.
Sagittal suture is in an anteroposterior diameter or right or left occiput anterior or posterior position.
Rotation does not exceed 45°.
Low Forceps
Leading point of fetal skull is at station 2 cm or more and not on the pelvic floor.
Without rotation: Rotation is 45° or less (right or left occiput anterior to occiput anterior, or right or left occiput posterior to occiput posterior).
With rotation: Rotation is greater than 45°.
Mid Forceps
Station above +2 cm but head is engaged.

Source: Reproduced with permission from Committee on Practice Bulletins—Obstetrics. ACOG Practice Bulletin No. 154: Operative vaginal delivery. *Obstet Gynecol.* 2015 Nov;126(5):e56-65. Copyright © 2015 The American College of Obstetricians and Gynecologists.

Operative Vaginal Delivery **OBSTETRICS**

Table 2.17. ACOG summary recommendations for operative vaginal delivery

The Following Recommendations and Conclusions Are Based On Good and Consistent Scientific Evidence (Level A):

- Forceps and vacuum extractors have low risk of complications and are acceptable for operative vaginal delivery.
- A vaginal birth is more likely to be achieved with forceps than with vacuum extractors; however, forceps are more likely to be associated with third- and fourth-degree perineal tears.
- Routine episiotomy with operative vaginal delivery is not recommended because poor healing and prolonged discomfort has been reported with mediolateral episiotomy and because of the association of midline episiotomies with increased risk of injury to the anal sphincter and extension into the rectum.

The Following Recommendations and Conclusions Are Based On Limited or Inconsistent Scientific Evidence (Level B):

- Episiotomy should not be performed routinely for all operative vaginal deliveries.
- Operative vaginal delivery is contraindicated if the fetal head is unengaged, the position of the fetal head is unknown, or a live fetus is known or strongly suspected to have a bone demineralization condition (e.g., osteogenesis imperfecta) or a bleeding disorder (e.g., alloimmune thrombocytopenia, hemophilia, or von Willebrand disease).
- A trial of operative vaginal delivery is an appropriate option in a situation where the obstetrician or obstetric care provider feels the chances of success are high, but he or she must be prepared to abandon the attempt if appropriate descent does not occur.
- Sequential use of vacuum extractor and forceps has been associated with increased rates of neonatal complications and should not routinely be performed.
- Cephalohematoma is more likely to occur as the duration of vacuum application increases.
- Midforceps and rotational forceps delivery are appropriate options in select clinical circumstances.

The Following Recommendations and Conclusions Are Based Primarily On Consensus and Expert Opinion (Level C):

- Vacuum extraction has been discouraged for gestational age less than 34 weeks, although a safe lower limit for gestational age has not been established.
- For the fetus who manifests signs of compromise in the second stage of labor, the timely and skilled use of instrumental vaginal delivery has the potential to decrease the exposure to intrauterine insults and could decrease the contribution of intrapartum factors leading to neonatal encephalopathy and hypoxic-ischemic encephalopathy.
- Neonatal care providers should be made aware of the mode of delivery in order to observe for potential complications associated with operative vaginal delivery.

Source: Reproduced with permission from Committee on Practice Bulletins—Obstetrics. ACOG Practice Bulletin No. 154: Operative vaginal delivery. *Obstet Gynecol.* 2015 Nov;126(5):e56-65. Copyright © 2015 The American College of Obstetricians and Gynecologists.

Table 2.18. Relative risks based upon delivery method

Delivery Method	Neonatal Death	Intracranial Hemorrhage	Other[a]
Spontaneous vaginal delivery	1/5000	1/1900	1/216
Cesarean delivery during labor	1/1250	1/952	1/71
Cesarean delivery after vacuum/forceps	N/R	1/333	1/38
Cesarean delivery with no labor	1/1250	1/2040	1/105
Vacuum alone	1/3333	1/860	1/122
Forceps alone	1/2000	1/664	1/76
Vacuum and forceps	1/1666	1/280	1/58

N/R, not reported.

[a]Facial nerve/brachial plexus injury, convulsions, central nervous system depression, mechanical ventilation.

Source: Data from Towner D, Castro MA, Eby-Wilkens E, Gilbert WM. Effect of mode of delivery in nulliparous women on neonatal intracranial brain injury. *N Engl J Med.* 1999;341:1709-14.

OBSTETRICS

Operative Vaginal Delivery

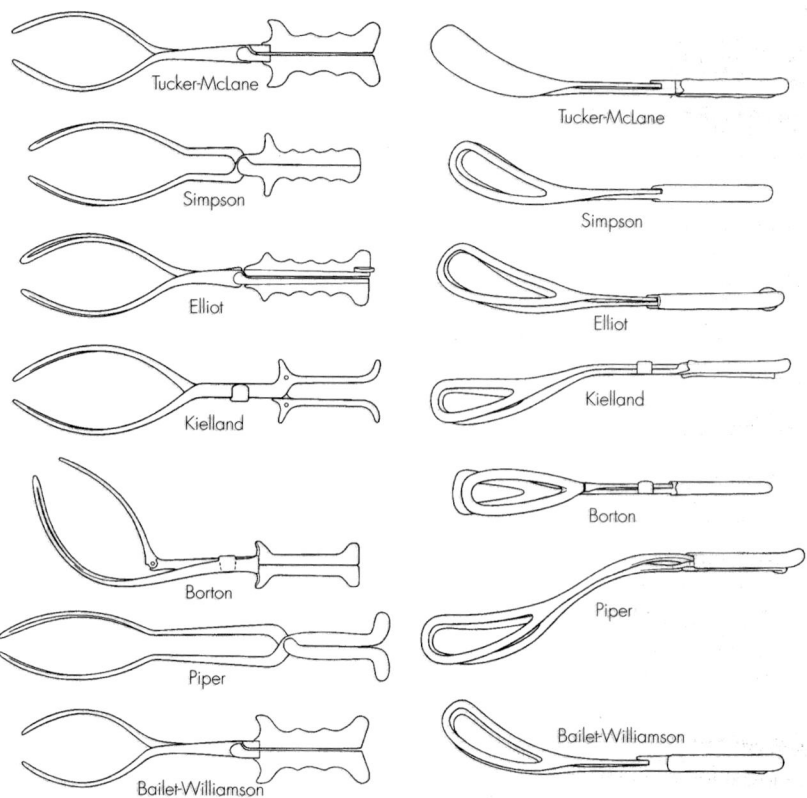

Figure 2.6. Types of forceps
Source: From Zuspan FP, Quilligan EJ. Forceps. In: *Douglas-Stromme Operative Obstetrics, 5th Ed*. Norwalk, CT: Appleton & Lange; 1988. Reproduced with the permission of the publisher.

Operative Vaginal Delivery **OBSTETRICS**

Vacuum Extraction
Fast Facts
- Use same indications as forceps, but ease of application has clouded judgment of some physicians.
- All cups are approximately 6 cm in diameter.
- Can result in fetal injuries similar to forceps, higher incidence of scalp injuries.
- Cephalohematoma in 14–16% of vacuum deliveries (vs. 2% with forceps).
- Subgaleal hematoma in 26–45/1000 vacuum deliveries.
- Retinal hemorrhages in 38% (vs. 17% with forceps).

Application and Delivery
- Know the fetal position exactly.
- Check manufacturer's recommendations.
- Position cup symmetrically over sagittal suture 3 cm anterior to posterior fontanelle: "flexion point."
- Apply low suction (100 mm Hg), increase pressure to 500 mm Hg, and pull along pelvic curve.
- Check that no vaginal or cervical tissue is trapped by cup.
- Descent of the head must occur with each pull.
- Delivery should be accomplished with 3–5 pulls.
- Maximum of 2 "pop-offs."
- Head should be completely delivered within 15 minutes of first application.
- Do not use for rotation.
- Avoid rocking movements or excessive torque.

Table 2.19. Classification and use of vacuum delivery cups

Soft cups—Indicated for outlet and low OA <45° assisted deliveries	Kiwi ProCup and Kiwi OmniCup
	Silc, Gentle Vac, and Secure Cups
	Silastic. Reusable and Vac-U-Nate cups
	Standard MityVac and Soft Touch cups
Rigid "anterior" cups—Indicated for outlet and low OA <45° assisted deliveries	M-Style MityVac cup
	Flex cup
	Malmstrom, Bird, and O'Neil cups
Rigid "posterior" cups—Indicated for OA >45°, OP, and OT assisted deliveries	Kiwi OmniCup
	M-Select Mityvac cup
	Bird and O'Neil Posterior cups

OA, occiput-anterior; OP, occiput-posterior; OT, occiput-transverse.

Source: Reproduced with permission from McQuivery RW. Vacuum-assisted delivery: a review. *J Matern Fetal Neonatal Med.* 2003;16:171-79. Copyright © 2003 Taylor & Francis.

Operative Vaginal Delivery

The center of the cup should be over the sagittal suture and about 3 cm in front of the posterior fontanelle. The cup is generally placed as far posteriorly as possible.

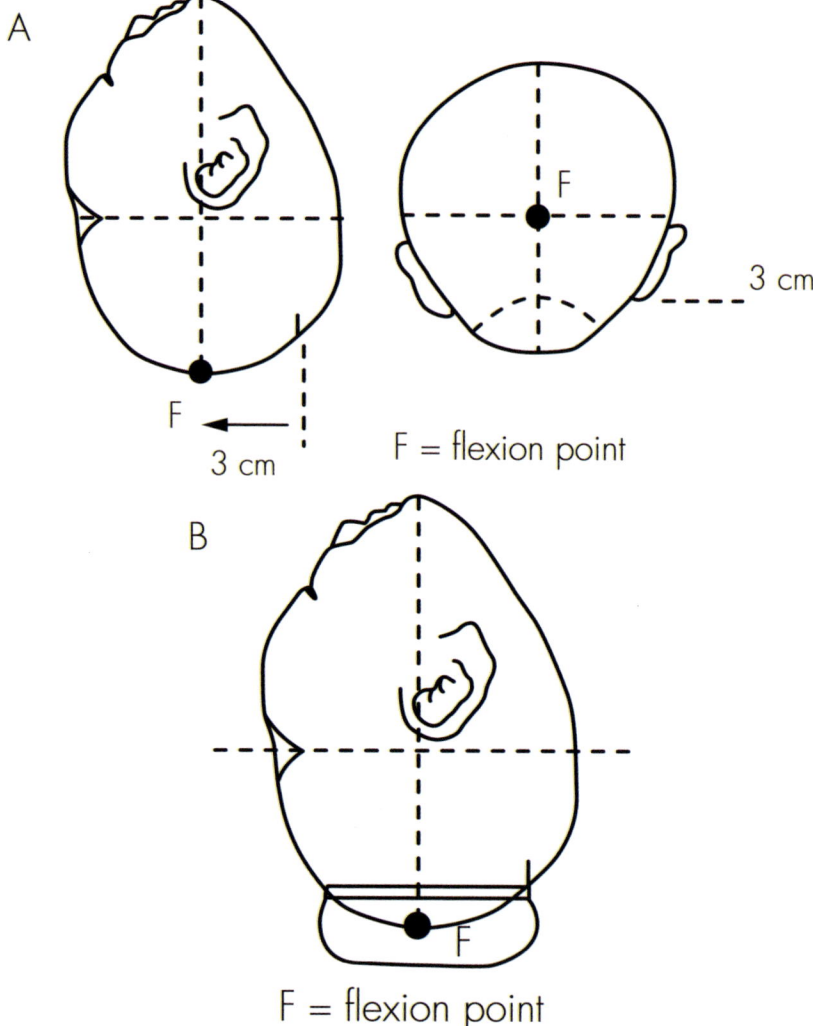

F = flexion point

F = flexion point

(A) During normal delivery condition, the mentocervical diameter emerges on the sagittal suture approximately 3 cm in front of the posterior fontanelle. **(B)** The center of the extraction cup has been placed over the flexion point, and axis traction is applied.

(continued)

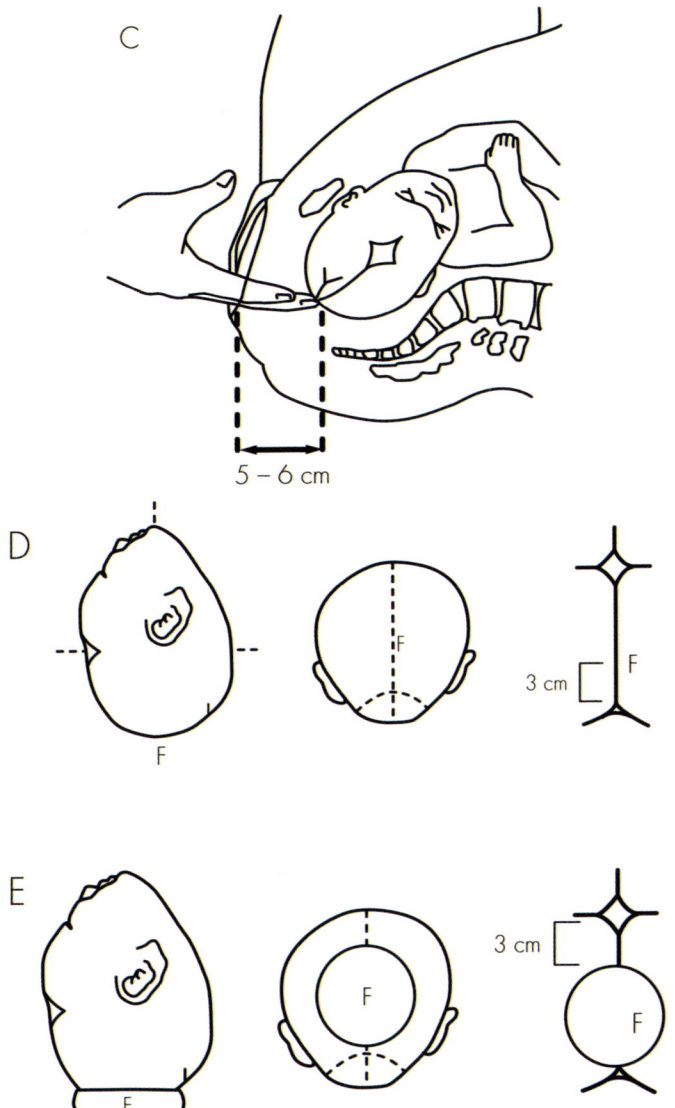

(C) Locating the flexion point and calculating the distance from the posterior fourchette using the examining finger.
(D) The flexion point is situated on the sagittal suture 3 cm forward of the posterior fontanelle. **(E)** The center of the vacuum cup should be placed over the flexion point with the sagittal suture in the midline.

Figure 2.7. Proper placement of the vacuum cup
Source: Reproduced with permission from Vacca A. Vacuum-assisted delivery: improving patient outcomes and protecting yourself against litigation. *OBG Management.* 2004 Feb. Suppl:S1–S7.

CESAREAN DELIVERY
Fast Facts
- Origin of term remains mysterious
- Method of delivery of Julius Caesar (certainly a myth)
- *Lex cesarea*: Roman law requiring removal of fetus from dead mother
- Derived from Latin verb *caedere*, "to cut"
  - In 2011, approximately 1/3 births were cesarean deliveries
  - Safe reduction in the cesarean delivery rate is supported by ACOG and SMFM given the increased maternal and neonatal complications of cesarean delivery

Indications
- Be precise; be specific
- Write a detailed preoperative note

Table 2.20. Indications for cesarean delivery

Fetal
Abnormal or indeterminate fetal status
Malpresentation (breech, transverse lie)
Twins (nonvertex first twin, possibly for nonvertex second twin)
Maternal HSV infection
Fetal congenital anomalies
Maternal-fetal

Labor abnormalities
  ◦ Active phase arrest
  ◦ Arrest of descent
  ◦ Failed induction
  ◦ Inefficient uterine contractility unresponsive to therapy

Placental abruption (certain cases)
Placenta previa/invasive placentation
Pelvic malformation (absolute pelvic disproportion)
Estimated fetal weight >4500 g in patients with diabetes or 5000 g in nondiabetic patients
Maternal
Obstructive benign/malignant tumors
Severe vulvar condylomata
Cervical carcinoma
Abdominal cerclage
Prior vaginal colporrhaphy
Vaginal delivery contraindicated (medical indications eg active HSV, HIV with viral load >1,000 copies/mL)

HSV, herpes simplex virus.

Table 2.21. Risk of adverse maternal and neonatal outcomes by mode of delivery

	Risk	
Outcome	Vaginal delivery	Cesarean delivery
Maternal		
Overall severe morbidity and mortality[a]	8.6%	9.2%[a]
	0.9%	2.7%
Maternal mortality[b]	3.6:100,000	13.3:100,000
Amniotic fluid embolism	3.3–7.7:100,000	15.8:100,000
Third- or fourth-degree perineal laceration	1.0–3.0%	NA (scheduled delivery)
Placental abnormalities	Increased with prior cesarian vs. vaginal delivery, and risk continues to increase with each subsequent cesarean delivery	
Urinary incontinence	No difference between cesarean and vaginal delivery at 2 yr	
Postpartum depression	No difference between cesarean and vaginal delivery	
Neonatal		
Laceration	NA	1.0–2.0%
Respiratory morbidity	<1.0%	1.0–4.0% (without labor)
Shoulder dystocia	1.0–2.0%	0%

NA, not available

[a]Defined as ≥1 of following: death, postpartum bleeding, genital tract injury; wound disruption, wound infection, or both; systemic infection.

[b]Defined as any 1 of following: death, hemorrhage requiring hysterectomy or transfusion; uterine rupture; anesthetic complications; shock; cardiac arrest; acute renal failure; assistant ventilation venous thromboembolic event; major infection; in-hospital wound disruption, wound hematoma, or both.

Source: Reproduced with permission from American College of Obstetricians and Gynecologists; Society for Maternal-Fetal Medicine, Caughey AB, Cahill AG, Guise JM, Rouse DJ. Safe prevention of the primary cesarean delivery. *Am J Obstet Gynecol.* 2014 Mar;210(3):179-93. Copyright © 2014 The American College of Obstetricians and Gynecologists.

Safe Prevention of Primary Cesarean Delivery

Table 2.22. Recommendations for safe prevention of primary cesarean delivery

Recommendations	Grade of Recommendations
First stage of labor	
A prolonged latent phase (e.g., >20 hr in nulliparous women and >14 hr in multiparous women) should not be indication for cesarean delivery.	1B Strong recommendation, moderate-quality evidence
Slow but progressive labor in first stage of labor should not be indication for cesarean delivery.	1B Strong recommendation, moderate-quality evidence
Cervical dilation of 6 cm should be considered threshold for active phase of most women in labor. Thus, before 6 cm of dilation is achieved, standards of active-phase progress should not be applied.	1B Strong recommendation, moderate-quality evidence
Cesarean delivery for active-phase arrest in first stage of labor should be reserved for women ≥6 cm of dilation with ruptured membranes who fail to progress despite 4 hr of adequate uterine activity, or at least 6 hr of oxytocin administration with inadequate uterine activity and no cervical change.	1B Strong recommendation, moderate-quality evidence
Second stage of labor	
A specific absolute maximum length of time spent in second stage of labor beyond which all women should undergo operative delivery has not been identified.	1C Strong recommendation, low-quality evidence
Before diagnosing arrest of labor in second stage, if maternal and fetal conditions permit, allow for the following: • At least 2 hr of pushing in multiparous women (1B) • At least 3 hr of pushing in nulliparous women (1B) Longer duration may be appropriate on individualized basis (e.g., with use of epidural analgesia or with fetal malposition) as long as progress is being documented (1B).	1B Strong recommendation, moderate-quality evidence
Operative vaginal delivery in second stage of labor by experienced and well-trained physicians should be considered safe, acceptable alternative to cesarean delivery. Training in, and ongoing maintenance of, practical skills related to operative vaginal delivery should be encouraged.	1B Strong recommendation, moderate-quality evidence
Manual rotation of fetal occiput in setting of fetal malposition in second stage of labor is reasonable intervention to consider before moving to operative vaginal delivery or cesarean delivery. To safely prevent cesarean deliveries in setting of malposition, it is important to assess fetal position in second stage of labor, particularly in setting of abnormal fetal descent.	1B Strong recommendation, moderate-quality evidence
Fetal heart rate monitoring	
Amnioinfusion for repetitive variable fetal heart rate decelerations may safely reduce rate of cesarean delivery.	1A Strong recommendation, high-quality evidence
Scalp stimulation can be used as means of assessing fetal acid-base status when abnormal or indeterminate (formerly, nonreassuring) fetal heart patterns (e.g., minimal variability) are present and is safe alternative to cesarean delivery in this setting.	1C Strong recommendation, low-quality evidence

(continued)

Cesarean Delivery

Recommendations	Grade of Recommendations
Induction of labor	
Before 41 0/7 wk of gestation, induction of labor generally should be performed based on maternal or fetal medical indications. Inductions at ≥41 0/7 wk of gestation should be performed to reduce risk of cesarean delivery and risk of perinatal morbidity and mortality.	1A Strong recommendation, high-quality evidence
Cervical ripening method should be used when labor is induced in women with unfavorable cervix.	1B Strong recommendation, moderate-quality evidence
If maternal and fetal status allow, cesarean deliveries for failed induction of labor in latent phase can be avoided by allowing longer durations of latent phase (up to ≥24 hr) and requiring that oxytocin be administered for at least 12–18 hr after membrane rupture before deeming induction failure.	1B Strong recommendation, moderate-quality evidence
Fetal malpresentation	
Fetal presentation should be assessed and documented beginning at 36 0/7 wk of gestation to allow for external cephalic version to be offered.	1C Strong recommendation, low-quality evidence
Suspected fetal macrosomia	
Cesarean delivery to avoid potential birth trauma should be limited to estimated fetal weights of at least 5000 g in women without diabetes and at least 4500 g in women with diabetes. Prevalence of birth weight ≥5000 g is rare, and patients should be counseled that estimates of fetal weight, particularly late in gestation, are imprecise.	2C Weak recommendation, low-quality evidence
Excessive maternal weight gain	
Women should be counseled about IOM maternal weight guidelines in attempt to avoid excessive weight gain.	1B Strong recommendation, moderate-quality evidence
Twin gestations	
Perinatal outcomes for twin gestations in which first twin is in cephalic presentation are not improved by cesarean delivery. Thus, women with either cephalic/cephalic-presenting twins or cephalic/noncephalic-presenting twins should be considered to attempt vaginal delivery.	1B Strong recommendation, moderate-quality evidence
Other	
Individuals, organizations, and governing bodies should work to ensure that research is conducted to provide better knowledge base to guide decisions regarding cesarean delivery and to encourage policy changes that safely lower rate of primary cesarean delivery.	1C Strong recommendation, low-quality evidence

ICM, Institute of Medicine

Source: Reproduced with permission from American College of Obstetricians and Gynecologists; Society for Maternal-Fetal Medicine, Caughey AB, Cahill AG, Guise JM, Rouse DJ. Safe prevention of the primary cesarean delivery. *Am J Obstet Gynecol.* 2014 Mar;210(3):179-93.Copyright © 2014 The American College of Obstetricians and Gynecologists.

Cesarean Section Operative Techniques

Table 2.23. Summary of operative techniques in cesarean delivery

Variable	PKM	JCM	MLM	MMLM
Skin incision	Pfannenstiel[a]	Joel-Cohen[b]	Joel-Cohen[b]	Pfannenstiel[a]
Subcutaneous layer closure	Sharp dissection	Blunt dissection	Blunt dissection	Blunt dissection
Fascia opening	Sharp extension	Blunt extension	Blunt extension	Blunt extension
Peritoneal opening	Sharp entry	Blunt entry	Blunt entry	Blunt entry
Uterine incision	Sharp superficial, then blunt entry	Sharp superficial, then blunt entry	Sharp superficial, then blunt entry	Sharp superficial, then blunt entry
Placenta removal	Manual	Spontaneous	Manual	Spontaneous
Uterine closure	Single layer, interrupted	Single layer, interrupted	Single layer, running	Single layer, running
Peritoneal closure	Closed	Not closed	Not closed	Closed
Fascia closure	Interrupted	Interrupted	Continuous	Continuous
Subcutaneous closure	Not sutured	Not sutured	Not sutured	Not sutured
Skin closure	Continuous suture	Continuous suture	Mattress suture	Continuous suture

CD, cesarean delivery; JCM, Joel-Cohen method; MLM, Misgav-Ladach method; MMLM, Modified Misgav-Ladach method; PKM, Pfannenstiel-Kerr method.

[a]Pfannenstiel skin incision is slightly curved, 2–3 cm or 2 fingers above the symphysis pubis, with the midportion of the incision within the shaved area of the pubic hair.

[b]Joel-Cohen incision is straight, 3 cm below the line that joins the anterior superior iliac spines, slightly more cephalad than Pfannenstiel.

Source: Reproduced with permission from Dahlke JD, Mendez-Figueroa H, Rouse DJ, et al. Evidence-based surgery for cesarean delivery: an updated systematic review. *Am J Obstet Gynecol*. 2013 Oct;209(4):294-306. Copyright © 2013 Elsevier.

Uterine Incision for Cesarean Section
- Most common:
  - Low transverse (see figure A below) or Kerr (see figure D below)
- Low vertical (see figure B below)
  - Premature fetus with malpresentation or poorly developed lower segment
  - Usually extends into active segment
- Classical (see figure C below)
  - Often used for delivery of premature infants as needed
  - Impacted transverse lie, cervical carcinoma

Druzin Splint Maneuver
- Malpresentations in premature fetus often associated with difficult delivery.
- Choose correct uterine incision.
- Druzin splint technique as detailed below to allow atraumatic delivery.
- Breech or transverse lie
- Intact membranes helpful
- If fails, then uterine relaxants and version/extraction.

Cesarean Delivery OBSTETRICS

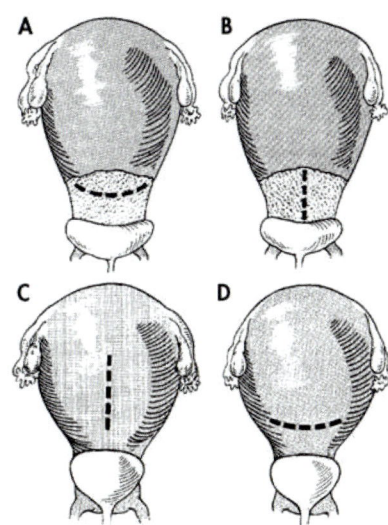

Figure 2.8. Location of uterine incision in types of cesarean delivery
(A) Low transverse. (B) Low vertical. (C) Classical. (D) Kerr.
  Source: Scott JR. Cesarean delivery. In: Scott JR, DiSaia PD, Hammond CB, Spellacy WN, ed. *Danforth's Obstetrics and Gynecology, 7th Ed.* Philadelphia: Lippincott; 1994. Reproduced with the permission of the publisher.

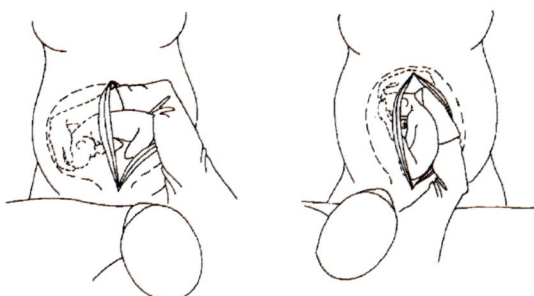

Figure 2.9. Druzin splint maneuver
  Source: Druzin ML. Atraumatic delivery in cases of malpresentation of the very low birth weight fetus at cesarean section: the splint technique. *Am J Obstet Gynecol.* 1986;154(4):941-42. Reproduced with the permission of the publisher, Mosby Year Book: St. Louis. Copyright © 1986 Elsevier.

Table 2.24. Maternal morbidity of women who had cesarean delivery without labor

Morbidity	First CD[a]	Second CD	Third CD	Fourth CD	Fifth CD	Sixth CD	P Value[b]
No.	6201	15,808	6324	1452	258	89	—
Placenta accreta	15 (0.24)	49 (0.31)	36 (0.57)	31 (2.13)	6 (2.33)	6 (6.74)	< .001
Hysterectomy	40 (0.65)	67 (0.42)	57 (0.90)	35 (2.41)	9 (3.49)	8 (8.99)	< .001
Any blood transfusion	251 (4.05)	242 (1.53)	143 (2.26)	53 (3.65)	11 (4.26)	14 (15.73)	.61
Blood transfusion >4 U	65 (1.05)	76 (0.48)	49 (0.77)	23 (1.59)	6 (2.33)	9 (10.11)	< .001
Cystotomy	8 (0.13)	15 (0.09)	18 (0.28)	17 (1.17)	5 (1.94)	4 (4.49)	< .001
Bowel injury	7 (0.11)	9 (0.06)	8 (0.13)	5 (0.34)	0 (0.00)	1 (1.12)	.02
Ureteral injury	2 (0.03)	2 (0.01)	1 (0.02)	1 (0.07)	1 (0.39)	1 (1.12)	.008
Placenta previa	398 (6.42)	211 (1.33)	72 (1.14)	33 (2.27)	6 (2.33)	3 (3.37)	< .001
Ileus	41 (0.66)	71 (0.45)	43 (0.68)	13 (0.90)	4 (1.55)	3 (3.37)	.01
Postoperative ventilator	62 (1.0)	33 (0.21)	15 (0.24)	10 (0.69)	2 (0.78)	1 (1.12)	< .001
Intensive care admission	115 (1.85)	90 (0.57)	34 (0.54)	23 (1.58)	5 (1.94)	5 (5.62)	.007
Operative time, min	50.6 (24.0)	54.9 (23.2)	60.7 (25.6)	64.5 (32.7)	67.9 (32.6)	79.9 (53.4)	< .001[c]
Hospital stay, d	5.6 (7.2)	3.9 (4.2)	3.8 (4.0)	4.2 (5.2)	4.1 (5.0)	5.5 (7.8)	< .001[c]
Wound infection	95 (1.53)	148 (0.94)	97 (1.53)	19 (1.31)	9 (3.45)	3 (3.37)	.09
Endometritis	371 (5.98)	404 (2.56)	178 (2.81)	43 (2.96)	4 (1.55)	6 (6.74)	< .001
Wound dehiscence	23 (0.37)	17 (0.11)	10 (0.16)	3 (0.21)	2 (0.78)	0	.18
Deep venous thrombosis	17 (0.27)	24 (0.15)	9 (0.14)	3 (0.21)	0	1 (1.12)	.42
Pulmonary embolus	13 (0.21)	18 (0.11)	5 (0.08)	4 (0.28)	1 (0.39)	1 (1.12)	.85
Reoperation	26 (0.42)	35 (0.22)	16 (0.25)	6 (0.41)	1 (0.39)	3 (3.37)	.57
Maternal death	12 (0.19)	11 (0.07)	3 (0.05)	1 (0.07)	0	0	.02

Data are presented as n (%).

CD, cesarean delivery.

[a] Primary cesarean delivery.

[b] P values are from Cochran-Armitage test for trend unless otherwise indicated.

[c] From Spearman rank correlation test. Reprinted with permission from Silver, et al.

Reproduced with permission from Clark EA, Silver RM. Long-term maternal morbidity associated with repeat cesarean delivery. *Am J Obstet Gynecol.* 2011 Dec;205(6 Suppl):S2-10. Copyright © 2011 Elsevier.

Table 2.25. Placenta previa and accreta by number of cesarean deliveries

Cesarean Delivery	Previa	Previa[a]: Accreta[b] n (%)	No Previa[c]: Accreta[b] n (%)
First[d]	398	13 (3.3)	2 (0.03)
Second	211	23 (11)	26 (0.2)
Third	72	29 (40)	7 (0.1)
Fourth	33	20 (61)	11 (0.8)
Fifth	6	4 (67)	2 (0.8)
≥Sixth	3	2 (67)	4 (4.7)

[a] Percentage of placenta accreta in women with placenta previa.
[b] Increased risk with increasing number of cesarean deliveries, $P < .001$.
[c] Percentage of accreta in women without placenta previa.
[d] Primary cesarean.

Source: Reproduced with permission from Silver RM, Landon MB, Rouse DJ, et al. Maternal morbidity associated with multiple cesarean deliveries. *Obstet Gynecol* 2006;107:1226-32. Copyright © 2006 The American College of Obstetricians and Gynecologists.

VAGINAL BIRTH AFTER CESAREAN
Candidates for a TOLAC
- One or two previous Low transverse cesarean deliveries with a singleton gestation
- One previous cesarean delivery and a twin gestation
- Previous low vertical uterine incision
- Previous cesarean delivery with an unknown scar type unless there is a high suspicion for previous classical cesarean uterine incision
- Best candidates are those women with at least a 60% chance of successful VBAC

Contraindications to a TOLAC
- Previous classical or T-incision
- Prior uterine rupture
- Extensive transfundal uterine surgery
- Contraindication to vaginal delivery such as placenta previa

Predicting Success
- Success rates vary with indications of previous cesarean delivery.
  - Non-recurrent indications (breech): 75–86% success, similar to women without a prior C/S
  - Previous arrest disorder: 50–80%
- Individualized patient VBAC success rates can be estimated using the NIH VBAC calculator:
  - https://mfmunetwork.bsc.gwu.edu/PublicBSC/MFMU/VGBirthCalc/vagbirth.html

Clinical Practice Guidelines Regarding VBAC

Table 2.26. Comparison of clinical practice guidelines for VBAC

Society	VBAC Counseling	Facilities and Personnel	Other Recommendations
The College	VBAC should be offered to most women with one previous cesarean delivery with Low transverse incision; consider those with two previous Low transverse cesarean deliveries.	Safest where staff can provide immediate emergency cesarean delivery, but patients should be allowed to accept increased risk when such resources are not available.	Twins, macrosomia, postdatism, low vertical incision, and unknown type of uterine incision should not preclude.
RCOG	Women with one prior low segment cesarean delivery should be able to discuss option of VBAC; final decision between woman and her obstetrician.	Should be conducted in suitably staffed and equipped delivery suite with continuous intrapartum care and monitoring and available resources for immediate cesarean delivery and advanced neonatal resuscitation.	Caution with twins and macrosomia (uncertainty due to underpowered studies).
SOGC	VBAC should be offered to women with one previous cesarean delivery with Low transverse incision.	In hospital where a timely cesarean is available; an approximate timeframe of 30 min should be considered adequate for urgent laparotomy.	Twins, macrosomia, and postdatism are not contraindications.
AAFP	VBAC should be offered to women with one previous cesarean delivery with Low transverse incision.	Should not be restricted only to those facilities with available surgical teams present throughout labor because there is no evidence that these additional resources result in improved outcome.	Not addressed.
AHRQ	VBAC is a reasonable choice for the majority of women with prior cesarean delivery.	Not addressed.	Not addressed.

VBAC, Vaginal Birth After Cesarean Delivery; The College, American College of Obstetricians and Gynecologists; RCOG, Royal College of Obstetricians and Gynaecologists; SOGC, Society of Obstetricians and Gynaecologists of Canada; AAFP, American Academy of Family Physicians; AHRQ, Agency for Healthcare Research and Quality.

Source: Reproduced with permission from Scott JR. Vaginal birth after cesarean delivery: a common-sense approach. *Obstet Gynecol.* 2011 Aug;118(2 Pt 1):342-50. Copyright © 2011 The American College of Obstetricians and Gynecologists.

Table 2.27. Composite maternal risks from elective repeat cesarean delivery and trial of labor after previous cesarean delivery

Maternal Risks	ERCD (%)	TOLAC (%)	
		One CD	Two or more CDs
Endometritis	1.5–2.1	2.9	3.1
Operative injury	0.42–.6	0.4	0.4
Blood transfusion	1–1.4	0.7–1.7	3.2
Hysterectomy	0–0.4	0.2–0.5	0.6
Uterine rupture	0.02–0.04	0.02	0

CD, cesarean delivery; ERCD, elective repeat cesarean delivery; TOLAC, trial of labor after cesarean delivery; VBAC, vaginal birth after cesarean.

Data from Landon 2004; Landon 2006; Macones 2005; Hibbard 2001; Rossi 2008.

Source: Reproduced with permission from American College of Obstetricians and Gynecologists. ACOG Practice Bulletin No. 115: Vaginal birth after previous cesarean delivery. *Obstet Gynecol.* 2010 Aug;116(2 Pt 1):450-63. Copyright © 2010 The American College of Obstetricians and Gynecologists.

Table 2.28. Composite neonatal morbidity elective repeat cesarean delivery and trial of labor after previous cesarean delivery

Neonatal Risks	ERCD (%)	TOLAC (%)	Comment
Antepartum stillbirth*[1]			
37–38 weeks	0.08	0.38	
39 weeks or greater	0.01	0.16	
HIE[1]	0–0.13	0.08	Secondary analysis (Spong 2007 had three cases of HIE in cesarean delivery group)
Neonatal death[1]	0.05	0.08	Not significant
Perinatal death[2]	0.01	0.13	Increase seen due to intrapartum hypoxia
Neonatal admission[3]	6.0	6.6	Not significant
Respiratory morbidity[4]	1–5	0.1–1.8	
Transient tachypnea[5]	6.2	3.5	
Hyperbilirubinemia[5]	5.8	2.2	

*Excludes malformations.

ERCD, elective repeat cesarean delivery; HIE, hypoxic ischemic encephalopathy; TOLAC, trial of labor after previous cesarean delivery.

If uterine rupture, risk of HIE 6.2% (95% confidence interval, 1.8–10.6%), risk of neonatal death 1.8% (95% CI, 0–4.2%).

[1] Landon 2004.
[2] Smith 2002.
[3] Tan 2007.
[4] Signore 2006.
[5] Hook 1997.

Source: Reproduced with permission from American College of Obstetricians and Gynecologists. ACOG Practice Bulletin No. 115: Vaginal birth after previous cesarean delivery. *Obstet Gynecol.* 2010 Aug;116 (2 Pt 1):450-63. Copyright © 2010 The American College of Obstetricians and Gynecologists.

Table 2.29. Incidence and relative risk of uterine rupture during a second delivery among women with a prior cesarean delivery

Type of Delivery	No. of Women	Incidence (Per 1,000)	Relative Risk (95% Confidence Interval)
Repeated cesarean delivery without labor	6,980	1.6	1.0
Spontaneous onset of labor	10,789	5.2	3.3 (1.8–6.0)
Induction of labor without prostaglandins	1960	7.7	4.9 (2.4–9.7)
Induction of labor with prostaglandins	366	24.5	15.6 (8.1–30.0)

[a] Incidence is expressed as the number of cases of uterine rupture per 1000 women who delivered a second singleton infant after a prior cesarean delivery. Women who had repeated cesarean delivery served as the reference group.

Source: Reproduced with permission from Lydon-Rochelle M, Holt VL, Easterling TR, Martin DP. The risk of uterine rupture during labor among women with a prior cesarean delivery. *N Engl J Med.* 2001;345:3. Copyright © 2001 Massachusetts Medical Society.

CARE OF THE NEONATE
Neonatal Resuscitation

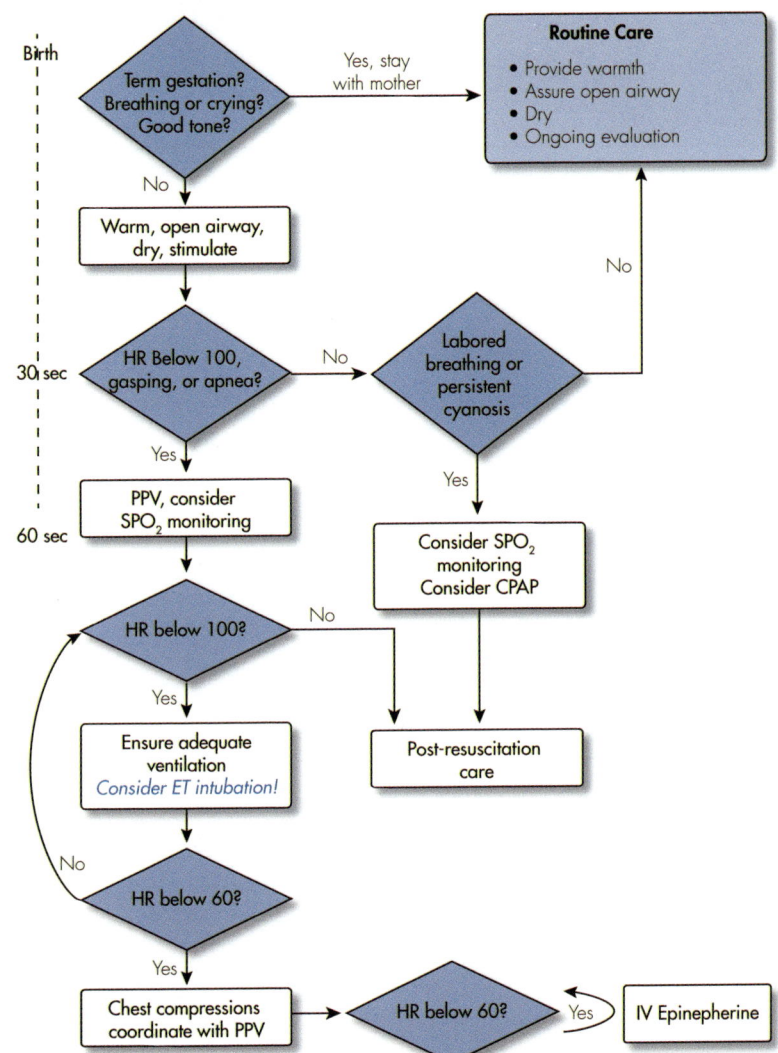

Figure 2.10. Algorithm for neonatal resuscitation

Source: Reproduced with permission from Perlman JM, et al. Neonatal resuscitation: 2010 international consensus on cardiopulmonary resuscitation and emergency cardiovascular care science with treatment recommendations. *Pediatrics.* 2010;126(5):e1319-e1344. Copyright © 2010 AAP.

Table 2.30. Apgar score

Feature	0	1	2
Appearance	Blue, pale	Body pink, extremities blue	Pink
Pulse	Absent	<100 beats/min	>100 beats/min
Grimace (tone)	None	Grimace	Cough, sneeze
Activity	Limp	Some tone	Active
Respirations	Absent	Crying	Good cry

Source: From Apgar V. A proposal for a new method of evaluation of the newborn infant. *Curr Res Anesth Analg.* 1953;32:260-67.

ANTEPARTUM FETAL SURVEILLANCE

Table 2.31. Indications for antepartum fetal surveillance

Maternal Conditions
• Pregestational diabetes mellitus
• Hypertension
• Systemic lupus erythematosus
• Chronic renal disease
• Antiphospholipid syndrome
• Hyperthyroidism (poorly controlled)
• Hemoglobinopathies (sickle cell, sickle cell–hemoglobin C, or sickle cell–thalassemia disease)
• Cyanotic heart disease

Pregnancy-related Conditions
• Gestational hypertension
• Preeclampsia
• Decreased fetal movement
• Gestational diabetes mellitus (poorly controlled or medically treated)
• Oligohydramnios
• Fetal growth restriction
• Late term or postterm pregnancy
• Isoimmunization
• Previous fetal demise (unexplained or recurrent risk)
• Monochorionic multiple gestation (with significant growth discrepancy)

Data from Liston R, Sawchuck D, Young D. Fetal health surveillance: antepartum and intrapartum consensus guideline. Society of Obstetrics and Gynaecologists of Canada, British Columbia Perinatal Health Program [published erratum appears in *J Obstet Gynaecol Can*. 2007;29:909]. *J Obstet Gynaecol Can*. 2007;29:S3-56. (Level III).

Source: Reproduced with permission from American College of Obstetricians and Gynecologists. Practice Bulletin No. 145: Antepartum fetal surveillance. *Obstet Gynecol*. 2014; 124:182. Copyright © 2014 The American College of Obstetricians and Gynecologists.

Nonstress Test
- Can be used in an outpatient setting to assess fetal well-being.
- After 32-week gestation, a reactive nonstress test (NST) includes two 15-beat accelerations lasting 15 seconds during a 20-minute period.
- A nonreactive NST can be caused by a sleep cycle, maternal medications, smoking, an abnormal CNS, or fetal hypoxia.
- A reactive NST is associated with a perinatal mortality of 5/1000.
- A nonreactive NST is associated with a perinatal mortality of 30–40/1000, but has a 75–90% false positive rate.
- If the NST is nonreactive, vibroacoustic stimulation (VAS) can be applied to the fetal head for 3 seconds to wake the fetus from a sleep cycle. Reactivity after VAS is as reassuring as spontaneous reactive NST.

Contraction Stress Test

- The contraction stress test (CST) was the first test used to assess antepartum fetal well-being.
- During the CST the FHR response to the stress of contractions (either spontaneous or induced with Pitocin) is assessed.
- CST are limited by a high (>30%) false positive rate, time required to perform the test, and need for access to labor and delivery if the induced contractions cause FHR abnormalities that necessitate delivery.
- A negative CST, however, has been shown to be more reassuring than a reactive NST.
- CST can be used to follow up nonreactive NST.

Table 2.32. Interpretation of contraction stress test

Interpretation	Description	Incidence (%)
Negative	No late decelerations appearing anywhere on the tracing with adequate uterine contractions (three in 10 mins)	80
Positive	Late decelerations that are consistent and persistent, present with the majority (>50%) of contractions without excessive uterine activity; if persistent late decelerations seen before the frequency of contractions is adequate, test interpreted as positive	3–5
Suspicious	Inconsistent late decelerations	5
Hyperstimulation	Uterine contractions closer than every 2 mins or lasting >90 secs, or five uterine contractions in 10 mins; if no late decelerations seen, test interpreted as negative	5
Unsatisfactory	Quality of the tracing inadequate for interpretation or adequate uterine activity cannot be achieved	5

Source: Adapted from Manning FA. Biophysical profile scoring. In Nijhuis J, ed. *Fetal Behaviour.* New York: Oxford University Press; 1992. Reproduced with permission of Oxford University Press.

Table 2.33. Biophysical profile

Biophysical Variable	Normal (Score = 2)	Abnormal (Score = 0)
Fetal breathing movements	At least one episode of >30 secs duration in 30 mins observation	Absent or no episode of <30 secs duration in 30 minutes
Gross body movement	At least three discrete body/limb movements in 30 mins (episodes of active continuous movement considered a single movement)	Up to two episodes of body/limb movements in 30 mins
Fetal tone	At least one episode of active extension with return to flexion of fetal limb(s) or trunk; opening and closing of hand considered normal tone	Either slow extension with return to partial flexion or movement of limb in full extension or absent fetal movement
Reactive fetal heart rate	At least two episodes of acceleration of ≥15 bpm and 15 secs duration associated with fetal movement in 30 mins	Fewer than two accelerations or acceleration <15 bpm in 30 mins
Qualitative amniotic fluid volume	At least one pocket of amniotic fluid measuring 2 cm in two perpendicular planes	Either no amniotic fluid pockets or a pocket <2 cm in two perpendicular planes

bpm, beats per minute.

Source: Adapted from Manning FA. Biophysical profile scoring. In Nijhuis J, ed. *Fetal Behaviour.* New York: Oxford University Press; 1992. Reproduced with permission of Oxford University Press.

Modified Biophysical Profile
- Includes an NST combined with assessment of amniotic fluid volume.
- A normal result includes both a reactive NST and a maximum vertical pocket of amniotic fluid >2 cm.
- Biophysical profile (BPP) can be used for assessment as early as 26–28 weeks.
- If the BPP is <6, VAS can be applied and the BPP repeated.
- The risk of fetal death is increased by 14 × with absence of movement and by 18 × with absence of breathing.
- BPP may be artificially low within 24–96 hours of receiving steroids for fetal lung maturity.
- A lower BPP score is associated with a higher rate of cerebral palsy; increased risk of cerebral palsy with decreasing score.

Umbilical Artery Dopplers
- During normal pregnancies there is increased blood flow during diastole as gestation progresses.
- The ratio of systolic to diastolic blood flow (S/D ratio) reflects placental resistance.
- Recommended when fetal growth restriction is diagnosed.
- The S/D ratio is not affected by fetal hypoxia.
- Abnormally elevated S/D ratios are associated with IUGR and possibly chromosomal and fetal anomalies.
- Absent end-diastolic flow is associated with an increase in perinatal morbidity and mortality. Reverse end-diastolic flow is predictive of poor fetal outcome including a 36% mortality rate.
- If the S/D ratio shows absent or reverse end-diastolic flow, increased fetal monitoring is indicated. Delivery is not mandatory but can be considered in the clinical context of the gestational age, fetal and maternal health, and results of other monitoring tests.

Table 2.34. Management based on biophysical profile score

Test Score Result	Interpretation	PMN Within 1 Week Without Intervention	Management ACOG (2014)	Management SOGC (2007)
10/10 **8/10 Normal Fluid 8/8 (NST not done)**	Risk of fetal asphyxia extremely rare	1/1,000		Intervention for obstetric and maternal factors.
8/10 (abnormal fluid)	Probable chronic fetal compromise	89/1,000	Uncomplicated, isolated persistent oligohydramnios deliver at 36 to 37 weeks.	Determine that there is evidence of renal tract function and intact membranes. If so, delivery of the term fetus is indicated. In the preterm fetus >34 weeks, intensive surveillance may be preferred to maximize fetal maturity.
6/10 (normal fluid)	Equivocal test, possible fetal asphyxia	Variable	At or beyond 37 0/7 weeks of gestation, further evaluation and consideration of delivery. Less than 37 0/7 weeks repeat BPP in 24 hours	Repeat test within 24 hr
6/10 (abnormal fluid)	Probable fetal asphyxia	89/1,000		Delivery of the term fetus. In the preterm fetus >34 weeks, intensive surveillance may be preferred to maximize fetal maturity.
4/10	High probability of fetal asphyxia	91/1,000	Delivery is usually indicated. Pregnancies at less than 32 0/7 weeks of gestation, management should be individualized, and extended monitoring may be appropriate.	Deliver for fetal indications.
2/10	Fetal asphyxia almost certain	125/1,000	Deliver for fetal indications.	Deliver for fetal indications.
0/10	Fetal asphyxia certain	600/1,000	Deliver for fetal indications.	Deliver for fetal indications.

Sources: Data from Manning FA. Dynamic ultrasound-based fetal assessment: the fetal biophysical profile score. *Clin Obstet Gynecol.* 1995; 38(1):26-44; American College of Obstetricians and Gynecologists. Practice Bulletin No. 145: Antepartum fetal surveillance. *Obstet Gynecol.* 2014; 124:182; Liston R, Sawchuck D, Young D; Society of Obstetrics and Gynaecologists of Canada; British Columbia Perinatal Health Program. Fetal health surveillance: antepartum and intrapartum consensus guideline. *J Obstet Gynaecol Can.* 2007 Sep;29(9 Suppl 4):S3-56.

Risk of Stillbirth and Antenatal Testing Guidelines

Table 2.35. Maternal risk factors and estimated risk of stillbirth and reported strategies for antepartum fetal surveillance

Condition	Prevalence	Estimated Rate of Stillbirth	Odds Ratio	GA to Initiate Testing	Testing Mode and Schedule
All pregnancies	—	6.4/1,000	1.0	—	—
Low-risk pregnancies	80%	4.0–5.5/1,000	0.86	—	—
Diabetes					
Treated with diet (A1)	2.5–5%	6–10/1,000	1.2–2.2	Not indicated	—
Treated with insulin	2.4%	6–35/1,000	1.7–7.0	A2, B, C, D without HTN, renal disease, or FGR: 32 wk	CST/wk, midweek NST
				32 wk	NST or BPP 2x/wk
				34 wk	NST 2x/wk + AFI/wk
				R, F: 26 wk	CST/wk, midweek NST
				Any class with HTN, renal disease, FGR: 26 wk	CST/wk, midweek NST
				28 wk	NST or BPP 2x/wk
Hypertensive disorder					
Chronic hypertension	6–10%	6–25/1,000	1.5–2.7	26 wk	NST, AFI 2x/wk
				33 wk	MBPP 2x/wk
				With SLE or FGR or DM or PIH: 26 wk	NST, AFI 2x/wk
Pregnancy-induced hypertension					
Mild	5.8–7.7%	9–51/1,000	1.2–4.0	At diagnosis	MBPP 2x/wk
Severe	1.3–3.3%	12–29/1,000	1.8–4.4	At diagnosis	NST/day with BPP if nonreactive; AFI 2x/wk
Growth restricted fetus	2.5–10%	10–47/1,000	7–11.8	Suspected: at diagnosis	NST, AFI/wk
					UAD 1–2x/wk
				Confirmed	MBPP 2x/wk
					UAD 1–2x/wk

(continued)

Condition	Prevalence	Estimated Rate of Stillbirth	Odds Ratio	GA to Initiate Testing	Testing Mode and Schedule
Multiple gestation	2 – 3.5%				
Twins	2.7%	12/1,000	1.0–2.8	Concordant growth: 32 wk	NST, AFI/wk
				Discordant growth: at diagnosis	MBPP 2x/wk
Triplets	0.14%	34/1,000	2.8–3.7	28 wk	BPP, 2x/wk
Oligohydramnios	2%	14/1,000	4.5	At diagnosis	NST, AFI 2x/wk
PPROM				At diagnosis	NST/day
					BPP/day
Postterm pregnancy (compared to 40 wk)					
41 wk	9%	1.6/1,000	1.5	41 wk	BPP 2x/wk
				41 wk	MBPP/wk
≥42 wk	5%	2 – 3.5/1,000	1.8–2.9	42 wk	MBPP 2x/wk
Previous stillbirth	0.5–1.0%	9 – 20/1,000	1.4–3.2	32 wk	MBPP 2x/wk or BPP/wk or CST/wk
				34 wk or 1 wk prior to previous stillbirth	MBPP/wk
Decreased fetal movement	4 – 15%	13/1,000	2.5–5.6	At diagnosis	MBPP
SLE	<1%	40–150/1,000	6 – 20	26 wk	CST, BPP, or NST/wk
Renal disease	<1%	15–200/1,000	2.2–30	30–32	BPP 2x/wk
Cholestasis of pregnancy	<0.1%	12–30/1,000	1.8–4.4	34 wk	MBPP/wk
Advanced maternal age (reference <35 yr)					
35–39 yr	15–18%	11–14/1,000	1.8–2.2	ID	ID
40 yr +	2%	11–21/1,000	1.8–3.3	ID	ID
Black women compared with white women	15%	12–14/1,000	2.0–2.2	ID	ID
Maternal age <20	4%	7 – 13/1,000	1.1–1.6	ID	ID
Nulliparity	40%	3.8 (Sweden)	1.2 (Sweden)	ID	ID
Very high (10–14) or extremely high (≥15) parity	0.1%	14–22/1,000	2.0–2.2	ID	ID
Assisted reproductive technology	1%	12/1,000	2.6	ID	ID
Abnormal serum markers					
First trimester PAPP-A <5th Percentile	5%	9/1,000	2.2–4.0	ID	ID
2 or more abnormal second trimester quad screen markers	0.1–2%	8 – 18/1,000	4.3–9.2	ID	ID

(continued)

Antepartum Fetal Surveillance — OBSTETRICS

Condition	Prevalence	Estimated Rate of Stillbirth	Odds Ratio	GA to Initiate Testing	Testing Mode and Schedule
Obesity (prepregnancy)					
BMI 25–29.9 kg/m^2	21%	12–15/1,000	1.9–2.7	ID	ID
BMI ≥30 kg/m^2	20%	13–18/1,000	2.1–2.8	ID	ID
Low educational attainment (<12 yr vs. 12 yr +)	30%	10–13/1,000	1.6–2.0	ID	ID
Smoking >10 cigarettes/day	10–20%	10–15/1,000	1.7–3.0	ID	ID
Thrombophilia	1–5%	18–40/1,000	2.8–5.0	ID	ID
Thyroid disorders	0.2–2%	12–20/1,000	2.2–3.0	ID	ID

GA, gestational age; CST, contraction stress test; w, week; HTN, hypertension; FGR, fetal growth restriction; NST, nonstress test; BPP, biophysical profile; AFI, amniotic fluid index; mBPP, modified biophysical profile; SLE, systemic lupus erythematosus; DM, diabetes mellitus; PIH, pregnancy-induced hypertension; yr, years; ID, insufficient data; BMI, body mass index.

Source: Reproduced with permission from Signore C, Freeman RK, Spong CY. Antenatal testing—a reevaluation: executive summary of a Eunice Kennedy Shriver National Institute of Child Health and Human Development workshop. *Obstet Gynecol.* 2009;113(3):687-701. Copyright © 2009 The American College of Obstetricians and Gynecologists.

OBSTETRICS

TRAUMA IN PREGNANCY

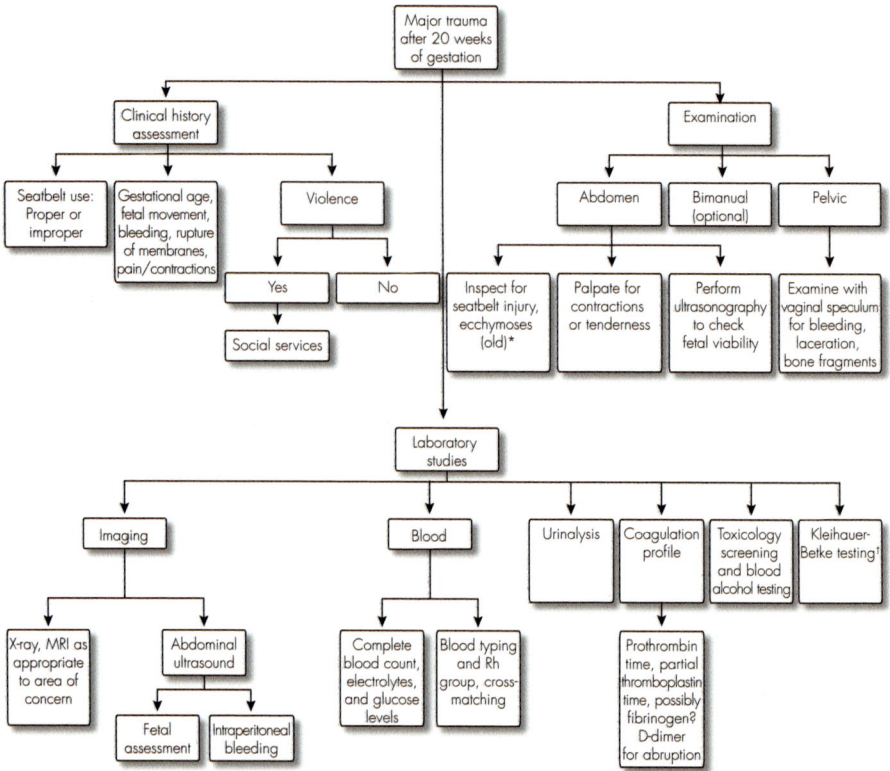

Figure 2.11. Clinical assessment of the trauma patient more than 20 weeks of gestation
Source: Reproduced with permission from Brown HL. Trauma in pregnancy. *Obstet Gynecol*. 2009 Jul;114(1):147-60. Copyright © 2009 The American College of Obstetricians and Gynecologists.

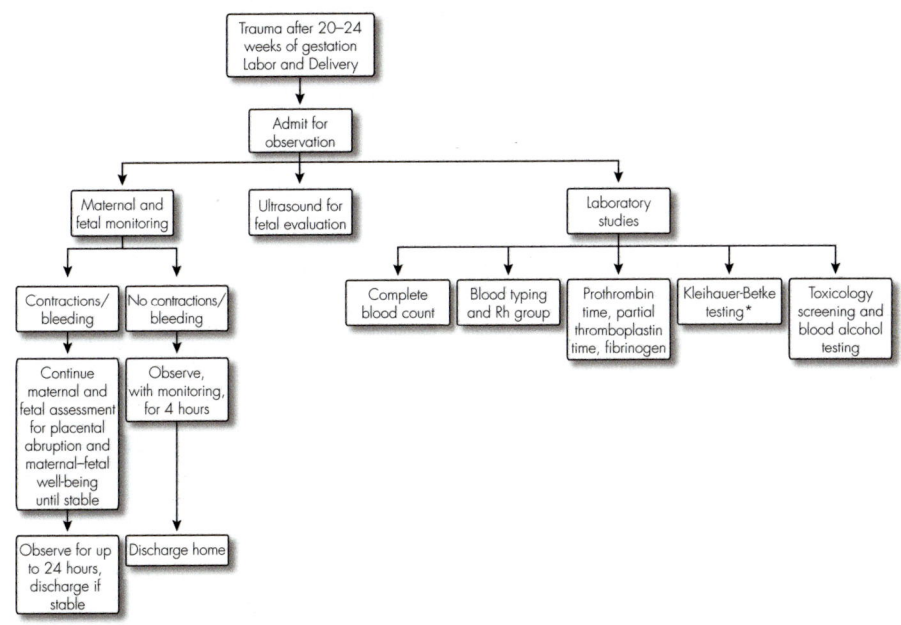

Figure 2.12. Labor and delivery observation after maternal trauma
Source: Reproduced with permission from Brown HL. Trauma in pregnancy. *Obstet Gynecol.* 2009 Jul;114(1):147-60. Copyright © 2009 The American College of Obstetricians and Gynecologists.

GUIDELINES FOR DIAGNOSTIC IMAGING IN PREGNANCY
Fast Facts
- Diagnostic X-ray is a frequent source of patient anxiety.
- No single diagnostic X-ray procedure is enough to threaten the well-being of the embryo or fetus.
- Risk of fetal anomalies, growth restriction, or spontaneous abortion not increased at exposure level of <5 rad.

Table 2.36. Summary of key points from the imaging guidelines

Topic	Key Points
Risk of teratogenesis after diagnostic CT	Teratogenesis in the fetus is not a major concern after diagnostic pelvic CT studies
Risk of carcinogenesis after diagnostic CT	Carcinogenesis in the fetus is a key concern after diagnostic pelvic CT studies; hence, CT of the fetus should be avoided in all trimesters of pregnancy unless absolutely necessary
Pregnancy termination after diagnostic irradiation	It is exceptionally unlikely that any single diagnostic radiological study would deliver a radiation dose sufficient to justify pregnancy termination
CT contrast media and pregnancy	Use of iodinated contrast seems safe in pregnancy and should be administered in the usual fashion. This is preferable to repeating a CT study because the initial examination was nondiagnostic due to the lack of intravenous contrast administration
MRI in pregnancy	Although most studies evaluating MRI safety during pregnancy show no ill effects, it is good practice to avoid MRI during pregnancy, particularly for elective studies or during the first trimester
MRI contrast media and pregnancy	Intravenous gadolinium is contraindicated in pregnancy and should be used only if absolutely essential
Contrast media and lactation	Lactating women who receive iodinated contrast or gadolinium can continue breast-feeding without interruption
Imaging of suspected pulmonary embolism	Computed tomographic pulmonary angiogram is the preferred modality for imaging of suspected pulmonary embolism
Imaging of suspected acute appendicitis	Ultrasonography is the preferred modality for imaging of suspected acute appendicitis except in later pregnancy (more than 35 wk), when MRI or CT may be required
Imaging of suspected renal colic	Ultrasonography is the preferred modality for imaging of suspected colic; if the ultrasound examination is negative, CT may be required
Imaging of trauma	Ultrasonography may be sufficient for the initial imaging evaluation of a pregnant patient who has sustained trauma, but CT should be performed if serious injury is suspected
Imaging of suspected cephalopelvic disproportion	On the rare occasion that pelvimetry is required to assess cephalopelvic disproportion, pelvimetry can be performed with minimal risk using low-dose CT

CT, computed tomography; MRI, magnetic resonance imaging.

Source: Reproduced with permission from Chen MM, Coakley FV, Kaimal A, Laros RK Jr. Guidelines for computed tomography and magnetic resonance imaging use during pregnancy and lactation. *Obstet Gynecol*. 2008 Aug;112(2 Pt 1):333-40. Copyright © 2008 The American College of Obstetricians and Gynecologists.

Diagnostic Imaging in Pregnancy — OBSTETRICS

Table 2.37. Effects of gestational age and radiation dose on radiation-induced teratogenesis

Gestational Period	Effects	Estimated Threshold Dose*
Before implantation (0–2 wk after conception)	Death of embryo or no consequence (all or none)	50–100 mGy
Organogenesis (2–8 wk after conception)	Congenital anomalies (skeleton, eYes, genitals)	200 mGy
	Growth retardation	200–250 mGy
Fetal period		
8–15 wk	Severe mental retardation (high risk)†	60–310 mGy
	Intellectual deficit	25 IQ point loss per gray
	Microcephaly	200 mGy
16–25 wk	Severe mental retardation (low risk)	250–280 mGy

*Data based on results of animal studies, epidemiologic studies of survivors of the atomic bombings in Japan, and studies of groups exposed to radiation for medical reasons (e.g., radiation therapy for carcinoma of the uterus).

†Because this is a period of rapid neuronal development and migration.

Source: Reproduced with permission from Patel SJ, Reede DL, Katz DS, Subramaniam R, Amorosa JK. Imaging the pregnant patient for nonobstetric conditions: algorithms and radiation dose considerations. *Radiographics*. 2007 Nov-Dec;27(6):1705-22. Copyright © 2007 RSNA.

Table 2.38. Estimated fetal radiation absorption per procedure or event

Clinical Suspicion	Procedure	Estimated Fetal Absorption (mGy) Per Procedure	Estimated Fetal Absorption (rad) Per Procedure
Pneumonia	X-ray chest	<0.01	<0.001
Pulmonary embolism	CT scan	0.06–0.96	0.006–0.096
	VP scan	0.1–0.37	0.01–0.037
Appendicitis	Ultrasound	Nonionizing radiation	Nonionizing radiation
	CT scan abdomen	8–49	0.8–4.9
	MRI	Nonionizing radiation	Nonionizing radiation
Nephrolithiasis	Ultrasound	Nonionizing radiation	Nonionizing radiation
	X-ray abdomen	1–4.2	0.1–0.42
	Pyelogram	1.7–10	0.17–1
	CT scan abdomen	8–49	0.8–4.9
	MRI	Nonionizing radiation	Nonionizing radiation
Breast nodule	Ultrasound	Nonionizing radiation	Nonionizing radiation
	Mammogram	0.07–0.2	0.007–0.02
Colon pathology	X-ray abdomen	1–4.2	0.1–0.42
	Barium enema	7	0.7

(continued)

Clinical Suspicion	Procedure	Estimated Fetal Absorption (mGy) Per Procedure	Estimated Fetal Absorption (rad) Per Procedure
Trauma			
Spine injury	X-ray lumbar spine	6	0.6
	X-ray thoracic/cervical spine	<0.01	<0.001
	X-ray skull	<0.01	<0.001
Pelvic injury	X-ray pelvis	1.1–4	0.11–0.4
	CT scan pelvis	20–79	2.0–7.9
Abdominal injury	Ultrasound (FAST)	Nonionizing radiation	Nonionizing radiation
	CT scan abdomen	8–49	0.8–4.9
	MRI	Nonionizing radiation	Nonionizing radiation
Background radiation	None	1 mSv	0.1 rem[a]
Commercial flight	Round trip Toronto-Frankfurt	0.1 mSv	0.01 rem[a]
	100 hr of commercial flying	1 mSv	0.1 rem[a]

General considerations: (1) All estimates have wide variation of estimation due to more exposure in more advanced pregnancies and different scanning techniques. (2) Procedures have different sensitivity and specificity, and therefore, estimated fetal exposure of ionizing radiation is not the only consideration to undertake an imaging procedure. The clinical maternal condition indicates the appropriate mode of examination for the pregnant patient. (3) MRI might have some fetal health hazards based on thermal and acoustical effects of MRI. These effects seem more theoretical and are not proven by limited available studies on MRI and pregnancy outcome.

American College of Radiology states, however, that answers to the following questions should be documented before proceeding with MRI in pregnancy: (a) MRI will give information that cannot be acquired via other proven harmless means (ultrasonography). (b) Information given by MRI will affect care of patient or fetus during pregnancy. (c) Referring physician does not think it is prudent to wait until patient is no longer pregnant to obtain these data (Kanal E, Barkovich AJ, Bell C, et al. ACR guidance document for safe MR practices: 2007. *Am J Roentgenol.* 2007;188: 1447-74).

CT, computed tomography; FAST, focused assessment with sonography for trauma; MRI, magnetic resonance imaging; VP, ventilation perfusion scan.

[a] 1 rem is comparable but not equivalent to 1 rad.

Source: Reproduced with permission from Groen RS, Bae JY, Lim KJ. Fear of the unknown: ionizing radiation exposure during pregnancy. *Am J Obstet Gynecol.* 2012 Jun;206(6):456-62. Copyright © 2012 Elsevier.

INTRAPARTUM FETAL EVALUATION
Fetal Heart Rate Patterns

Table 2.39. Electronic fetal monitoring definitions

Pattern	Definition

Baseline
- The mean FHR rounded to increments of 5 beats per minute during a 10-minute segment, excluding:
  - Periodic or episodic changes
  - Periods of marked FHR variability
  - Segments of baseline that differ by more than 25 beats per minute.
- The baseline must be for a minimum of 2 minutes in any 10-minute segment, or the baseline for that time period is indeterminate. In this case, one may refer to the prior 10-minute window for determination of baseline.
- Normal FHR baseline: 110–160 beats per minute.
- Tachycardia: FHR baseline is greater than 160 beats per minute.
- Bradycardia: FHR baseline is less than 110 beats per minute.

Baseline variability
- Fluctuations in the baseline FHR that are irregular in amplitude and frequency.
- Variability is visually quantitated as the amplitude of peak-to-trough in beats per minute.
  - Absent—amplitude range undetectable
  - Minimal—amplitude range detectable but 5 beats per minute or fewer
  - Moderate (normal)—amplitude range 6–25 beats per minute
  - Marked—amplitude range greater than 25 beats per minute

Acceleration
- A visually apparent abrupt increase (onset to peak in less than 30 seconds) in the FHR.
- At 32 weeks of gestation and beyond, an acceleration has a peak of 15 beats per minute or more above baseline, with a duration of 15 seconds or more but less than 2 minutes from onset to return.
- Before 32 weeks of gestation, an acceleration has a peak of 10 beats per minute or more above baseline, with a duration of 10 seconds or more but less than 2 minutes from onset to return.
- Prolonged acceleration lasts 2 minutes or more but less than 10 minutes in duration.
- If an acceleration lasts 10 minutes or longer, it is a baseline change.

Early deceleration
- Visually apparent usually symmetrical gradual decrease and return of the FHR associated with a uterine contraction.
- A gradual FHR decrease is defined as from the onset to the FHR nadir of 30 seconds or more.
- The decrease in FHR is calculated from the onset to the nadir of the deceleration.
- The nadir of the deceleration occurs at the same time as the peak of the contraction.
- In most cases, the onset, nadir, and recovery of the deceleration are coincident with the beginning, peak, and ending of the contraction, respectively.

Late deceleration
- Visually apparent usually symmetrical gradual decrease and return of the FHR associated with a uterine contraction.
- A gradual FHR decrease is defined as from the onset to the FHR nadir of 30 seconds or more.
- The decrease in FHR is calculated from the onset to the nadir of the deceleration.
- The deceleration is delayed in timing, with the nadir of the deceleration occurring after the peak of the contraction.
- In most cases, the onset, nadir, and recovery of the deceleration occur after the beginning, peak, and ending of the contraction, respectively.

(continued)

OBSTETRICS Intrapartum Fetal Evaluation

Pattern Definition

Variable deceleration
- Visually apparent abrupt decrease in FHR.
- An abrupt FHR decrease is defined as from the onset of the deceleration to the beginning of the FHR nadir of less than 30 seconds.
- The decrease in FHR is calculated from the onset to the nadir of the deceleration.
- The decrease in FHR is 15 beats per minute or greater, lasting 15 seconds or greater, and less than 2 minutes in duration.
- When variable decelerations are associated with uterine contractions, their onset, depth, and duration commonly vary with successive uterine contractions.

Prolonged deceleration
- Visually apparent decrease in the FHR below the baseline.
- Decrease in FHR from the baseline that is 15 beats per minute or more, lasting 2 minutes or more but less than 10 minutes in duration.
- If a deceleration lasts 10 minutes or longer, it is a baseline change.

Sinusoidal pattern
- Visually apparent, smooth, sine wave–like undulating pattern in FHR baseline with a cycle frequency of 3–5 per minute that persists for 20 minutes or more.

When variable decelerations are associated with uterine contractions, their onset, depth, and duration commonly vary with successive uterine contractions.

Source: Adapted from Macones GA, Hankins GD, Spong CY, Hauth J, Moore T. The 2008 National Institute of Child Health and Human Development workshop report on electronic fetal monitoring: update on definitions, interpretation, and research guidelines. *Obstet Gynecol.* 2008 Sep;112(3):661-66. Copyright © 2008 The American College of Obstetricians and Gynecologists.

Table 2.40. Three-tiered fetal heart rate interpretation system

Category I

*Category I fetal heart rate (FHR) tracings include **all** of the following:*
- Baseline rate: 110–160 beats per minute (bpm)
- Baseline FHR variability: moderate
- Late or variable decelerations: absent
- Early decelerations: present or absent
- Accelerations: present or absent

Category II

Category II FHR tracings include all FHR tracings not categorized as Category I or Category III. Category II tracings may represent an appreciable fraction of those encountered in clinical care. Examples of Category II FHR tracings include any of the following:

Baseline rate
- Bradycardia not accompanied by absent baseline variability
- Tachycardia

Baseline FHR variability
- Minimal baseline variability
- Absent baseline variability not accompanied by recurrent decelerations
- Marked baseline variability

Accelerations
- Absence of induced accelerations after fetal stimulation

Periodic or episodic decelerations
- Recurrent variable decelerations accompanied by minimal or moderate baseline variability
- Prolonged deceleration >2 minutes but <10 minutes
- Recurrent late decelerations with moderate baseline variability
- Variable decelerations with other characteristics, such as slow return to baseline, "overshoots," or "shoulders"

Category III

Category III FHR tracings include either:
- Absent baseline FHR variability and any of the following:
  - Recurrent late decelerations
  - Recurrent variable decelerations
  - Bradycardia
- Sinusoidal pattern

Source: Reproduced with permission from Macones GA, Hankins GD, Spong CY, Hauth J, Moore T. The 2008 National Institute of Child Health and Human Development workshop report on electronic fetal monitoring: update on definitions, interpretation, and research guidelines. *Obstet Gynecol.* 2008 Sep;112(3):661-66. Copyright © 2008 The American College of Obstetricians and Gynecologists.

Management of Intrapartum Fetal Heart Rate Tracings

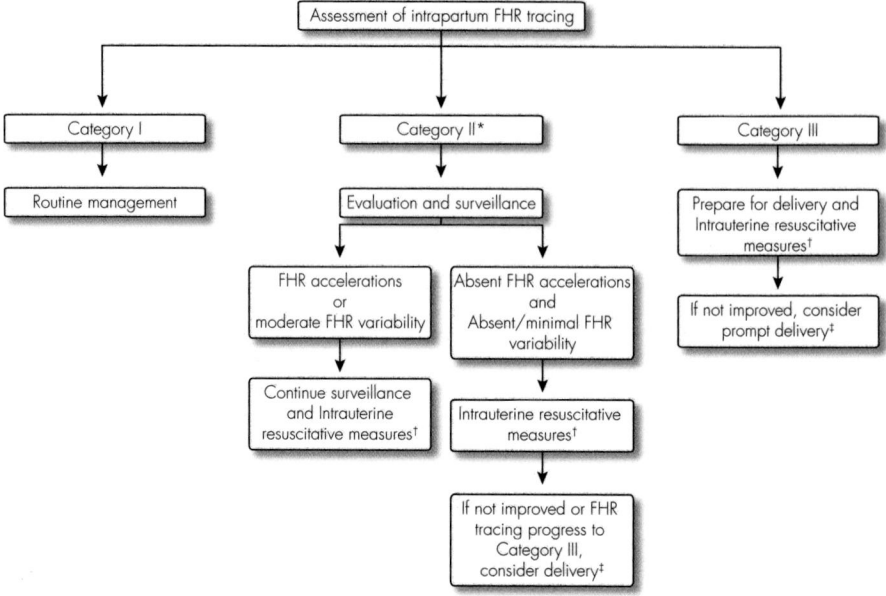

Figure 2.13. Intrauterine resuscitation measures
Source: Reproduced with permission from American College of Obstetricians and Gynecologists. ACOG Practice Bulletin No. 116: Management of intrapartum fetal heart rate tracings, November 2010 (Reaffirmed 2013). *Obstet Gynecol.* 2010 Nov;116(5):1232-40. Copyright © 2010 The American College of Obstetricians and Gynecologists.

Intrapartum Fetal Evaluation   **OBSTETRICS**

Table 2.41. Various intrauterine resuscitative measures for category II or category III tracings or both

Goal	Associated Fetal Heart Rate Abnormality*	Potential Intervention(s)†
Promote fetal oxygenation and improve uteroplacental blood flow	Recurrent late decelerations	Initiate lateral positioning (either left or right)
	Prolonged decelerations or bradycardia	Administer maternal oxygen administration
	Minimal or absent fetal heart rate variability	Administer intravenous fluid bolus
		Reduce uterine contraction frequency
Reduce uterine activity	Tachysystole with Category II or III tracing	Discontinue oxytocin or cervical ripening agents Administer tocolytic medication (e.g., terbutaline)
Alleviate umbilical cord compression	Recurrent variable decelerations	Initiate maternal repositioning
	Prolonged decelerations or bradycardia	Initiate amnioinfusion
		If prolapsed umbilical cord is noted, elevate the presenting fetal part while preparations are underway for operative delivery

*Evaluation for the underlying suspected cause(s) is also an important step in management of abnormal FHR tracings.

†Depending on the suspected underlying cause(s) of FHR abnormality, combining multiple interventions simultaneously may be appropriate and potentially more effective than doing individually or serially (Simpson KR, James DC. Efficacy of intrauterine resuscitation techniques in improving fetal oxygen status during labor. *Obstet Gynecol.* 2005;105:1362–68).

Source: Reproduced with permission from American College of Obstetricians and Gynecologists. ACOG Practice Bulletin No. 116: Management of intrapartum fetal heart rate tracings, November 2010 (Reaffirmed 2013). *Obstet Gynecol.* 2010 Nov;116(5):1232-40. Copyright © 2010 The American College of Obstetricians and Gynecologists.

Data from Young BK, Katz M, Klein SA, Silverman F. Fetal blood and tissue pH with moderate bradycardia. *Am J Obstet Gynecol.* 1979;135:45-7; Chauhan SP, Roach H, Naef RW 2nd, Magann EF, Morrison JC, Martin JN Jr. Cesarean section for suspected fetal distress: does the decision-incision time make a difference? *J Reprod Med.* 1997;42:347-52; Schauberger CW, Chauhan SP. Emergency cesarean section and the 30-minute rule: definitions. *Am J Perinatol.* 2009;26:221-26; and Schifrin BS, Hamilton-Rubinstein T, Shields JR. Fetal heart rate patterns and the timing of fetal injury. *J Perinatol.* 1994;14:174-81.

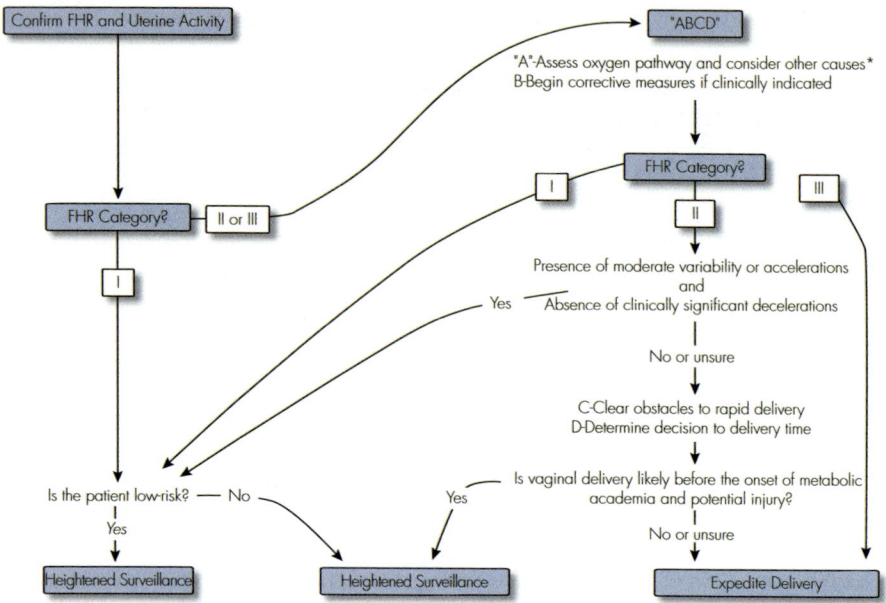

Figure 2.14. A standardized ABCD approach to EFM management
Source: Reproduced with permission from Miller DA, Miller LA. Electronic fetal heart rate monitoring: applying principles of patient safety. *Am J Obstet Gynecol.* 2012 Apr;206(4):278-83. Copyright © 2010 The American College of Obstetricians and Gynecologists.

Intrapartum Fetal Evaluation — OBSTETRICS

Table 2.42. A simplified ABCD checklist

Step	"A" Assess Oxygen Pathway	"B" Begin Corrective Measures *If Indicated*	Variable	"C" Clear Obstacles to Rapid Delivery	"D" Determine Decision to Delivery Time
Lungs	Respiratory rate Airway and breathing	Supplemental oxygen	Facility	Consider: *OR availability* *Equipment*	Consider *Facility response time* *Location and availability of OR*
Heart	Heart rate and rhythm	Position changes Fluid bolus Correct hypotension	Staff	Consider notifying: *Obstetrician* *Surgical assistant* *Anesthesiologist* *Neonatologist* *Pediatrician* *Nursing staff*	Consider: *Availability* *Training* *Experience*
Vasculature	Blood pressure Volume status		Mother	Consider: *Informed consent* *Anesthesia options* *Laboratory tests* *Blood products* *Intravenous access* *Urinary catheter* *Abdominal prep* *Transfer to OR*	Surgical considerations (prior abdominal or uterine surgery) Medical considerations (obesity, hypertension, diabetes, SLE) Obstetric considerations (parity, pelvimetry, placental location)
Uterus	Contraction strength Contraction frequency Baseline uterine tone Exclude uterine rupture	Stop or reduce stimulant Consider uterine relaxant	Fetus	Consider: *Fetal number* *Gestational age* *Estimated weight* *Position* *Presentation* *Anomalies*	Consider factors such as: *Estimated fetal weight* *Gestational age* *Presentation* *Position*
Placenta	Placental separation Bleeding vasa previa		Labor	Confirm: *Adequate UC monitoring*	Consider factors such as: *Arrest disorder* *Protracted labor* *Remote from delivery* *Poor expulsive efforts*
Cord	Vaginal exam Exclude cord prolapse	Consider amnioinfusion			

OR, operating room; SLE, systemic lupus erythematosis; UC, uterine contraction.

Source: Reproduced with permission from Miller DA, Miller LA. Electronic fetal heart rate monitoring: applying principles of patient safety. *Am J Obstet Gynecol.* 2012 Apr;206(4):278-83. Copyright © 2012 Elsevier.

AMNIOINFUSION
Fast Facts
- Reduction in C/S rate for fetal distress by reducing variable decelerations.
- Not shown to reduce the risk of meconium aspiration syndrome or other complications of meconium stained fluid (Fraser 2005).

Candidates for Amnioinfusion
- Term labor with recurrent variable decelerations and decreased amniotic fluid.
- Cephalic presentation.
- Previous cesarean delivery or previous myomectomy not an absolute contraindication.
- Chorioamnionitis is a relative contraindication.

Technique
- Document fetal presentation.
- Place fetal scalp electrode and intrauterine pressure catheter (preferably double lumen catheter).
- Initial bolus of 250–500 cc of normal saline (warmed) with maintenance infusion (3 cc/min).
- Rebolus as needed.
- Measure intrauterine pressure every 30 minutes or continuously (second intrauterine pressure catheter or double lumen).

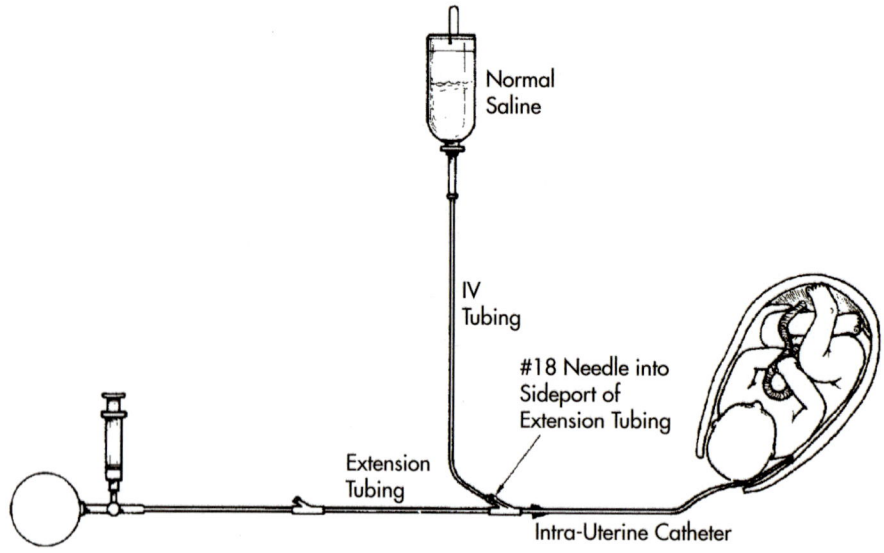

Figure 2.15. Typical setup for amnioinfusion
Source: Miyazaki FS, Nevarez F. Saline amnioinfusion for relief of repetitive variable decelerations: a prospective randomized study. *Am J Obstet Gynecol.* 1985;153(3):301-306. Reproduced with the permission of the publisher, Mosby Year Book: St. Louis. Copyright © 1985 Elsevier.

Umbilical Cord Gas Assessment

Table 2.43. Umbilical cord gas values for arterial and venous blood in term newborns

Value	Yeomans (1985)[a] (N = 146)	Ramin (1989)[a] (N = 1292)	Riley (1993)[b] (N = 3522)
Arterial Blood in Term Newborns (Mean ± One Standard Deviation)			
pH	7.28 ± 0.05	7.28 ± 0.07	7.27 ± 0.069
PCO_2 (mm Hg)	49.2 ± 8.4	49.9 ± 14.2	50.3 ± 11.1
HCO_3^- (meq/L)	22.3 ± 2.5	23.1 ± 2.8	22.0 ± 3.6
Base excess (meq/L)	—[c]	−3.6 ± 2.8	−2.7 ± 2.8
Venous Blood in Term Newborns (Mean ± One Standard Deviation)			
PH	7.35 ± 0.05	—	7.34 ± 0.063
PCO_2 (mm Hg)	38.2 ± 5.6	—	40.7 ± 7.9
HCO_3^- (meq/L)	20.4 ± 4.1	—	21.4 ± 2.5
Base excess (meq/L)	—	—	−2.4 ± 2.0

[a]Data are from infants of selected patients with uncomplicated vaginal deliveries.
[b]Data are from infants of unselected patients with vaginal deliveries.
[c]Data were not obtained.

Table 2.44. Umbilical cord gas values for arterial blood in preterm newborns

Value	Ramin (1989)[a] (N = 77)	Dickinson (1992)[b] (N = 949)	Riley (1993)[c] (N = 11015)
Arterial Blood in Preterm Newborns (Mean ± One Standard Deviation)			
pH	7.29 ± 0.07	7.27 ± 0.07	7.28 ± 0.089
PCO_2 (mm Hg)	49.2 ± 9.0	51.6 ± 9.4	50.2 ± 12.3
HCO_3^- (meq/L)	23.0 ± 3.5	23.9 ± 2.1	22.4 ± 3.5
Base excess (meq/L)	−3.3 ± 2.4	−3.0 ± 2.5	−2.7 ± 3.0

[a]Data are from infants of selected patients with uncomplicated vaginal deliveries.
[b]Data are from infants of unselected patients with vaginal deliveries.

ABRUPTIO PLACENTAE
Fast Facts
- Premature separation of the normally-implanted placenta.
- Abruption represents 30% of third trimester bleeding, seen in 1% of all births.
- Occurs most often between 24–26 weeks.

Table 2.45. Evidence and strength of association linking major risk factors with placental abruption

Risk Factors	Strength	RR or OR
Maternal age and parity	+	1.1–3.7
Cigarette smoking	+ +	1.4–2.5
Cocaine and drug use	+ + +	5.0–10.0
Multiple gestations	+ +	1.5–3.0
Chronic hypertension	+ +	1.8–5.1
Mild and severe preeclampsia	+ +	0.4–4.5
Chronic hypertension with preeclampsia	+ + +	7.8
Premature rupture of membranes	+ +	1.8–5.1
Oligohydramnios	+	2.5–10.0
Chorioamnionitis	+ +	2.0–2.5
Dietary or nutritional deficiency	+/−	0.9–2.0
Male fetus	+/−	0.9–1.3

RR, relative risk; OR, odds ratio.

These estimates are the ranges of RR or OR found in independent studies.

Source: Reproduced with permission from Yeo, L, Ananth CV, Vintzileos AM. Placental abruption. In: Sciarra J, editor. *Gynecology and Obstetrics, Vol 2*, 2003. Hagerstown, MD: Lippincott Williams & Wilkins.

Recurrence Risk
- 5–16%.
- Increases to 25% after 2 previous abruptions.

Classic Signs and Symptoms
- Painful vaginal bleeding.
- Abdominal pain.
- Uterine hypertonicity and tenderness.
- Fetal distress or fetal death (usually with at least a 50% abruption).

Management
- Consider expectant management or tocolytic with mild abruption and premature fetus.
- Moderate to severe abruptions indicate need for delivery.
- Amniotomy useful in augmenting labor in anticipation of vaginal delivery.
- Close fetal monitoring.
- Perinatal mortality has been reduced by appropriate intervention with cesarean.
- Lab studies: CBC, type and cross, prothrombin time/partial thromboplastin time, and fibrinogen.
- Replace blood products and coagulation factors aggressively.

Ultrasonographic Criteria for Diagnosis of Placental Abruption
- 24% sensitive, 96% specific, 88% positive predictive value, 53% negative predictive value.

Table 2.46. Ultrasonographic criteria for diagnosis of placental abruption

1. Preplacental collection under the chorionic plate (between the placenta and amniotic fluid)
2. Jello-like movement of the chorionic plate with fetal activity
3. Retroplacental collection
4. Marginal hematoma
5. Subchorionic hematoma
6. Increased heterogeneous placental thickness (more than 5 cm in a perpendicular plane)
7. Intra-amniotic hematoma

Source: Reproduced with permission from Yeo, L, Ananth CV, Vintzileos AM. Placental abruption. In: Sciarra J, editor. *Gynecology and Obstetrics, Vol 2*, 2003. Hagerstown, MD: Lippincott Williams & Wilkins.

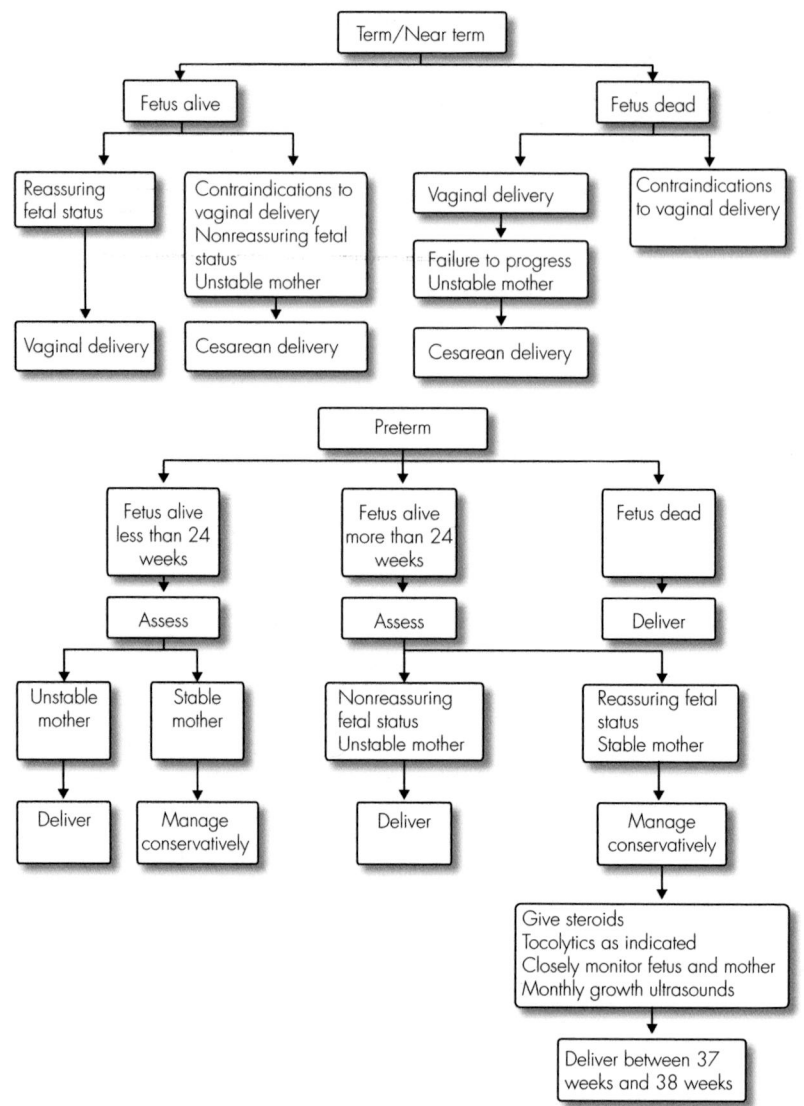

Figure 2.16. Management of abruption

Algorithm for the management of placental abruption in term or near term and preterm births. In all cases, complete blood count and coagulation indices should be checked; blood or blood volume should be replaced; coagulopathy should be corrected; and intake, output, and renal function should be monitored.

Source: Reproduced with permission from Oyelese Y, Ananth CV. Placental abruption. *Obstet Gynecol*. 2006;108(4):1005-16. Copyright © 2008 The American College of Obstetricians and Gynecologists.

PLACENTA PREVIA
Fast Facts
Definitions based on ultrasound assessment of placental location:
- Complete Previa—Placental edge covers the internal os or reaches the internal os and is not a measurable distance away.
- Partial Previa—Placenta partially covers a dilated internal os (would apply only rarely).
- Low Lying placenta—Placental edge does not reach the internal os, but is 20 mm from the os.
  - Placenta Previa represents 20% of third trimester bleeding
  - In the United States, 0.03% maternal mortality
  - Incidence 1/250 live births
  - Bleeding is maternal
  - Often presents as painless, bright-red bleeding
  - May be associated with contractions

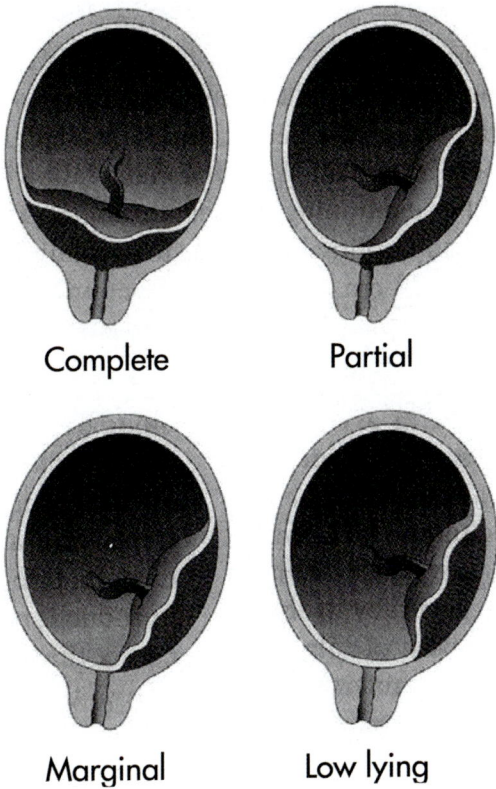

Figure 2.17. Types of placenta previa
Source: Reproduced with permission from Oyelese Y, Smulian JC. Placenta Previa, Placenta Accreta, and Vasa Previa. *Obstet Gynecol.* 2006;107(4):927-41. Copyright © 2006 The American College of Obstetricians and Gynecologists.

Risk Factors
- Previous cesarean delivery (RR 4.5 with one prior c/s, 44.9 with 4 prior C/D)
- Grand multiparity
- Intrauterine surgery, smoking, multifetal gestation, advanced maternal age

Management
- Transvaginal ultrasound for accurate diagnosis.
- Cervical length surveillance may help identify women at higher risk of bleeding (higher risk associated with TVCL 3 cm).
- No vaginal exams.
- Serial ultrasound for interval growth, resolution of partial previa.
- Use of tocolytic drugs during an episode of vaginal bleeding is controversial. Consider MgSO4 as first choice.
- Hospitalization usually after first bleed, but depends on clinical situation.
- β-Methasone if bleeding and or contractions occur between 24 and 34 weeks.
- Delivery by cesarean if a placenta previa persists at term. Consider administration of corticosteroids and delivery by 36 weeks.
  - If placenta is not covering the os, may consider vaginal delivery, but monitor closely for postpartum hemorrhage, which is more likely the closer the placenta edge comes to the os
- High risk for accreta, hemorrhage (especially if previous C/D).
- Discuss blood products, risk of hysterectomy.
- See section on uterine packing (see page 139).

Table 2.47. Studies of second-trimester transvaginal sonography in the prediction of placenta previa at delivery

Author	Gestational Age at Sonogram (wk)	Number of Women	Incidence of Placenta Previa at First- or Second-trimester Sonography (n [%])	Incidence at Delivery (n [%])
Becker 2001	20–23	8650	99 (1.1)	28 (0.32)
Taipale 1998	18–23	3969	57 (1.5)	5 (0.14)
Hill 1995	9–13	1252	77 (6.2)	4 (0.31)
Mustafa 2002	20–24	203	8 (3.9)	4 (1.9)
Lauria 1996	15–20	2910	36 (1.2)	5 (0.17)
Rosati 2000	10–16	2158	105 (4.9)	8 (0.37)

Source: Reproduced with permission from Oyelese Y, Sumulian, JC. Placenta Previa, Placenta Accreta, and Vasa Previa. *Obstet Gynecol.* 2006;107:927–941. Copyright © 2006 The American College of Obstetricians and Gynecologists.

Placenta Previa

OBSTETRICS

Evaluation

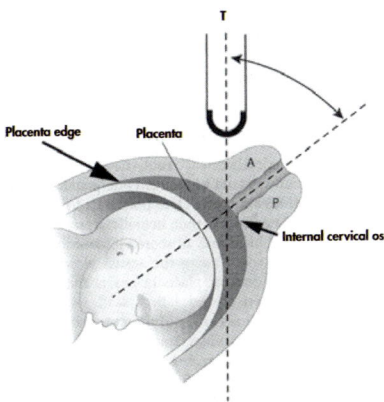

Figure 2.18. Diagram demonstrating the technique for transvaginal sonography of placenta previa

T, transvaginal transducer; A, anterior lip of cervix; P, posterior lip of cervix. Complete placenta Previa is shown completely covering the internal os (arrow). The transvaginal transducer lies within the vagina, about 2 cm from the anterior lip of the cervix. The angle between the transducer and the cervical canal is 32 degrees, demonstrating why the probe does not enter the cervix. Illustration: John Yanson.

Source: Oyelese Y, Sumulian, JC. Placenta Previa, Placenta Accreta, and Vasa Previa. *Obstet Gynecol.* 2006;107:927-41. Copyright © 2006 The American College of Obstetricians and Gynecologists.

POSTPARTUM HEMORRHAGE

Definition
- ~500 cc blood loss in first 24 hours after delivery

Etiology and Risk Factors
- Atony
- Grand multiparity
- Uterine overdistention
- Prolonged labor with Pitocin augmentation
- Chorioamnionitis
- General anesthesia
- MgSO4 therapy for seizure prophylaxis
- Rapid labor
- Retained placental tissue
- Usually delayed postpartum hemorrhage
- Placenta accreta (especially multiple prior cesarean deliveries or other uterine surgery)
- Preterm delivery
- Succenturiate lobe
- Cord avulsion
- Genital tract laceration
- Precipitous labor and delivery
- Improper episiotomy repair
- Operative vaginal delivery
- Uterine inversion—don't pull on that cord!

Table 2.48. Maternal adaptation to blood loss

Mild Blood Loss: 20–25% of Blood Volume (1,200 –1,500 mL)
Tachycardia (95–105 beats per minute [bpm]) Vasoconstriction—cold, pale extremities Mean arterial pressure drops by 10 –15% (70 –75 mm Hg)
Moderate Blood Loss: 25–35% of Blood Volume (1,500 –2,000 mL)
Tissue hypoxia Tachycardia (105–120 bpm), restlessness Mean arterial pressure drop of 25–30% (50–60 mm Hg) Oliguria (less than .5 mL/kg of actual weight)
Severe Blood Loss: More Than 30% of Blood Volume or More Than 2,000 mL
Hemorrhagic shock Tissue hypoxia Tachycardia (more than 120 bpm) Hypotension (mean arterial pressure less than 50 mm Hg) Altered consciousness Anuria Disseminated intravascular coagulation

Source: Reproduced with permission from Brown HL. Trauma in pregnancy. *Obstet Gynecol.* 2009 Jul;114(1):147-60. Copyright © 2009 The American College of Obstetricians and Gynecologists.

Postpartum Hemorrhage — OBSTETRICS

Table 2.49. Blood component therapy

Component	Contents	Volume	Anticipated Effect (Per Unit)
Packed red blood cells	RBC, WBC, plasma	300 mL	Increase in hemoglobin by 1 g/dL
Platelets^a	Platelets, RBC, WBC, plasma	50 mL	Increase in platelet count by 7500/mm^3
Fresh frozen plasma	Fibrinogen, antithrombin III, clotting factors, plasma	250 mL	Increase in fibrinogen by 10 mg/dL
Cryoprecipitate	Fibrinogen, factor VIII, von Willebrand factor, factor XIII	40 mL	Increase in fibrinogen by 10 mg/dL
Tranexamic acid*	Antifibrinolytic	Initial dose 1 g IV, may repeat after 30 minutes and may be followed by 1 g/hr.	
rFVIIa*	Factor VIIa	90 µg/kg may repeat x 1 in 14 to 30 min if no response	There have been associated complications of VTE and therefore should be used in cases of severe PPH

Source: Modified from Martin SR, Strong TH Jr. Transfusion of blood components and derivatives in the obstetric intensive care patient. In: Foley MR, Strong TH Jr, Garite TJ. *Obstetric Intensive Care Manual.* 2004. McGraw-Hill Medical Publishing Division; Abdul-Kadir R, et al. Evaluation and management of postpartum hemorrhage: consensus from and international expert panel. *Transfusion.* 2014;54(7):1756-68.

Table 2.50. Duke University obstetric bleeding emergency transfusion algorithm

Transfusion Management
Patient with in-date type and screen available
4 units type-specific packed red blood cells (pRBCs)
4 units type-specific or AB thawed plasma
5 units of cryoprecipitate
Patient with in-date type and screen not available
4 units of O negative pRBCs
4 units of thawed AB plasma
5 units of cryoprecipitate

Laboratory and Assessment

- Hemostasis panel immediately and at 30-minute intervals until patient stable
- Obstetrician and anesthesiologist make joint assessment of cumulative estimated blood loss every 30 minutes
- Notify transfusion services when the emergency is over and patient stable
- Monitor laboratory ever 4–6 hours for 24 hours to include hemoglobin, platelet count, prothrombin time, international normalized ratio, and fibrinogen

Acknowledgement: Evelyn Lockhart, MD, Duke Transfusion Services.
Source: © Duke University, 2016.

Table 2.51. Uterotonic therapy

Agent	Dose	Route	Dosing Frequency	Side Effects	Contraindications
Oxytocin (Pitocin)	10–80 units in 1000 mL of crystalloid solution	First line: IV Second line: IM or IU	Continuous	Nausea, emesis, water intoxication	None
Methylergonovine (Methergine)	0.2 mg	First line: IM Second line: IU or PO	Every 2–4 hr	Hypertension, hypotension, nausea, emesis	Hypertension, preeclampsia
15-methyl prostaglandin $F_2\alpha$ (Hemabate)	0.25 mg	First line: IM Second line: IU	Every 15–90 mins (8 dose maximum)	Nausea, emesis, diarrhea, flushing, chills	Active cardiac, pulmonary, renal, or hepatic disease
Prostaglandin E2 (Dinoprostone)	20 mg	PR	Every 2 hr	Nausea, emesis, diarrhea, fever, chills, headache	Hypotension
Misoprostol[a] (Cytotec)	600–1000 mcg	First line: PR Second line: PO	Single dose	Nausea, emesis, diarrhea, fever, chills	None

IM, intramuscular; IU, intrauterine; IV, intravenous; PO, per oral; PR, per rectum.

[a]Off-label use, not FDA-approved

Source: Reproduced with permission from Francois K. Managing uterine atony and hemorrhagic shock. *Cont Ob/Gyn*. 2006;Feb:52-59. *Contemporary Ob/Gyn* is a copyrighted publication of Advanstar Communications Inc. All rights reserved.

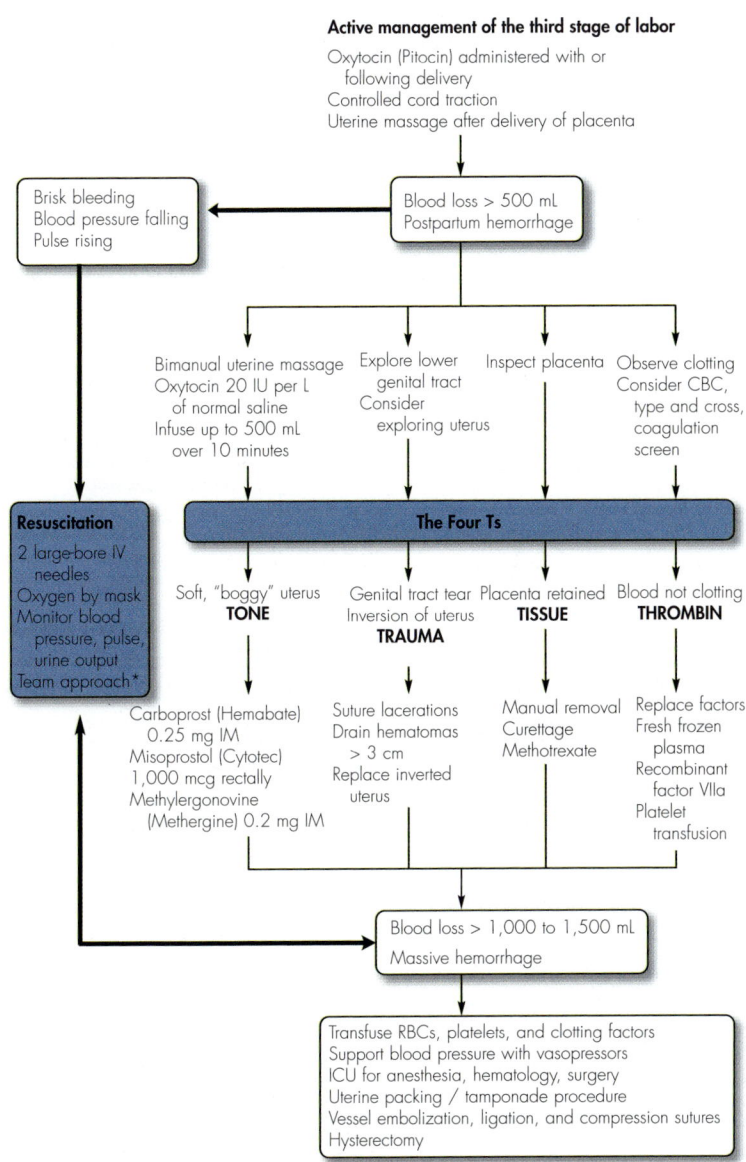

Figure 2.19. Management algorithm for postpartum hemorrhage
Source: Reproduced with permission from Anderson JM and Etches DE. Prevention and Management of Postpartum Hemorrhage. *Am Fam Physician.* 2007; 75:875-82. Copyright © 2007 American Academy of Family Physicians.

Hemorrhage after vaginal birth	Hemorrhage after cesarean delivery
This sequence of steps applies (1) after vaginal delivery (including the left hand-side interventions) and (2) after cesarean delivery, with the abdominal incision still open (including the right hand-side interventions).	
Administer oxytocin	
Perform uterine massage	
Administer additional uterotonics (methergine, misoprostol, carboprost [Hemabate])	
Bring 2 units of packed RBCs and 2 units of fresh frozen plasma (FFP) to point of care. Transfuse based on the clinical condition. Consider transfusing RBCs and FFP at a 1:1 ratio until clotting parameters are evaluated. Obtain Stat clotting studies. Start an additional intravenous line.	
Move the patient to the operating room	• Inspect the broad ligament and posterior uterus • Check for retained placental tissue
Repair any tears	• Place uterine devascularization sutures • Ligate the uterine artery • Ligate uterine vessels below the insertion of the fallopian tube
• Perform dilation and curettage to rule out, or treat, retained placental tissue • Perform ultrasonography to assess the uterine cavity for retained placental tissue	Place uterine compression suture(s), such as a B-Lynch suture
Place an intrauterine balloon	Consider bilateral ligation of the internal iliac artery
If indicated, call for additional specialists: second anesthesiologist, gyn surgeon, interventional radiologist, blood bank director	
Selective embolization by interventional radiology	Hysterectomy
Exploratory laparotomy—follow steps (along the right-hand side of this table) for treating hemorrhage after cesarean delivery	Pelvic packing
Adapted from California Maternal Quality Care Collaborative (www.CMQCC.org [http://www.CMQCC.org]).	

Figure 2.20. Sequential interventions for managing postpartum hemorrhage

Source: Reproduced with permission from Barbieri RL. Have you made best use of the Bakri balloon in PPH? *OBG Management*. 2011; 23(7):6-9. © Copyright Frontline Medical Communications. All rights reserved. Reproduced with permission.

Postpartum Hemorrhage **OBSTETRICS**

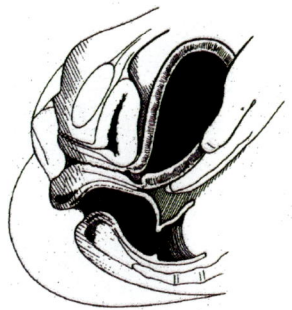

Grasp and elevate the uterus with the left hand and tilt it to expose the vessels.

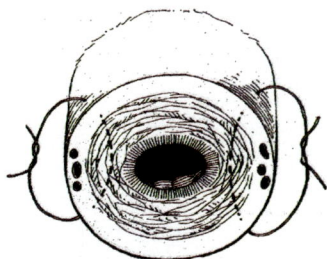

A coronal view of lower uterine segment is shown. Insert the suture into the substance of the cervix without entering the uterine cavity and medial to the blood vessels.

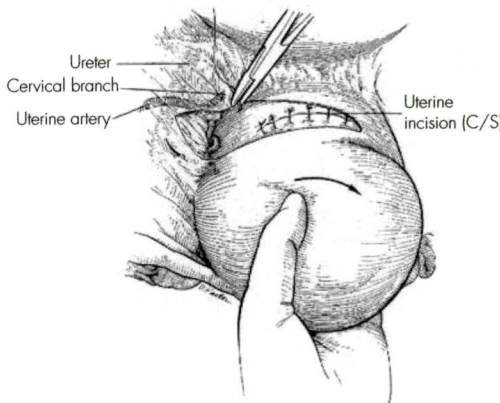

The ligation, 2–3 cm inferior to the uterine incision, includes 2–3 cm of myometrium in the suture.

Figure 2.21. Uterine artery ligation
  Source: Reproduced from O'Leary JA. Stop OB hemorrhage with uterine artery ligation. *Cont Ob/Gyn Special Issue: Update on Surgery.* 1986. Reproduced with the permission of David A. Factor, medical illustrator. *Cont Ob/Gyn* is a copyrighted publication of Advanstar Communications Inc. All rights reserved.

OBSTETRICS — Postpartum Hemorrhage

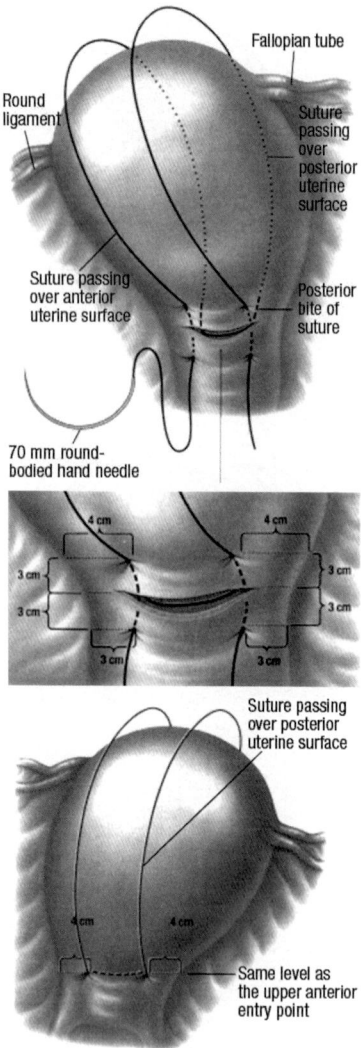

Figure 2.22. B-Lynch suture for postpartum hemorrhage
Source: Reproduced from Chez RA, B-Lynch C. The B-Lynch suture for control of massive postpartum hemorrhage. *Cont Ob/Gyn.* 1998 Aug:93-98. Reproduced with permission of Mr. Philip Wilson, F.M.A.A., R.M.I.P. *Cont Ob/Gyn* is a copyrighted publication of Advanstar Communications Inc. All rights reserved.

Tamponade in the Treatment of Postpartum Hemorrhage

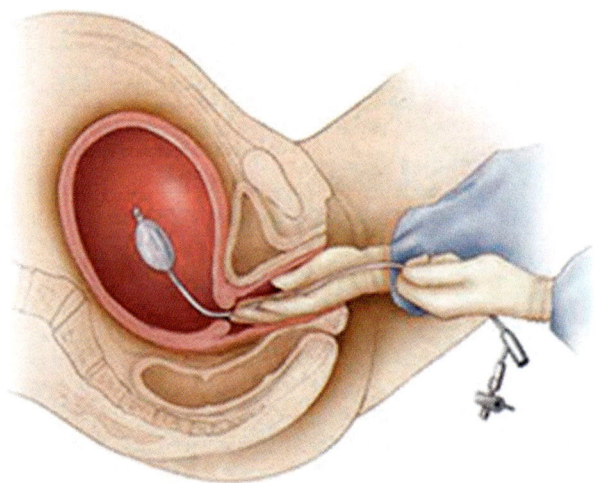

Figure 2.23. Manual insertion of a Bakri balloon
Source: Reproduced with permission from Barbieri RL. Have you made best use of the Bakri balloon in PPH? *OBG Management*. 2011; 23(7):6-9. © Copyright Frontline Medical Communications. All rights reserved. Artist: Molly Borman-Pullen.

Tips from Dr. Barbieri on Bakri Balloon Use

Place the Bakri balloon early in the PPH treatment algorithm.
Have 3 clinicians place the balloon.
Teamwork is a key to success here: The Bakri balloon is most quickly and elegantly inserted and inflated when three clinicians team up, as follows:
- Clinician #1 scans the uterus, assessing for retained products of conception and providing real-time imaging as the balloon is placed and inflated. This team member provides feedback to the others about correct placement and filling of the balloon.
- Clinician #2 inserts the balloon into the uterus by placing her hand into the vagina and guiding the balloon into the proper intrauterine position. (Most often, Clinician #2 is the delivering clinician.) This technique is performed in a manner similar to how one places an intrauterine pressure catheter. Clinician #2 stabilizes the balloon in position by maintaining her hand in the vagina. She ensures that the balloon does not "pop" out of the lower uterus as the balloon is filled.
- Clinician #3 simultaneously begins to instill sterile fluid into the balloon. This team member can be a nurse, medical assistant, or surgical technician.

Instill at least 150 mL of fluid.
Place a pack in the upper vagina to stabilize the balloon in position.
Check the hemoglobin concentration, platelet count, and coagulation status.
Practice your team's response to PPH with simulation.

Source: From Barbieri RL. Have you made best use of the Bakri balloon in PPH? *OBG Management*. 2011; 23(7):6–9. © Copyright Frontline Medical Communications.

UTERINE INVERSION

Fast Facts
- 1/25,000 deliveries
- More common in multigravida pregnancies
- Often iatrogenic

Presentation
- Placenta appears at introitus with mass attached.
- Shock with bradycardia secondary to vagal response.
- Excessive hemorrhage.

Treatment
- Treat for shock and blood loss.
- Call for assistance (especially anesthesia).
- Administer uterine relaxants.
- Terbutaline 0.25 mg IV (may repeat × 1)
- Nitroglycerine 100–250 mcg IV up to total of 1000 mcg (watch blood pressure).
- Replace uterus.
- "Last out; first in."
- Pressure applied around, not at, leading point.
- May require general anesthesia (halothane).
- Do not remove placenta if firmly attached until uterus replaced.
- Exploratory laparotomy with replacement if all else fails.

OBSTETRICS

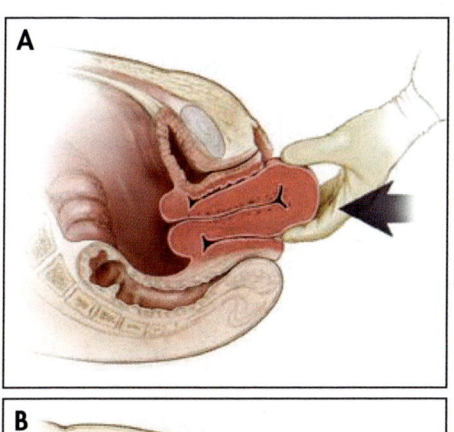

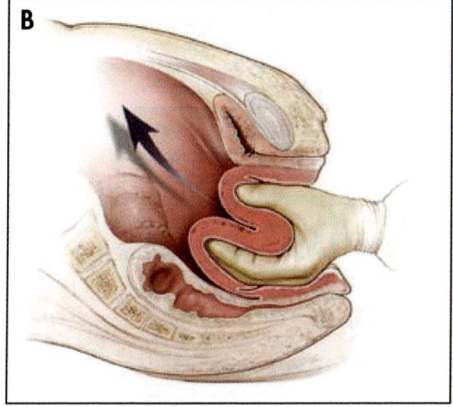

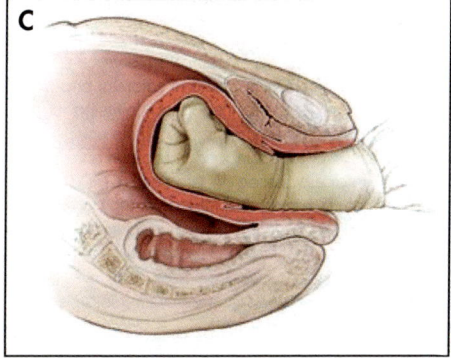

Figure 2.24. Reduction of uterine inversion
(A) The protruding fundus is grasped with fingers directed toward the posterior fornix. **(B, C)** The uterus is returned to position by pushing it through the pelvis and into the abdomen with steady pressure towards the umbilicus.
Source: Reproduced with permission from Anderson JM and Etches DE. Prevention and management of postpartum hemorrhage. *Am Fam Physician.* 2007; 75:875-82. Copyright © 2007 American Academy of Family Physicians.

CERVICAL INSUFFICIENCY
Indications for Cerclage in Women with Singleton Pregnancies
History
- History of one or more second-trimester pregnancy losses related to painless cervical dilation and in the absence of labor or abruption placentae.
- Prior cerclage due to painless cervical dilation in the second trimester.

Physical Examination
- Painless cervical dilation in the second trimester.

Ultrasonographic Finding with a History of Prior Preterm Birth
- Current singleton pregnancy, prior spontaneous preterm birth at less than 34 weeks of gestation, and short cervical length (less than 25 mm) before 24 weeks of gestation.

    Source: Reproduced with permission from American College of Obstetricians and Gynecologists. ACOG Practice Bulletin No. 142: Cerclage for the management of cervical insufficiency. *Obstet Gynecol*. 2014 Feb;123(2 Pt 1):372–9.

Summary of ACOG Recommendations and Conclusions
The Following Recommendations Are Based on Good or Consistent Scientific Evidence (Level A)
- Cerclage placement may be effective in women with a current singleton pregnancy, prior spontaneous preterm birth at less than 34 weeks of gestation, and short cervical length (less than 25 mm) before 24 weeks of gestation.
- Cerclage placement in women without a prior spontaneous preterm birth and a cervical length less than 25 mm detected between 16 weeks and 24 weeks of gestation has not been associated with a significant reduction in preterm birth.

The Following Recommendations Are Based on Limited or Inconsistent Scientific Evidence (Level B)
- Activity restriction, bed rest, and pelvic rest have not been proved to be effective for the treatment of cervical insufficiency and their use is discouraged.
- Cerclage methods currently used include modifications of the McDonald and Shirodkar techniques. The superiority of one suture type or surgical technique over another has not been established.
- Cerclage may increase the risk of preterm birth in women with a twin pregnancy and an ultrasonographically detected cervical length less than 25 mm and is not recommended.
- Neither antibiotics nor prophylactic tocolytics have been shown to improve the efficacy of cerclage, regardless of timing or indication.
- A history-indicated cerclage can be considered in a patient with a history of unexplained second-trimester delivery in the absence of labor or abruptio placentae.

The Following Recommendations Are Based Primarily on Consensus and Expert Opinion (Level C)

- Cerclage should be limited to pregnancies in the second trimester before fetal viability has been achieved.
- Transabdominal cervicoisthmic cerclage generally is reserved for patients in whom a cerclage is indicated but cannot be placed because of anatomical limitations, or in the case of failed transvaginal cervical cerclage procedures that resulted in second-trimester pregnancy loss.
- After clinical examination to rule out uterine activity, or intraamniotic infection, or both, physical examination-indicated cerclage placement (if technically feasible) in patients with singleton gestations who have cervical change of the internal os may be beneficial.
- In patients with no complications, transvaginal McDonald cerclage removal is recommended at 36–37 weeks of gestation.
- For patients who elect cesarean delivery at or beyond 39 weeks of gestation, cerclage removal at the time of delivery may be performed; however, the possibility of spontaneous labor between 37 weeks and 39 weeks of gestation must be considered.
- In most cases, removal of a McDonald cerclage in the office setting is appropriate.

Source: Reproduced with permission from American College of Obstetricians and Gynecologists. ACOG Practice Bulletin No. 142: Cerclage for the management of cervical insufficiency. *Obstet Gynecol*. 2014 Feb;123(2 Pt 1):372–9.

McDonald Cerclage

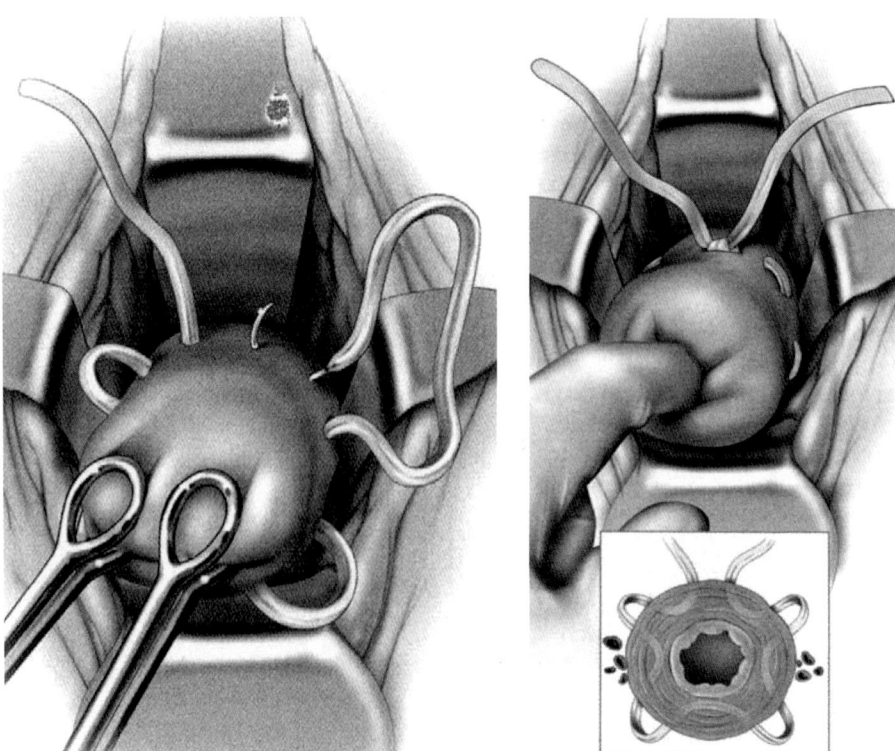

Figure 2.25. McDonald cerclage
A weighted speculum and right angle retractors are used to optimized visualization of the surgical field. Starting at the vesicocervical reflection, a purse-string suture is placed in four to six passes circumferentially around the cervix. Each pass should be deep enough to contain sufficient cervical stroma to avoid "pulling through," but not too deep as to enter the endocervical canal. Taking care to avoid the uterine vessels laterally, place the suture high on the posterior aspect of the cervix, as this is the most likely site of suture displacement. The suture is tied anteriorly, tight enough to be closed at the internal os. Successive knots are placed, and the ends are left long enough to facilitate later removal.

Source: Reproduced with permission from Berghella V, Baxter J, Pereira L. Cerclage: should we be doing them? *Cont Ob/Gyn.* 2005; Dec:34-41. *Contemporary Ob/Gyn* is a copyrighted publication of Advanstar Communications Inc. All rights reserved.

Modified Shirodkar Cerclage

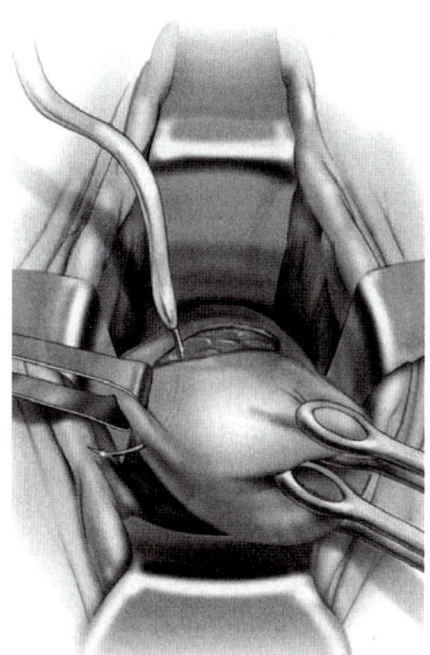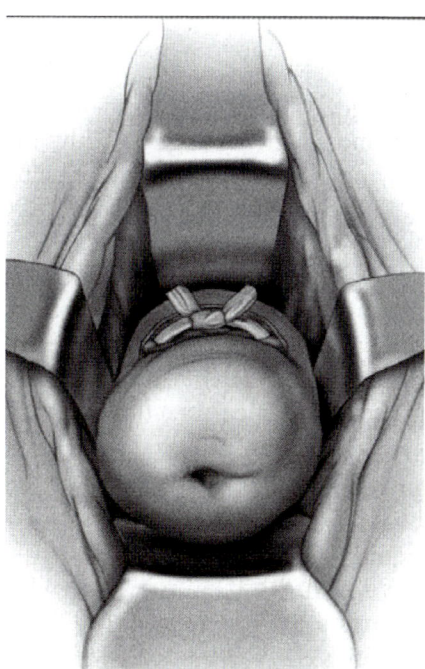

Figure 2.26. Modified Shirodkar cerclage
The initial transverse incision is made in the anterior cervicovaginal epithelium at the reflection of the bladder. The vesicovaginal fascia is reflected cephalad to the level of the internal os, similarly to when beginning a vaginal hysterectomy. A similar incision is made posteriorly. An Allis clamp is placed laterally with the jaws in the anterior and posterior incisions as high on the cervix as possible to minimize the cephalad dissection. Lateral traction is placed on the submucosal tissue to avoid the uterine vasculature. The suture is driven by successive passes with an atraumatic needle on each side just distal to the Allis clamp above the insertion of the cardinal ligaments. After ensuring that the suture tape lies flat posteriorly, the suture is then tied anteriorly, light enough as to be closed at the internal os. Successive knots are placed to facilitate identification and later removal. The mucosal incisions are closed over only if active bleeding is noted.

Source: Reproduced with permission from Berghella V, Baxter J, Pereira L. Cerclage: Should we be doing them? *Cont Ob/Gyn.* 2005; Dec:34-41. *Contemporary Ob/Gyn* is a copyrighted publication of Advanstar Communications Inc. All rights reserved.

Transabdominal Cerclage

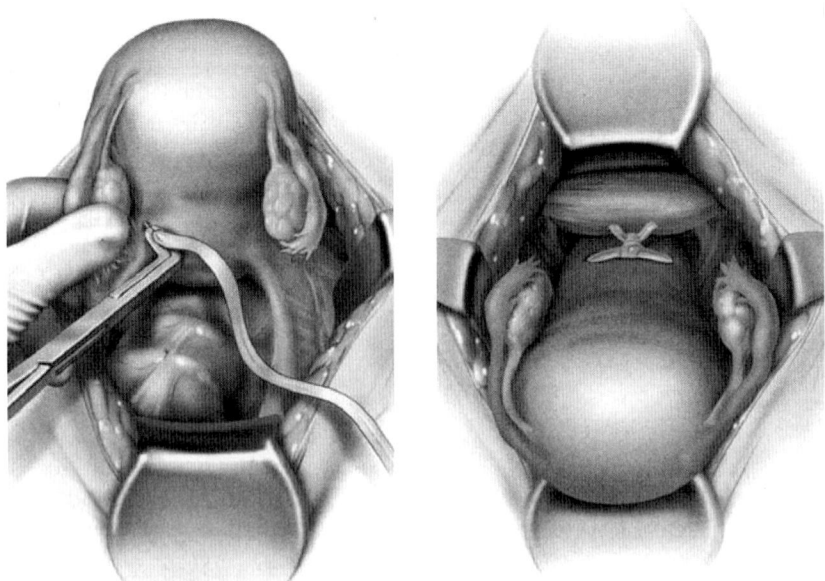

Figure 2.27. Transabdominal cerclage
While the surgeon digitally places the uterine vessels laterally, a 5-mm Mersilene suture is guided through the broad ligament at the level of the internal os by blunt perforation with a right-angle clamp. This is completed on each side and the suture is tied anteriorly.
  Source: Reproduced with permission from Berghella V, Baxter J, Pereira L. Cerclage: should we be doing them? *Cont Ob/Gyn.* 2005; Dec:34-41. *Contemporary Ob/Gyn* is a copyrighted publication of Advanstar Communications Inc. All rights reserved.

Physical Exam Indicated Cerclage (Emergency/Rescue Cerclage)

Fast Facts
- Method to perform cerclage in face of cervical dilation
- Heroic measure

Inclusion Criteria
- Intact membranes
- No evidence of chorioamnionitis
- Advanced dilation
- History compatible with incompetent cervix (not preterm labor)
- No gross fetal anomalies
- Extreme prematurity

Cervical Insufficiency

Preparation
- Informed consent
- General or regional anesthesia
- Perineal and vaginal prep

Technique
- Steep Trendelenburg position
- Insert Foley into bladder
- Backfill bladder with 1/2 NS in 250 cc increments
- Membranes usually recede after 800–1000 cc
- Place cerclage (McDonald or Shirodkar)

Postoperative Care
- Empty bladder
- Perioperative antibiotics (cefazolin) and tocolytics (indomethicin × 3 doses) have been shown to have some benefit (Miller 2014)

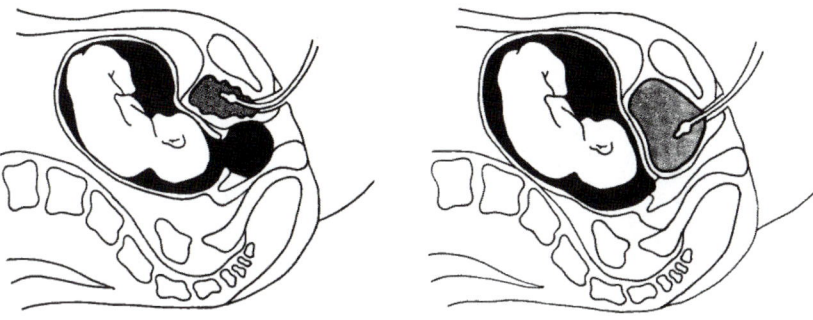

Figure 2.28. Technique to reduce prolapsed membranes before performing cerclage
Source: Scheerer LJ, Lam F, Bartolucci L, et al. A new technique for reduction of prolapsed fetal membranes for emergency cervical cerclage. *Obstet Gynecol*. 1989;74(3):408-410. Copyright © 1989 The American College of Obstetricians and Gynecologists.

OBSTETRICS

PRETERM LABOR

Fast Facts
- Preterm birth causes 85% of all perinatal morbidity and mortality
- 11.38% of all pregnancies (National vital statistics report 2013)
- Spontaneous preterm labor (70–80%)
- Indicated preterm delivery (20–30%)

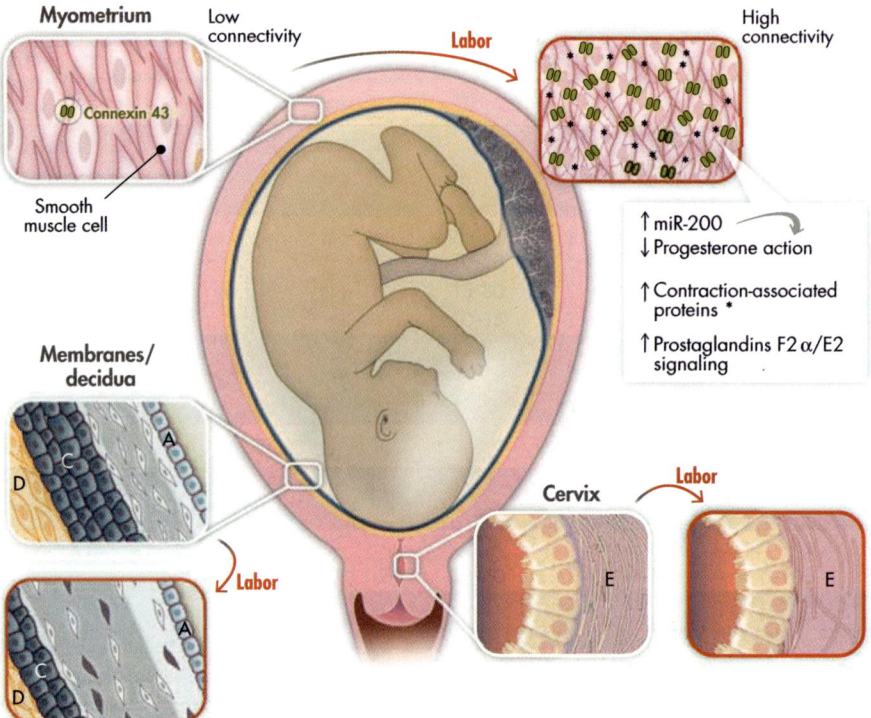

Figure 2.29. Pathways to preterm delivery
Source: Reproduced with permission from Romero R, Dey SK, Fisher SJ. Preterm labor: one syndrome, many causes. *Science*. 2014;345(6198):760-65. Reprinted with permission from American Association for the Advancement of Science (AAAS).

Diagnosis
- Estimated gestational age <37 completed weeks
- Uterine activity with either
  - Cervical dilation >2 cm or 80% effacement OR
  - Documented cervical change

Preterm Labor **OBSTETRICS**

Prevention

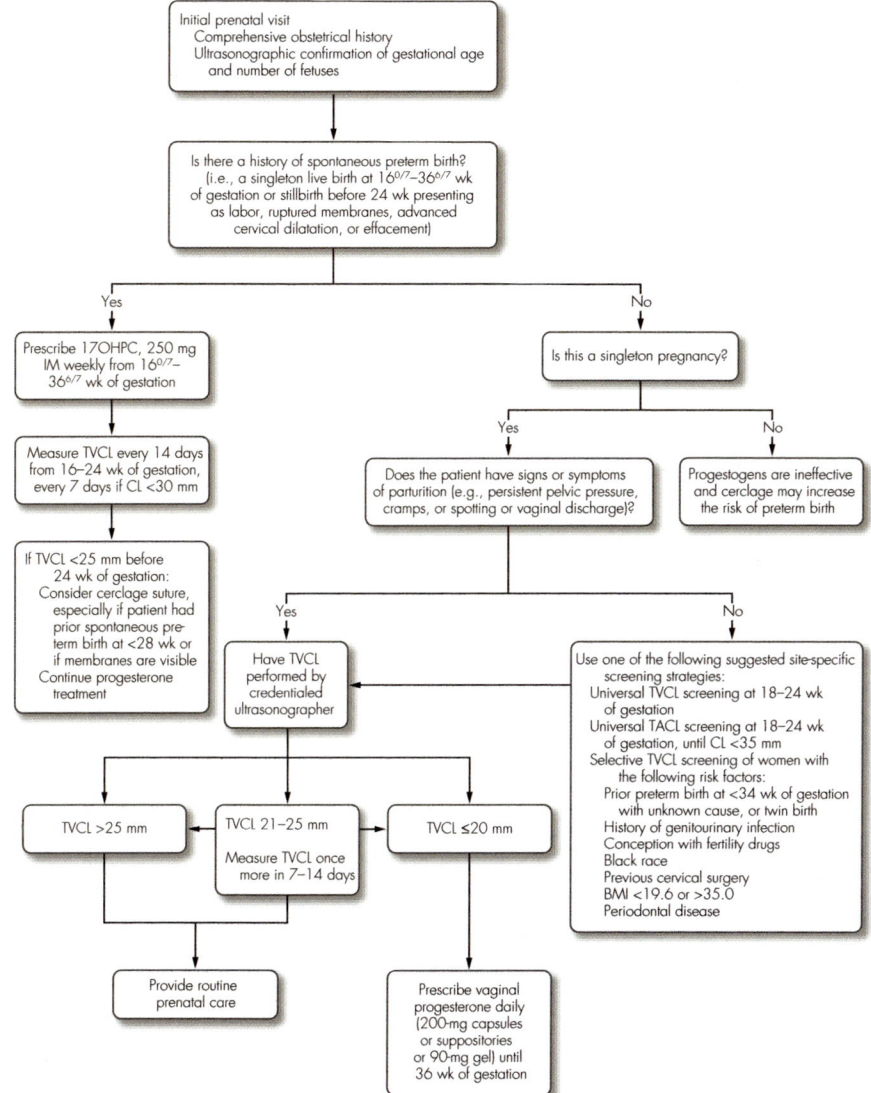

Figure 2.30. Algorithm for the screening and treatment of pregnant women to reduce the risk of preterm birth
The definition of spontaneous preterm birth includes a stillbirth before 24 weeks of gestation because many stillbirths at this gestational age represent the intrapartum death of previable neonates.

(continued)

The symptoms of parturition are symptoms of preterm cervical change, not of active labor; they may occur in normal pregnancy. Measurement of cervical length (CL) is appropriate when these symptoms persist for more than 1 day. There is no evidence-based treatment protocol for twin or triplet pregnancies.

If the transvaginal cervical length (TVCL) is less than 25 mm before 24 weeks of gestation, continued treatment with 17OHPC 17 alpha-hydroxy-progesterone caproate (17OHPC) is appropriate, although some experts recommend switching to vaginal progesterone when progressive cervical shortening occurs in such women.

If the TVCL is 20 mm or less and there has been no previous preterm birth, the role of cervical cerclage is uncertain. The choice of suggested screening strategies depends on the population of women cared for in the practice or clinic.

The risk factors associated with selective TVCL screening represent factors associated with a relative risk of preterm birth of 1.5 or more as compared with the risk in the general population of pregnant women, but the list is not prescriptive or all-inclusive.

BMI denotes body mass index (the weight in kilograms divided by the square of the height in meters), IM intramuscular, and TACL transabdominal cervical length. Gestation is represented in weeks^{days}/7.

Source: Reproduced with permission from Iams JD. Clinical practice: prevention of preterm parturition. *N Engl J Med.* 2014 Jan 16;370(3):254-61. Copyright © 2014 Massachusetts Medical Society. All rights reserved.

Table 2.52. Current Society for Maternal-Fetal Medicine recommendations regarding use of progestogens to prevent preterm birth

Population	Recommendation Regarding Use of Progestogens
Asymptomatic	
Singletons without prior SPTB and unknown or normal TVU CL	No evidence of effectiveness
Singletons with prior SPTB	17P 250 mg IM weekly from 16–20 wk until 36 wk
Singletons without prior SPTB but CL ≤20 mm at ≤24 wk	Vaginal progesterone 90-mg gel or 200-mg suppository daily from diagnosis of short CL until 36 wk
Multiple gestations	No evidence of effectiveness
Symptomatic	
PTL	No evidence of effectiveness
PPROM	No evidence of effectiveness

17P, 17-alpha-hydroxy-progesterone caproate; CL, cervical length; IM, intramuscularly; PPROM, preterm premature rupture of membranes; PTL, preterm labor; SPTB, spontaneous preterm birth; TVU, transvaginal ultrasound.

Source: Reproduced with permission from Society for Maternal-Fetal Medicine Publications Committee, with assistance of Vincenzo Berghella. Progesterone and preterm birth prevention: translating clinical trials data into clinical practice. *Am J Obstet Gynecol.* 2012 May;206(5):376-86. Copyright © 2012 Elsevier.

Preterm Labor

OBSTETRICS

Predicting Preterm Delivery
- Home uterine activity monitoring of unproven benefit.
- Fetal fibronectin screening has a strong negative predictive value between 24 and 34 weeks.
- Cervical length on sonogram may be predictive of preterm delivery.
- Prophylactic treatment of mother for group B *streptococcus* is appropriate pending culture results to prevent neonatal infection, but not to prevent preterm delivery.
- Tocolytic therapy may at least provide for administration of corticosteroids or transport to tertiary center for delivery.

Table 2.53. Predicted probability of delivery before week 32 by cervical length (millimeters) and gestational age in weeks at time of measurement

Cervical length, mm	Week of pregnancy													
	15	16	17	18	19	20	21	22	23	24	25	26	27	28
0	76.3	73.7	70.9	67.9	64.7	61.4	58.0	54.5	51.0	47.5	44.0	40.5	37.2	33.9
5	67.9	64.8	61.5	58.1	54.6	51.1	47.6	44.0	40.6	37.2	34.0	30.9	28.0	25.2
10	58.1	54.7	51.2	47.6	44.1	40.7	37.3	34.1	31.0	28.0	25.3	22.7	20.3	18.1
15	47.7	44.2	40.7	37.4	34.1	31.0	28.1	25.3	22.7	20.4	18.2	16.2	14.3	12.7
20	37.4	34.2	31.1	28.1	25.4	22.8	20.4	18.2	16.2	14.4	12.7	11.2	9.9	8.7
25	28.2	25.4	22.8	20.4	18.2	16.2	14.4	12.7	11.3	9.9	8.7	7.7	6.7	5.9
30	20.5	18.3	16.3	14.4	12.8	11.3	9.9	8.7	7.7	6.7	5.9	5.2	4.5	3.9
35	14.5	12.8	11.3	10.0	8.8	7.7	6.8	5.9	5.2	4.5	4.0	3.5	3.0	2.6
40	10.0	8.8	7.7	6.8	5.9	5.2	4.5	4.0	3.5	3.0	2.6	2.3	2.0	1.7
45	6.8	5.9	5.2	4.5	3.9	3.4	3.0	2.6	2.3	2.0	1.7	1.5	1.3	1.1
50	4.6	4.0	3.5	3.0	2.6	2.3	2.0	1.7	1.5	1.3	1.2	1.0	0.9	0.8
55	3.0	2.7	2.3	2.0	1.8	1.5	1.3	1.2	1.0	0.9	0.8	0.7	0.6	0.5
60	2.0	1.8	1.5	1.3	1.2	1.0	0.9	0.8	0.7	0.6	0.5	0.4	0.4	0.3

Source: Reproduced with permission from Berghella V, Roman A, Daskalakis C, et al. Gestational age at cervical length measurement and incidence of preterm birth. *Obstet Gynecol.* 2007 Aug;110(2 Pt 1):311-17. Copyright © 2007 The American College of Obstetricians and Gynecologists.

Table 2.54. Determining risk of preterm delivery in parous women at 24 weeks gestation

Technique for Determining Risk	% Risk Based On History of Delivery			
	18–26 wk	27–31 wk	32–36 wk	37 wk
	Risk of delivery at <35 wk			
By obstetric history	15	15	14	3
FFN (+)	49	48	46	13
FFN (−)	13	13	12	2
CL (cm) at 24 wk				
≤2.5	31	32	31	8
26–3.5	16	16	16	4
>3.5	8	8	8	2
	Risk of spontaneous preterm delivery at <35 wk			
FFN (−) by CL (cm)				
≤2.5	25	25	25	6
2.6–3.5	14	14	13	3
>3.5	7	7	7	1
FFN (+) by CL (cm)				
≤2.5	64	64	63	25
2.6–3.5	64	45	45	14
>3.5	28	28	27	7

FNN, fetal fibronectin; CL, cervical length.

Source: Modified from Iams JD, Goldberg RL, Mercer BM, Moawad A, Thom E, Meis PJ, et al. The Preterm Prediction Study: recurrence risk of spontaneous preterm birth. *Am J Obstet Gynecol.* 1998;178:1038-39.

Fetal Fibronectin Testing

Table 2.55. Predictive value of FFN testing in women with signs and symptoms of preterm labor

Negative predictive value	99.2%	124 out of 125 women with a normal (negative) fetal fibronectin test result **will not** deliver within the next 14 days.
Positive predictive value	16.7%	1 out of 6 women with an elevated (positive) fetal fibronectin test result **will deliver preterm within 14 days. However, almost 1 out of 2 women with an elevated (positive) fetal fibronectin test result will** spontaneously give birth before 37 wk.

Source: Peaceman AM, Andrews WW, Thorp JM, et al. Fetal fibronectin as a predictor of preterm birth in patients with symptoms: a multicenter trial. *Am J Obstet Gynecol.* 1997 Jul;177(1):13-18.

Table 2.56. Predictive value of FFN testing in women with risk factors for preterm delivery but no symptoms

Negative predictive value	93.9%	15 out of 16 women with a normal (negative) fetal fibronectin test result **will not spontaneously give birth before 37 wk.**
Positive predictive value	46.3%	Almost 1 out of 2 women with an elevated (positive) fetal fibronectin test result **will** spontaneously give birth before 37 wk.

Source: Nageotte MP, Casal D, Senyei AE. Fetal fibronectin in patients at increased risk for premature birth. *Am J Obstet Gynecol.* 1994;170(1 Pt 1):20-25.

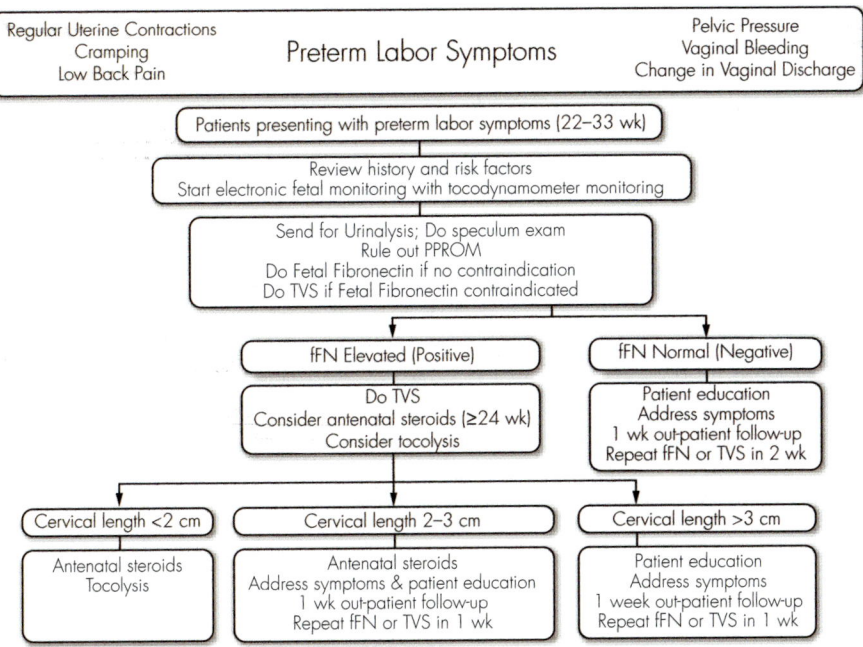

Figure 2.31. Triage protocol for PTL symptoms
Source: Reproduced, courtesy of Cytyc Corporation and affiliates. Algorithm provided by Herman L. Hedriana, MD, Sutter Medical Center Sacramento.

Antenatal Steroids

- A single course of corticosteroids is recommended for pregnant women between 24 weeks and 34 weeks of gestation and may be considered for pregnant women starting at 23 weeks of gestation, who are at risk of preterm delivery within 7 days (ACOG 2016).
- A single course of repeat antenatal corticosteroids should be considered in women whose prior course of antenatal steroids was administered at least 7 days previously and who remain at risk of preterm birth before 34 weeks of gestation (ACOG 2016). Repeat courses are not recommended.
- A single course of corticosteroids is recommended for pregnant women with preterm premature rupture of membranes between 24 0/7 weeks and 34 0/7 weeks of gestation and may be considered for pregnant women as early as 23 0/7 weeks of gestation who are at risk of preterm delivery.
  - Weekly administration of steroids is not recommended. There is a lack of data on administration of a rescue course of corticosteroids in the context of preterm premature rupture of membranes (ACOG 2016).

Dose

- β-Methasone
  - 12 mg IM given in 2 doses 24 hours apart. Twelve-hour dosing may be equally effective
- Dexamethasone
  - 6 mg IM given in 4 doses, one every 12 hours

    Source: Brownfoot FC, Gagliardi DI, Bain E, Middleton P, Crowther CA. Different corticosteroids and regimes for accelerating fetal lung maturation for women at risk of preterm birth. *Cochrane Database Syst Rev.* 2013;8:CD006764.

Tocolytics for Preterm Labor

Table 2.57. Common tocolytic agents

Agent or Class	Maternal Side Effects	Fetal or Newborn Adverse Effects	Contraindications
Calcium channel blockers	Dizziness, flushing, and hypotension; suppression of heart rate, contractility, and left ventricular systolic pressure when used with magnesium sulfate; and elevation of hepatic transaminases	No known adverse effects	Hypotension and preload-dependent cardiac lesions, such as aortic insufficiency
Nonsteroidal antiinflammatory drugs	Nausea, esophageal reflux, gastritis, and emesis; platelet dysfunction is rarely of clinical significance in patients without underlying bleeding disorder	In utero constriction of ductus arteriosus,* oligohydramnios,* necrotizing enterocolitis in preterm newborns, and patent ductus arteriosus in newborn†	Platelet dysfunction or bleeding disorder, hepatic dysfunction, gastrointestinal ulcerative disease, renal dysfunction, and asthma (in women with hypersensitivity to aspirin)
Beta-adrenergic receptor agonists	Tachycardia, hypotension, tremor, palpitations, shortness of breath, chest discomfort, pulmonary edema, hypokalemia, and hyperglycemia	Fetal tachycardia	Tachycardia-sensitive maternal cardiac disease and poorly controlled diabetes mellitus
Magnesium sulfate	Causes flushing, diaphoresis, nausea, loss of deep tendon reflexes, respiratory depression, and cardiac arrest; suppresses heart rate, contractility and left ventricular systolic pressure when used with calcium channel blockers; and produces neuromuscular blockade when used with calcium-channel blockers	Neonatal depression‡	Myasthenia gravis

*Greatest risk associated with use for longer than 48 hours.

†Data are conflicting regarding this association.

‡The use of magnesium sulfate in doses and duration for fetal neuroprotection alone does not appear to be associated with an increased risk of neonatal depression when correlated with cord blood magnesium levels (Johnson LH, Mapp DC, Rouse DJ, Spong CY, Mercer BM, Leveno KJ, et al. Association of cord blood magnesium concentration and neonatal resuscitation. Eunice Kennedy Shriver National Institute of Child Health and Human Development Maternal-Fetal Medicine Units Network. *J Pediatr.* 2011;DOI: 10.1016/j.jpeds.2011.09.016. [PubMed]).

Source: Reproduced with permission from Hearne AE, Nagey DA. Therapeutic agents in preterm labor: tocolytic agents. *Clin Obstet Gynecol.* 2000 Dec;43(4):787-801.

Magnesium Sulfate for Neuroprotection

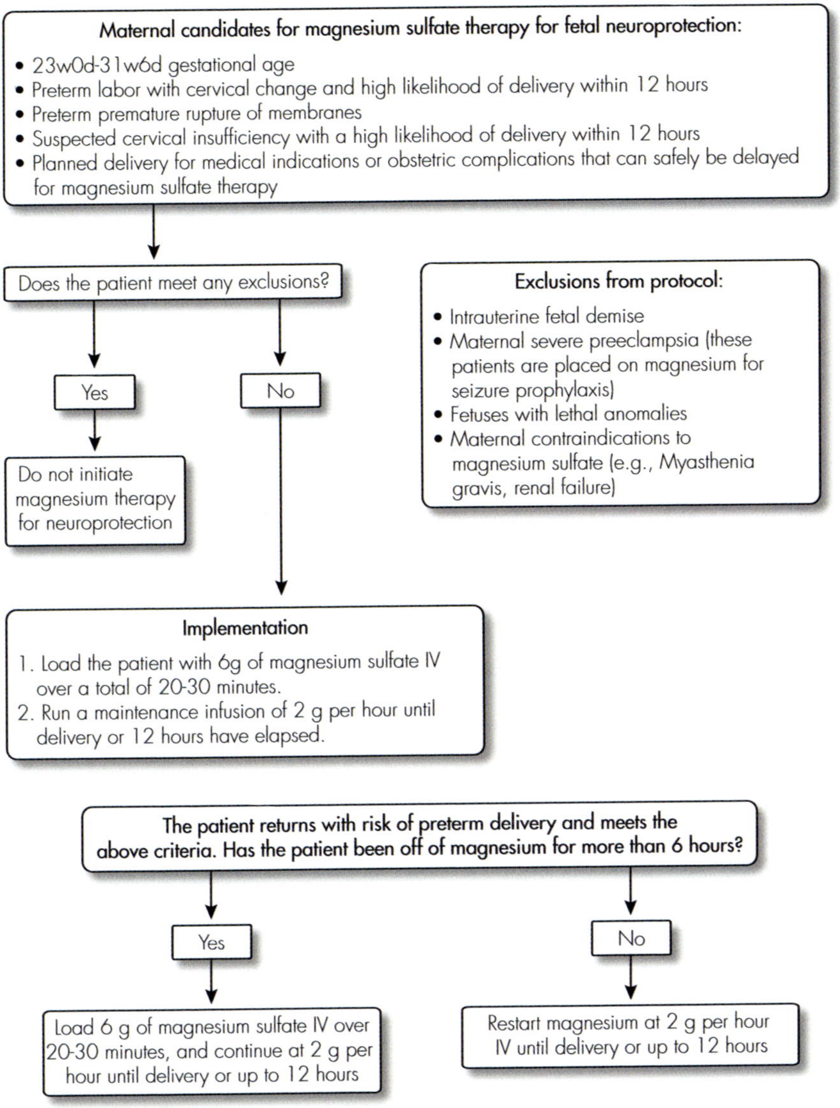

Maternal candidates for magnesium sulfate therapy for fetal neuroprotection:
- 23w0d-31w6d gestational age
- Preterm labor with cervical change and high likelihood of delivery within 12 hours
- Preterm premature rupture of membranes
- Suspected cervical insufficiency with a high likelihood of delivery within 12 hours
- Planned delivery for medical indications or obstetric complications that can safely be delayed for magnesium sulfate therapy

Does the patient meet any exclusions?

- Yes → Do not initiate magnesium therapy for neuroprotection
- No → Implementation

Exclusions from protocol:
- Intrauterine fetal demise
- Maternal severe preeclampsia (these patients are placed on magnesium for seizure prophylaxis)
- Fetuses with lethal anomalies
- Maternal contraindications to magnesium sulfate (e.g., Myasthenia gravis, renal failure)

Implementation
1. Load the patient with 6g of magnesium sulfate IV over a total of 20-30 minutes.
2. Run a maintenance infusion of 2 g per hour until delivery or 12 hours have elapsed.

The patient returns with risk of preterm delivery and meets the above criteria. Has the patient been off of magnesium for more than 6 hours?

- Yes → Load 6 g of magnesium sulfate IV over 20-30 minutes, and continue at 2 g per hour until delivery or up to 12 hours
- No → Restart magnesium at 2 g per hour IV until delivery or up to 12 hours

Figure 2.32. Algorithm for selection of candidates and administration of magnesium sulfate for fetal neuroprotection
Source: Reproduced with permission from Reeves SA, Gibbs RS, Clark SL. Magnesium for fetal neuroprotection. *Am J Obstet Gynecol.* 2011 Mar;204(3):202. Copyright © 2011 Elsevier.

Table 2.58. Inclusion criteria, treatment regimens, and outcomes of large randomized control trials of magnesium neuroprotection and cerebral palsy

Author	No.	Inclusion Criteria	Magnesium Sulfate Treatment Protocol	Death and CP RR (95% CI)	CP RR (95% CI)
Crowther (2003)	1,255	GA <30 weeks Likely PTB <24 hours	4-g load, 1 g/hour	0.83 (0.66–1.03)	0.83 (0.54–1.27)
Marret (2007)	688	GA <33 weeks	4-g load only	0.80 (0.58–1.1)	0.70 (0.41–1.19)
Rouse (2008)	2,241	GA 24–31 weeks High risk of PTB	6-g load, 2 g/hour	0.97 (0.77–1.23)	0.55 (0.32–0.95)

CI, confidence interval; CP, cerebral palsy; GA, gestational age; PTB, preterm birth; RR, relative risk.

Source: Reproduced with permission from American College of Obstetricians and Gynecologists Committee on Obstetric Practice; Society for Maternal-Fetal Medicine. Committee Opinion No. 455: Magnesium sulfate before anticipated preterm birth for neuroprotection. *Obstet Gynecol.* 2010 Mar;115(3):669-71. Copyright © 2010 The American College of Obstetricians and Gynecologists.

PERIVIABLE BIRTH

Table 2.59. General guidance regarding obstetric interventions for threatened and imminent periviable birth by best estimate of gestational age

	20 0/7 Weeks To 21 6/7 Weeks	22 0/7 Weeks To 22 6/7 Weeks	23 0/7 Weeks To 23 6/7 Weeks	24 0/7 Weeks To 24 6/7 Weeks	25 0/7 Weeks To 25 6/7 Weeks
Neonatal assessment for resuscitation*	Not recommended 1A	Consider 2B	Consider 2B	Recommended 1B	Recommended 1B
Antenatal corticosteroids	Not recommended 1A	Not recommended 1A	Consider 2B	Recommended 1B	Recommended 1B
Tocolysis for preterm labor to allow for antenatal corticosteroid administration	Not recommended 1A	Not recommended 1A	Consider 2B	Recommended 1B	Recommended 1B
Magnesium sulfate for neuroprotection	Not recommended 1A	Not recommended 1A	Consider 2B	Recommended 1B	Recommended 1B
Antibiotics to prolong latency during expectant management of PPROM if delivery is not considered imminent	Consider 2C	Consider 2C	Consider 2B	Recommended 1B	Recommended 1B
Intrapartum antibiotics for group B *streptococci* prophylaxis[†]	Not recommended 1A	Not recommended 1A	Consider 2B	Recommended 1B	Recommended 1B
Cesarean delivery for fetal indication[‡]	Not recommended 1A	Not recommended 1A	Consider 2B	Consider 1B	Recommended 1B

PROM, premature rupture of membranes.

*Many of the other decisions on this table will be linked to decisions regarding resuscitation and support and should be considered in that context; b Group B *streptococci* carrier, or carrier status unknown; c For example, persistently abnormal fetal heart rate patterns or biophysical testing, malpresentation. Many of the other decisions on this table will be linked to decisions regarding resuscitation and support and should be considered in that context.

[†] Group B *streptococci* carrier, or carrier status unknown.

[‡] For example, persistently abnormal fetal heart rate patterns or biophysical testing, malpresentation.

Many of the other decisions on this table will be linked to decisions regarding resuscitation and support and should be considered in that context; b Group B *streptococci* carrier, or carrier status unknown; c For example, persistently abnormal fetal heart rate patterns or biophysical testing, malpresentation.

Many of the other decisions on this table will be linked to decisions regarding resuscitation and support and should be considered in that context; b Group B *streptococci* carrier, or carrier status unknown.; c For example, persistently abnormal fetal heart rate patterns or biophysical testing, malpresentation.

Source: Reproduced with permission from American College of Obstetricians and Gynecologists and the Society for Maternal-fetal medicine, Ecker JL, Kaimal A, Mercer BM, Blackwell SC, deRegnier RA, Farrell RM, Grobman WA, Resnik JL, Sciscione AC. #3: Periviable birth. *Am J Obstet Gynecol*. 2015 Nov;213(5):604-614. Copyright © 2015 The American College of Obstetricians and Gynecologists

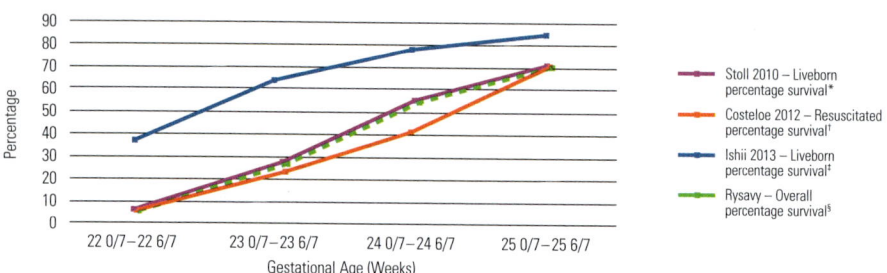

Figure 2.33. Percentage of survival by gestational age
Source: Reproduced with permission from American College of Obstetricians and Gynecologists and the Society for Maternal-fetal medicine, Ecker JL, Kaimal A, Mercer BM, Blackwell SC, deRegnier RA, Farrell RM, Grobman WA, Resnik JL, Sciscione AC. #3: periviable birth. *Am J Obstet Gynecol.* 2015 Nov;213(5):604-614. With permission from Elsevier. Copyright © 2015 The American College of Obstetricians and Gynecologists.

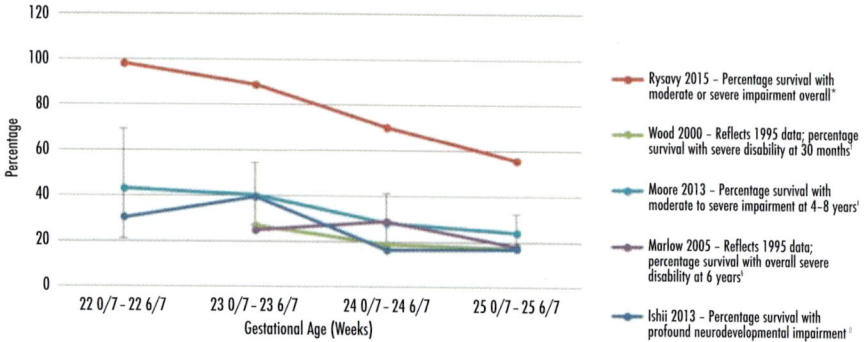

Figure 2.34. Percentage with severe or moderate disability by gestational age among surviving newborns

*Rysavy (2015).
†Wood (2000).
‡Moore (2013).
§Marlow (2005).
‖Ishii (2013).

Source: Reproduced with permission from American College of Obstetricians and Gynecologists and the Society for Maternal-fetal medicine, Ecker JL, Kaimal A, Mercer BM, Blackwell SC, deRegnier RA, Farrell RM, Grobman WA, Resnik JL, Sciscione AC. #3: periviable birth. *Am J Obstet Gynecol.* 2015 Nov;213(5):604-614. With permission from Elsevier. Copyright © 2015 The American College of Obstetricians and Gynecologists.

PRETERM PREMATURE RUPTURE OF MEMBRANES (PPROM)
Fast Facts
- 3% of pregnancies in the US
- 90% of term and 50% of preterm patients will enter labor within 24 hours
- At least 50% of patients with PPROM will deliver within 1 week
- Clinically evident intraamniotic infection present in 15–25% of PPROM patients
- Rate of fetal malpresentation increased
- Abruptio placentae occurs in 2–5%
- Risk of antenatal fetal demise 1–2%
- Risk of pulmonary hypoplasia variable
- Rarely lethal if PPROM occurs after 23–24 weeks
- Affects 10–20% of infants with PPROM prior to 24 weeks. Risk depends gestational age at rupture and remaining amniotic fluid level
- PPROM associated with amniocentesis has better outcome than spontaneous PPROM

Risk Factors
- Intraamniotic infection
- Lower socioeconomic classes, teenagers, smokers, single mothers, previous STD in pregnancy
- Second and third trimester bleeding, cervical cerclage, prior cervical conization
- Low BMI, nutritional deficiencies (copper, ascorbic acid)
- Connective tissue disorders (Ehlers-Danlos Syndrome)
- Pulmonary disease
- Uterine overdistention
- Prior PROM (16–32% recurrence risk)
- Short cervical length

Diagnosis/Evaluation
- History
- Sterile speculum exam (SSE)
  - Pooling
  - Ferning
  - Nitrazine positive (this may be falsely positive with blood, semen, alkaline antiseptic, BV, or anything the elevates the vaginal pH >6)
- Rupture of membrane kits including ROM Plus are available; false positive test results have been reported
- Vaginal/cervical cultures
- For definitive diagnosis, one can use the "tampon test" and inject indigo carmine into the amnion via amniocentesis; if a vaginal tampon turns blue, rupture can be confirmed
- Ultrasound for presentation, careful monitoring for cord prolapse if the infant is nonvertex
- Evaluate for chorioamnionitis

Table 2.60. Management of PROM based on gestational age

Early Term and Term (37 0/7 Weeks of Gestation or More)
Proceed to delivery
GBS prophylaxis as indicated
Late Preterm (34 0/7–36 6/7 Weeks of Gestation)
Same as for early term and term
Preterm (24 0/7–33 6/7 Weeks of Gestation)*†
Expectant management
Antibiotics recommended to prolong latency if there are no contraindications
Single-course corticosteroids
GBS prophylaxis as indicated
Less Than 24 Weeks of Gestation‡
Patient counseling
Expectant management or induction of labor
Antibiotics are not recommended before viability
GBS prophylaxis is not recommended before viability
Corticosteroids are not recommended before viability
Tocolysis is not recommended before viability
Magnesium sulfate for neuroprotection is not recommended before viability

GBS, group B streptococci.
*Unless fetal pulmonary maturity is documented.
†Magnesium sulfate for neuroprotection in accordance with one of the larger studies.
‡The combination of birth weight, gestational age, and sex provide the best estimate of chances of survival and should be considered in individual cases.

Source: Reproduced with permission from Practice Bulletin No. 160: Premature rupture of membranes. *Obstet Gynecol.* 2016 Jan;127(1):e39-51. Copyright © 2016 The American College of Obstetricians and Gynecologists.

Summary of Recommendations and Conclusions

The Following Recommendations Are Based on Good and Consistent Scientific Evidence (Level A)

- Patients with PROM before 34 0/7 weeks of gestation should be managed expectantly if no maternal or fetal contraindications exist.
- To reduce maternal and neonatal infections and gestational-age dependent morbidity, a 7-day course of therapy with a combination of erythromycin and ampicillin or amoxicillin is recommended during expectant management of women with PPROM who are less than 34 0/7 weeks of gestation.
- Women with PPROM and a viable fetus who are candidates for intrapartum GBS prophylaxis should receive intrapartum GBS prophylaxis to prevent vertical transmission regardless of earlier treatments.
- A single course of corticosteroids is recommended for pregnant women between 24 0/7 weeks and 34 0/7 weeks of gestation and may be considered for pregnant women as early as 23 0/7 weeks of gestation who are at risk of preterm delivery.

- Women with PPROM before 32 0/7 weeks of gestation who are thought to be at risk of imminent delivery should be considered candidates for fetal neuroprotective treatment with intravenous magnesium sulfate.

The Following Recommendations and Conclusions Are Based on Limited and Inconsistent Scientific Evidence (Level B)

- For women with PROM at 37 0/7 weeks of gestation or more, if spontaneous labor does not occur near the time of presentation in those who do not have contraindications to labor, labor should be induced.
- At 34 0/7 weeks or greater gestation, delivery is recommended for all women with ruptured membranes.
- In the setting of ruptured membranes with active labor, therapeutic tocolysis has not been shown to prolong latency or improve neonatal outcomes. Therefore, therapeutic tocolysis is not recommended.

The Following Conclusion Is Based Primarily on Consensus and Expert Opinion (Level C)

- The outpatient management of PPROM with a viable fetus has not been sufficiently studied to establish safety and, therefore, is not recommended.

Source: Reproduced with permission from ACOG Practice Bulletin No. 160: Premature rupture of membranes. *Obstet Gynecol*. 2016 Jan;127(1):e39-51. Copyright © 2016 The American College of Obstetricians and Gynecologists.

MULTIPLE GESTATION
Fast Facts
- Dizygotic: fertilization of 2 separate ova by 2 sperm.
- Monozygotic: division of single ovum fertilized by single sperm.
- In 2009, the rate of twin birth was 33.3/1,000 and the rate of triplet birth was 153.4/100,000.

Placentation
- Dizygotic twins (2/3 of U.S. twins) have separate chorion/amnion.
- Type of Monozygotic twins (1/3 of U.S. twins) dependent on timing of embryonic division.

Table 2.61. Timing of embryonic division in monozygotic twinning

0–72 hr	diamniotic, dichorionic (30%)
4–8 days	monochorionic, diamniotic (68%)
8–13 days	monochorionic, monoamniotic (2%)
>13 days	conjoined twins

Maternal Complications of Twin Gestation
- Gestational diabetes
- Increased risk of hypertension (6.5% of singletons, 12.7% of twins, 20.0% of triplets)
- Six times more likely to be hospitalized with pregnancy complications
- Hyperemesis
- Pyelonephritis
- Postpartum hemorrhage
- Preterm labor
- Acute fatty liver
- Thromboembolism

Antepartum Management
- High risk for preterm labor
- Serial sonogram for growth
- NST as indicated
- May be useful in multiple gestations to assess fetal well-being and predict cord compression

Multiple Gestation — OBSTETRICS

Table 2.62. Morbidity and mortality in multiple pregnancies

Characteristic	Singleton	Twins	Triplets	Quadruplets
Mean birth	3,296 g	2,336 g	1,660 g	1,291 g weight[*]
Mean gestational age[*]	38.7 weeks	35.3 weeks	31.9 weeks	29.5 weeks
Percentage less than 32 weeks of gestation[*]	1.6	11.4	36.8	64.5
Percentage less than 37 weeks of gestation[*]	10.4	58.8	94.4	98.3
Rate of cerebral palsy (per 1,000 live births)[†]	1.6	7	28	—
Infant mortality rate[‡] (per 1,000 live births)	5.4	23.6	52.5	96.3[§]

[*]Martin (2011).
[†]Petterson (1993).
[‡]Luke (2006).
[§]Quadruplet and quintuplet data combined.

Source: American College of Obstetricians and Gynecologists; Society for Maternal-Fetal Medicine. ACOG Practice Bulletin No. 144: Multifetal gestations: twin, triplet, and higher-order multifetal pregnancies. *Obstet Gynecol.* 2014 May;123(5):1118-32. Copyright © 2014 The American College of Obstetricians and Gynecologists.

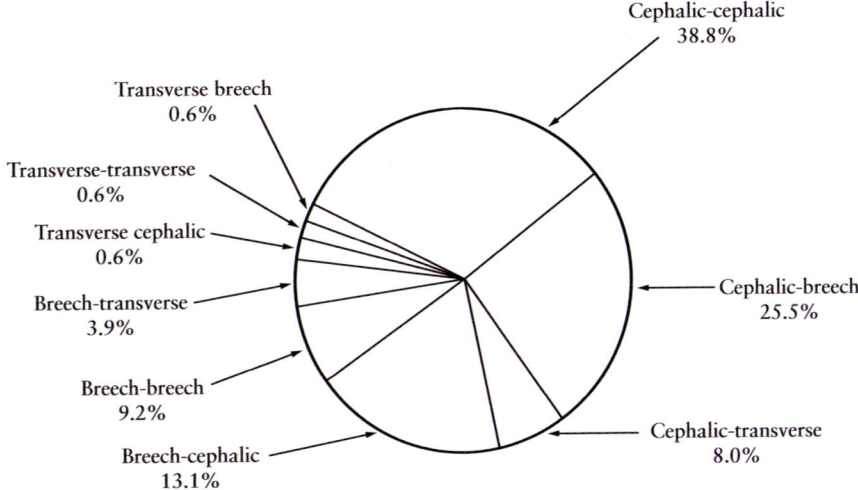

Figure 2.35. Presentation of twins presenting in labor or at term
Source: Reproduced with permission from Thompson SA, Lyons TL, Makowski EL. Outcomes of twin gestations at the University of Colorado Health Sciences Center, 1973–1983. *J Reprod Med.* 1987;32 (5):328-39.

Twin-to-Twin Transfusion Syndrome
- Monochorionic-diamniotic twin pregnancies.
  - 10 to 15% will be complicated by twin to twin transfusion syndrome (TTTS)
  - Also at risk for selective intrauterine growth restriction and twin anemia-polycythemia sequence (TAPS)
- Consider monitoring every 2 weeks by ultrasound assessment.

Table 2.63. Staging for twin-twin transfusion syndrome

Stage 1	Monochorionic-diamniotic gestation with oligohydramnios (MVP less than 2 cm) and polyhydramnios (MVP greater than 8 cm)
Stage 2	Absent (empty) bladder in donor
Stage 3	Abnormal Doppler ultrasonography findings*
Stage 4	Hydrops
Stage 5	Death of one or both twins

MVP, maximum vertical pocket.

*Defined as the presence of one or more of the following: umbilical artery absent or reversed diastolic flow, ductus venosus absent or reversed diastolic flow, or umbilical vein pulsatile flow.

Data from Quintero (1999).

Source: Reprinted by permission from Macmillan Publishers Ltd. Quintero RA, Morales WJ, Allen MH, Bornick PW, Johnson PK, Kruger M. Staging of twin-twin transfusion syndrome. *J Perinatol.* 1999 Dec;19(8 Pt 1):550-55.

Management of Multiple Gestation Delivery
- In twins between 32 0/7 and 38 6/7 weeks with a vertex presenting twin, planned cesarean delivery is not associated with decreased neonatal morbidity or mortality nor with increased maternal complications if the patient has access to a practitioner experienced in vaginal breech delivery of the second twin (Barrett 2013).
- Timing of delivery depends on chorionicity.
- Uncomplicated dichorionic-diamniotic twins: delivery at 38 weeks.
- Uncomplicated monochorionic-diamniotic twins: delivery between 34 and 37 6/7 weeks.
- Uncomplicated monochorionic-monoamniotic twins: delivery at 32–34 weeks.

Table 2.64. Number of cesarean sections needed to prevent one instance of composite morbidity and mortality

Presentation	Birth Wt	Number of Cesarean Sections Needed to Prevent One Instance of Composite Morbidity and Mortality
Vtx/Non-vtx	500–1499 g	7
Vtx/Non-vtx	1500–4000 g	25

Source: Meyer, MC. Translating data to dialogue: how to discuss mode of delivery with you patient with twins. *Am J Obstet Gynecol.* 2006;195(4):899-906.

Multiple Gestation OBSTETRICS

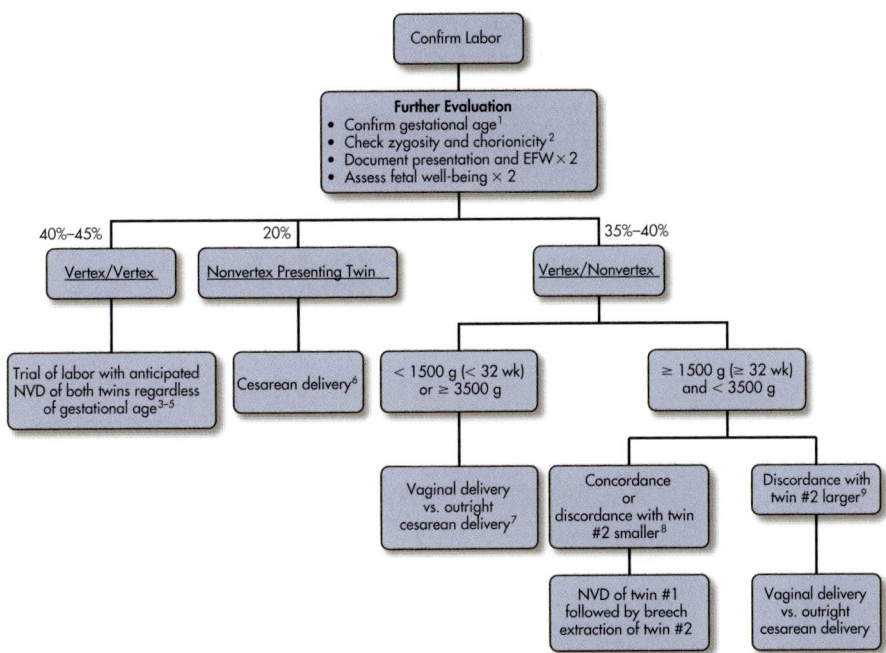

Figure 2.36. Algorithm for route of delivery of twin pregnancy

EFW, estimated fetal weight; NVD, natural vaginal delivery.

[1]There is considerable controversy about the intrapartum management of twin pregnancies, which is due primarily to an absence of well-designed clinical trials and to conflicting recommendations in the literature.

[2]Many authorities recommend that monoamniotic twin pregnancies be delivered by elective cesarean as early as 32 to 34 weeks of gestation due to the risk of fetal demise secondary to cord entanglement.

[3]Continuous electronic fetal monitoring of both fetuses is required throughout labor and delivery. Intravenous access should be attained and blood readily available, if needed. Anesthesiology should be notified and regional anesthesia recommended. Cesarean delivery may be indicated for the usual obstetric indications (such as nonreassuring fetal testing, placenta previa, or elective repeat cesarean after prior cesarean delivery). It is generally recommended that a neonatologist be present at delivery, because a second twin is more likely to require resuscitation. If a vaginal delivery is to be attempted, ultrasound equipment should be available throughout labor and delivery to document the fetal heart rate of the second twin, if necessary, and to confirm presentation (note that presentation of the second twin may change in up to 20% of cases after delivery of twin 1). With the possible exception of concordant, vertex/vertex, and diamniotic twin pregnancies in labor at term, all twin pregnancies should be delivered in the operating room with the availability of urgent cesarean delivery.

[4]Internal podalic version and breech extraction of twin 2 is an acceptable option. An obstetrician skilled in operative vaginal delivery and vaginal breech delivery is a prerequisite for any such a delivery.

[5]In the setting of reassuring intrapartum fetal heart rate monitoring, there is no urgency to deliver a cephalically presenting second twin, because delivery interval per se does not appear to affect perinatal outcome. However, a delivery interval of >15 min is associated with an increased risk of cesarean delivery. For this reason, active rather than expectant management of the second twin (artificial rupture of membranes, oxytocin augmentation, and/or breech extraction) is generally recommended.

(continued)

[6]There is no place for external cephalic version of twin 1.

[7]Several studies have suggested that vaginal breech delivery of fetuses, <1500 g is safe, whereas others suggest a poorer neonatal outcome for second twins delivered vaginally when in a nonvertex presentation. Provided an obstetrician skilled in breech extraction is present, preterm status with weight, <1500 g for second twin does not contravene a trial of labor.

[8]Discordance is often defined as ≥25% difference between twins (= EFW of larger fetus − smaller fetus/EFW of larger fetus x 100, expressed as a percentage).

[9]Twin discordance does not represent an absolute contraindication to a vaginal trial of labor, though weak evidence may support consideration of an outright cesarean in cases with extreme discordance in order to avoid a combined delivery, particularly when the nonpresenting twin is ≥40% larger than the second twin.

Source: Reprinted with permission from Christopher D, et al. *Rev Obstet Gynecol.* 2011;4(3-4):109-116. Copyright © MedReviews®, LLC. All rights reserved.

INTRAUTERINE GROWTH RESTRICTION
Fast Facts
- Intrauterine growth restriction is defined as a fetus failing to meet its growth potential.
- Often a cut off of fetal growth less than the 10th percentile for growth is used.
- Many fetuses that measure less than the 10th percentile for growth are constitutionally small.
- Small for gestational age (SGA) is a term that applies to infants after birth who weigh less than the 10th percentile.

Table 2.65. Risk factors associated with fetal intrauterine growth restriction

Fetal	Placental	Maternal
Chromosomal abnormalities	Small placenta	Extremes of under and/or malnutrition
Multifactorial congenital malformations	Circumvallate placenta	Vascular/renal disease
Multiple gestations	Chorioangiomata	Congenital or acquired thrombophylic disorder
Infection		Drugs/lifestyle
		High altitude or significant hypoxic disorder

Source: Reproduced with permission from Resnick R. Intrauterine growth restriction. *Obstet Gynecol.* 2002;99(3): 490-96. Copyright © 2002 The American College of Obstetricians and Gynecologists.

Table 2.66. Evaluation and management of the IUGR fetus

	Constitutionally Small Fetus	Fetus with Structural and/or Chromosome Abnormality; Fetal Infection	Substrate Deprivation; Uteroplacental Insufficiency
Growth rate and pattern	Usually below but parallel to normal; symmetric	Markedly below normal; symmetric	Variable; usually asymmetric
Anatomy	Normal	Usually abnormal	Normal
Amniotic fluid volume	Normal	Normal or hydramnios; decreased in the presence of renal agenesis or urethral obstruction	Low
Additional evaluation	None	Karyotype; specific testing for viral DNA in amniotic fluid as indicated	Fetal lung maturity testing as indicated
Additional laboratory evaluation of fetal well-being	Normal BPP/UAV	BPP variable; normal UAV	BPP score decreases; UAV evidence of vascular resistance
Continued surveillance and timing of delivery	None; anticipate term delivery	Dependent upon etiology	BPP and UAV; delivery timing requires balance of gestational age and BPP/UAV findings; fetal lung maturity testing often helpful

IUGR, intrauterine growth restriction; BPP, biophysical profile; UAV, umbilical artery velocimetry.

Source: Reproduced with permission from Resnick R. Intrauterine growth restriction. *Obstet Gynecol.* 2002;99(3):490-96. Copyright © 2002 The American College of Obstetricians and Gynecologists.

Table 2.67. Timing of delivery in cases of intrauterine growth restriction

Diagnosis	Gestational Age
Isolated fetal growth restriction	38 0/7 – 39 6/7 wk
Growth restriction with additional risk factors (e.g., oligohydramnios, abnormal umbilical artery Doppler velocimetry, maternal risk factors, comorbidities)	34 0/7 – 37 6/7

ACOG Practice Bulletin No. 134: Fetal growth restriction. *Obstet Gynecol.* 2013 May;121(5):1122-33.

- If delivery is considered prior to 34 weeks, antenatal corticosteroids should be administered.
- If delivery is considered prior to 32 weeks, antenatal corticosteroids should be administered AND Magnesium sulfate for neuroprotection should be considered.

ASTHMA IN PREGNANCY
Fast Facts
- No predictable effect on asthma.
- 1/3 improved, 1/3 worsened, 1/3 unchanged.
- Mild asthmatics at low risk.
- Severe asthmatics should have high-risk follow-up.
- Mortality of asthma is that of mechanical ventilatory fatigue.
- All pregnant patients with asthma should be monitored with peak flow meters by establishing their personal baseline when asymptomatic and following their peak flows when symptomatic.
- Administer flu vaccine annually.
- Administer pneumococcal vaccine (PPSV23) if not previously vaccinated.

Table 2.68. Medical management of asthma in pregnancy

Type	Management Preferred	Management Alternative
Mild intermittent asthma	No daily medications; albuterol as needed	
Mild persistent asthma	Low-dose inhaled corticosteroid	Cromolyn, leukotriene receptor antagonist, or theophylline (serum level 5–12 mcg/mL)
Moderate persistent asthma	Low-dose inhaled corticosteroid and salmeterol or medium-dose inhaled corticosteroid or (if needed) medium-dose inhaled corticosteroid and salmeterol	Low-dose or (if needed) medium-dose inhaled corticosteroid and either leukotriene receptor antagonist or theophylline (serum level 5–12 mcg/mL)
Severe persistent asthma	High-dose inhaled corticosteroid and salmeterol and (if needed) oral corticosteroid	High-dose inhaled corticosteroid and theophylline (serum level 5–12 mcg/mL) and oral corticosteroid if needed

Albuterol 2–4 puffs as needed for peak expiratory flow rate or forced expiratory volume in 1 sec less than 80%, asthma exacerbations, or exposure to exercise or allergens; oral corticosteroid burst if inadequate response to albuterol regardless of asthma severity.

Source: Adapted from National Institutes of Health, National Heart, Lung, and Blood Institute. National Asthma Education Program (NAEPP). Working group on managing asthma during pregnancy. Recommendations for Pharmacologic Treatment, Update 2004. NIH publication No. 05-5236, March 2005.

Table 2.69. NAEPP asthma classification

	Mild Intermittent	Mild Persistent	Moderate Persistent	Severe Persistent
Symptoms	<2 times/wk Asymptomatic between exacerbations	>2 times/wk but <1 time a day	Daily Exacerbations occur <2 times/wk	Continual Frequent exacerbations
Pulmonary function tests	Normal PEFR between exacerbations FEV_1 or PEFR >80% of predicted PEFR variability <20%	FEV_1 or PEFR >80% of predicted PEFR variability 20–30%	FEV_1 or PEFR 60–80% of predicted PEFR variability >30%	FEV_1 or PEFR <60% of predicted PEFR variability >30%
Nocturnal awakening	≤2 times/mo	>2 times/mo	>1 time/wk	Nightly awakenings
Interference with daily activities	None	Mild	Some interference with normal activities but rare severe exacerbation	Limitations of physical activity
Treatment	Inhaled short-acting β_2-agonist (albuterol)	Inhaled short-acting β_2-agonist + daily antiinflammatory (low-dose inhaled corticosteroid or cromolyn)	Inhaled β_2-agonist + daily medication (medium-dose inhaled corticosteroid **OR** low-medium dose inhaled corticosteroid **AND** long-acting bronchodilator)	Inhaled short-acting β_2-agonist + daily medication (inhaled high-dose corticosteroid **AND** long-acting bronchodilator **AND** oral corticosteroid)

NAEPP, National Asthma Education and Prevention Program; PEFR, peak expiratory flow rate; FEV1, forced expiratory volume in 1 sec.

Source: Adapted from National Institutes of Health, National Heart, Lung, and Blood Institute. National Asthma Education Program. Working group on managing asthma during pregnancy. Recommendations for Pharmacologic Treatment, Update 2004. NIH publication No. 05-5236, March 2005.

Table 2.70. Dosages of commonly used asthma medications in pregnancy

Medication	Dosage Range	FDA Category[a]	Class of Asthma
Albuterol (Proventil, Ventolin)	2 puffs q4–6hrs prn	B	All
Salmeterol (Serevent)	2 puffs q12 hrs or hs	C	Moderate to severe
Cromolyn (Intal)	2 puffs qid	B	Mild persistent to severe
Beclomethasone (Beclovent, Vancenase, Qvar)	2–4 puffs (42 mcg) tid or qid double strength (84 mcg) 2 puffs bid	C	Mild persistent to severe
Triamcinolone (Azmacort, Nasacort)	2–4 puffs (100 mcg) tid or qid	C	Mild persistent to severe
Budesonide (Pulmicort, Rhinocort)	200 or 400 pg/inhalation, 1–2 inhalations bid	C	Mild persistent to severe
Flunisolide (Aerobid)	2–4 puffs (250 mcg) bid	C	Mild persistent to severe
Fluticasone (Flovent, Advair)	44,110,220 mcg/puffs, 1 inhalation bid	C	Mild persistent to severe
Montelukast (Singular)	10 mg hs	B	Severe, possibly moderate
Zafirlukast (Accolate)	20 mg bid	B	Severe, possibly moderate

[a]B, no evidence to risk in humans; C, risk cannot be ruled out.

Source: Reproduced with permission from Sakornbut E. How to treat pregnant patients with asthma. *Cont Ob/Gyn.* 2003;April:26-43. *Cont Ob/Gyn* is a copyrighted publication of Advanstar Communications Inc. All rights reserved.

Asthma

Table 2.71. Drugs for treating an acute severe asthma exacerbation in pregnancy

Medication	Dosage
Inhaled beta-agonists	
Albuterol	Nebulizer: 2.5–5.0 mg (0.5–1.0 mL of a 0.5% solution, diluted with 2–3 mL normal saline) given every 20 mins for three doses MDI with a holding chamber: 90 mcg/puff given as 4–8 puffs every 20 mins up to 4 hr
Metaproterenol	Nebulizer: 15 mg (0.3 mL of a 5% solution, diluted with 2–3 mL normal saline)
Subcutaneous beta-agonists	
Terbutaline	0.25 mg every 20 mins for three doses
Epinephrine	0.3 mg of 1:1000 solution every 20 mins for three doses
Corticosteroids	
Methylprednisolone	60–80 mg IV every 6–8 hr or 125 mg IV bolus followed by inhaled/subcutaneous beta-agonist or oral steroids, depending on initial response
Hydrocortisone	2.0 mg/kg IV bolus every 4 hr or 2.0 mg/kg IV bolus followed by 0.5 mg/kg/hr continuous infusion
Anticholinergics	
Ipratropium bromide	Nebulizer: 0.5 mg (one vial 0.02% solution) every 30 mins for three doses
	MDI: 18 mcg/puff given as 4–8 puffs as needed
Other	
Magnesium sulfate	2 g IV bolus over 2 min, followed immediately by inhaled beta-agonist
Heliox	80% helium/20% oxygen mixture (or alternative ways to prepare heliox depending on a given hospital pharmacy of 70%/30% or 60%/40%) through a nonrebreather mask

Source: Reproduced with permission from Sakornbut E. How to treat pregnant patients with asthma. *Cont Ob/Gyn.* 2003;April:26-43. *Cont Ob/Gyn* is a copyrighted publication of Advanstar Communications Inc. All rights reserved.

MATERNAL HEART DISEASE
Pregnancies Complicated by Maternal Congenital Heart Disease

Table 2.72. Maternal cardiovascular and offspring risk scores and modified WHO classification of maternal risk

Predictor	Risk Points (Maternal Risk)	Risk Points (Offspring Risk)
CARPREG		
Prior cardiac event (heart failure, transient ischaemic attack, stroke, arrhythmia)	1	–
NYHA functional class III/IV or cyanosis (SpO$_2$<90%)	1	1
Left heart obstruction (mitral valve area <2 cm² or aortic valve area <1.5 cm² or peak LVOT gradient >30 mm Hg (echocardiography))	1	0.75
Reduced systemic ventricular systolic function (EF <40%)	1	–
Multiple gestation	–	3
Smoking	–	1
Heparin/warfarin during pregnancy	–	1
ZAHARA		
Prior arrhythmia	1.50	–
NYHA functional class III/IV	0.75	–
Left heart obstruction (peak LVOT gradient >50 mm Hg or aortic valve area <1.0 cm²)	2.50	–
Mechanical valve prosthesis	4.25	2.50
Systemic atrioventricular valve regurgitation (moderate/severe)	0.75	–
Pulmonary atrioventricular valve regurgitation (moderate/severe)	0.75	–
Cardiac medication before pregnancy	1.50	0.75
Cyanotic heart disease (corrected and uncorrected)	1.00	0.75
Twin or multiple gestation	–	1.75
Smoking during pregnancy	–	0.50

(continued)

Maternal Congenital Heart Disease

Modified WHO classification

Conditions in which maternal risk is WHO class I
- Uncomplicated, small, or mild pulmonary stenosis
- Successfully repaired simple lesions (atrial or ventricular septal defect, patent ductus arteriosus, anomalous pulmonary venous drainage)

WHO class II (if otherwise well and uncomplicated)
- Unoperated atrial or ventricular septal defect, repaired tetralogy of Fallot

WHO class II–III (depending on individual)
- Native or tissue valvular heart disease not considered WHO I or IV; repaired coarctation; Marfan syndrome without aortic dilatation, bicuspid valve with aorta <45 mm; mild ventricular impairment

WHO class III
- Mechanical valve; systemic RV; Fontan circulation; unrepaired cyanotic heart disease; other complex congenital heart disease; Marfan syndrome with aorta 40–45 mm; bicuspid aortic valve with aorta 45–50 mm

Conditions in which pregnancy risk is WHO class IV (contraindicated)
- Pulmonary hypertension/Eisenmenger syndrome; systemic ventricular EF <30% or systemic ventricular dysfunction with NYHA class III–IV; severe mitral stenosis, severe symptomatic aortic stenosis, Marfan syndrome with aorta >45 mm; bicuspid aortic valve with aorta >50 mm; native severe coarctation

CARPREG risk score: For each CARPREG predictor that is present, a predictor-specific number of points is assigned for maternal cardiovascular risk or offspring risk, according to the table. The risk score (either maternal or offspring) is the total number of points. The risk of maternal cardiovascular complication is 5% with 0 points, 27% with 1 point, and 75% with ≥1 point. The risk of offspring complications is higher with a higher risk score; no percentages are assigned to the score.

ZAHARA risk score: For each ZAHARA predictor that is present, a predictor-specific number of points is assigned to the pregnancy, according to the table. The risk of maternal cardiovascular complications is 2.9% with <0.50 points, 7.5% with 0.51–1.50 points, 17.5% with 1.51–2.50 points, 43.1% with 2.51–3.50 points, and 70% with >3.51 points. The risk of offspring complications is 19.9% with <0.50 risk points, 33.3% with 0.50–0.99 risk points, 46.7% with 1.0–1.49 risk points, and 59.6% with ≥1.50 risk points.

Modified WHO classification: Class I: no detectable increased risk of maternal mortality and no/mild increase in morbidity; class II: small increased risk of maternal mortality or moderate increase in morbidity; class III: significantly increased risk of maternal mortality or severe morbidity; class IV: extremely high risk of maternal mortality or severe morbidity, pregnancy is contraindicated.

CARPREG, cardiac disease in pregnancy; LVOT, LV outflow tract; NYHA, New York Heart Association; SpO_2, oxygen saturation as measured by pulse oximetry; ZAHARA, Zwangerschap bij Aangeboren HARtAfwijkingen (pregnancy in congenital heart disease).

Source: Reproduced from Balci A, et al. Prospective validation and assessment of cardiovascular and offspring risk models for pregnant women with congenital heart disease. *Heart*. 2014;100:1373-81. Reproduced with permission from BMJ Publishing Group Ltd.

Maternal Valvular Heart Disease

Table 2.73. Recommendations for the evaluation and care of women of childbearing age with mechanical valve prostheses who are taking anticoagulants

Before Conception
Clinical evaluation of cardiac functional status and previous cardiac events
Echocardiographic assessment of ventricular and valvular function and pulmonary pressure
Discussion of risks associated with pregnancy
Discussion of risks and benefits associated with anticoagulant therapy
Family or pregnancy planning

Conception
Change to therapeutic, adjusted-dose unfractionated heparin (titrated to a midinterval therapeutic activated partial-thromboplastin time or antifactor Xa level) from time of confirmed pregnancy through week 12

Completion of First Trimester
Warfarin therapy, week 12–36

Week 36[a]
Discontinue warfarin
Change to unfractionated heparin titrated to a therapeutic activated partial-thromboplastin time or antifactor Xa level

Delivery
Restart heparin therapy 4–6 hr after delivery if no contraindications
Resume warfarin therapy the night after delivery if no bleeding complications

[a]If labor begins while the woman is receiving warfarin, anticoagulation should be reversed and cesarean delivery should be performed.

Source: Reproduced with permission from Reimold SC, Rutherford JD. Valvular heart disease in pregnancy. *N Engl J Med*. 2003;349(1):52-59. Copyright © 2003 Massachusetts Medical Society. All rights reserved.

Table 2.74. Classification of valvular heart lesions according to maternal, fetal, and neonatal risk

Low Maternal and Fetal Risk	High Maternal and Fetal Risk	High Maternal Risk	High Neonatal Risk
Asymptomatic aortic stenosis with a low mean outflow gradient (<50 mm Hg) in the presence of normal left ventricular systolic function	Severe aortic stenosis with or without symptoms	Reduced left ventricular systolic function (left ventricular ejection fraction <40%)	Maternal age <20 yr or >35 yr
	Aortic regurgitation with NYHA class III or IV symptoms		Use of anticoagulant therapy throughout pregnancy
Aortic regurgitation of NYHA class I or II with normal left ventricular systolic function	Mitral stenosis with NYHA class II, III, or IV symptoms	Previous heart failure	Smoking during pregnancy
	Mitral regurgitation with NYHA class III or IV symptoms	Previous stroke or transient ischemic attack	Multiple gestations
Mitral regurgitation of NYHA class I or II with normal left ventricular systolic function	Aortic-valve disease, mitral-valve disease, or both, resulting in severe pulmonary hypertension (pulmonary pressure >75% of systemic pressures)		
Mitral-valve prolapse with no mitral regurgitation or with mild-to-moderate mitral regurgitation and with normal left ventricular systolic function	Aortic-valve disease, mitral-valve disease, or both, with left ventricular systolic dysfunction (ejection fraction <0.40)		
Mild-to-moderate mitral stenosis (mitral-valve area >1.5 cm², gradient <5 mm Hg) without severe pulmonary hypertension	Maternal cyanosis		
	Reduced functional status (NYHA class III or IV)		
Mild-to-moderate pulmonary-valve stenosis			

Source: Reproduced with permission from Reimold SC, Rutherford JD. Valvular heart disease in pregnancy. *N Engl J Med.* 2003;349(1):52-59. Copyright © 2003 Massachusetts Medical Society. All rights reserved.

Table 2.75. Fetal effects of, maternal indications for, and risks associated with drugs used in the treatment of maternal valvular heart disease

Drug	Fetal Effects	Indications in Pregnant Patients with Valve Disease	Risk Category[a]
Diuretics			
Furosemide	Increased urinary sodium and potassium levels	To decrease congestion associated with valvular heart disease	C_m
Antihypertensive Agents			
Beta-blockers	Possible decreased heart rate, possible lower birth weight	Hypertension, supraventricular arrhythmias, to control heart rate in women with clinically significant mitral stenosis	D_m
Methyldopa	No major adverse effects	Hypertension	C
Vasodilator Agents			
Angiotensin-converting enzyme inhibitors	Urogenital defects, death, intrauterine growth retardation	Not indicated during pregnancy and should be discontinued	D_m
Hydralazine	No major adverse effects	For vasodilation in cases of aortic regurgitation and ventricular dysfunction	C_m
Nitrates	Possible bradycardia	Rarely used to decrease venous congestion	$B-C_m$
Anticoagulant and Antithrombotic Agents			
Warfarin	Hemorrhage, developmental abnormalities when used between wk 6–12 of gestation	For anticoagulation of mechanical heart valves, valvular heart disease with associated atrial fibrillation during wk 12–36 of pregnancy	D_m
Unfractionated heparin	Hemorrhage, no congenital defects	For anticoagulation of mechanical heart valves, valvular heart disease with associated atrial fibrillation during wk 6–12 and after wk 36 of pregnancy	C_m
Low-molecular-weight heparin	Hemorrhage	Not currently indicated during pregnancy	D_m
Aspirin	Hemorrhage, prolongation of labor, low birth weight (when taken in high doses)	Low-dose aspirin (81 mg/day) occasionally used as an adjunct in patients with previous embolic events or prosthetic-valve thrombosis	C
Antiarrhythmic Agents			
Digoxin	No major adverse effects	For suppression of supraventricular arrhythmias	C
Adenosine	No major adverse effects	For immediate conversion of supraventricular arrhythmias	C_m
Quinidine	High doses may be oxytocic	Occasionally used for suppression of atrial or ventricular arrhythmias	C_m
Procainamide	No major adverse effects	Occasionally used for suppression of atrial or ventricular arrhythmias	C_m
Amiodarone	Hypothyroidism, intrauterine growth retardation, premature birth	Rarely used during pregnancy because of side effects; may be used to suppress atrial or ventricular arrhythmias in high-risk patients	C_m

(continued)

Drug	Fetal Effects	Indications in Pregnant Patients with Valve Disease	Risk Category[a]
Antibiotics for Prophylaxis Against Endocarditis[b]			
Ampicillin	No major adverse effects	Given along with gentamicin to high-risk patients to prevent endocarditis	B
Vancomycin	No major adverse effects	Given along with gentamicin to high-risk patients with allergy to penicillin to prevent endocarditis	C_m
Gentamicin	No major adverse effects	Given along with ampicillin or vancomycin to high-risk patients to prevent endocarditis	C

[a]The risk categories are defined as follows. For drugs in category B, either studies of animal reproduction have not demonstrated a fetal risk but there have been no controlled studies in pregnant women or studies of animal reproduction have shown an adverse effect (other than a decrease in fertility) that was not confirmed in controlled studies in women in the first trimester of pregnancy (and there is no evidence of a risk in later trimesters). For drugs in category C, either studies in animals have revealed adverse effects on the fetus and there have been no controlled studies in pregnant women or no studies in women or animals are available; these drugs should be given only if the potential benefit justifies the potential risk to the fetus. For drugs in category D, there is evidence of risk to the human fetus, but the benefits from use in pregnant women may be acceptable despite the risk. A subscript m indicates that the manufacturer has rated the risk.

[b]Antibiotic prophylaxis against endocarditis may be used at the discretion of the treating physician at the time of delivery in high-risk patients. High-risk patients include those with prosthetic cardiac valves, previous bacterial endocarditis, surgically constructed systemic pulmonary shunts or conduits, or complex cyanotic congenital heart disease. Ampicillin should be given intramuscularly or intravenously in a dose of 2 g within 30 mins before delivery; 1 g should be given orally, intramuscularly, or intravenously 6 hr later. Vancomycin should be given intravenously in a dose of 1 g over a period of 1 to 2 hr, beginning 30 mins before delivery. Gentamicin should be given in a dose of 1.5 mg per kilogram of body weight (not to exceed 120 mg) within 30 mins before delivery.

Source: Reproduced with permission from Reimold SC, Rutherford JD. Valvular heart disease in pregnancy. N Engl J Med. 2003;349(1):52-59. Copyright © 2003 Massachusetts Medical Society. All rights reserved.

DIABETES IN PREGNANCY
Screening for Gestational Diabetes
- ACOG and the NICHD
- GCT: Nonfasting 50 g oral glucose challenge test
- Venous plasma glucose measured 1 hour later
    - Value of ≥140 mg/dL indicates need for 3 hour OGTT (~80% sensitivity).
    - Value of ≥130 mg/dL will improve sensitivity to 90% but will necessitate OGTT on 25% of women.
    - The International Association of Diabetes in Pregnancy Study Group (IADPSG) recommends a one-step testing algorithm for Gestational diabetes.

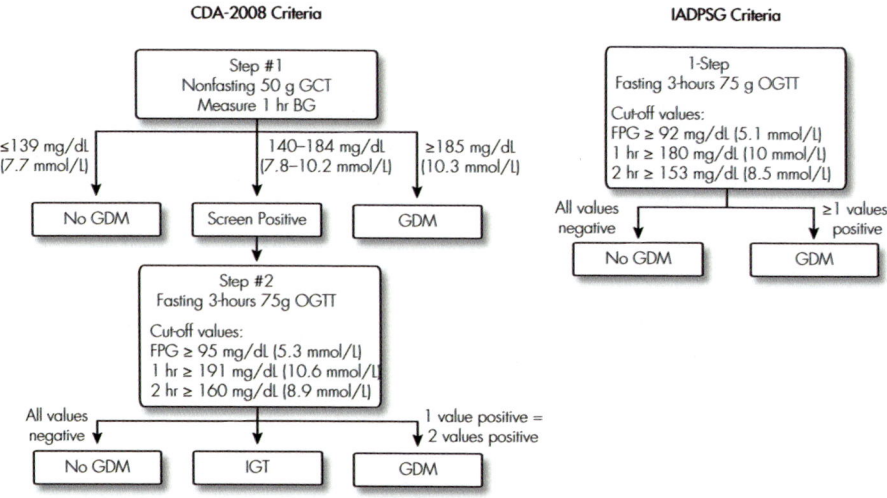

Figure 2.37. CDA 2008 and IADPSG algorithms for diagnosis of GDM
Source: Mayo K, Melamed N, Vandenberghe H, Berger H. The impact of adoption of the International Association of Diabetes in Pregnancy Study Group criteria for the screening and diagnosis of Gestational diabetes. *Am J Obstet Gynecol.* 2015;212(2):224;e1-224;e9. Copyright © 2015 Elsevier.

- National Diabetes Data Group (NDDG) diagnostic thresholds for OGTT are: plasma glucose levels of 105 mg/dL, 190 mg/dL, 165 mg/dL and 145 mg/dL for fasting, 1-hour, 2-hour, and 3-hour post 100 g glucose load (2 abnormal values = GDM)
- Carpenter and Coustan diagnostic thresholds for OGTT are 95 mg/dL, 180 mg/dL, 155 mg/dL and 140 mg/dL for fasting, 1-hour, 2-hour, and 3-hour post 100 g glucose load (2 abnormal values = GDM)

Table 2.76. Arguments in favor and against use of IADPSG threshold OGTT values for diagnosing GDM

Arguments in Favor
• Previous OGTT thresholds were set in such a way that about 2.5% of population would classify as GDM, irrespective of relationship of glucose values with perinatal outcome
• Striking increase in obesity and type 2 diabetes in general population may well correspond to GDM incidence of about 20%
• Treatment of GDM improves perinatal outcome
• Treatment of GDM is generally easy with insulin treatment in only 8–20% of women
• Adequate diagnosis is cost-effective

Arguments Against
• OGTT has poor reproducibility
• Even with very strict threshold values, only a minority of fetal macrosomia will be identified
• GDM is related to childhood obesity, but mainly in case of maternal obesity
• Overdiagnosis of GDM may well result in overtreatment
• Stricter OGTT criteria will result in increasing workload

GDM, Gestational diabetes mellitus; IADPSG, International Association of Diabetes and Pregnancy Study Groups; OGTT, oral glucose tolerance test.

Source: Reproduced with permission from Visser GH, de Valk HW. Is the evidence strong enough to change the diagnostic criteria for Gestational diabetes now? *Am J Obstet Gynecol.* 2013 Apr;208(4):260-64. Copyright © 2013 Elsevier.

Management
- For an excellent review, see Landon MB, Gabbe SG. Gestational diabetes mellitus. *Obstet Gynecol*. 2011;118(6):1379–93.

Diet (Ideal Body Weight)
- Ideal body weight (IBW): 100 lb @ 5 feet, plus 5 lb/inch >5 feet
- Daily kcal: 36 kcal/kg or 15 kcal/lb of IBW + 100 kcal/trimester
- Nutrients
- 40–50% carbohydrate
- 12–20% protein
- 30–35% fat

Glucose Monitoring
- Desired ranges
- Fasting 60–90 mg/dL
- 2 hours postprandial ≤ 120 mg/dL
- 2 am to 6 am above 60 mg/dL

Insulin
- Usually begun for fasting >105 mg/dL consistently.
- Anticipated eventual insulin requirements for gestational diabetic listed below.
- Distribution:
  - A.M. 2/3 Total: 2/3 NPH, 1/3 Reg
  - P.M. 1/3 Total: 1/2 NPH, 1/2 Reg
- Insulin dependent diabetes mellitus requires individualization (see following page).

Table 2.77. Pharmacokinetic profiles of insulin analogs and human insulins

Insulin	Onset of Action, min	Peak, hr	Duration, hr
Analog			
Long-acting			
• detemir	48–120	NA	<24
• glargine	66	NA	<24
Rapid-acting			
• aspart	10–20	1–3	3–5
• lispro	15–30	0.5–2.5	3–6.5
• glulisine	10–15	1–1.5	3–5
Premixed			
• 70% aspart protamine suspension/30% aspart	10–20	1–4 (2.4)*	<24
• 75% lispro protamine suspension/25% lispro	10–30	1–6.5 (2.6)*	<24
Human			
Intermediate-acting			
• NPH	60–120	6–14	16–>24
Short-acting			
• regular	30–60	1–5	6–10
Premixed			
• 70% NPH/30% regular	30–60	1.5–16 (4.4)*	18–24

NA, not applicable (i.e., no pronounced peak); NPH, neutral protamine Hagedorn.
*Data reported as range (mean).

Source: Reproduced with permission from Freeman JS. Insulin analog therapy: improving the match with physiologic insulin secretion. *J Am Osteopath Assoc.* 2009;109(1):26-36. Copyright © 2013 American Osteopathic Association. Reproduced with the consent of the American Osteopathic Association.

Diabetes in Pregnancy — OBSTETRICS

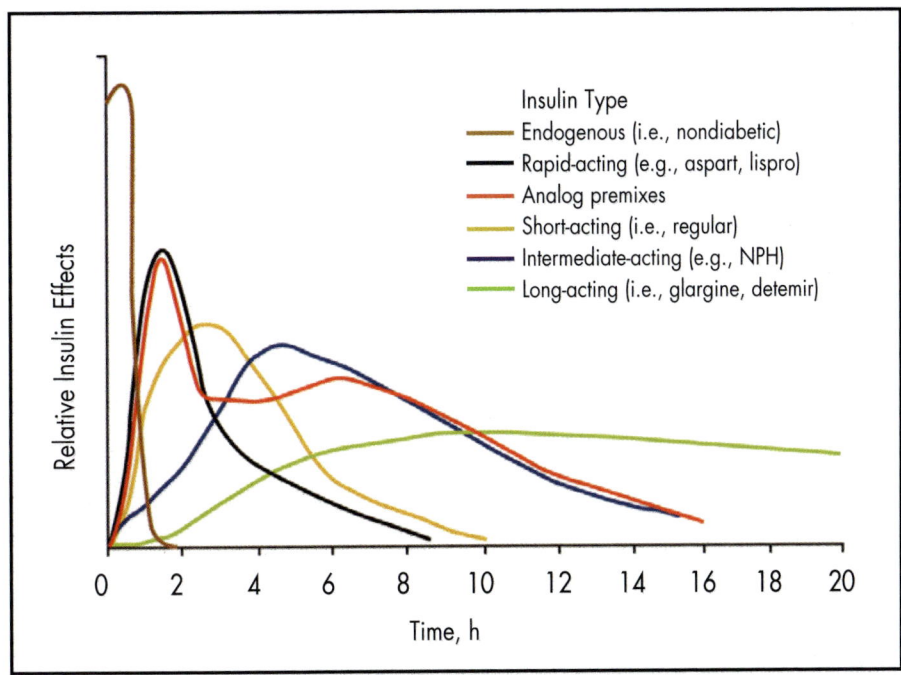

Figure 2.38. Pharmacokinetic profiles of human insulins compared with insulin analogs and endogenous insulin
Source: Reproduced with permission from Freeman JS. Insulin analog therapy: improving the match with physiologic insulin secretion. *J Am Osteopath Assoc.* 2009;109(1):26-36. Copyright © 2013 American Osteopathic Association. Reproduced with the consent of the American Osteopathic Association.

Table 2.78. Anticipated insulin dosage as a function of gestational age

Gestational Age (wk)	Anticipated Insulin Dose
6–18	0.7 units/kg
18–26	0.8 units/kg
26–36	0.9 units/kg
36–40	1.0 units/kg

Oral Hypoglycemics

- Glyburide is pregnancy category C.
- If elevated values, start with glyburide 2.5 mg PO with morning meal. Add 2.5 mg increments every week if level not achieved.
- If 10 mg is exceeded, change to twice daily dosing.
- If 20 mg is reached, change to insulin.
- Up to 85% will be well controlled on Glyburide (Jacobson 2005).

Insulin Management during Labor and Delivery (Coustan 2004; Jovanovic 1980)
- Usual dose of intermediate-acting insulin is given at bedtime.
- Morning dose of insulin is withheld.
- Intravenous infusion of normal saline is begun.
- Once active labor begins or glucose levels decrease to less than 70 mg/dL, the infusion is changed from saline to 5% dextrose and delivered at a rate of 100–150 cc/hr (2.5 mg/kg/min) to achieve a glucose level of approximately 100 mg/dL.
- Glucose levels are checked hourly using a bedside meter allowing for adjustment in the insulin or glucose infusion rate.
- Regular (short-acting) insulin is administered by intravenous infusion at a rate of 1.25 units/hr if glucose levels exceed 100 mg/dL.

Management of Diabetes in Active Labor
- Usual dose of intermediate-acting insulin is given at bedtime.
- Morning dose of insulin is withheld.
- Intravenous infusion of normal saline is begun.
- Once active labor begins or if FSBG is <150 mg/dL, give D5 normal saline at 125 mL/hr.
- Glucose levels are checked hourly using a bedside meter allowing for adjustment in the insulin or glucose infusion rate.
- Check ketones Q void.
- Use the following insulin scale to ensure normoglycemia at delivery.

Table 2.79. Insulin drip sliding scale for patients in labor

FSBG	Insulin Drip
<70	0
70–90	0.5 units/hr for DM I
91–110	1 units/hr for DM I
111–130	2 units/hr for DM I/DM II/GDM
131–150	3 units/hr
151–170	4 units/hr
171–200	5 units/hr
>200	Check urine ketones and call physician

DM I, type 1 diabetes; DM II, type II diabetes; GDM, Gestational diabetes.

Source: Personal communication Jeffrey Clayton Faig, MD, FACOG, FACP. Clinical Professor, Obstetrics and Gynecology—Maternal Fetal Medicine. Stanford University Medical Center.

Insulin-Dependent Diabetes and Pregnancy
Management of Insulin-Dependent Diabetics in Pregnancy
- ✓ HgBA1C preconception and during first trimester.
- Rate of malformations 22% for HgBA1C >8.5.
- Fetal cardiac echocardiogram at 22 weeks.
- Ophthalmology evaluation during first and third trimesters.
- 24 hour urine for creatinine clearance, total protein.
- Antenatal testing 2x/week starting at 32 weeks.
- Follow fetal growth in the third trimester and consider cesarean delivery if EFW >4500 g.

Table 2.80. Management of DKA during pregnancy

Evaluation	Therapy
Laboratory assessment	Arterial blood gas, then glucose, ketones, electrolytes q2 hr
Insulin	Low dose, intravenous regular insulin
	Loading dose: 0.2–0.4 units/kg
	Maintenance 2.0–10 units/hr
Fluids	Isotonic NaCl
	Total replacement in first 12 hr = 4–6 L
	500–1000 mL/hr for 2–4 hr
	250 mL/hr until 80% replaced
Glucose	Begin D5-NS when plasma glucose reaches 250 mg/dL
Potassium	If initially normal or reduced then add 40–60 mEq/L
	If initially elevated then give 20–30 mEq/L once levels begin to decline
Bicarbonate	Add one amp (44 mEq) to 1 L of 0.45 NS if pH is <7.10

Source: Landon MB. Diabetes mellitus and other endocrine diseases. In: Gabbe SG, Niebyl JR, Simpson JL, ed. *Obstetrics: Normal and Problem Pregnancies, 2nd Ed.* New York: Churchill Livingstone; 1991. Reproduced with the permission of the publisher.

Table 2.81. White classification of diabetes

Class	Onset	Duration	Vascular Disease
A	Any	Any	None
B	>20 yr old	<10 yr	None
C	10–19 yr old	10–19 yr	None
D	<10 yr old	>20 yr	Benign retinopathy
F	Any	Any	Nephropathy
R	Any	Any	Proliferative retinopathy
H	Any	Any	Heart disease
RT	Any	Any	Renal transplant

Source: Hare JW, White P. Gestational diabetes and the White classification. *Diabetes Care.* 1980;3:394-96.

HYPERTENSIVE DISORDERS OF PREGNANCY
Classification of Hypertensive Disorders of Pregnancy
Chronic Hypertension
- Hypertension present and observable before pregnancy or prior to 20th week of gestation.
- Hypertension defined as blood pressure >140 mm Hg systolic or 90 mm Hg diastolic.
- Persistence of hypertension beyond the usual postpartum period.
- Use of antihypertensive medications before pregnancy.

Table 2.82. Diagnostic criteria for preeclampsia

Blood pressure	• Greater than or equal to 140 mm Hg systolic or greater than or equal to 90 mm Hg diastolic on two occasions at least 4 hours apart after 20 weeks of gestation in a woman with a previously normal blood pressure • Greater than or equal to 160 mm Hg systolic or greater than or equal to 110 mm Hg diastolic; hypertension can be confirmed within a short interval (minutes) to facilitate timely antihypertensive therapy
and	
Proteinuria	• Greater than or equal to 300 mg per 24 hour urine collection (or this amount extrapolated from a timed collection) or • Protein/creatinine ratio greater than or equal to 0.3* • Dipstick reading of 1+ (used only if other quantitative methods not available)
Or, in the absence of proteinuria, new-onset hypertension with the new onset of any of the following:	
Thrombocytopenia	• Platelet count less than 100,000/microliter
Renal insufficiency	• Serum creatinine concentrations greater than 1.1 mg/dL or a doubling of the serum creatinine concentration in the absence of other renal disease
Impaired liver function	• Elevated blood concentrations of liver transaminases to twice normal concentration
Pulmonary edema	
Cerebral or visual symptoms	

*Each measured as mg/dL.
Source: Reproduced with permission from American College of Obstetricians and Gynecologists. Task Force on Hypertension in Pregnancy. *Hypertension in pregnancy.* Copyright © 2013 The American College of Obstetricians and Gynecologists.

Table 2.83. Severe features of preeclampsia (any of these findings)

- Systolic blood pressure of 160 mm Hg or higher, or diastolic blood pressure of 110 mm Hg or higher on two occasions at least 4 hours apart while the patient is on bed rest (unless antihypertensive therapy is initiated before this time)
- Thrombocytopenia (platelet count less than 100,000/microliter)
- Impaired liver function as indicated by abnormally elevated blood concentrations of liver enzymes (to twice normal concentration), severe persistent right upper quadrant or epigastric pain unresponsive to medication and not accounted for by alternative diagnoses, or both
- Progressive renal insufficiency (serum creatinine concentration greater than 1.1 mg/dL or a doubling of the serum creatinine concentration in the absence of other renal disease)
- Pulmonary edema
- New-onset cerebral or visual disturbances

Source: Reproduced with permission from American College of Obstetricians and Gynecologists. Task Force on Hypertension in Pregnancy. *Hypertension in pregnancy.* Copyright © 2013 The American College of Obstetricians and Gynecologists.

Hypertensive Disorders of Pregnancy — OBSTETRICS

Table 2.84. Risk factors for preeclampsia

- Primiparity
- Previous preeclamptic pregnancy
- Chronic hypertension or chronic renal disease or both
- History of thrombophilia
- Multifetal pregnancy
- In vitro fertilization
- Family history of preeclampsia
- Type I diabetes mellitus or type II diabetes mellitus
- Obesity
- Systemic lupus erythematosus
- Advanced maternal age (older than 40 years)

Source: Reproduced with permission from American College of Obstetricians and Gynecologists. Task Force on Hypertension in Pregnancy. *Hypertension in pregnancy.* Copyright © 2013 The American College of Obstetricians and Gynecologists.

Table 2.85. Preconception risk factors for preeclampsia

20–30%	Previous preeclampsia
50%	Previous preeclampsia at 28 wk
15–25%	Chronic hypertension
40%	Severe hypertension
25%	Renal disease
20%	PreGestational diabetes mellitus
10–15%	Class B/C diabetes
35%	Class F/R diabetes
10–40%	Thrombophilia
10–15%	Obesity/insulin resistance
10–20%	Age >35 years
10–15%	Family history of preeclampsia
6–7%	Nulliparity/primipaternity

Source: Reproduced with permission from Sibai BM. Preeclampsia: 3 preemptive tactics. *OBG Management.* 2005;17(2):20-32.© Copyright Frontline Medical Communications.

Table 2.86. Pregnancy-related risk factors for preeclampsia

Magnitude of Risk Depends On the Number of Factors	
2-fold normal	Unexplained midtrimester elevations of serum AFP, HCG, inhibin-A
10–30%	Abnormal uterine artery Doppler velocimetry
0–30%	Hydrops/hydropic degeneration of placenta
10–20%	Multifetal gestation (depends on number of fetuses and maternal age)
10%	Partner who fathered preeclampsia in another woman
8–10%	Gestational diabetes mellitus
8–10%	Limited sperm exposure (teenage pregnancy)
6–7%	Nulliparity/primipaternity
Limited data	Donor insemination, oocyte donation
Limited data	Unexplained persistent proteinuria or hematuria
Unknown	Unexplained fetal growth restriction

Source: Reproduced with permission from Sibai BM. Preeclampsia: 3 preemptive tactics. *OBG Management.* 2005;17(2):20-32.© Copyright Frontline Medical Communications.

Preeclampsia Superimposed upon Chronic Hypertension
- Prognosis worse than in either condition alone.
- Overdiagnosis is appropriate and unavoidable.
- Consider this diagnosis in following findings:
  - A sudden exacerbation of hypertension, or need to escalate the antihypertensive drug dose especially when previously well controlled with these medications
  - Sudden increase in liver enzymes to abnormal levels
  - Decrease in platelet count to <100,000/microliter
  - Symptoms such as right upper quadrant pain or severe headache
  - Pulmonary congestion or edema
  - New renal insufficiency (creatinine level doubling or increasing to or above 1.1 mg/dL in women without other renal disease)
  - Sudden, substantial, and sustained increase in protein excretion

Table 2.87. Complication rates in women with superimposed preeclampsia vs. women without hypertension

Complication	Without Hypertension (Per 1000 Cases)	Preeclampsia Superimposed On Chronic Hypertension (Per 1000 Cases)
Abruptio placentae	9.6	30.6
Thrombocytopenia	1.6	11.5
Disseminated intravascular coagulation	2.9	17.4
Pulmonary edema	0.2	6.4
Blood transfusion	1.5	16.3
Mechanical ventilation.	0.2	17.0

[a]US women, 1988–1997.

Source: Reproduced with permission from Sibai BM. Preeclampsia: 3 preemptive tactics. *OBG Management.* 2005;17(2):20-32.© Copyright Frontline Medical Communications.

Hypertensive Disorders of Pregnancy

OBSTETRICS

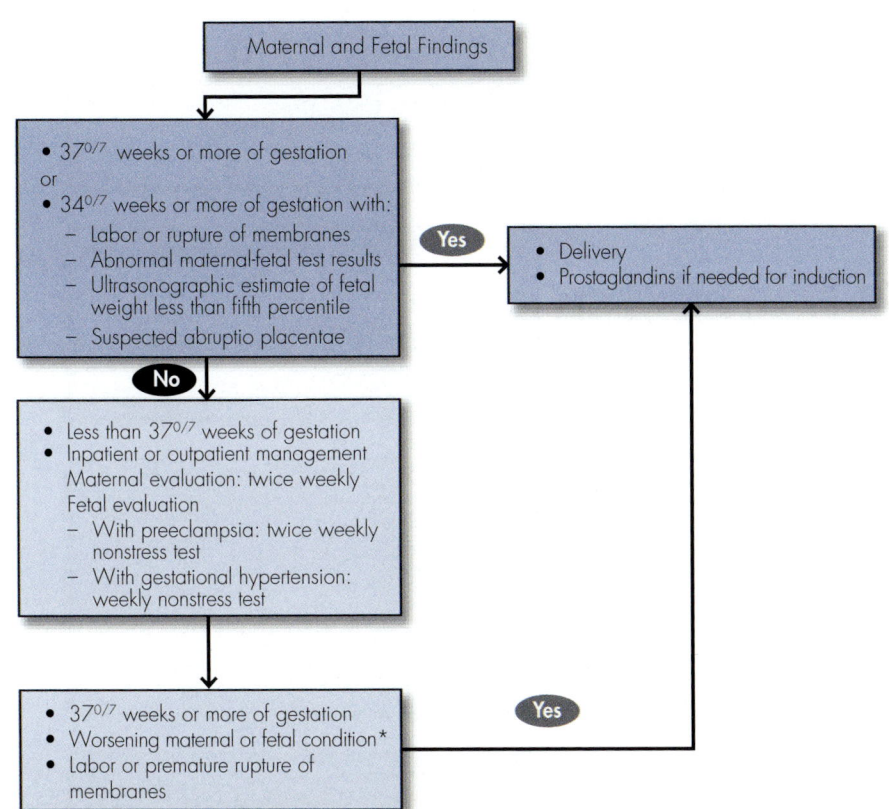

Figure 2.39. Management of gestational hypertension or preeclampsia without severe features
Source: Reproduced with permission from American College of Obstetricians and Gynecologists. Task Force on Hypertension in Pregnancy. Hypertension in pregnancy. Copyright © 2013 The American College of Obstetricians and Gynecologists.

OBSTETRICS

Hypertensive Disorders of Pregnancy

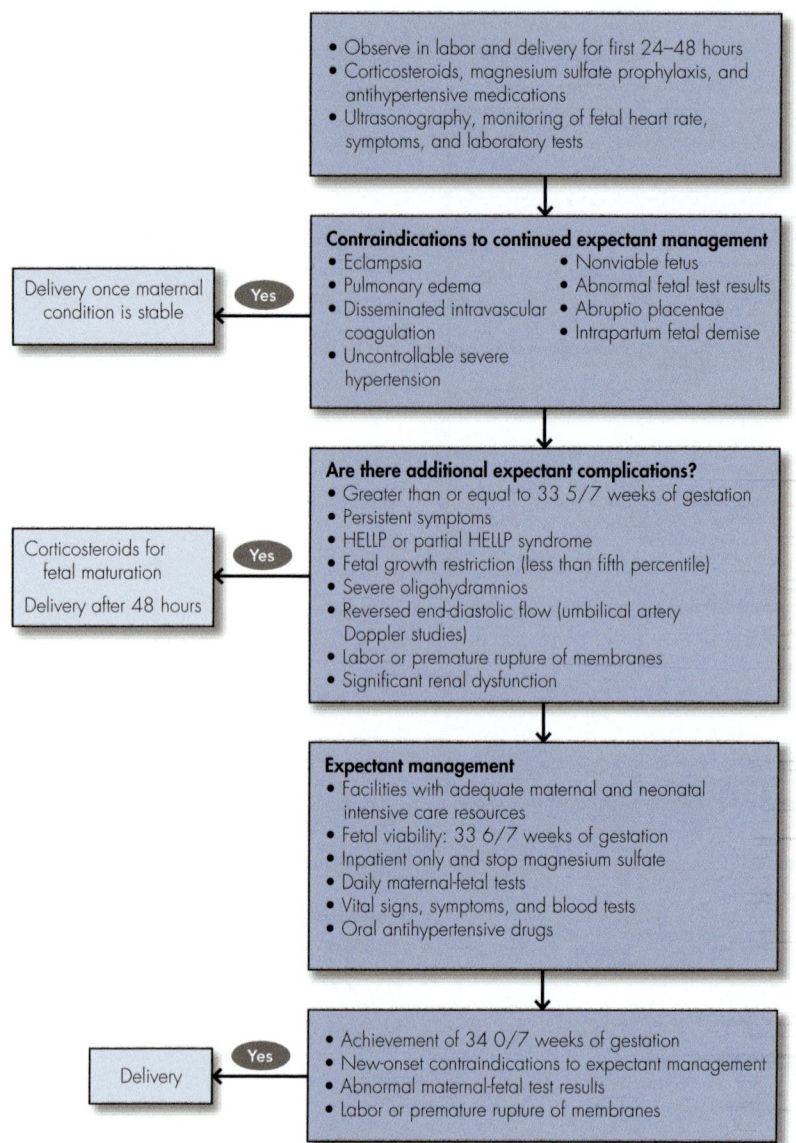

Figure 2.40. Management of severe preeclampsia at less than 34 weeks gestation
Source: Reproduced with permission from American College of Obstetricians and Gynecologists. Task Force on Hypertension in Pregnancy. Hypertension in pregnancy. Copyright © 2013 The American College of Obstetricians and Gynecologists.

Hypertensive Disorders of Pregnancy

Table 2.88. Order set for severe intrapartum or postpartum hypertension initial first-line management with labetalol

- Notify physician if systolic blood pressure (BP) measurement is greater than or equal to 160 mm Hg or if diastolic BP measurement is greater than or equal to 100 mm Hg.
- Institute fetal surveillance if undelivered and fetus is viable.
- If severe BP elevations persist for 15 minutes or more, administer labetalol (20 mg intravenously [IV] over 2 minutes).
- Repeat BP measurement in 10 minutes and record results.
- If either BP threshold is still exceeded, administer labetalol (40 mg IV over 2 minutes). If BP is below threshold, continue to monitor BP closely.
- Repeat BP measurement in 10 minutes and record results.
- If either BP threshold is still exceeded, administer labetalol (80 mg IV over 2 minutes). If BP is below threshold, continue to monitor BP closely.
- Repeat BP measurement in 10 minutes and record results.
- If either BP threshold is still exceeded, administer hydralazine (10 mg IV over 2 minutes). If BP is below threshold, continue to monitor BP closely.
- Repeat BP measurement in 20 minutes and record results.
- If either BP threshold is still exceeded, obtain emergency consultation from maternal-fetal medicine, internal medicine, anesthesia, or critical care subspecialists.
- Give additional antihypertensive medication per specific order.
- Once the aforementioned BP thresholds are achieved, repeat BP measurement every 10 minutes for 1 hour, then every 15 minutes for 1 hour, then every 30 minutes for 1 hour, and then every hour for 4 hours.
- Institute additional BP timing per specific order.

*Please note there may be adverse effects and contraindications.

Source: Reproduced with permission from American College of Obstetricians and Gynecologists. Committee on Obstetric Practice. Committee Opinion No. 623: Emergent therapy for acute-onset, severe hypertension during pregnancy and the postpartum period. *Obstet Gynecol.* 2015 Feb;125(2):521-25. Copyright © 2015 The American College of Obstetricians and Gynecologists.

Table 2.89. Order set for severe intrapartum or postpartum hypertension initial first-line management with hydralazine

- Notify physician if systolic blood pressure (BP) is greater than or equal to 160 mm Hg or if diastolic BP is greater than or equal to 110 mm Hg.
- Institute fetal surveillance if undelivered and fetus is viable.
- If severe BP elevations persist for 15 minutes or more, administer hydralazine (5 mg or 10 mg intravenously [IV] over 2 minutes).
- Repeat BP measurement in 20 minutes and record results.
- If either BP threshold is still exceeded, administer hydralazine (10 mg IV over 2 minutes). If BP is below threshold, continue to monitor BP closely.
- Repeat BP measurement in 20 minutes and record results.
- If either BP threshold is still exceeded, administer labetalol (20 mg IV over 2 minutes). If BP is below threshold, continue to monitor BP closely.
- Repeat BP measurement in 10 minutes and record results.
- If either BP threshold is still exceeded, administer labetalol (40 mg IV over 2 minutes) and obtain emergency consultation from maternal-fetal medicine, internal medicine, anesthesia, or critical care subspecialists.
- Give additional antihypertensive medication per specific order.
- Once the aforementioned BP thresholds are achieved, repeat BP measurement every 10 minutes for 1 hour, then every 15 minutes for 1 hour, then every 30 minutes for 1 hour, and then every hour for 4 hours.
- Institute additional BP timing per specific order.

*Please note there may be adverse effects and contraindications.

Source: Reproduced with permission from American College of Obstetricians and Gynecologists. Committee on Obstetric Practice. Committee Opinion No. 623: Emergent therapy for acute-onset, severe hypertension during pregnancy and the postpartum period. *Obstet Gynecol.* 2015 Feb;125(2):521-25. Copyright © 2015 The American College of Obstetricians and Gynecologists.

Hypertensive Disorders of Pregnancy — OBSTETRICS

Table 2.90. Order set for severe intrapartum or postpartum hypertension initial first-line management with oral nifedipine

- Notify physician if systolic blood pressure (BP) is greater than or equal to 160 mm Hg or if diastolic BP is greater than or equal to 110 mm Hg.
- Institute fetal surveillance if undelivered and fetus is viable.
- If severe BP elevations persist for 15 minutes or more, administer nifedipine† (10 mg orally).
- Repeat BP measurement in 20 minutes and record results.
- If either BP threshold is still exceeded, administer nifedipine capsules (20 mg orally). If BP is below threshold, continue to monitor BP closely.
- Repeat BP measurement in 20 minutes and record results.
- If either BP threshold is still exceeded, administer nifedipine capsules (20 mg orally). If BP is below threshold, continue to monitor BP closely.
- Repeat BP measurement in 20 minutes and record results.
- If either BP threshold is still exceeded, administer labetalol (40 mg intravenously over 2 minutes) and obtain emergency consultation from maternal-fetal medicine, internal medicine, anesthesia, or critical care subspecialists.
- Give additional antihypertensive medication per specific order.
- Once the aforementioned BP thresholds are achieved, repeat BP measurement every 10 minutes for 1 hour, then every 15 minutes for 1 hour, then every 30 minutes for 1 hour, and then every hour for 4 hours.
- Institute additional BP timing per specific order.

*Please note there may be adverse effects and contraindications.

†Capsules should be administered orally and not punctured or otherwise administered sublingually.

Source: Reproduced with permission from American College of Obstetricians and Gynecologists. Committee on Obstetric Practice. Committee Opinion No. 623: Emergent therapy for acute-onset, severe hypertension during pregnancy and the postpartum period. *Obstet Gynecol.* 2015 Feb;125(2):521-25. Copyright © 2015 The American College of Obstetricians and Gynecologists.

Table 2.91. Magnesium sulfate toxicity

MgSO4 Overdose	**Toxicity**
EKG changes	5–10 mEq/L
Loss of deep tendon reflexes	10 mEq/L
Respiratory suppression	15 mEq/L
Cardiovascular collapse	>25 mEq/L

Treatment of toxicity is: 1 gm Ca^{+2} gluconate IV push.

Table 2.92. Laboratory evaluation of preeclampsia

Test	Rationale
Hemoglobin and hematocrit	Hemoconcentration supports the diagnosis of preeclampsia and is an indicator of severity. Values may be decreased, however, if hemolysis accompanies the disease.
Platelet count	Thrombocytopenia suggests preeclampsia.
Quantification of protein excretion	Pregnancy hypertension with proteinuria should be considered preeclampsia (pure or superimposed) until it is proven otherwise.
Serum creatinine level	Abnormal or rising creatinine levels, especially in association with oliguria, suggest severe preeclampsia.
Serum Uric acid level	Increased Uric acid levels suggest the diagnosis of preeclampsia.
Serum transaminase levels	Rising serum transaminase levels suggest severe preeclampsia with hepatic involvement.
Serum albumin, lactic acid dehydrogenase, blood smear and coagulation profile	For women with severe disease, these values indicate the extent of endothelial leak (hypoalbuminemia), presence of hemolysis (LDH level, peripheral smear), and possible coagulopathy including thrombocytopenia.

LDH, lactate dehydrogenase.

Source: National High Blood Pressure Education Program Working Group Report on High Blood Pressure in Pregnancy, NIH Publication No. 00–3029, July 2000.

Table 2.93. Antihypertensive agents used for urgent blood pressure control in pregnancy

Drug	Dose	Comments
Labetalol	10–20 mg IV, then 20–80 mg every 20–30 min to a maximum dose of 300 mg or Constant infusion 1–2 mg/min IV	Considered a first-line agent Tachycardia is less common and fewer adverse effects Contraindicated in patients with asthma, heart disease, or congestive heart failure
Hydralazine	5 mg IV or IM, then 5–10 mg IV every 20–40 min or Constant infusion 0.5–10 mg/hr	Higher or frequent dosage associated with maternal hypotension, headaches, and fetal distress—may be more common than other agents
Nifedipine	10–20 mg orally, repeat in 30 minutes if needed; then 10–20 mg every 2–6 hours	May observe reflex tachycardia and headaches

IM, intramuscularly; IV, intravenously.

Source: Reproduced with permission from American College of Obstetricians and Gynecologists. Task Force on Hypertension in Pregnancy. *Hypertension in pregnancy.* Copyright © 2013 The American College of Obstetricians and Gynecologists.

Hypertensive Disorders of Pregnancy — OBSTETRICS

Table 2.94. Common oral antihypertensive agents in pregnancy

Drug	Dosage	Comments
Labetalol	200–2,400 mg/d orally in two to three divided doses	Well tolerated. Potential bronchoconstrictive effects. Avoid in patients with asthma and congestive heart failure
Nifedipine	30–120 mg/d orally of a slow-release preparation	Do not use sublingual form
Methyldopa	0.5–3 g/d orally in two to three divided doses	Childhood safety data up to 7 years of age. May not be as effective in control of severe hypertension
Thiazide diuretics	Depends on agent	Second-line agent
Angiotensin-converting enzyme inhibitors/angiotensin receptor blockers		Associated with fetal anomalies. Contraindicated in pregnancy and preconception period

Source: Reproduced with permission from American College of Obstetricians and Gynecologists. Task Force on Hypertension in Pregnancy. *Hypertension in pregnancy.* Copyright © 2013 The American College of Obstetricians and Gynecologists.

Eclampsia

Table 2.95. Signs and symptoms of eclampsia[a]

Condition	Frequency (%) In Women with Eclampsia	Remarks
Signs		
Hypertension	85	Should be documented on at least 2 occasions more than 6 hr apart
Severe: 160/110 mm Hg or more	20–54	
Mild: 140–160/90–110 mm Hg	30–60	
No hypertension	16	
Proteinuria	85	
At least 1+ on dipstick	48	
At least 3+ on dipstick	14	
No proteinuria	15	
Symptoms		
At least 1 of the following:	33–75	Clinical symptoms may occur before or after a convulsion
Headache	30–70	Persistent, occipital, or frontal
Right upper quadrant or epigastric pain	12–20	
Visual changes	19–32	Blurred vision, photophobia
Altered mental changes	4–5	

[a]Summary of 5 series.

Source: Reproduced with permission from Sibai BM. Managing an eclamptic patient. *OBG Management.* 2005:37-50. © Copyright Frontline Medical Communications.

Table 2.96. Usual times of onset of eclampsia[a]

Onset	Frequency (%)	Remarks
Antepartum	38–53	Maternal and perinatal mortality, and the incidence of complications and underlying disease, are higher in antepartum eclampsia, especially in early cases
<20 wk	1.5	
21 to 27 wk	7.5	
>28 wk	91	
Intrapartum	18–36	Intrapartum eclampsia more closely resembles postpartum disease than antepartum cases
Postpartum	11–44	Late postpartum eclampsia occurs more than 48 hr but less than 4 wk after delivery
<48 hr	7–39	
>48 hr	5–26	

[a]Summary of 5 series.

Source: Reproduced with permission from Sibai BM. Managing an eclamptic patient. *OBG Management.* 2005:37-50. © Copyright Frontline Medical Communications.

Table 2.97. Maternal complications associated with preeclampsia

Complication	Rate (%)	Remarks
Death	0.5–2.0	Risk of death is higher: Older than 30 yr of age; No prenatal care; African Americans; Onset of preeclampsia or eclampsia before 28 wk gestation
Intracerebral hemorrhage	<1	Usually related to several risk factors
Aspiration pneumonia	2–3	Heightened risk of maternal hypoxemia and acidosis
Disseminated coagulopathy	3–5	Regional anesthesia is contraindicated in these patients, and there is a heightened risk of hemorrhagic shock
Pulmonary edema	3–5	Heightened risk of maternal hypoxemia and acidosis
Acute renal failure	5–9	Usually seen in association with abruptio placentae, maternal hemorrhage, and prolonged maternal hypotension
Abruptio placentae	7–10	Can occur after a convulsion; suspect it if fetal bradycardia or late decelerations persist
HELLP syndrome	10–15	

HELLP, hemolysis, elevated liver enzymes, and low platelets.

Source: Reproduced with permission from Sibai BM. Managing an eclamptic patient. *OBG Management.* 2005:37-50. © Copyright Frontline Medical Communications.

Table 2.98. Management of eclamptic seizure

Avoid Maternal Injury
Insert padded tongue blade
Avoid inducing gag reflex
Elevate padded bedside rails
Use physical restraints as needed

Maintain Oxygenation to Mother and Fetus
Apply face mask with or without oxygen reservoir at 8–10 L/min
Monitor oxygenation and metabolic status via
    Transcutaneous pulse oximetry
    Arterial blood gases (sodium bicarbonate administered accordingly)
Correct oxygenation and metabolic status before administering anesthetics that may depress myocardial function

Minimize Aspiration
Place patient in lateral decubitus position (which also maximizes uterine blood flow and venous return)
Suction vomitus and oral secretions
Obtain chest X-ray after the convulsion is controlled to rule out aspiration

Source: Reproduced with permission from Sibai BM. Managing an eclamptic patient. *OBG Management.* 2005:37-50. © Copyright Frontline Medical Communications.

Table 2.99. Evaluation and management of women at risk for preeclampsia recurrence

Preconception

- Identify risk factors (i.e., type 2 diabetes mellitus, obesity, hypertension, and family history).
- Review outcome of previous pregnancy (abruptio placentae, fetal death, fetal growth restriction, and gestational age at delivery).
- Perform baseline metabolic profile and urinalysis.
- Optimize maternal health.
- Supplement with folic acid.

First Trimester

- Perform the following:
  - Ultrasonography for assessment of gestational age and fetal number
  - Baseline metabolic profile and complete blood count
  - Baseline urinalysis
- Continue folic acid supplementation.
- Offer first-trimester combined screening.
- For women with prior preeclampsia that led to delivery before 34 weeks of gestation or occurring in more than one pregnancy, offer low-dose aspirin late in the first trimester and discuss the risks and benefits of low-dose aspirin with other women.

Second Trimester

- Counsel patient about signs and symptoms of preeclampsia beginning at 20 weeks of gestation; reinforce this information with printed handouts.
- Monitor for signs and symptoms of preeclampsia.
- Monitor blood pressure at prenatal visits, with nursing contacts, or at home.
- Perform ultrasonography at 18–22 weeks of gestation for fetal anomaly evaluation and to rule out molar gestation.
- Hospitalize for severe gestational hypertension, severe fetal growth, or recurrent preeclampsia.

Third Trimester

- Monitor for signs and symptoms of preeclampsia.
- Monitor blood pressure at prenatal visits, with nursing contacts, or at home.
- Perform the following as indicated by clinical situation:
  - Laboratory testing
  - Serial ultrasonography for fetal growth and amniotic fluid assessment
  - Umbilical artery Doppler with nonstress test, biophysical profile, or both
- Hospitalize for severe gestational hypertension or recurrent preeclampsia.

Source: Reproduced with permission from American College of Obstetricians and Gynecologists. Task Force on Hypertension in Pregnancy. *Hypertension in pregnancy.* Copyright © 2013 The American College of Obstetricians and Gynecologists.

Postpartum Hypertension

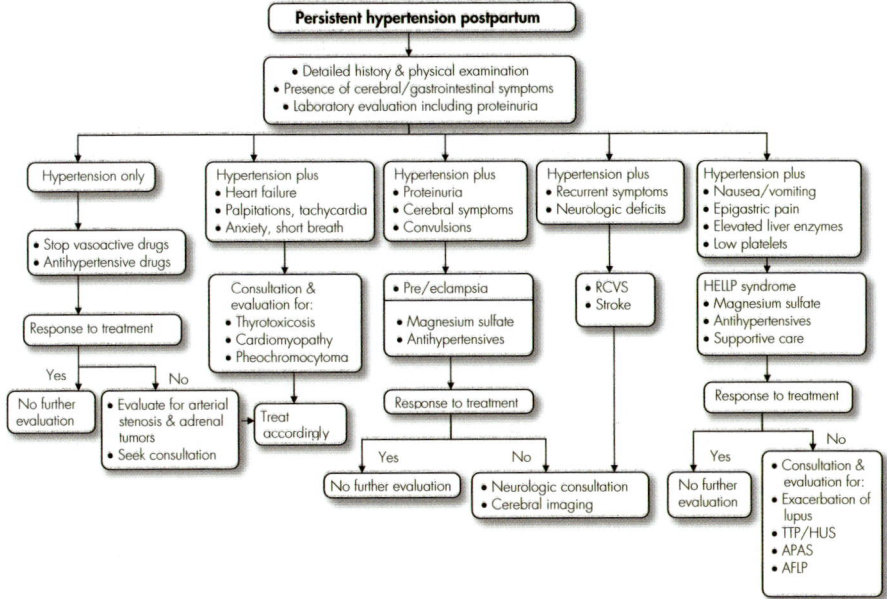

Figure 2.41. Recommended evaluation and management of women with postpartum hypertension

AFLP, acute fatty liver of pregnancy; APAS, antiphospholipid antibody syndrome; HELLP, hemolysis, elevated liver enzymes, and low platelet; HUS, hemolytic uremic syndrome; RCVS, reversible cerebral vasoconstriction syndrome; TTP, thrombotic thrombocytopenic purpura.

Source: Reproduced with permission from Sibai BM. Etiology and management of postpartum hypertension-preeclampsia. *Am J Obstet Gynecol.* 2012 Jun;206(6):470-75. Copyright © 2012 Elsevier.

Table 2.100. Etiology and differential diagnosis of postpartum hypertension

Etiology	Key Findings to Consider
New-onset hypertension-preeclampsia	Onset 3–6 d postpartum without headaches
Volume overload	Large volume of fluids, regional analgesia, delayed mobilization
Medications/drugs	Nonsteroidal analgesics, ergot derivatives
Ibuprofen, indomethacin	Peripheral and cerebral vasoconstriction, headaches
Phenylpropanolamine, ephedrine	Peripheral and cerebral vasoconstriction, headaches
Ergotamine, ergonovine	Vasoconstriction, headaches, nausea, vomiting, seizures
Persistence of GH-preeclampsia	Preexisting condition antepartum/in labor
Late-onset eclampsia	Headaches, visual changes, seizures, absent neurologic deficits
HELLP syndrome	Nausea/vomiting, epigastric pain, low platelets, increased liver enzymes
Preexisting/undiagnosed hypertension	Hypertension prior to pregnancy, or <20 wk
Preexisting renal disease	Proteinuria or hematuria <20 wk
Hyperthyroidism	Palpitations tachycardia, sweating, dry skin, heart failure
Primary hyperaldosteronism	Refractory hypertension, hypokalemia, metabolic alkalosis
Pheochromocytoma	Paroxysmal hypertension, headaches, chest pain, hyperglycemia
Renal artery stenosis	Hypertension that is refractory to treatment
Cerebral vasoconstriction syndrome	Sudden thunderclap headaches, visual changes, neurologic deficits
Cerebral venous thrombosis/stroke	Onset 3–7 d, gradual or acute headaches, seizures, neurologic deficits
TTP/hemolytic uremic syndrome	Hemolysis, severe thrombocytopenia, neurologic symptoms, normal liver enzymes

GH, gestational hypertension; HELLP, hemolysis, elevated liver enzymes, and low platelet; TTP, thrombotic thrombocytopenic purpura.

Source: Reproduced with permission from Sibai BM. Etiology and management of postpartum hypertension-preeclampsia. *Am J Obstet Gynecol.* 2012 Jun;206(6):470-75. Copyright © 2012 Elsevier.

Acute Fatty Liver, HELLP, Hepatitis, Etc.

Table 2.101. Frequency of various signs and symptoms among imitators of preeclampsia–eclampsia

Signs and Symptoms	HELLP Syndrome	AFLP	TTP	HUS	Exacerbation of SLE
Hypertension	85	50	20–75	80–90	80 with APA, nephritis
Proteinuria	90–95	30–50	With hematuria	80–90	100 with nephritis
Fever	Absent	25–32	20–50	NR	Common during flare
Jaundice	5–10	40–90	Rare	Rare	Absent
Nausea and vomiting	40	50–80	Common	Common	Only with APA
Abdominal pain	60–80	35–50	Common	Common	Only with APA
Central nervous system	40–60	30–40	60–70	NR	50 with APA

AFLP, acute fatty liver of pregnancy; APA, antiphospholipid antibodies with or without catastrophic antiphospholipid syndrome; Common, reported as the most common presentation; HELLP, hemolysis, elevated liver enzymes, low platelets; HUS, hemolytic uremic syndrome; NR, values are not reported; SLE, systemic lupus erythematosus; TTP, thrombotic thrombocytopenic purpura.

Data are in percentages.

Source: Reproduced with permission from Sibai BM. Imitators of preeclampsia. *Obstet Gynecol.* 2007 Apr;109(4):956-66. Copyright © 2007 The American College of Obstetricians and Gynecologists.

Table 2.102. Frequency and severity of laboratory findings among imitators of preeclampsia–eclampsia

Laboratory Findings	HELLP Syndrome	AFLP	TTP	HUS	Exacerbation of SLE
Thrombocytopenia (less than 100,000/mm³)	More than 20,000	More than 50,000	20,000 or less	More than 20,000	More than 20,000
Hemolysis (%)	50–100	15–20	100	100	14–23 with APA
Anemia (%)	Less than 50%	Absent	100	100	14–23 with APA
DIC (%)	Less than 20	50–100	Rare	Rare	Rare
Hypoglycemia (%)	Absent	50–100	Absent	Absent	Absent
VW factor multimers (%)	Absent	Absent	80–90	80	Less than 10
ADAMTS13 less than 5% (%)	Absent	Absent	33–100	Rare	Rare
Impaired renal function (%)	50	90–100	30	100	40–80
LDH (IU/L)	600 or more	Variable	More than 1000	More than 1000	With APA
Elevated ammonia (%)	Rare	50	Absent	Absent	Absent
Elevated bilirubin (%)	50–60	100	100	NA	Less than 10
Elevated transaminases (%)	100	100	Usually mild*	Usually mild*	With APA

AFLP, acute fatty liver of pregnancy; ADAMTS, von Willebrand factor-cleaving metalloprotease; APA, antiphospholipid antibodies; DIC, disseminated intravascular coagulopathy; HELLP, hemolysis, elevated liver enzymes, low platelets; HUS, hemolytic uremic syndrome; LDH, lactic dehydrogenase; NA, values are not available; SLE, systemic lupus erythematosus; TTP, thrombotic thrombocytopenic purpura; VW, von Willebrand.

*Levels less than 100 IU/L.

Source: Reproduced with permission from Sibai BM. Imitators of preeclampsia. *Obstet Gynecol.* 2007 Apr;109(4):956-66. Copyright © 2007 The American College of Obstetricians and Gynecologists.

Table 2.103. Characteristics of common liver disease in pregnancy

	Fatty Liver of Pregnancy	Acute Viral Hepatitis	HELLP Syndrome/ Preeclampsia/ Eclampsia	Cholestasis of Pregnancy	Hemolytic Uremic Syndrome	Thrombotic Thrombocytopenic Purpura
Onset (I/II/III trimester)	II/III, most greater than 35 weeks, rare reports less than 30 weeks	Any	II/III (after 20 weeks)	III, rare reports II	Any	Any, 60% less than 24 weeks
Clinical findings	Malaise, nausea/emesis, jaundice, mental status changes, abdominal pain, ± hemorrhage, ± preeclampsia	Malaise, nausea/emesis, jaundice, abdominal pain	Malaise, hypertension, proteinuria, nausea, abdominal pain, rare jaundice ± seizures ± oliguria ± coagulopathy	Pruritus (worst in PM, palms and soles) ± jaundice	Hypertension, acute renal failure, nausea/emesis, may have fever and neurologic findings, hallmarks microangiopathic anemia, severe thrombocytopenia	Often neurologic findings, fever and renal dysfunction, hallmarks microangiopathic anemia, severe thrombocytopenia
Laboratory Transaminases (units/mL)	↑ Usually less than 500	↑ Commonly greater than 1,000	Normal-↑ 50× (more if liver hematoma)	↑(usually less than 300)	Usually normal ↑ (unconjugated)	Usually normal ↑ (unconjugated)

(continued)

OBSTETRICS — Hypertensive Disorders of Pregnancy

	Fatty Liver of Pregnancy	Acute Viral Hepatitis	HELLP Syndrome/ Preeclampsia/ Eclampsia	Cholestasis of Pregnancy	Hemolytic Uremic Syndrome	Thrombotic Thrombocytopenic Purpura
Bilirubin (mg/dL)	↑	±↑	↑occasionally (usually less than 2–3 times)	Often ↑(usually less than 5)	Usually normal	Usually normal
Prothrombin time	↑	±↑	Normal unless DIC/intrauterine fetal distress/ abruptio placentae	Usually normal; may be ↑	Usually normal	Usually normal
Alkaline phosphatase		↑occasionally	↑ (up to 4 times normal)			
Other	↑ Ammonia, very ↓ antithrombin III, ↓ platelets, ↓ fibrinogen, ↑ WBC, ↑ creatinine, proteinuria, ↓ glucose	+ hepatitis serology, ↓ antithrombin III	Moderately ↓ antithrombin III, proteinuria, ↓ platelets, ↑ creatinine, ↑ Uric acid	↑serum bile acids	Normal antithrombin III, usually normal fibrinogen, ↑WBC, ↓ platelets (often less than 20,000), normal–slightly ↑ creatinine, ± proteinuria	Normal antithrombin III, usually normal fibrinogen, ↑ WBC, ↓ platelets (often less than 20,000), normal–slightly ↑ creatinine, ± proteinuria
Liver histopathology	Centrilobular microvesicular fat, cholestasis	Marked inflammation and necrosis	Periportal fibrin deposits, hemorrhagic hepatocellular necrosis, inflammation	Centrilobular cholestasis, no inflammation	Unknown	Unknown
Treatment	Immediate delivery, supportive	Supportive	MgSO$_4$ seizure prophylaxis, delivery (delayed in very selected preterm cases), antihypertensive treatment	Ursodeoxycholic acid, corticosteroids, cholestyramine all of reported benefit, vitamin K	Plasma exchange, FFP infusion pending initiation of plasma exchange, corticosteroids/ antiplatelet agents	Plasma exchange, FFP infusion pending initiation of plasma exchange, corticosteroids/ antiplatelet agents

DIC, disseminated intravascular coagulation; FFP, fresh frozen plasma; MgSO$_4$, magnesium sulfate; WBC, white blood cell count.

Reproduced with permission from Ko HH, Yoshida E. Acute fatty liver of pregnancy. *Can J Gastroenterol.* 2006;20(1):25-30.

INTRAUTERINE FETAL DEMISE

Inspect fetus and placenta:
- Weight, head circumference, and length of fetus
- Weight of placenta
- Photographs of fetus and placenta
- Frontal and profile photographs of whole body, face, extremities, palms, and any abnormalities
- Document finding and abnormalities

↓

Obtain consent from parents for cytologic specimens:
- Obtain cytologic specimens with sterile techniques and instruments
- Acceptable cytologic specimens (at least one)
  - Amniotic fluid obtained by amniocentesis at time of prenatal diagnosis of demise: particularly valuable if delivery is not expected imminently
  - Placental block (1 × 1) cm taken from below the cord insertion site on the unfixed placenta
  - Umbilical cord segment (1.5 cm)
  - Internal fetal tissue specimen, such as costochondral junction or patella; skin is not recommended
- Place specimens in a sterile tissue culture medium of lactated Ringer's solution and keep at room temperature when transported to cytology laboratory

↓

Obtain parental consent for fetal autopsy

↓   ↓

Fetal autopsy and placental pathology (may include fetal whole-body X-ray) | If no consent is given for autopsy, send placenta alone for pathology

Figure 2.42. Flowchart for fetal and placental evaluation following fetal demise
Source: Reproduced with permission from ACOG Practice Bulletin No. 102: Management of stillbirth. *Obstet Gynecol.* 2009 Mar;113(3):748-61. Copyright © 2009 The American College of Obstetricians and Gynecologists.

Table 2.104. Estimate of stillbirth risk for selected maternal risk factors

Condition	Prevalence	Estimated Rate of Stillbirth	OR*
All pregnancies		6.4/1000	1.0
Low-risk pregnancies	80%	4.0–5.5/1000	0.86
Hypertensive disorders			
Chronic hypertension	6%–10%	6–25/1000	1.5–2.7
Pregnancy-induced hypertension			
Mild	5.8%–7.7%	9–51/1000	1.2–4.0
Severe	1.3%–3.3%	12–29/1000	1.8–4.4
Diabetes			
Treated with diet	2.5%–5%	6–10/1000	1.2–2.2
Treated with insulin	2.4%	6–35/1000	1.7–7.0
SLE	<1%	40–150/1000	6–20
Renal disease	<1%	15–200/1000	2.2–30
Thyroid disorders	0.2%–2%	12–20/1000	2.2–3.0
Thrombophilia	1%–5%	18–40/1000	2.8–5.0
Cholestasis of pregnancy	<0.1%	12–30/1000	1.8–4.4
Smoking >10 cigarettes	10%–20%	10–15/1000	1.7–3.0
Obesity (prepregnancy)			
BMI 25–29.9 kg/m^2	21%	12–15/1000	1.9–2.7
BMI >30	20%	13–18/1000	2.1–2.8
Low educational attainment (<12 yr vs. 12 yr+)	30%	10–13/1000	1.6–2.0
Previous growth-restricted infant (<10%)	6.7%	12–30/1000	2–4.6
Previous stillbirth	0.5%–1.0%	9–20/1000	1.4–3.2
Multiple gestation			
Twins	2.7%	12/1000	1.0–2.8
Triplets	0.14%	34/1000	2.8–3.7
Advanced maternal age (reference <35 yr)			
35–39 yr	15%–18%	11–14/1000	1.8–2.2
40 yr+	2%	11–21/1000	1.8–3.3
Black women compared with white women	15%	12–14/1000	2.0–2.2

*OR of the factor present compared to the risk factor absent.

Source: Reproduced with permission from Fretts RC. Etiology and prevention of stillbirth. *Am J Obstet Gynecol.* 2005 Dec;193(6):1923-35. Copyright 2005 Elsevier.

Table 2.105. Elements of the stillbirth evaluation

Key Components	Details	Comments
Patient history	Family history • Recurrent spontaneous abortions • Venous thromboembolism or pulmonary embolism • Congenital anomaly or abnormal karyotype • Hereditary condition or syndrome • Developmental delay • Consanguinity	
	Maternal history • Prior venous thromboembolism or pulmonary embolism • Diabetes mellitus • Chronic hypertension • Thrombophilia • Systemic lupus erythematosus • Autoimmune disease • Epilepsy • Severe anemia • Heart disease • Tobacco, alcohol, drug, or medication abuse	
	Obstetric history • Recurrent miscarriages • Previous child with anomaly, hereditary condition, or growth restriction • Previous gestational hypertension or preeclampsia • Previous Gestational diabetes mellitus • Previous placental abruption • Previous fetal demise	
	Current pregnancy • Maternal age • Gestational age at fetal death • Medical conditions complicating pregnancy 　○ Hypertension 　○ Gestational diabetes mellitus 　○ Systemic lupus erythematosus 　○ Cholestasis • Pregnancy weight gain and body mass index • Complications of multifetal gestation, such as twin-twin transfusion syndrome, twin reversed arterial perfusion syndrome, and discordant growth • Placental abruption • Abdominal trauma • Preterm labor or rupture of membranes • Gestational age at onset of prenatal care • Abnormalities seen on an ultrasound image • Infections or chorioamnionitis	

(continued)

Key Components	Details	Comments
Fetal autopsy	If patient declines, external evaluation by a trained perinatal pathologist. Other options include photographs, X-ray imaging, ultrasonography, magnetic resonance imaging, and sampling of tissues, such as blood or skin.	Provides important information in approximately 30% of cases
Fetal karyotype	Amniocentesis before delivery provides the greatest yield (84%). Umbilical cord proximal to placenta if amniocentesis declined (30%). Fluorescence in situ hybridization may be useful if fetal cells cannot be cultured.	Abnormalities found approximately 8%
Placental examination	Includes evaluation for signs of viral or bacterial infection. Discuss available tests with pathologist.	Provides additional information in 30% of cases. Infection is more common in preterm stillbirth (19% versus 2% at term)

Maternal evaluation at time of demise	• Complete blood count
	• Fetal-maternal hemorrhage screen: Kleihauer–Betke test or comparable test for fetal cells in maternal circulation
	• Human parvovirus B-19 immunoglobulin G and immunoglobulin M antibody
	• Syphilis
	• Lupus anticoagulant
	• Anticardiolipin antibodies
	• Thyroid-stimulating hormone
	• Thrombophilia (selected cases only)
	  ◦ Factor V Leiden
	  ◦ Prothrombin gene mutation
	  ◦ Antithrombin III
	  ◦ Fasting homocysteine
		Routine testing for thrombophilias is controversial and may lead to unnecessary interventions. Consider in cases with severe placental pathology and or growth restriction, or in the setting of a personal or family history of thromboembolic disease

Postpartum	Protein S and protein C activity (selected cases) Parental karyotype (if appropriate)	
In selected cases	Indirect Coombs test	If not performed previously in pregnancy
	Glucose screening (oral glucose tolerance test, hemoglobin A1C)	In the large for gestational age baby
	Toxicology screen	In cases of placental abruption or when drug use is suspected
Unproven benefit	Antinuclear antibody test	Many times is an incidental finding and may lead to unnecessary interventions
	Serology for toxoplasmosis, rubella, cytomegalovirus, herpes simplex virus	Rarely helpful, infection causing death is made by history and examining the baby, placenta, and cord
Developing technology	Comparative genomic hybridization Testing for single-gene mutations Testing for confined placental mosaicism and nucleic acid-based testing for infection	The value of these has not yet been established

Source: Reproduced with permission from ACOG Practice Bulletin No. 102: Management of stillbirth. *Obstet Gynecol.* 2009 Mar;113(3):748-61. Copyright © 2009 The American College of Obstetricians and Gynecologists.

NONIMMUNE HYDROPS
Evaluation

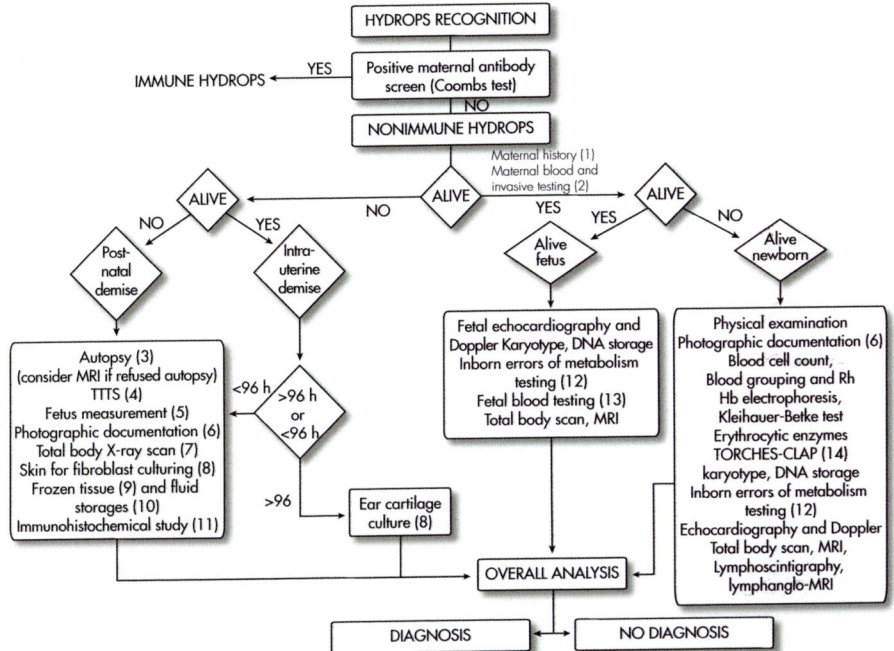

Figure 2.43. Algorithm for the evaluation of nonimmune hydrops

(1) *Maternal history.* Consider collagen-vascular diseases, organ transplant, blunt abdominal trauma, coagulopathies, sexually transmitted disorders, thyroid disorders, diabetes mellitus, viral infections, teratogenics through occupation, pets or place of living, and jaundice in other family member. Consider maternal medication use: indomethacin, sodium diclofenac, or potentially teratogenic drugs during pregnancy; prior administration of blood product; risks of illicit drug use. Determine ethnicity and chances for hemoglobinopathies in the population from which parents originate. Exclude immune hydrops. Check history of previous pregnancies: jaundice in previous child, twin-to-twin tranfusion syndrome (TTTS; see point 4), genetic disorders in earlier fetuses and children, chromosomal abnormalities, inborn errors of metabolism (see point 12), congenital malformations, cardiac defects, fetal death, polydramnios, torches-clap (see point 14).

(2) *Maternal blood and invasive testing.* Blood cell count, blood grouping and Rh, hgb electrophoresis, Kleihauer-Betke test, erythrocytic enzymes (include at least G6PD, pyruvate kinase, and glucose phosphate isomerase), torches-clap, serum alpha-fetoprotein, maternal anti-ssa/ssb antibodies, karyotype, DNA storage, inborn errors of metabolism, total body scan, and MRI.

(3) *Autopsy.* The value of autopsy can not be overestimated. If consent to autopsy is refused, a total body MRI may be a noninvasive and acceptable alternative for the family involved.

(4) *TTTS.* Twin-to-twin transfusion syndrome, including acardiac parasitic twin.

(5) *Fetal measurements.* Length, weight, and skull circumference are obligatory. Foot length can be used to determine gestational age. Other useful measurements can be inner canthal distance, outer canthal distances, philtrum length, and ear length. In severe hydrops, some of the obtained values may be unreliable.

(continued)

(6) *Photographic documentation.* A full body picture, facial pictures in two directions, and pictures of any other structure that seems abnormal can be an important tool in diagnosis. Digital photographs are advisable, as such pictures can be more easily used in consultations.

(7) *Total body X-ray scan.* A total body radiograph in two directions is useful and will allow diagnosis of most skeletal dysplasias and dysostoses. Detailed views of the hands and feet should be made if the suspicion of a skeletal dysplasia or dysostosis is high.

(8) *Skin for fibroblast culturing.* A skin specimen (diameter 3–5 mm) should be collected and placed in culture medium. If culture media are unavailable, the skin specimen can be placed in sterile saline for a short time only. Do not allow specimen to freeze. It is our experience ear cartilage is usually the tissue that remains the longest viable. If there is intrauterine demise and delivery will be induced using prostaglandins, it is advisable to obtain amnion cells before induction of the delivery, as growth of fibroblasts is usually very poor after prostaglandins.

(9) *Frozen tissue storage.* Include specimen from muscle, heart, brain, liver, intestine, kidney, peripheral nerve, bone marrow, conjunctiva, amniocytes, and placenta. The specimens should be frozen as soon as possible at −70°C if available, or otherwise at −20°C. Tissue specimens should be stored in a nonfixed way and not treated with a preservative.

(10) *Fluid storages.* Parental informed consent. Include plasma, blood, urine, visceral effusion, bile, cerebrospinal fluid. Use filter paper for adjunctive storage; the specimen should be allowed to dry. Post-mortem blood specimen collection is possible during many hours after demise by intracardiac puncture. Urine may be obtained by swabbing the bladder. Bile collection is obtained by direct gallbladder puncture. Cerebrospinal fluid collection is obtained by anterior fontanel puncture.

(11) *Immunohistochemical studies.* Routine staining on five microtome sections, using as monoclonal antibodies at least a cd 31 antibody, a cd 34 antibody, a smooth muscle actin antibody, and podoplanin (d2-40) is advisable. Inclusion of specimens from the nuchal region is useful.

(12) *Inborn errors of metabolism testing.* Consider lysosomal storage diseases: lysosomal enzyme and molecular analysis in cultured amniocytes or cell line from trophoblast. Hydrops fetalis has been described in Gaucher disease type II, Morquio disease, Hurler syndrome, Sly syndrome, Farber disease, gm1 gangliosidosis, i-cell disease, Niemann-pick disease type A and type C, infantile sialic acid storage disorder, alpha-neuroaminidase deficiency, multiple sulfatase deficiency, and Wolman disease. Consider also nonlysosomal diseases, including glycogenosis type IV, long-chain hydroxy-acyl coa dehydrogenase deficiency, CDG type1A, CDG type i/ix, hypothyroidism, carnitine deficiency, and Smith-Lemli-Opitz syndrome.

(13) *Fetal blood testing.* Consider fetal karyotype, fetal complete blood count, hemoglobin electrophoresis, torches-clap, fetal albumin, and inborn errors of metabolism.

(14) *Torches-clap.* Toxoplasma gondii, rubella virus, cytomegalovirus, herpes simplex virus, enterovirus, syphilis, chickenpox [varicella-zoster] virus, lyme disease [borrelia burgdoferi], AIDS, parvovirus B19.

Source: Reproduced with permission from Bellini C, Hennekam RCM, Bonioli E. A diagnostic flow chart for NONIMMUNE HYDROPS fetalis. *Am J Med Gen.* 2009;149A(5):852-53. Copyright © 2009 Wiley-Liss, Inc.

Table 2.106. Etiologies of nonimmune hydrops fetalis

Cause	Cases	Mechanism
Cardiovascular	17–35%	Increased central venous pressure
Chromosomal	7–16%	Cardiac anomalies, lymphatic dysplasia, abnormal myelopoiesis
Hematologic	4–12%	Anemia, high output cardiac failure; hypoxia (alpha thalassemia)
Infectious	5–7%	Anemia, anoxia, endothelial cell damage, and increased capillary permeability
Thoracic	6%	Vena caval obstruction or increased intrathoracic pressure with impaired venous return
Twin-twin transfusion	3–10%	Hypervolemia and increased central venous pressure
Urinary tract abnormalities	2–3%	Urinary ascites; nephrotic syndrome with hypoproteinemia
Gastrointestinal	0.5–4%	Obstruction of venous return; gastrointestinal obstruction and infarction with protein loss and decreased colloid osmotic pressure
Lymphatic dysplasia	5–6%	Impaired venous return
Tumors, including chorioangiomas	2–3%	Anemia, high output cardiac failure, hypoproteinemia
Skeletal dysplasias	3–4%	Hepatomegaly, hypoproteinemia, impaired venous return
Syndromic	3–4%	Various
Inborn errors of metabolism	1–2%	Visceromegaly and obstruction of venous return, decreased erythropoiesis and anemia, and/or hypoproteinemia
Miscellaneous	3–15%	
Unknown	15–25%	

Source: Reproduced with permission from Society for Maternal-Fetal Medicine (SMFM), Norton ME, Chauhan SP, Dashe JS. Society for maternal-fetal medicine (SMFM) clinical guideline #7: nonimmune hydrops fetalis. *Am J Obstet Gynecol.* 2015 Feb;212(2):127-39. Copyright © 2015 Elsevier.

Table 2.107. Therapy for selected etiologies of nonimmune hydrops

Recommendations	Grading of Recommendations
• We recommend that initial evaluation of hydrops include an antibody screen (indirect Coombs test) to verify that it is nonimmune, targeted sonography with echocardiography to evaluate for fetal and placental abnormalities, MCA Doppler evaluation for anemia, and fetal karyotype or chromosomal microarray analysis, regardless of whether structural fetal anomalies are identified	1C Strong recommendation, low-quality evidence
• We recommend that fetal therapy decisions be based on underlying etiology, in particular whether there is a treatable cause and the gestational age that NIHF develops or is first identified	1C Strong recommendation, low-quality evidence
• As prematurity is likely to worsen prognosis, we recommend that preterm delivery be undertaken only for obstetric indications	1C Strong recommendation, low-quality evidence
• We recommend that pregnancies with NIHF due to nonlethal or potentially treatable etiologies be considered candidates for corticosteroid therapy and antepartum surveillance, and that they be delivered at a center that has capability to stabilize and treat critically ill neonates	1C Strong recommendation, low-quality evidence
• We recommend that in most cases, development of mirror syndrome is an indication for delivery	1C Strong recommendation, low-quality evidence

MCA, middle cerebral artery; NIHF, nonimmune hydrops fetalis.

Source: Reproduced with permission from Society for Maternal-Fetal Medicine (SMFM), Norton ME, Chauhan SP, Dashe JS. Society for maternal-fetal medicine (SMFM) clinical guideline #7: nonimmune hydrops fetalis. *Am J Obstet Gynecol.* 2015 Feb;212(2):127-39. Copyright © 2015 Elsevier.

ISOIMMUNIZATION

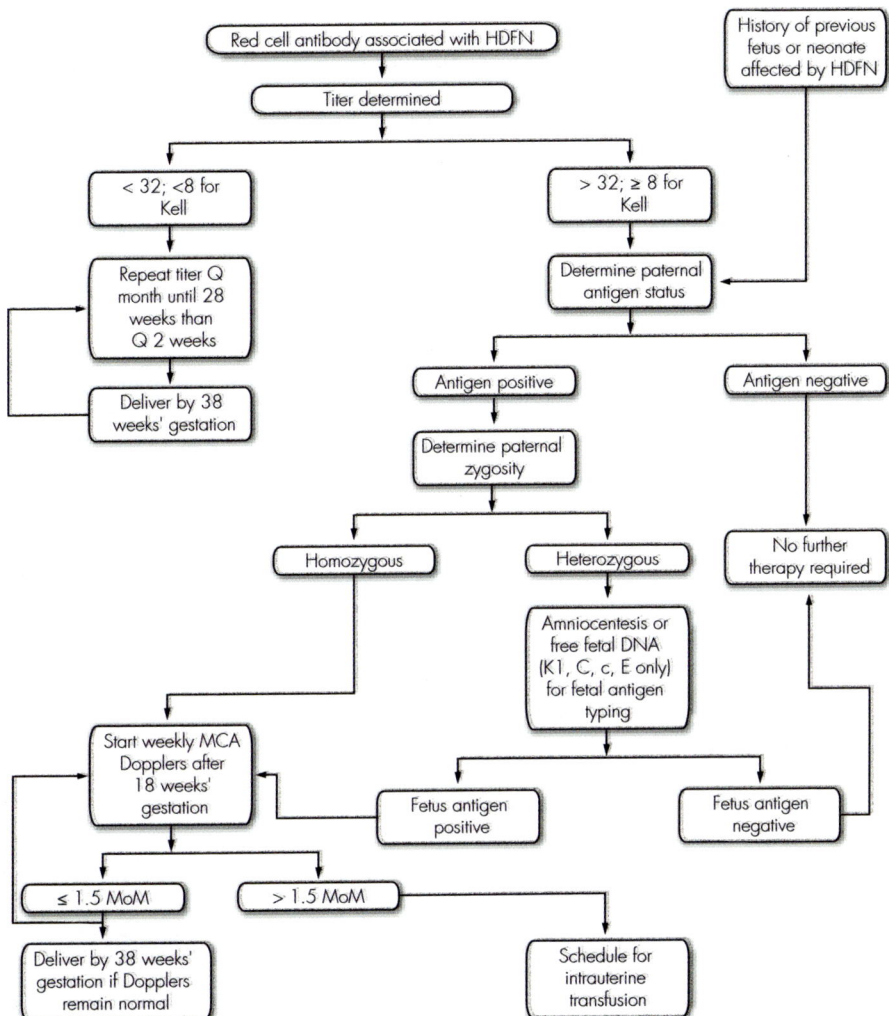

Figure 2.44. Evaluation of obstetric patients with a positive indirect Coombs test result
Source: Reproduced with American College of Obstetricians and Gynecologists. *PROLOG Obstetrics, 7th Ed.* Washington, DC: American College of Obstetricians and Gynecologists; 2013. Copyright © 2013 The American College of Obstetricians and Gynecologists.

Table 2.108. Non-Rhesus-D antibodies associated with hemolytic disease of the fetus and newborn

Antigen System	Specific Antigen	Antigen System	Specific Antigen	Antigen System	Specific Antigen
Infrequently associated with severe disease					
Colton	-Coa	MNS	-Mta	Rhesus	-HOFM
	-Co3		-MUT		-LOCR
Diego	-ELO		-Mur		-Riv
	-Dia		-Mv		-Rh29
	-Dib		-s		-Rh32
	-Wra		-sD		-Rh42
	-Wrb		-S		-Rh46
Duffy	-Fya		-U		-STEM
Kell	-Jsa		-Vw		-Tar
	-Jsb	Rhesus	-Bea	Other antigens	-HJK
	-k (K2)		-C		-JFV
	-Kpa		-Ce		-JONES
	-Kpb		-Cw		-Kg
	-K11		-Cx		-MAM
	-K22		-ce		-REIT
	-Ku		-Dw		-Rd
	-Ula		-E		
Kidd	-Jka		-Ew		
MNS	-Ena		-Evans		
	-Far		-e		
	-Hil		-G		
	-Hut		-Goa7		
	-M		-Hr		
	-Mia		-Hro		
	-Mit		-JAL		
Associated with mild disease					
Dombrock	-Doa	Gerbich	-Ge2	Scianna Other	-Sc2
	-Gya		-Ge3		-Vel
	-Hy		-Ge4		-Lan
	-Joa		-Lsa		-Ata
Duffy	-Fyb	Kidd	-Jkb		-Jra
	-Fy3		-Jk3		

Source: Reproduced with permission from Moise KJ. Fetal anemia due to non-Rhesus-D red-cell alloimmunization. *Semin Fetal Neonatal Med.* 2008 Aug;13(4):207-214. Copyright © 2008 Elsevier.

Middle Cerebral Artery Doppler Evaluation

- Ultrasound measurement of the MCA peak systolic blood flow velocity can be used to predict fetal anemia instead of the DOD-450.
- MCA Dopplers are 88% sensitive and 82% specific for fetal anemia, whereas DOD-450 was 76% sensitive 77% specific for fetal anemia (Oepkes 2006).

Managing the Sensitized Pregnancy

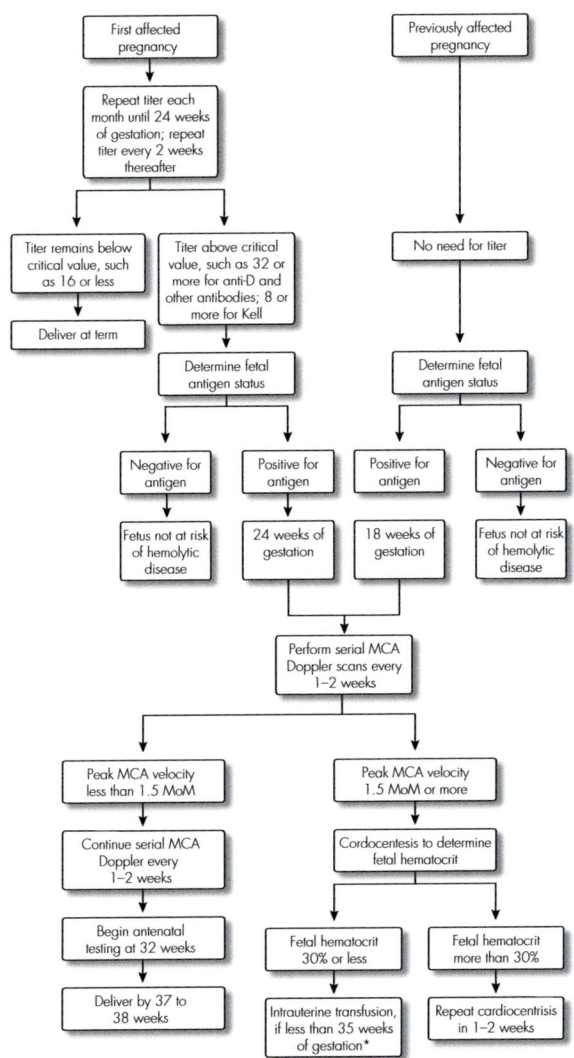

Figure 2.45. Algorithm for the clinical management of the red cell alloimmunized pregnancy
MCA, middle cerebral artery; MoM, multiples of the median.
* After 35 weeks, in utero transfusion is considered riskier than late preterm delivery for neonatal treatment of severe anemia.

Source: Reproduced from Moise KJ Jr., Argoti PS. Management and prevention of red cell alloimmunization in pregnancy: a systematic review. *Obstet Gynecol.* 2012; 120:1132-9. Copyright © 2012 The American College of Obstetricians and Gynecologists.

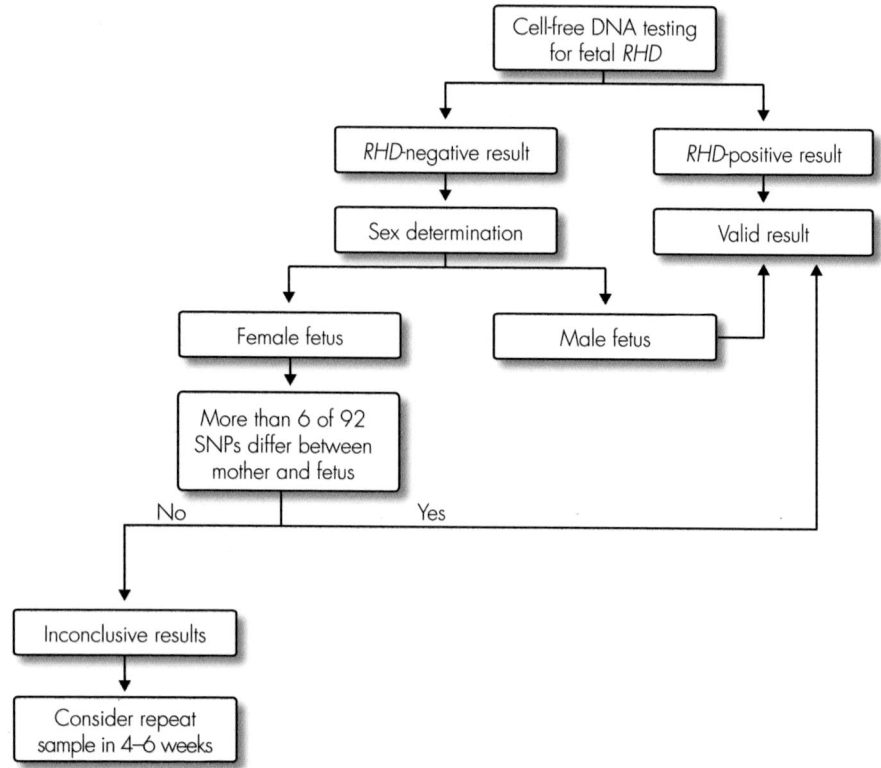

Figure 2.46. Algorithm for determining the results of cell-free fetal DNA testing to determine the fetal RHD status

Cell-free fetal DNA testing is widely used in Europe to determine fetal Rh status. This testing is available in the US with an accuracy of 97.1%, sensitivity 97.2%, and specificity of 96.8%.

Source: Reproduced with permission from Moise KJ Jr, Argoti PS. Management and prevention of red cell alloimmunization in pregnancy: a systematic review. *Obstet Gynecol.* 2012; 120:1132. Copyright © 2012 The American College of Obstetricians and Gynecologists.

SYSTEMIC LUPUS ERYTHEMATOSUS (SLE) AND APS IN PREGNANCY

Diagnosis

Table 2.109. Classification criteria for systemic lupus erythematosus: clinical and immunologic criteria used in the SLICC classification system

ACR Criteria for the Classification of Systemic Lupus Erythematosus[1,2]		SLICC Criteria for the Classification of Systemic Lupus Erythematosus[3]	
(4 Of 11 Criteria)*		(4 of 17 Criteria, Including at Least One Clinical Criterion and One Immunologic Criterion;• OR Biopsy-proven Lupus Nephritis◊)	
Criterion	Definition	Criterion	Definition
Clinical criteria			
Malar rash	Fixed erythema, flat or raised, over the malar eminences, tending to spare the nasolabial folds	Acute cutaneous lupus	Lupus malar rash (do not count if malar discoid); bullous lupus; toxic epidermal necrolysis variant of SLE; maculopapular lupus rash; photosensitive lupus rash (in the absence of dermatomyositis); **OR** subacute cutaneous lupus (nonindurated psoriaform and/or annular polycyclic lesions that resolve without scarring, although occasionally with postinflammatory dyspigmentation or telangiectasias)
Photosensitivity	Skin rash as a result of unusual reaction to sunlight, by patient history or clinician observation		
Discoid rash	Erythematosus raised patches with adherent keratotic scaling and follicular plugging; atrophic scarring may occur in older lesions	Chronic cutaneous lupus	Classic discoid rash; localized (above the neck); generalized (above and below the neck); hypertrophic (verrucous) lupus; lupus panniculitis (profundus); mucosal lupus; lupus erythematosus tumidus; chilblains lupus; **OR** discoid lupus/lichen planus overlap
		Nonscarring alopecia	Diffuse thinning or hair fragility with visible broken hairs (in the absence of other causes, such as alopecia areata, drugs, iron deficiency, and androgenic alopecia)
Oral ulcers	Oral or nasopharyngeal ulceration, usually painless, observed by a clinician	Oral or nasal ulcers	Palate, buccal, tongue, **OR** nasal ulcers (in the absence of other causes, such as vasculitis, Behçet's disease, infection [herpes virus], inflammatory bowel disease, reactive arthritis, and acidic foods)
Arthritis	Nonerosive arthritis involving two or more peripheral joints, characterized by tenderness, swelling, or effusion	Joint disease	Synovitis involving two or more joints, characterized by swelling or effusion **OR** Tenderness in two or more joints and at least 30 minutes of morning stiffness
Serositis	Pleuritis—Convincing history of pleuritic pain or rubbing heard by a clinician or evidence of pleural effusion **OR** Pericarditis—Documented by EKG, rub, or evidence of pericardial effusion	Serositis	Typical pleurisy for more than 1 day, pleural effusions, or pleural rub, **OR** Typical pericardial pain (pain with recumbency improved by sitting forward) for more than 1 day, pericardial effusion, pericardial rub, or pericarditis by electrocardiography in the absence of other causes, such as infection, uremia, and Dressler's syndrome

(continued)

ACR Criteria for the Classification of Systemic Lupus Erythematosus[1,2]		SLICC Criteria for the Classification of Systemic Lupus Erythematosus[3]	
(4 Of 11 Criteria)*		(4 of 17 Criteria, Including at Least One Clinical Criterion and One Immunologic Criterion;• OR Biopsy-proven Lupus Nephritis◊)	
Criterion	Definition	Criterion	Definition
Renal disorder	Persistent proteinuria greater than 500 mg/24 hours or greater than 3+ if quantitation not performed **OR**	Renal	Urine protein-to-creatinine ratio (or 24-hour urine protein) representing 500 mg protein/24 hours, **OR**
	Cellular casts—May be red cell, hemoglobin, granular, tubular, or mixed		Red blood cell casts
Neurologic disorder	Seizures **OR** psychosis—In the absence of offending drugs or known metabolic derangements (uremia, ketoacidosis, or electrolyte imbalance)	Neurologic	Seizures; psychosis; mononeuritis multiplex (in the absence of other known causes, such as primary vasculitis); myelitis; peripheral or cranial neuropathy (in the absence of other known causes, such as primary vasculitis, infection, and diabetes mellitus); **OR** acute confusional state (in the absence of other causes, including toxic/metabolic, uremia, drugs)
Hematologic disorder	Hemolytic anemia—With reticulocytosis **OR**	Hemolytic anemia	Hemolytic anemia
	Leukopenia—Less than 4000/mm³ total on two or more occasions **OR**	Leukopenia or lymphopenia	Leukopenia (<4000/mm³ at least once) (in the absence of other known causes, such as Felty's syndrome, drugs, and portal hypertension), **OR**
	Lymphopenia—Less than 1500/mm³ on two or more occasions **OR**		Lymphopenia (<1000/mm at least once) (in the absence of other known causes, such as glucocorticoids, drugs, and infection)
	Thrombocytopenia—Less than 100,000/mm³ (in the absence of offending drugs)	Thrombocytopenia	Thrombocytopenia (<100,000/mm³) at least once in the absence of other known causes, such as drugs, portal hypertension, and thrombotic thrombocytopenic purpura
Immunologic criteria			
ANA	An abnormal titer of antinuclear antibody by immunofluorescence or an equivalent assay at any point in time and in the absence of drugs known to be associated with "drug-induced lupus" syndrome	ANA	ANA level above laboratory reference range

(continued)

ACR Criteria for the Classification of Systemic Lupus Erythematosus[1,2]		SLICC Criteria for the Classification of Systemic Lupus Erythematosus[3]	
(4 Of 11 Criteria)*		(4 of 17 Criteria, Including at Least One Clinical Criterion and One Immunologic Criterion;• OR Biopsy-proven Lupus Nephritis[☐])	
Criterion	Definition	Criterion	Definition
Immunologic disorders	Anti-DNA—Antibody to native DNA in abnormal titer **OR**	Anti-dsDNA	Anti-dsDNA antibody level above laboratory reference range (or >twofold the reference range if tested by ELISA)
	Anti-Sm—Presence of antibody to Sm nuclear antigen **OR**	Anti-Sm	Presence of antibody to Sm nuclear antigen
	Positive finding of antiphospholipid antibody based on an abnormal serum level of IgG or IgM anticardiolipin antibodies, on a positive test result for lupus anticoagulant using a standard method, or on a false-positive serologic test for syphilis known to be positive for at least 6 months and confirmed by Treponema pallidum immobilization or fluorescent treponemal antibody absorption test	Antiphospholipid	Antiphospholipid antibody positivity as determined by any of the following: positive test result for lupus anticoagulant; false-positive test result for rapid plasma reagin; medium- or high-titer anticardiolipin antibody level (IgA, IgG, or IgM); or positive test result for antibeta 2-glycoprotein I (IgA, IgG, or IgM)
		Low complement	Low C3; low C4; **OR** low CH50
		Direct Coombs test	Direct Coombs test in the absence of hemolytic anemia

ACR, American College of Rheumatology; SLICC, Systemic Lupus International Collaborating Clinics; SLE, systemic lupus erythematosus; EKG, electrocardiogram; ANA, antinuclear antibodies; Anti-Sm, anti-Smith antibody; IgG, immunoglobulin G; IgM, immunoglobulin M; Anti-dsDNA, anti-double-stranded DNA; ELISA, enzyme-linked immunosorbent assay, IgA, immunoglobulin A.

*For the ACR criteria, no distinction is made between clinical and immunologic criteria in determining whether the required number has been met. The classification is based upon 11 criteria. For the purpose of identifying patients in clinical studies, a person is said to have SLE if any 4 or more of the 11 criteria are present, serially or simultaneously, during any interval of observation.

•For the SLICC criteria, criteria are cumulative and need not be presently concurrently. A patient is classified as having SLE if he or she satisfies four of the clinical and immunologic criteria used in the SLICC classification criteria, including at least one clinical criterion and one immunologic criterion.

☐Alternatively, according to the SLICC criteria, a patient is classified has having SLE if he or she has biopsy-proven nephritis compatible with SLE in the presence of ANAs or anti-dsDNA antibodies.

[1] Tan (1982).
[2] Hochberg (1997).
[3] Petri (2012).

Source: Reproduced with permission from Petri M, Orbai AM, Alarcón GS, et al. Derivation and validation of the Systemic Lupus International Collaborating Clinics classification criteria for systemic lupus erythematosus. *Arthritis Rheum.* 2012 Aug;64(8):2677-86. Copyright © 2012 The American College of Rheumatology.

Common Complaints of Lupus Patients
- Arthritis or rheumatism for >3 months
- Fingers that become cold, pale, numb, or uncomfortable in the cold
- Mouth sores for ≥2 weeks
- Prominent facial rash for >1 month
- Photosensitivity
- Pleurisy
- Rapid hair loss
- Seizures or convulsions

Initial Labs in Pregnancy
- Antinuclear antibody screen and titer
- Anti-double-stranded DNA
- Anti-Ro(SS-A), Anti-La(SS-B) antibodies
- Lupus anticoagulant and anticardiolipin antibodies (see below) C3 and C4, or CH50
- Chemistry panel, electrolytes
- Thyroid function tests (as indicated)
- Anti-platelet antibodies
- 24-hour urine for creatinine clearance, total protein and or urine protein/creatinine ration
- Uric acid

Pregnancy
- Studies are inconsistent, but as a rule of thumb 1/3 get better, 1/3 get worse, and 1/3 remain stable.
- Patients should be counseled to get pregnant when their disease has been in remission for 4–6 months.
- Monitor for disease flare and hypertensive complications of pregnancy (especially in women with a history of lupus nephritis).
- Patients are best managed in collaboration with a rheumatology.

Table 2.110. Revised classification criteria for the antiphospholipid syndrome

Antiphospholipid antibody syndrome is present if at least one of the clinical criteria and one of the laboratory criteria that follow are met.[a]

Clinical Criteria

1. Vascular thrombosis[b]

One or more clinical episodes[c] of arterial, venous, or small vessel thrombosis[d] in any tissue or organ. Thrombosis must be confirmed by objective validated criteria (i.e., unequivocal findings of appropriate imaging studies or histopathology). For histopathologic confirmation, thrombosis should be present without significant evidence of inflammation in the vessel wall.

2. Pregnancy morbidity

(a) One or more unexplained deaths of a morphologically normal fetus at or beyond the 10th wk of gestation, with normal fetal morphology documented by ultrasound or by direct examination of the fetus, or

(b) One or more premature births of a morphologically normal neonate before the 34th wk of gestation because of: (i) eclampsia or severe preeclampsia defined according to standard definitions, or (ii) recognized features of placental insufficiency,[e] or

(c) Three or more unexplained consecutive spontaneous abortions before the 10th wk of gestation, with maternal anatomic or hormonal abnormalities and paternal and maternal chromosomal causes excluded.

In studies of populations of patients who have more than one type of pregnancy morbidity, investigators are strongly encouraged to stratify groups of subjects according to a, b, or c above.

Laboratory Criteria[f]

1. Lupus anticoagulant present in plasma, on two or more occasions at least 12 wk apart, detected according to the guidelines of the International Society on Thrombosis and Haemostasis (Scientific Subcommittee on LAs/phospholipid-dependent antibodies).

2. Anticardiolipin antibody of IgG and/or IgM isotype in serum or plasma, present in medium or high titer (i.e. >40 IgG antiphospholipid or IgM antiphospholipid, or > the 99th percentile), on two or more occasions, at least 12 wk apart, measured by a standardized enzyme-linked immunosorbent assay.

3. Anti-β_2 glycoprotein-I antibody of IgG and/or IgM isotype in serum or plasma (in titer > the 99th percentile), present on two or more occasions, at least 12 wk apart, measured by a standardized enzyme-linked immunosorbent assay, according to recommended procedures.

[a]Classification of antiphospholipid antibody syndrome should be avoided if less than 12 wk or more than 5 yr separate the positive antiphospholipid test and the clinical manifestation.

[b]Coexisting inherited or acquired factors for thrombosis are not reasons for excluding patients from APS trials. However, two subgroups of APS patients should be recognized, according to: (a) the presence and (b) the absence of additional risk factors for thrombosis. Indicative (but not exhaustive) such cases include: age (>55 in men and >65 in women), the presence of any of the established risk factors for cardiovascular disease (hypertension, diabetes mellitus, elevated LDL or low HDL cholesterol, cigarette smoking, family history of premature cardiovascular disease, body mass index ≥30 kg m^{-2}, microalbuminuria, estimated glomerular filtration rate <60 mL min^{-1}), inherited thrombophilias, oral contraceptives, nephrotic syndrome, malignancy, immobilization, and surgery. Thus, patients who fulfill criteria should be stratified according to contributing causes of thrombosis.

[c]A thrombotic episode in the past could be considered as a clinical criterion, provided that thrombosis is proved by appropriate diagnostic means and that no alternative diagnosis or cause of thrombosis is found.

[d]Superficial venous thrombosis is not included in the clinical criteria.

[e]Generally accepted features of placental insufficiency include: (i) abnormal or Nonreassuring fetal surveillance test(s), e.g., a nonreactive nonstress test, suggestive of fetal hypoxemia, (ii) abnormal Doppler flow velocimetry waveform analysis suggestive of fetal hypoxemia (e.g., absent end-diastolic flow in the umbilical artery), (iii) oligohydramnios (e.g., an amniotic fluid index of 5 cm or less), or (iv) a postnatal birth weight less than the 10th percentile for the gestational age.

[f]Investigators are strongly advised to classify APS patients in studies into one of the following categories: (I) more than one laboratory criteria present (any combination), (IIa) LA present alone, (IIb) aCL antibody present alone, (IIc) anti-β2 glycoprotein-I antibody present alone.

Source: Reproduced with permission from Miyakis S, Lockshin MD, Atsumi T, et al. International consensus statement on an update of the classification criteria for definite antiphospholipid syndrome (APS). J Throm Haemost. 2006;4:295-306. Copyright © 2006 International Society on Thrombosis and Haemostasis.

Table 2.111. Treatment of pregnant women with APS

	Antepartum	Postpartum
APS with prior arterial or venous thrombosis	LMWH	Warfarin
APS with prior arterial or venous thrombosis and APS-defining pregnancy morbidity	LMWH and low-dose ASA	Warfarin
APS based on laboratory criteria for aPL and APS-defining pregnancy morbidity of ≥1 fetal losses ≥10 weeks of gestation or ≥3 unexplained consecutive spontaneous pregnancy losses <10 weeks of gestation, but no history of arterial or venous thrombosis	LMWH and low-dose ASA	LMWH and low-dose ASA
APS based on laboratory criteria for aPL and APS-defining pregnancy morbidity of ≥1 preterm deliveries of a morphologically normal infant before 34 weeks of gestation due to severe preeclampsia, eclampsia, or other findings consistent with placental insufficiency. No history of arterial or venous thrombosis.	Low-dose ASA LMWH with low-dose ASA in cases of ASA failure or when placental examination shows extensive decidual inflammation and vasculopathy and/or thrombosis	None LMWH with low-dose ASA
Laboratory criteria for aPL but no clinical criteria for APS	Low-dose ASA	None

APS, antiphospholipid syndrome; aPL, antiphospholipid antibodies; ASA, aspirin; LMWH, low-molecular-weight heparin.

Graphic 91501 Version 2.0

Source: Reproduced with permission from park L, Lockwood CJ, Lockshin MD. Pregnancy in women with antiphospholipid syndrome. In: Post, TW, ed. *UpToDate*. Waltham, MA: UpToDate (accessed on February 19, 2016). Copyright © 2016 UpToDate, Inc. For more information, visit www.uptodate.com.

THROMBOEMBOLIC DISORDERS
Fast Facts
- Venous thromboembolism (VTE) occurs in 0.05–0.3% of pregnancies.
- PE occurs in 15–24% of untreated DVT cases with mortality rate of 15%.
- PE occurs in 4.5% treated cases with mortality rate of 1%.

Table 2.112. Risk of venous thromboembolism with different thrombophilias

	Prevalence in General Population (%)	VTE Risk Per Pregnancy (No History) (%)	VTE Risk Per Pregnancy (Previous VTE) (%)	Percentage of All VTE	References
Factor V Leiden heterozygote	1–15	0.5–1.2	10	40	1–4
Factor V Leiden homozygote	<1	4	17	2	1–4
Prothrombin gene heterozygote	2–5	<0.5	>10	17	1–4
Prothrombin gene homozygote	<1	2–4	>17	0.5	1–4
Factor V Leiden/prothrombin double heterozygote	0.01	4–5	>20	1–3	1–4
Antithrombin III activity (<60%)	0.02	3–7	40	1	1, 5, 6
Protein C activity (<50%)	0.2–0.4	0.1–0.8	4–17	14	1, 5, 7
Protein S free antigen (<55%)	0.03–0.13	0.1	0–22	3	1, 8–10

VTE, venous thromboembolism.

1. Franco (2001).
2. Gerhardt (2000).
3. Zotz (2003).
4. Haverkate (1995).
5. Carraro (2003).
6. Friederich (1997).
7. Vossen (2004).
8. Paidas (2005).
9. Dykes (2001).
10. Goodwin (2002).

Source: Reproduced with permission from American College of Obstetricians and Gynecologists Women's Health Care Physicians. ACOG Practice Bulletin No. 138: Inherited thrombophilias in pregnancy. *Obstet Gynecol.* 2013 Sep;122(3):706-717. Copyright © 2013 The American College of Obstetricians and Gynecologists.

Diagnosis
- Doppler ultrasound diagnostic study of choice in proximal DVT.
- Ventilation-perfusion scan or CT angiogram needed in cases of suspected pulmonary embolism.

Table 2.113. How to test for thrombophilias

Thrombophilia	Testing Method	Is Testing Reliable During Pregnancy?	Is Testing Reliable During Acute Thrombosis?	Is Testing Reliable with Anti-coagulation?
Factor V Leiden mutation	Activated protein C resistance assay (second generation)	Yes	Yes	No
	If abnormal: DNA analysis	Yes	Yes	Yes
Prothrombin G20210A mutation	DNA analysis	Yes	Yes	Yes
Protein C deficiency	Protein C activity (<60%)	Yes	No	No
Protein S deficiency	Functional assay (<55%)	No*	No	No
Antithrombin deficiency	Antithrombin activity (<60%)	Yes	No	No

*If screening in pregnancy is necessary, cutoff values for free protein S antigen levels in the second and third trimesters have been identified at less than 30% and less than 24%, respectively.

Source: Reproduced with permission from American College of Obstetricians and Gynecologists Women's Health Care Physicians. ACOG Practice Bulletin No. 138: Inherited thrombophilias in pregnancy. *Obstet Gynecol.* 2013 Sep;122(3):706-717. Copyright © 2013 The American College of Obstetricians and Gynecologists.

Thromboembolic Disorders — OBSTETRICS

Table 2.114. Anticoagulation regimen definitions

Anticoagulation Regimen	Definition
Prophylactic LMWH*	Enoxaparin, 40 mg SC once daily
	Dalteparin, 5,000 units SC once daily
	Tinzaparin, 4,500 units SC once daily
Therapeutic LMWH[†]	Enoxaparin, 1 mg/kg every 12 hours
	Dalteparin, 200 units/kg once daily
	Tinzaparin, 175 units/kg once daily
	Dalteparin, 100 units/kg every 12 hours
	May target an anti-Xa level in the therapeutic range of 0.6–1.0 units/mL for twice daily regimen; slightly higher doses may be needed for a once-daily regimen.
Minidose prophylactic UFH	UFH, 5,000 units SC every 12 hours
Prophylactic UFH	UFH, 5,000–10,000 units SC every 12 hours
	UFH, 5,000–7,500 units SC every 12 hours in first trimester
	UFH, 7,500–10,000 units SC every 12 hours in the second trimester
	UFH, 10,000 units SC every 12 hours in the third trimester, unless the aPTT is elevated
Therapeutic UFH[†]	UFH, 10,000 units or more SC every 12 hours in doses adjusted to target aPTT in the therapeutic range (1.5–2.5) 6 hours after injection
Postpartum anticoagulation	Prophylactic LMWH/UFH for 4–6 weeks or vitamin K antagonists for 4–6 weeks with a target INR of 2.0–3.0, with initial UFH or LMWH therapy overlap until the INR is 2.0 or more for 2 days
Surveillance	Clinical vigilance and appropriate objective investigation of women with symptoms suspicious of deep vein thrombosis or pulmonary embolism

aPTT, activated partial thromboplastin time; INR, international normalized ratio; LMWH, low-molecular-weight heparin; SC, subcutaneously; UFH, unfractionated heparin.

*Although at extremes of body weight, modification of dose may be required.

[†]Also referred to as weight adjusted, full treatment dose.

Source: Reproduced with permission from American College of Obstetricians and Gynecologists Women's Health Care Physicians. ACOG Practice Bulletin No. 138: Inherited thrombophilias in pregnancy. *Obstet Gynecol.* 2013 Sep;122(3):706-717. Copyright © 2013 The American College of Obstetricians and Gynecologists.

Table 2.115. Recommended thromboprophylaxis for pregnancies complicated by inherited thrombophilias

Clinical Scenario	Antepartum Management	Postpartum Management
Low-risk thrombophilia[†] without previous VTE	Surveillance without anticoagulation therapy	Surveillance without anticoagulation therapy or postpartum anticoagulation therapy if the patient has additional risks factors[‡]
Low-risk thrombophila with a family history (first-degree relative) of VTE	Surveillance without anticoagulation therapy	Postpartum anticoagulation therapy or intermediate-dose LMWH/UFH
Low-risk thrombophilia[†] with a single previous episode of VTE—Not receiving long-term anticoagulation therapy	Prophylactic or intermediate-dose LMWH/UFH or surveillance without anticoagulation therapy	Postpartum anticoagulation therapy or intermediate-dose LMWH/UFH
High-risk thrombophilia[§] without previous VTE	Surveillance without anticoagulation therapy, or prophylactic LMWH or UFH	Postpartum anticoagulation therapy

(continued)

Clinical Scenario	Antepartum Management	Postpartum Management
High-risk thrombophilia§ with a single previous episode of VTE or an affected first-degree relative—Not receiving long-term anticoagulation therapy	Prophylactic, intermediate-dose, or adjusted-dose LMWH/UFH regimen	Postpartum anticoagulation therapy, or intermediate or adjusted-dose LMWH/UFH for 6 weeks (therapy level should be at least as high as antepartum treatment)
No thrombophilia with previous single episode of VTE associated with transient risk factor that is no longer present—Excludes pregnancy- or estrogen-related risk factor	Surveillance without anticoagulation therapy	Postpartum anticoagulation therapy‖
No thrombophilia with previous single episode of VTE associated with transient risk factor that was pregnancy or estrogen-related	Prophylactic-dose LMWH or UFH‖	Postpartum anticoagulation therapy
No thrombophilia with previous single episode of VTE without an associated risk factor (idiopathic)—Not receiving long-term anticoagulation therapy	Prophylactic-dose LMWH or UFH‖	Postpartum anticoagulation therapy
Thrombophilia or no thrombophilia with two or more episodes of VTE—Not receiving long-term anticoagulation therapy	Prophylactic or therapeutic-dose LMWH or Prophylactic or therapeutic-dose UFH	Postpartum anticoagulation therapy or Therapeutic-dose LMWH/UFH for 6 weeks
Thrombophilia or no thrombophilia with two or more episodes of VTE—Receiving long-term anticoagulation therapy	Therapeutic-dose LMWH or UFH	Resumption of long-term anticoagulation therapy

LMWH, low-molecular-weight heparin; UFH, unfractionated heparin; VTE, venous thromboembolism.

*Postpartum treatment levels should be greater or equal to antepartum treatment. Treatment of acute VTE and management of antiphospholipid syndrome are addressed in other practice bulletins.

†Low-risk thrombophilia: factor V Leiden heterozygous; prothrombin G20210A heterozygous; protein C or protein S deficiency.

‡First-degree relative with a history of a thrombotic episode before age 50 years, or other major thrombotic risk factors (e.g., obesity or prolonged immobility).

§High-risk thrombophilia: antithrombin deficiency; double heterozygous for prothrombin G20210A mutation and factor V Leiden; factor V Leiden homozygous or prothrombin G20210A mutation homozygous.

‖Surveillance without anticoagulation therapy is supported as an alternative approach by some experts.

Source: Reproduced with permission from American College of Obstetricians and Gynecologists Women's Health Care Physicians. ACOG Practice Bulletin No. 138: Inherited thrombophilias in pregnancy. *Obstet Gynecol.* 2013 Sep;122(3):706-717. Copyright © 2013 The American College of Obstetricians and Gynecologists.

Thromboembolic Disorders — OBSTETRICS

Table 2.116. Prevalence and risk of reoccurrence of adverse pregnancy outcome without thrombophilia

Previous Pregnancy Complication	Prevalence of Pregnancy Complication (%)	Pregnancy Complication in Subsequent Pregnancy (%)	Fetal Death with Pregnancy Complication (%)
Fetal loss after or at 20 wk	0.5	8.5	8.5
Severe preeclampsia	2	26	13.5
HELLP	1	4	13.5
Eclampsia	0.5	3	13.5
Abruption	0.8	5	26
IUGR ≤ 5th percentile	5.3	16	20
One or more	8	61–85	—

Source: Reproduced with permission from Duhl AJ, Paidas MJ, Ural SH, et al. Antithrombotic therapy and pregnancy: consensus report and recommendations for prevention and treatment of venous thromboembolism and adverse pregnancy outcome. *Am J Obstet Gynecol.* 2007;197:457. Copyright © 2007 Elsevier.

Table 2.117. Relative risk of recurrent VTE in pregnancy

Disorder	Risk of VTE	Prophylaxis Intensity
Factor V Leiden heterozygote	3- to 9-fold	Low-dose prophylaxis
Factor V Leiden homozygote	49- to 80-fold	Adjusted-dose therapy
Prothrombin G20210A heterozygote	2- to 9-fold	Low-dose prophylaxis
Prothrombin G20210A homozygote	16-fold	Adjusted-dose therapy
Antithrombin III deficiency	25- to 50-fold	Adjusted-dose therapy
Protein C deficiency	3- to 15-fold	Low-dose prophylaxis
Protein S deficiency	2-fold	Low-dose prophylaxis
Hyperhomocysteinemia	2.5- to 4-fold	Low-dose prophylaxis
Antiphospholipid antibodies	5.3-fold	Adjusted-dose therapy
Compound heterozygote of Factor V Leiden and Prothrombin G20210A	150-fold	Adjusted-dose therapy

Source: Reproduced with permission from Duhl AJ, Paidas MJ, Ural SH, et al. Antithrombotic therapy and pregnancy: consensus report and recommendations for prevention and treatment of venous thromboembolism and adverse pregnancy outcome. *Am J Obstet Gynecol.* 2007;197:457. Copyright © 2007 Elsevier.

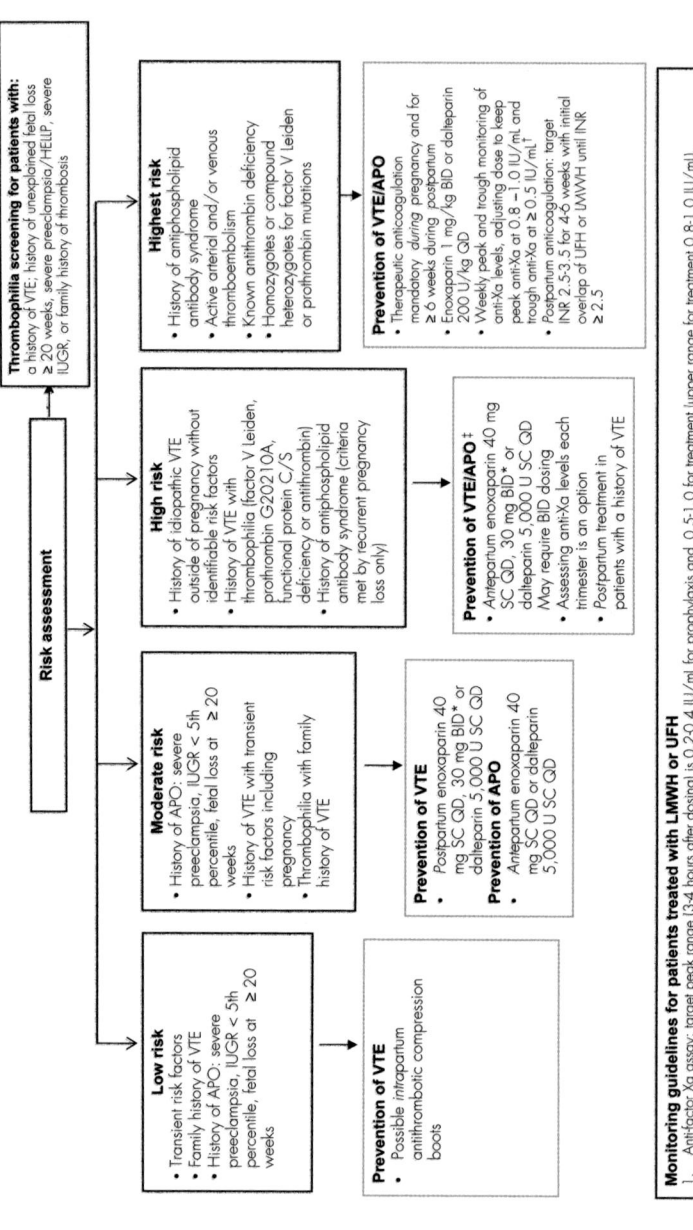

Figure 2.47. Risk assessment and prevention of VTE and adverse pregnancy outcome

Source: Reproduced with permission from Duhl AJ, Paidas MJ, Ural SH, et al. Antithrombotic therapy and pregnancy: consensus report and recommendations for prevention and treatment of venous thromboembolism and adverse pregnancy outcome. Am J Obstet Gynecol. 2007;197:457. Copyright © 2007 Elsevier.

THROMBOCYTOPENIA IN PREGNANCY

Fast Facts
- Defined as platelet count <150,000/mL.
- Repeat platelet count and obtain a CBC to exclude pancytopenia and lab artifact.
- Occurs in 8% of pregnancies.
- Obtaining antiplatelet antibodies is not recommended (does not help with the diagnosis or treatment).
- Regional anesthesia should not be given if maternal platelets are <50 K.
- Consultation with anesthesia recommended as platelet count threshold for regional anesthesia may vary.

Gestational Thrombocytopenia
- Most common cause of thrombocytopenia in pregnancy (2/3 of cases).
- Manifests itself usually in the third trimester and is usually mild (rarely <70 K).
- Usually not associated with fetal thrombocytopenia, thus there is no risk for fetal hemorrhage.
- Does not require any other testing than routine antepartum platelet count every 1–2 months.
- Can be difficult to distinguish from immune thrombocytopenic purpura since antibodies can also be present.
- Usually milder, occurs later in gestation, with no maternal history of thrombocytopenia
- Women are asymptomatic.
- No history of thrombocytopenia except in prior pregnancies.
- Resolves 2–12 weeks postpartum.

Immune Thrombocytopenia Purpura
- Occurs in 1:1,000 to 1:10,000 pregnancies.
- Caused by maternal IgG antiplatelet antibodies destroying maternal and fetal platelets.
- Maternal platelet count usually <100 K; maternal count correlates poorly with fetal count.
- 15% of infants to mothers with immune thrombocytopenia purpura will have counts <50 K; 5% with counts <20 K.
- Rate of intracranial hemorrhage is extremely low (<1%) as compared to neonatal alloimmune thrombocytopenia.
- Maternal treatment for fetal indications is not recommended.
- Obtain platelet counts frequently.
- Maternal therapy indicated for platelet count <50 K.
- Prednisone 1–2 mg/kg/d, PRN intravenous immunoglobulin and platelet transfusion.
- Obtaining fetal platelet count is probably not warranted.
- Mode of delivery should be based upon obstetric considerations only.
- C/S does not seem to decrease risk of intracranial hemorrhage.
- Diagnosis of exclusion.

Preeclampsia or HELLP
- Etiology in 20% of cases.
- Cause is unknown but platelet count rarely <20 K.
- Primary treatment in the setting of preeclampsia with severe features or HELLP syndrome is delivery.
- Consider increasing the platelet count to >50 K if considering cesarean delivery or regional anesthesia.

OBSTETRICS

Table 2.118. Characteristics of thrombocytopenia

Cause		Treatment
Gestational thrombocytopenia	75% (second/third trimester)	No treatment required, resolves spontaneously after delivery
Preeclampsia	15–20% (second/third trimester)	Delivery if ≥34 weeks. Platelet transfusions to support procedures
Immune thrombocytopenia	1–4% (first/second trimester)	IVIG or corticosteroids if platelets <30 k/uL. Splenectomy, azathioprine as second line
HELLP syndrome	Rare	Delivery if ≥34 weeks. Transfusions if platelets <20 k/uL. Plasmapheresis for refractory or atypical cases
Acute fatty liver of pregnancy (AFLP)	rare	Termination of pregnancy. Plasmapheresis for refractory or atypical cases
TTP	rare	Plasmapheresis and delivery if ≤34 weeks
SLE	rare	Platelets <95 k/uL indicate treating lupus flare
Antiphospholipid antibody syndrome	Rare (associated with thrombocytopenia in 30% of cases)	Anticoagulation therapy to prevent fetal loss. Treat as ITP if platelets <30–50 k/uL.
Type IIb VWD	rare	Platelet transfusions, factor replacement
Viral infections	rare	Screen for CMV, EBV, HCV, HIV, HBV
Bone marrow failure (congenital or acquired)	rare	Transfusion support until delivery

Source: Townsley DM. Hemotologic complications of pregnancy. *Semin Hematol.* 2013;50(3):222-31. Copyright © 2013 Elsevier.

EPILEPSY IN PREGNANCY

Fast Facts
- Epilepsy prevalence rate 6.8 per 1000 population.
- In the United States, 1.1 million women with epilepsy are in their active reproductive years.
- Epilepsy affects 0.5–1% of pregnant women.
- Most frequently encountered neurologic condition in obstetric practice after migraine.
- 80% of pregnant women with epilepsy use antiepileptic drugs.

Seizure Classification
- Generalized seizures (begins in both cerebral hemispheres)
  - Non-convulsive or Absence
  - Convulsive (Tonic, Clonic, Tonic-clonic, Myoclonic)
  - Partial seizures (begins in only one hemisphere)
  - Simple partial (no change in consciousness)
  - Complex partial (accompanied by a change in consciousness)
  - Secondary generalized

Table 2.119. Commonly used antiepileptic

Drug (FDA Pregnancy Category)	Associated Risks	Recommendations for Use During Pregnancy
Carbamazepine (C)	Cardiac malformations	Lower teratogenic potential than that of phenobarbital and valproate
Gabapentin (C)	No major congenital malformations associated with monotherapy	Limited data suggest a lower teratogenic risk, compared with traditional antiepileptic drugs[*]
Lamotrigine (C)	No distinctive pattern of major congenital malformation	
Levetiracetam (C)	Pyloric stenosis (in polytherapy with lamotrigine); spina bifida (in polytherapy with carbamazepine and valproate)	
Oxcarbazepine	Urogenital malformations	
Phenobarbital (D)	Cardiac malformations	Best avoided in women of childbearing age
	Increases risk of major congenital malformations to at least double that of the general population	
Phenytoin	Bradycardia and hypotension; fetal hydantoin syndrome	
Topiramate (D)	Hypospadias; oral clefts	Limited data suggest a lower teratogenic risk, compared with traditional antiepileptic drugs[*]
Valproate	Cardiac malformations; hypospadias; limb reduction defects; neural tube defects; porencephaly; spina bifida	Best avoided in women of childbearing age
	Increases risk of major congenital malformations to at least double that of the general population	

[*]Traditional antiepileptic drugs include carbamazepine, phenobarbital, phenytoin, and valproate.

Source: Reproduced with permission from Sethi NK, Wasterlain A and Harden CL. Pregnancy and epilepsy—managing both, in one patient. *OBG Management.* 2011; 23(6):18-24. © Copyright Frontline Medical.

Maternal Complications
- Repeat seizures (hypoxia)
- Status epilepticus (0–1.8% estimated risk)
- Seizures in labor
- Gestational hypertension
- Preterm labor (if a smoker)

Fetal Complications
- Miscarriage (2× normal)
- Congenital anomalies (2–3× normal)
- Hypoxia
- Small for gestational age (2× risk)
- Low birthweight
- Preterm delivery (if a smoker)
- Low IQ
- Abnormal behavior

Factors Contributing to Increased Seizures in Pregnancy
- High levels of estrogen
- Increased nausea and vomiting
- Changes in plasma volume
- Altered gastric motility
- Altered protein binding
- Increased metabolic capacity of the maternal liver
- Placental/fetal metabolism
- Poor compliance
- Increased life stressors

Seizures in Pregnancy
- Profound alterations in maternal acid-base equilibrium with grand mal seizure
- Maternal serum lactate concentration has been reported to rise tenfold, and pH drop as low as 6.9
- Changes in maternal acid-base equilibrium can be rapidly mediated through the placenta to the fetus

Congenital Malformations
- 6–8% risk of birth defects in infants born to women taking antiepileptic drugs (AEDs)
- 2–3 times the risk of the general population
- Increased risk associated with
  - Polytherapy—malformation incidence 25% with four or more AEDs
  - High peak drug levels
  - Not clearly associated with seizure frequency

Management of Antiepileptic Drugs in Pregnancy
- Consider withdrawal of antiepileptic drug therapy prior to conception if
  - No seizure activity during the past 2–5 years
  - A single type of seizure
  - A normal EEG with treatment
  - A normal neurologic exam
  - Completed 6 months prior to planned conception
- Associated with a recurrence risk
  - 25% if no risk factors
  - 50% if risk factors
  - 90% of recurrences occur first year

Consider Use of Monotherapy
- Single most effective drug at minimum effective dose
- Successful control in one third of patients undergoing planned polytherapy withdrawal
- Avoid arbitrary increases in drug doses for a decreased serum level
- Evaluate free fraction if marked decline in total level
- Increase dose if more seizures or marked decline in free fraction
- Avoid high peak levels (3 or 4 divided doses)

Antiepileptic Drug Monitoring in Pregnancy
- Levels before conception
- Beginning of each trimester
- During last month of pregnancy
- Through eighth postpartum week
- Monitoring schedule may need to be individualized

Folate Supplementation
- Deficiency strongly associated with increased risk of neural tube defects
- Supplementation provides risk reduction ranging from 60–100%
- Supplementation studies not conducted on women taking AEDs, and efficacy unclear
- Amount of folic acid supplementation extrapolated from general population

Folate Supplementation: Current Recommendations
- U.S. Public Health Service
- 0.4 mg/day for all women in United States capable of becoming pregnant
- 1996 American College of Obstetricians and Gynecologists
- 4 mg/day would "seem appropriate" for patients taking AEDs

Vitamin K Supplementation
- Vitamin K deficiency described in neonates born to women using AEDs
- Neonatal administration of 1 mg vitamin K
- May consider vitamin K 10 mg/day in last month of pregnancy (unproven benefit)

THYROID DISEASE IN PREGNANCY
Fast Facts
- Thyroid disease is the second most common endocrine disease in reproductive age women.
- The American College of Obstetricians and Gynecologists does not recommend routine screening of asymptomatic pregnant patients.
- See also pages 564-569 in the Reproductive Endocrinology section.

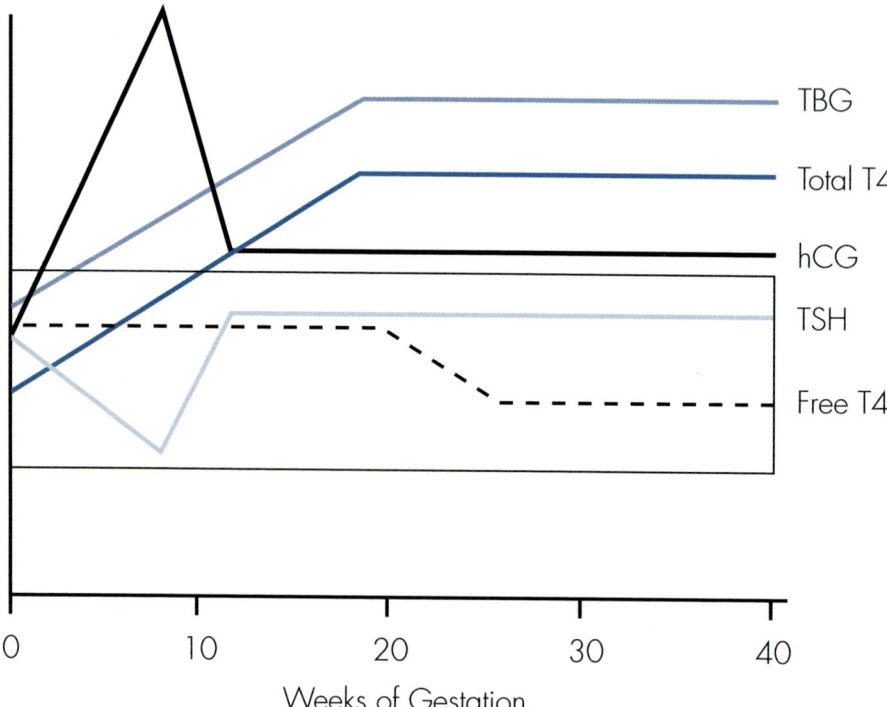

Figure 2.48. The pattern of changes in serum concentrations of thyroid function studies and hCG according to gestational age
TBG, thyroid-binding globulin; T4, thyroxine; TSH, thyroid-stimulating hormone.
  The shading area represents the normal range of thyroid-binding globulin, total thyroxine, thyroid-stimulating hormone, or free T in the nonpregnant woman.
  Source: Reproduced with permission from Casey BM, Leveno KJ. Thyroid disease in pregnancy. *Obstet Gynecol.* 2006;108(5):1283-92. Copyright © 2006 The American College of Obstetricians and Gynecologists.

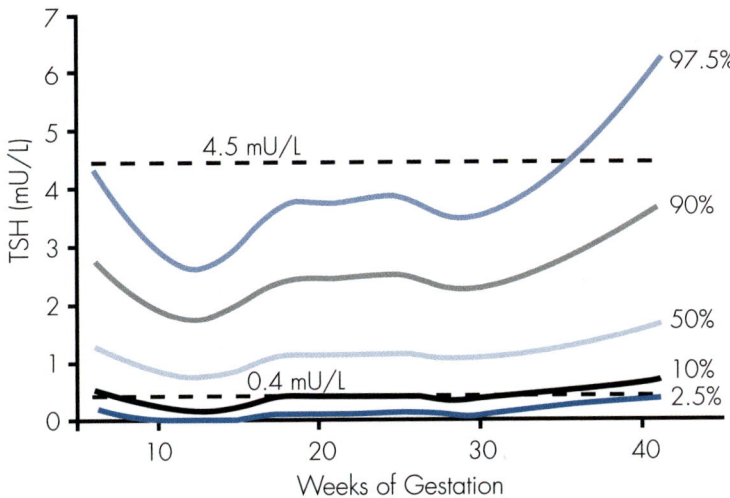

Figure 2.49. Gestational age-specific thyroid stimulating hormone nomogram
Gestational age-specific thyroid stimulating hormone (TSH) nomogram derived from 13,599 and 132 twin pregnancies as reported by Dashe and colleagues.
Source: Reproduced with permission from Dashe JS, Casey BM, Wells CE, et al. Thyroid-stimulating hormone in singleton and twin pregnancy: importance of gestational age-specific reference ranges. *Obstet Gynecol.* 2005 Oct;106(4):753-57. Copyright © 2006 The American College of Obstetricians and Gynecologists.

Table 2.120. Changes in thyroid function studies in normal pregnancy and in thyroid disease

Maternal Status	TSH	Free T4
Pregnancy	Varies by trimester*	No change
Overt hyperthyroidism	Decrease	Increase
Subclinical hyperthyroidism	Decrease	No change
Overt hypothyroidism	Increase	Decrease
Subclinical hypothyroidism	Increase	No change

t_4, thyroxine; TSH, thyroid-stimulating hormone.
*The level of TSH decreases in early pregnancy because of weak TSH receptor stimulation due to substantial quantities of human chorionic gonadotropin during the first 12 weeks of gestation. After the first trimester, TSH levels return to baseline values.

Source: Reproduced with permission from American College of Obstetricians and Gynecologists. ACOG Practice Bulletin No. 148: Thyroid disease in pregnancy. *Obstet Gynecol.* 2015;125:996-1005. Copyright © 2015 The American College of Obstetricians and Gynecologists.

Hyperthyroidism
Signs and Symptoms of Hyperthyroidism
- Nervousness
- Tremors
- Tachycardia
- Excessive sweating
- Heat intolerance
- Weight loss
- Goiter
- Insomnia
- Palpitations
- Hypertension

Graves' Disease Causes 95% of Hyperthyroidism in Pregnancy
- Autoantibodies, thyroid-stimulating immunoglobulin, and thyroid-stimulating hormone-binding inhibitory immunoglobulin act on the thyroid-stimulating hormone receptor to cause thyroid stimulation or inhibition.
- Thyroid-stimulating immunoglobulin and thyroid-stimulating hormone-binding inhibitory immunoglobulin can affect the fetal thyroid and cause fetal thyrotoxicosis or transient hypothyroidism in neonates of any woman with Graves' disease.

Inadequately Treated Maternal Thyrotoxicosis Can Contribute
- Preterm delivery
- Low birth weight
- Fetal loss
- Severe preeclampsia
- Heart failure

Management
- Measure free thyroxine, free thyroxine index (FTI), or total thyroxine every 2–4 weeks.
- Use free thyroxine levels if your lab has trimester specific normal ranges. If not, measure total thyroxine levels. Normal total thyroxine levels in the second and third trimesters are up to 1.5 × the normal range for the nonpregnant population.
- Keep thyroxine levels in the high normal range using the lowest dose of medication.
- Treat with either propylthiouracil (PTU) or methimazole.
- Methimazole has been associated with a higher risk of embyropathy when given in the first trimester.
- PTU has been associated with a risk of maternal hepatotoxicity and so is recommended in the first trimester only, after which methimazole is usually used.
- Both PTU and methimazole can lead to agranulocytosis (0.1% risk).
- Both medications decrease thyroid hormone synthesis. PTU also reduces peripheral conversion of thyroxine to triiodothyronine.
- PTU and methimazole both enter breast milk but are "compatible" with breastfeeding according to the American Academy of Pediatrics.
- β-blockers may be used to ameliorate the symptoms of thyrotoxicosis.

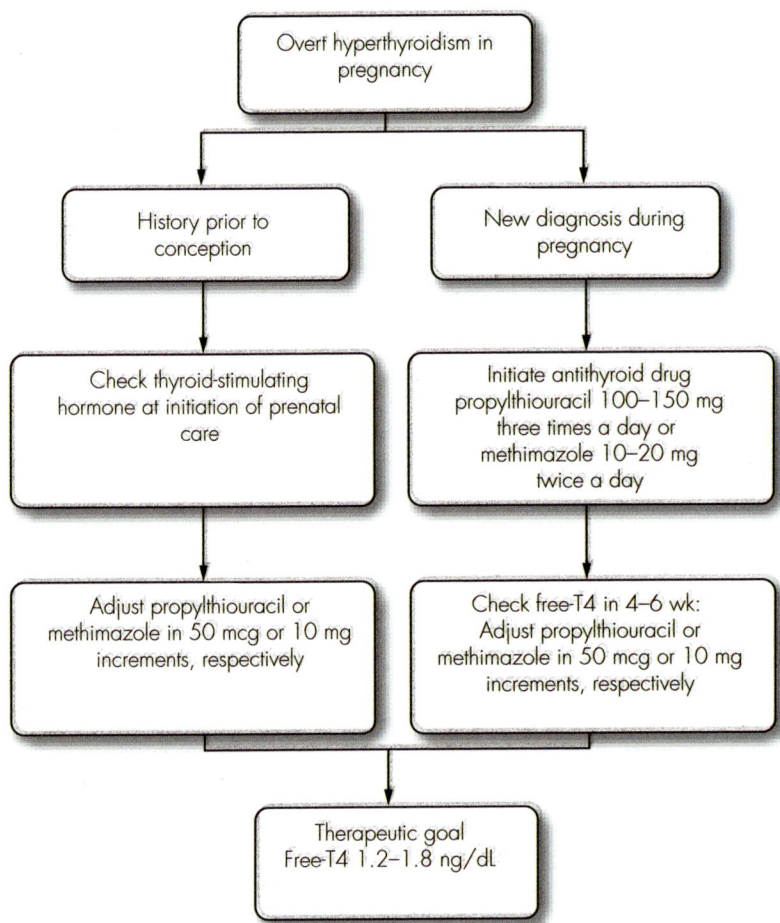

Figure 2.50. Management of hyperthyroidism in pregnancy
Source: Reproduced with permission from Casey BM, Leveno KJ: Thyroid Disease in Pregnancy. *Obstet Gynecol.* 2006;108(5):1283-92. Copyright © 2006 The American College of Obstetricians and Gynecologists.

Treatment of Thyroid Storm in Pregnant Women

Table 2.121. Diagnostic criteria for thyroid storm

Thermoregulatory Dysfunction		Cardiovascular Dysfunction	
Temperature (°F | °C)		Tachycardia	
99 to 99.9 | 37.2 to 37.7	5	99 to 109	5
100 to 100.9 | 37.8 to 38.2	10	110 to 119	10
101 to 101.9 | 38.3 to 38.8	15	120 to 129	15
102 to 102.9 | 38.9 to 39.4	20	130 to 139	20
103 to 103.9 | 39.4 to 39.9	25	≥140	25
≥104.0 | >40.0	30	Atrial fibrillation	10
Central Nervous System Effects		Heart Failure	
Mild	10	Mild	5
Agitation		Pedal edema	
Moderate	20	Moderate	10
Delirium		Bibasilar rales	
Psychosis			
Extreme lethargy			
Severe	30	Severe	15
Seizure		Pulmonary edema	
Coma			
		Precipitant history	
		Negative	0
		Positive	10
Gastrointestinal-hepatic dysfunction			
Moderate	10		
Diarrhea			
Nausea/vomiting			
Abdominal pain			
Severe	20		
Unexplained jaundice			

*A score of 45 or more is highly suggestive of thyroid storm; a score of 25 to 44 supports the diagnosis; and a score below 25 makes thyroid storm unlikely.

Source: Burch HB, Wartofsky L. Life-threatening thyrotoxicosis. Thyroid storm. *Endocrinol Metab Clin North Am.* 1993; 22:263.

Thyroid Disease in Pregnancy — OBSTETRICS

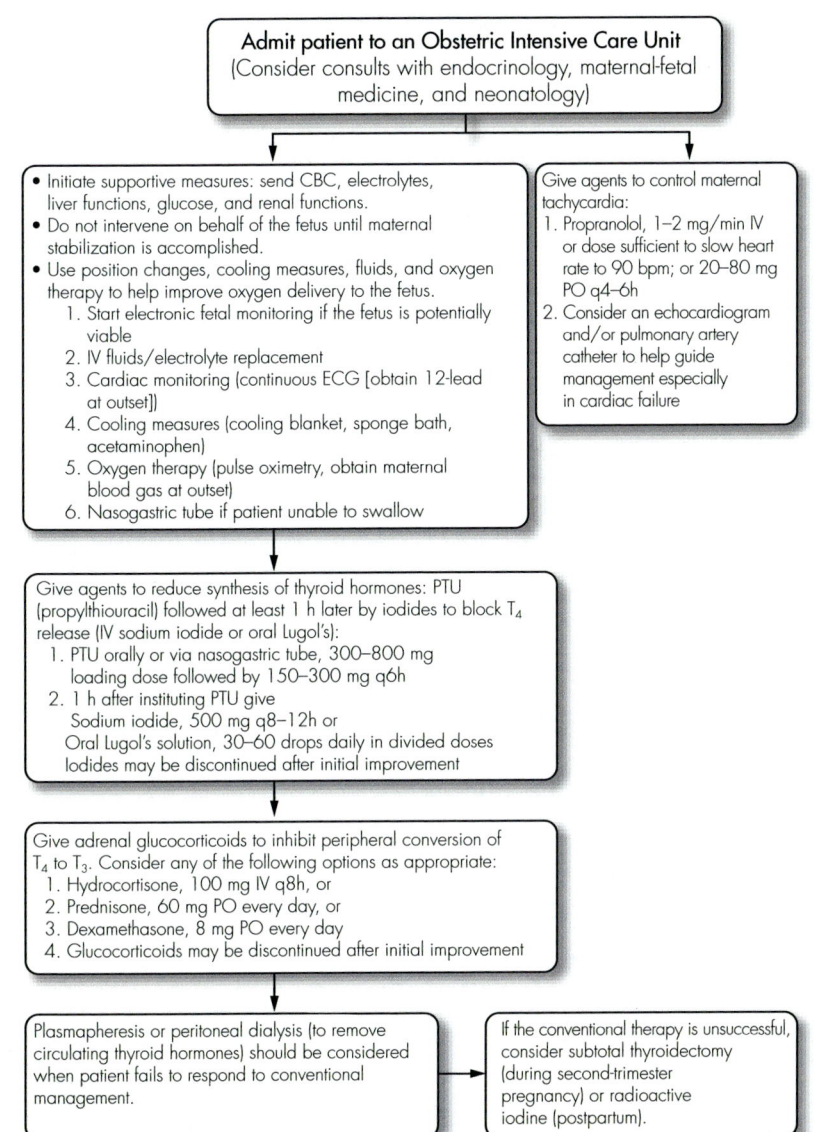

Figure 2.51. Management of thyroid storm
Source: Reproduced with permission from Belfort, MA. Critical care in OB: part 4 navigating a thyroid storm. *Cont Ob/Gyn.* 2006;51(10):38-47. *Cont Ob/Gyn* is a copyrighted publication of Advanstar Communications Inc. All rights reserved.

Hypothyroidism (see also pages 564-569)
Signs and Symptoms
- Fatigue
- Constipation
- Intolerance to cold
- Muscle cramps
- Hair loss
- Dry skin

Etiology
- Hashimoto's disease (chronic thyroiditis or chronic autoimmune thyroiditis)
- Subacute thyroiditis
- History of thyroidectomy
- History of radioactive iodine treatment
- Iodine deficiency
- Postpartum thyroiditis (autoimmune inflammation of the thyroid gland causing thyrotoxicosis followed by hypothyroidism within 1 year postpartum)
- Subclinical hypothyroidism (elevated TSH with normal FTI, asymptomatic)

Inadequately Treated Hypothyroidism Can Lead to
- Increased risk of preeclampsia
- Placental abruption
- Low birth weight
- Congenital cretinism (growth failure, mental retardation, other neuropsychologic defects)
- Trimester-specific ranges for TSH should be 0.1 to 2.5 mU/L (first trimester), 0.2 to 3.0 mU/L (second trimester), and 0.3 to 3.0 mU/L (third trimester)

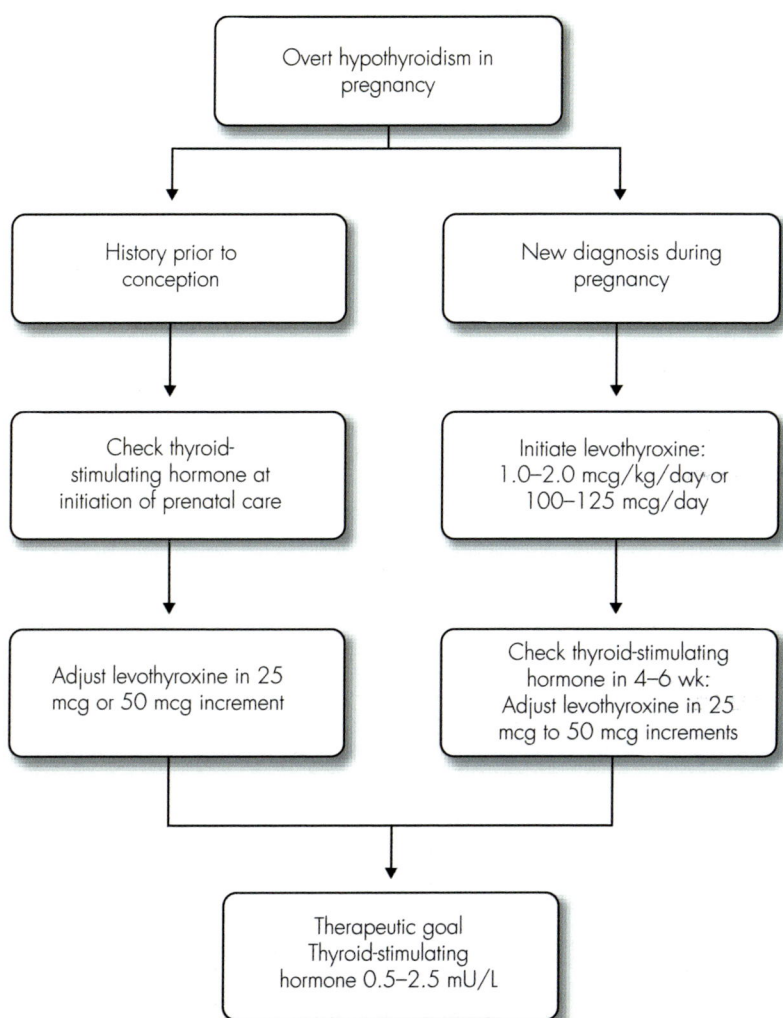

Figure 2.52. Management of hypothyroidism
Source: Reproduced with permission from Casey BM, Leveno KJ: Thyroid Disease in Pregnancy. *Obstet Gynecol.* 2006;108(5):1283-92. Copyright © 2006 The American College of Obstetricians and Gynecologists.

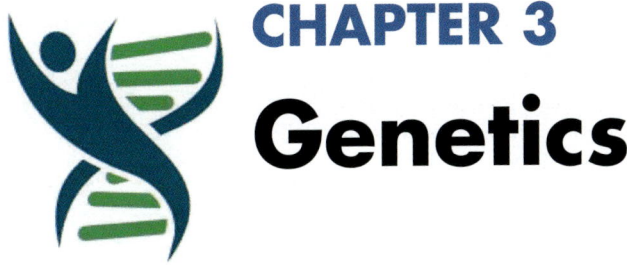

CHAPTER 3
Genetics

CARRIER SCREENING BASICS
Autosomal Recessive Inheritance
- Most disorders screened are autosomal recessive. Two carriers of the same disorder have a 25% risk with each pregnancy to have an affected child.

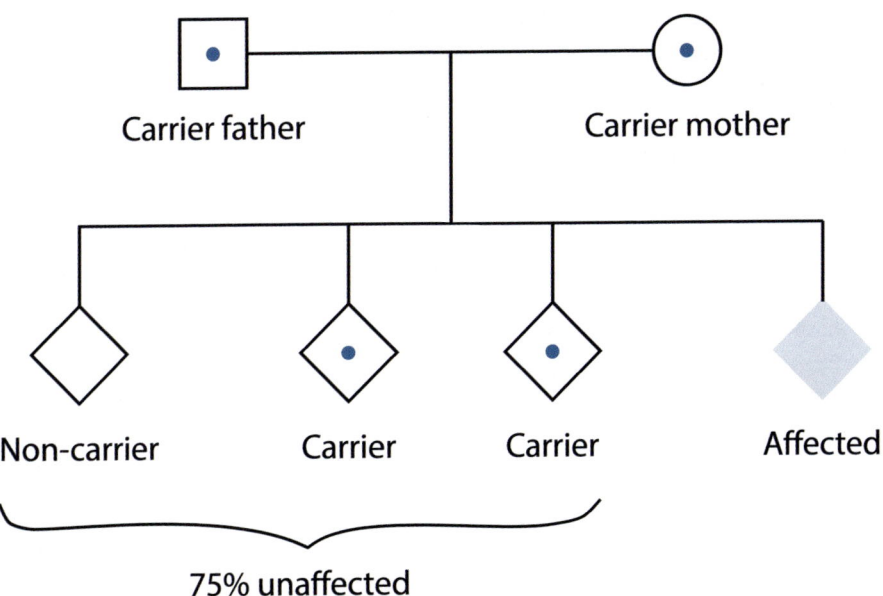

Figure 3.1. Outcomes in autosomal recessive genetic diseases

Possible Results of Carrier Screening
- Positive: The individual tested is a carrier
  - Next step: Test the reproductive partner
  - Exception: Fragile X syndrome, if a woman is a carrier, her pregnancies are at risk, no need to test her reproductive partner unless clinically indicated
- Negative: The individual is at reduced risk to be a carrier
  - There is a small residual risk to be a carrier even after a negative test
  - No additional testing is recommended
- Indeterminate/inconclusive
  - Test results may be indeterminate (e.g., Tay-Sachs enzyme)
  - May be due to specimen quality or quantity or failure of test due to other reasons; sample rerun may clarify

Benefits and Limitations of Carrier Screening
- Benefits
  - Identify at-risk couples.
  - Carrier identification allows for preconception planning as well as the option of prenatal diagnosis for the couple at risk.
  - Early identification of affected pregnancies allows condition-specific counseling and care.
  - Provide reassurance of reduced risk to have an affected child.
- Limitations
  - No test detects 100% of mutations; there is always a residual risk.

Candidates for Carrier Screening
- Women of reproductive age before conception
- Egg and sperm donors
- Pregnant couples

Screening Paradigms
- Screening can be based on ethnicity or screening can be offered to all patients regardless of ethnicity.
- Five professional organizations, including ACOG, ACMG, SMFM, NSGC, and the Perinatal Quality Foundation, recently issued a joint statement in the March 2015 issue of Obstetrics and Gynecology that helps clarify for physicians how to use expanded carrier screening and which patients can benefit from it.

PAN-ETHNIC CARRIER SCREENING OR EXTENDED CARRIER SCREENING (ECS)

Expanded Carrier Screening Incorporates the Following Concepts

1. All individuals, regardless of race or ethnicity, are offered screening for the same set of conditions.
2. Expanded carrier screening panels can include more than 100 genetic conditions, most of which are rare. Before testing, it is not practical or necessary to fully explain all of the clinical and test characteristics of each condition.
3. Pretest education and consent should broadly describe the types of conditions being screened for and their common features as well as the limitations of screening. Educating patients before testing may be done verbally or by using other informational approaches such as pamphlets, videos, or online resources. General concepts to be included in pretest counseling should include the following:
   a. Some conditions screened have less well-defined phenotypes.
   b. Because many conditions being screened are rare, disease prevalence, mutation frequencies, and detection rates may be imprecise and residual risk estimations may not be reliable.
   c. Screen-negative results reduce the likelihood of the carrier state for the conditions, but a residual risk of being a carrier always remains.
   d. Screening panels may change over time, and there may be differences in the conditions screened between laboratories. Despite this, carrier rescreening typically is not offered or recommended.
4. The majority of conditions on current expanded panels are autosomal-recessive. However, some may be X-linked or autosomal-dominant single-gene conditions.
5. Expanded screening panels include most of the conditions recommended in current guidelines. However, the molecular methods used in expanded carrier screening are not as accurate as methods recommended in current guidelines for the following conditions:
   a. Screening for hemoglobinopathies requires use of mean corpuscular volume and hemoglobin electrophoresis.
   b. Tay-Sachs disease carrier testing has a low detection rate in non-Ashkenazi populations using molecular testing for the three common Ashkenazi mutations. Currently, hexosaminidase A enzyme analysis on blood is the best method to identify carriers in all ethnicities.

Source: Reproduced with permission from Edwards JG, Feldman G, Goldberg J, et al. Expanded carrier screening in reproductive medicine-points to consider: a joint statement of the American College of Medical Genetics and Genomics, American College of Obstetricians and Gynecologists, National Society of Genetic Counselors, Perinatal Quality Foundation, and Society for Maternal-Fetal Medicine. *Obstet Gynecol.* 2015 Mar;125(3):653-62.

GENETICS — Ethnic-Specific Screening

ETHNIC-SPECIFIC SCREENING

- Non-Hispanic white individuals should be offered cystic fibrosis carrier screening.
- People of Eastern European Jewish descent (Ashkenazi Jews) should be offered screening for Tay-Sachs disease, Canavan disease, familial dysautonomia, and cystic fibrosis. Individuals can ask about screening for other disorders. Carrier screening is available for mucolipidosis IV, Niemann–Pick disease type A, Fanconi anemia group C, Bloom syndrome, and Gaucher disease.
- People of African, Mediterranean, and Southeast Asian heritage should be offered screening for thalassemias and sickle cell disease.

Table 3.1. Ethnic-specific genetic carrier screening
Disorders typically recommended based on a patient's ethnic background. Disorders may occur outside of high-risk ethnicities.

Ethnic Background	Disorder	Carrier Frequency
African American	Alpha thalassemia	1 in 30
	Beta thalassemia	1 in 75
	Sickle cell disease	1 in 10
Ashkenazi Jewish	Ashkenazi Jewish panel*	1 in 5
Asian	Alpha thalassemia	1 in 20
	Beta thalassemia	1 in 50
Cajun	Tay-Sachs disease	Increased
French Canadian	Tay-Sachs disease	1 in 251
Irish	Tay-Sachs disease	1 in 522, 3
Hispanic	Alpha thalassemia	Variable
	Beta thalassemia	1 in 32–75
	Sickle cell	1 in 30–200
Mediterranean	Alpha thalassemia	1 in 30–50
	Beta thalassemia	1 in 20–30
	Sickle cell disease	1 in 30–50
Middle Eastern	Alpha thalassemia	Variable
	Beta thalassemia	1 in 50
	Sickle cell disease	1 in 50–100
Sephardic Jewish	Alpha thalassemia	1 in 4–100
	Beta thalassemia	1 in 5–7
	Sephardic Jewish panel**	Increased

Courtesy of Good Start Genetics.

- **Ashkenazi Jewish disorders:** Recommended for Jewish individuals from Eastern Europe. Disorders range in severity and symptoms; however, all can have a serious impact on quality of life and life expectancy. May occur outside the Ashkenazi Jewish population at a reduced frequency. The 1-in-5-carrier frequency is based on the full extended screening panel.
- **Sephardic Jewish disorders:** Recommended for Jewish individuals from Spain, Portugal, the Middle East, or North Africa. Disorders range in severity and symptoms; however, all can have a serious impact on quality of life and life expectancy. May occur outside the Sephardic Jewish population at a reduced frequency.

Ethnic-Specific Screening

- Disorders at increased frequency (not all appropriate for routine carrier screening) include alpha-thalassemia, ataxia telangiectasia, beta-thalassemia, corticosterone methyloxidase type II deficiency, Costeff optical atrophy, cystic fibrosis, hereditary inclusion body myopathy, familial Mediterranean fever, glucose-6-phosphate-dehydrogenase (G6PD) deficiency, limb girdle muscular dystrophy, metachromatic leukodystrophy, polyglandular syndrome, pseudocholinesterase deficiency, spinal muscular atrophy, and Wolman syndrome.

Table 3.2. Genetic disorders in the Ashkenazi Jewish population

Disorder	Gene	Ashkenazi Jewish Carrier Frequency
Bloom's syndrome[2, 3]	BLM	1 in 134
Canavan disease[1, 2, 3]	ASPA	1 in 55
Cystic fibrosis[1, 2, 3]	CFTR	1 in 23
Dihydrolipoamide Dehydrogenase Deficiency[3]	DLD	1 in 107
Familial dysautonomia[1, 2, 3]	IKBKAP	1 in 31
Familial hyperinsulinism[3]	ABCC8	1 in 68
Fanconi anemia C[2, 3]	FANCC	1 in 100
Gaucher disease[2, 3]	GBA	1 in 15
Glycogen storage disease type 1a[3]	G6PC	1 in 64
Joubert syndrome type 2[3]	TMEM216	1 in 92
Maple syrup urine disease A/B[3]	BCKDHB/A	1 in 97
Mucolipidosis type IV[2, 3]	MCOLN1	1 in 89
Nemaline myopathy[c]	NEB	1 in 168
Niemann-Pick disease type A/B[b, c]	SMPD1	1 in 115
Spinal muscular atrophy[b, c]	SMN1	1 in 67
Tay-Sachs disease[a, b, c]	HEXA	1 in 27
Usher syndrome type 1F[c]	PCDH15	1 in 147
Usher syndrome type III[c]	CLRN1	1 in 120
Walker-Warburg syndrome[c]	FKTN	1 in 150

[a]ACOG recommended disorder.
[b]ACMG recommended disorder.
[c]Jewish advocacy organization recommended disorder.
[1]Andermann (1977).
[2]Van Bael (1996).
[3]Branda (2004).
Courtesy of Good Start Genetics.

Table 3.3. Current ACOG and ACMG screening guidelines

Screen	ACOG (Year of Publication)	ACMG (Year of Publication)
Cystic Fibrosis	Screening should be offered to all women of reproductive age (2001, reaffirmed 2011)	Screening should be considered by all couples for use for use before conception or prenatally (2001, reaffirmed 2013)
Spinal Muscular Atrophy	Preconception and prenatal screening is not recommended in the general population (2009)	Carrier testing should be offered to all couples regardless of race or ethnicity (2008, reaffirmed 2013)
Fragile X	Population carrier screening is not recommended (2010)	Population carrier screening is not recommended except as part of a well-defined clinical research protocol (2005)
Hemoglobinopathies	Individuals of African, Southeast Asian, and Mediterranean descent are at increased risk for being carriers of hemoglobinopathies and should be offered carrier screening and, if both parents are determined to be carriers, genetic counseling (2007)	Not currently addressed
Ashkenazi Jewish Descent	Individuals of AJ ancestry should be offered screening for four disorders—CF, TSD, Familial Dysautonomia (FD), and Canavan Disease (CD) and should be made aware of the availability of testing for five additional diseases—Fanconi Anemia Group C, Gaucher disease type I, Niemann-Pick disease type A, Bloom syndrome, and Mucolipidosis type IV (2009)	Screening should be offered for CF, TSD, Familial Dysautonomia, Canavan Disease, Fanconi anemia (Group C), Niemann-Pick (Type A), Bloom syndrome, Mucolipidosis IV, and Gaucher disease (2008)
Expanded Carrier Screening	Not currently addressed	The proper selection of appropriate disease-causing targets for general population-based carrier screening (i.e., absence of a family history of the disorder) should be developed using clear criteria, rather than simply including as many disorders as possible (2013)

Source: Adapted from Bajaj K, Gross SJ. Carrier screening: past, present, and future. *J Clin Med.* 2014;3(3):1033-42.

Table 3.4. Carrier frequency for cystic fibrosis, Fragile X, and spinal muscular atrophy

Disorder (*Gene*)	Ethnicity	Carrier Frequency
Cystic fibrosis (*CFTR*)	African American	1 in 61
	Ashkenazi Jewish	1 in 23
	Asian	1 in 94
	Caucasian	1 in 25
	Hispanic	1 in 58
Fragile X syndrome (*FMR1*)	All ethnicities	1 in 178 women
Spinal muscular atrophy (*SMN1*)	African American	1 in 72
	Ashkenazi Jewish	1 in 67
	Asian	1 in 59
	Caucasian	1 in 47
	Hispanic	1 in 68

Courtesy of Good Start Genetics.

CYSTIC FIBROSIS
Fast Facts
- Cystic fibrosis (CF) is an autosomal recessive, chronic disorder affecting epithelia of the respiratory, gastrointestinal, genitourinary, and hepatobiliary systems.
- Symptoms include, but are not limited to, obstructive lung disease, recurrent lung infection, meconium ileus, pancreatic insufficiency, recurrent pancreatitis, malnutrition, and male infertility.
- In severe cases, lung transplant may be necessary; pulmonary disease is the major cause of mortality.
- Average lifespan is into the late thirties.

Pathophysiology and Genetics
- Cystic Fibrosis Transmembrane Conductance Regulator (*CFTR*) on chromosome 7 encodes a chloride channel in the epithelia.
    - >1900 known variants reported in *CFTR* (Cystic Fibrosis Mutation Database, http://www.genet.sickkids.on.ca). Not all are pathogenic.
- Incidence in the United States: ~1/3,700, regardless of gender; varies by ethnic background (see carrier frequencies in Table 3.4.).
- Genitourinary symptoms include male infertility, specifically congenital bilateral absence of the vas deferens (CBAVD), presenting as obstructive azoospermia (see male subfertility, p. 475).

Table 3.5. *CFTR* mutations in men with congenital absence of the vas deferens

% Of Men with CBAVD	CFTR Mutations On Both Alleles
46%	2
28%	1
26%	0

Source: Adapted from Yu J, Chen Z, Ni Y, Li Z. *CFTR* mutations in men with congenital bilateral absence of the vas deferens (CBAVD): a systemic review and meta-analysis. Hum Reprod. Jan;27(1):25-35, 2012.

- Carrier screening for CF: molecular testing. ACOG recommends screening for at least 23 of the most common disease-causing mutations. Detection of more mutations will increase the detection rates.
    - Genotyping-based tests detect the most common mutations via SNP-based testing; these are limited to a predefined set of known, common mutations.
    - Sequencing-based tests detect a greater number of disease-causing mutations, including novel, pathogenic mutations, increasing sensitivity (detection rate). Depending on the application of the technology, it may identify variants of unknown significance.
- There is a genotype-phenotype correlation.
    - Nomenclature:
        - ΔF508: denotes a deletion ("delta") of phenylalanine ("F") at amino acid position 508.
        - c.1521_1523delCTT: denotes a deletion ("del") of nucleotides ("CTT") at positions 1521 through 1523 in the cDNA sequence.
        - R117H: denotes an amino acid change from arginine ("R") to histidine ("H") at amino acid position 117.

- Mutation information:
  - Some provide reliable There is a genotype-phenotype correlation for pancreatic function; however, the severity of pulmonary disease is more difficult to predict.
  - Inheritance of any two disease-causing mutations, one from each reproductive partner, can result in cystic fibrosis. It is <u>not</u> necessary to inherit two copies of the same mutation in order to have the disease.
- ΔF508 is the most common mutation in northern Europeans (75% of all CF mutations); known to cause severe/classic CF.

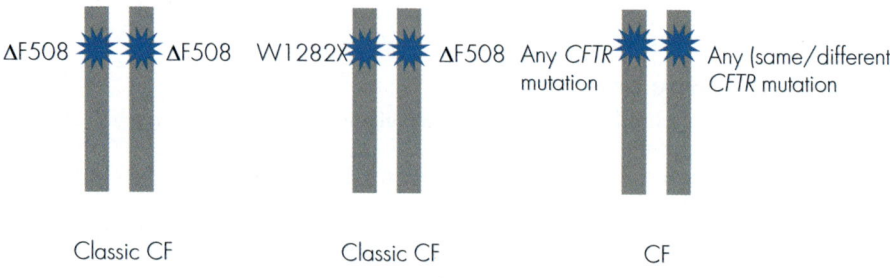

Figure 3.2. Cystic fibrosis genotype-phenotype correlation

- W1282X accounts for 46% of all CF mutations in Ashkenazi Jews.
- If a patient is positive **for** *R117H*, reflex tests should be performed on the same proband, looking for poly T tract (5T/7T/9T).
  - *R117H* is considered a classic disease-causing mutation <u>only</u> when in cis (same chromosome) with the 5T variant AND if there is a CF mutation on the other chromosome.
  - While 5T is known to be associated with CBAVD, other genetic modifiers (e.g., the TG tract in *CFTR*), make it difficult to predict the exact phenotype.

FRAGILE X

Fast Facts
- Fragile X syndrome is the most common cause of inherited intellectual disability.
- Fragile X Mental Retardation 1 (*FMR1*) encodes a protein (FMRP) that is found in many tissues throughout development and abundantly in neurons.
  - Large expansions of CGG repeats cause methylation and reduced/no expression of FMRP.
- X-linked inheritance: Fragile X syndrome is inherited from the mother. CGG repeats may expand when passed through the maternal line (maternal anticipation).
  - AGG interruptions:
    - In 45–69 length CGG repeats, the presence of AGG interruptions: may decrease the risk of expansion in offspring (Nolin 2013).

Table 3.6. Risk of expansion of Fragile X in next generation

# CGG Repeats	Type of Allele	Presentation in Proband	Risk of Expansion in Next Generation	
<45	Normal	n/a	n/a	
45–54	Intermediate	n/a	16% to expand to intermediate/premutation	
55–200	Premutation	FXPOI & FXTAS	Increases with premutation size[a]	
			55–59	4%
			60–69	5%
			70–79	31%
			80–89	58%
			90–99	80%
			100–200	98%
>200	Full Mutation	Fragile X syndrome	~100%	

[a]Nolin SL, Brown WT, Glicksman A, et al. Expansion of the Fragile X CGG repeat in females with premutation or intermediate alleles. *Am J Hum Genet.* 2003; 72:454.

*There have been occasional reports of expansion from 56 and 59 repeats to full mutations in one generation (Fernandez-Carvajal 2009).

Phenotype and Genotype
Full Mutations (>200 CGG Repeats): Fragile X Syndrome
- Symptoms include but are not limited to
  - Developmental: delayed motor/verbal milestones, intellectual disability
  - Behavioral: autistic-like behaviors, hyperactivity, anxiety, and autism
  - Physical: long face, prominent forehead and jaw, large ears, macroorchidism, joint hyperextensibility, mitral valve prolapse, and smooth skin
- Incidence
  - Males: 1 in 4,000 to 6,250 (de Vries 1997)
  - Women with a full mutation can be asymptomatic, mildly affected, or have Fragile X Syndrome.
  - Prevalence of females with Fragile X syndrome presumed to be approximately one half the male prevalence

Premutation (55–200 CGG Repeats) Carriers:
- Fragile X–associated Premature Ovarian Insufficiency (FXPOI).
  - 21% of premutation carriers develop POI (Sherman 2005).
- Fragile X–associated Tremor Ataxia Syndrome (FXTAS).
  - Late-onset, progressive ataxia and intention tremor; includes memory loss, muscle weakness, and autonomic dysfunction.
  - 8–16% risk in females (Saul 2012).
  - Up to 45% risk in males (Saul 2012).

Intermediate (45–54 CGG Repeats) Carriers:
- Clinically asymptomatic; not at risk for FXPOI or FXTAS.
- 16% risk for expansion to intermediate/premutation, depending on repeat size.
  - Unlikely to expand to a full mutation in one generation (Saul 2012).

Carrier Screening for Fragile X
- Triplet repeat analysis with Southern blot for confirmation.
- Recommended for individuals with a personal or family history of premature ovarian insufficiency (POI), diminished ovarian reserve, unexplained intellectual disability, unexplained autism, or Fragile X Syndrome

SPINAL MUSCULAR ATROPHY

Fast Facts
- Autosomal recessive neuromuscular disorder characterized by degeneration of anterior horn cells (lower motor neurons).
- Results in progressive muscle weakness.
- Bulbospinal variety of SMA is a triplet repeat (CAG) expansion disorder of the androgen receptor gene on the X chromosome.
- Incidence 1/10,000, regardless of gender
- Varies by ethnic background (see Table 3.4.).
- Symptoms and severity vary by age of onset; however, intellect and appearance are not affected.

Genotype and Phenotype
- Survival Motor Neuron 1 (*SMN1*) encodes a protein involved in small nuclear ribonuclear protein (snRNP) biogenesis and function.
- *SMN2*, directly adjacent to *SMN1*, differs by eight nucleotides. Also encodes SMN protein, at reduced levels compared to *SMN1*. *SMN1* is the disease-causing gene. Increased copy number of *SMN2* can decrease severity of SMA.
- 95–98% of disease is caused by a deletion in *SMN1*.
- 2–5% of affected individuals are compound heterozygotes.
- Carrier screening looks at exon 7 of *SMN1* to determine gene copy number.

Table 3.7. Types of SMA

Classification	% Of Cases	Onset	Clinical Presentation
SMA type 1 Werdnig-Hoffman	60%[a]	<6 months	Symmetric hypotonia; lack of motor development; unable to sit unsupported; difficulty sucking, swallowing, and breathing; death by age 2
SMA type 2 Dubowitz disease	27%[a]	6–12 months	Slow attainment of motor milestones, can sit unsupported, loss of skills with time, majority live into 20s
SMA type 3 Kugelberg-Welander	rare	>12 months	Independent walking, frequent falls, lose walking in teens or 30s, poor weight gain, sleep problems, scoliosis, normal life expectancy
SMA type 4	rare	Adult onset	Muscle weakness develops in teens or 20s, poor weight gain, sleep problems, scoliosis, normal life expectancy

[a]Ogino S, Wilson RB. Spinal muscular atrophy: molecular genetics and diagnostics. *Expert Rev Mol Diagn*. 2004 Jan;4(1):15-29.

Limitations of Carrier Screening Specific to SMA
- Routine carrier screening for SMA: copy number analysis of *SMN1*.
  - Copy number of *SMN1* (determined by the copy number of exon 7) is done by a PCR-based assay, such as multiplex ligation-dependent probe amplification (MLPA).
- ~6% of parents of an affected child will have a negative carrier screen.
- *De novo* mutations: Approximately 2% of affected individuals are born to a noncarrier parent. *De novo* mutations are typically paternal in origin (Wirth 1997; Smith 2007).
- While most individuals have one copy of *SMN1* on each chromosome, about 4% of people have two copies of *SMN1* on one chromosome (Ogino 2004).

GENETICS

- "2+0" silent carrier: normal carrier screening results because the carrier screen identifies 2 copies of the *SMN1* gene. However, this person is at risk for passing on the chromosome with no copies of the *SMN1* gene and is therefore at risk for having an affected child.
- 3 copies: reduced residual risk.

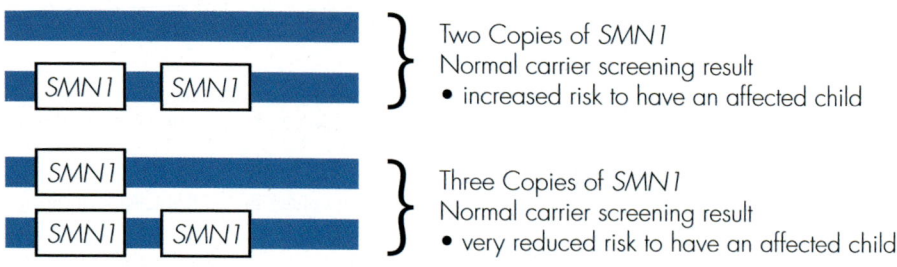

Figure 3.3. Risk of SMA is variable in patients with normal carrier screening result depending upon number of copies and gene location

HEMOGLOBINOPATHIES

Fast Facts
- Inherited disorders that affect the quantity or quality of hemoglobin
- Severe disease may result in transfusion dependency
- Carrier screening for hemoglobinopathies can be done with a complete blood count (CBC) with ferritin and a hemoglobin electrophoresis with quantitative A2

Alpha-Thalassemia
- Caused by mutations in the alpha-globin genes (*HBA1* & *HBA2*).
- Molecular testing, typically deletion/duplication analysis of *HBA1* and *HBA2*, may be appropriate for the partner of an alpha-thalassemia trait carrier.
- Severity depends on number of working alpha-globin genes.
  - Silent carrier (-Δ/Δ Δ) one mutation: asymptomatic. Normal MCV/MCH. Only detected by molecular analysis.
  - Alpha-trait (- Δ/- Δ) or (- -/Δ Δ) two mutations: mild anemia. Low MCV/MCH.
    - Carriers of mutations in *trans* (- Δ/- Δ) are more common in African American and Mediterranean populations. They are not at risk for having a child with Hb Barts hydrops fetalis.
    - Carriers of mutations in *cis* (- -/Δ Δ) are more common in Southeast Asian populations and are at risk for Hb Barts hydrops fetalis.
  - Hemoglobin H disease (- -/- Δ) three mutations: moderate anemia. Symptoms include splenomegaly, increased risk of infection, pregnancy complications. Low MCV/MCH.
  - Hb Barts Fetalis (- -/- -) four mutations: not compatible with life. Maternal complications with an affected pregnancy.

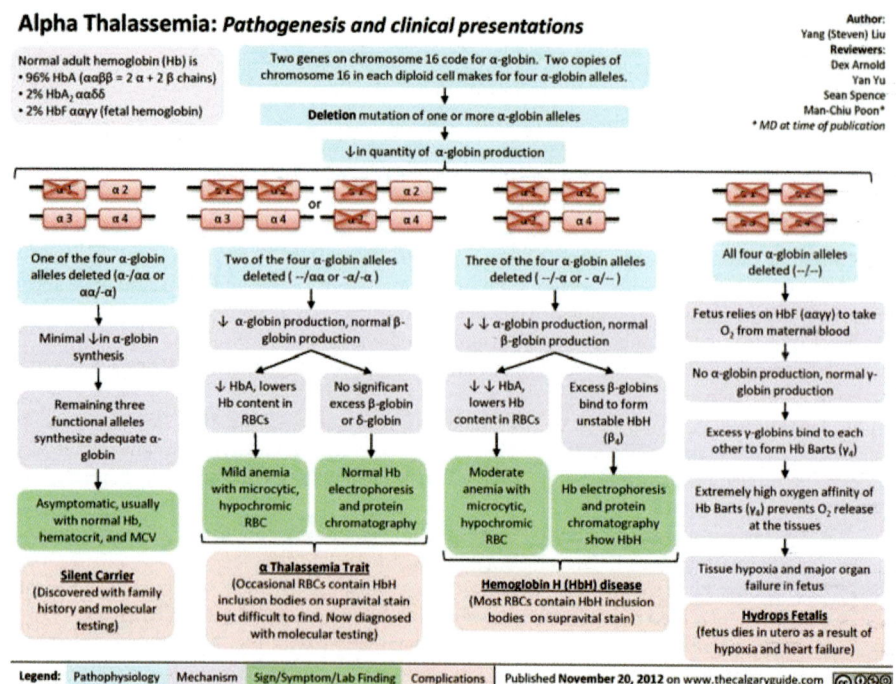

Figure 3.4. Summary of Alpha Thalassemia
Source: Reproduced with permission from *The Calgary Guide to Understanding Disease*, a collaborative student/faculty project of the University of Calgary. For this, and other materials which illuminate the connection between pathophysiology and clinical symptoms and signs, visit thecalgaryguide.com.

Beta-Thalassemia

- Caused by mutations in the beta-globin gene (*HBB*).
- Carriers typically have a low mean corpuscular volume (MCV) on CBC and elevated hemoglobin A2 on electrophoresis.
    - Partners of beta-thalassemia carriers should be screened for beta-thalassemia and sickle cell disease; heterozygous beta-thalassemia and sickle cell mutations cause sickle-beta-thalassemia, which could be clinically severe.
- Severity ranges from mild to severe, depending on residual beta-globin production.
    - Symptoms may include poor growth, skeletal abnormalities, risk for infection, and shortened lifespan.

Hemoglobinopathies

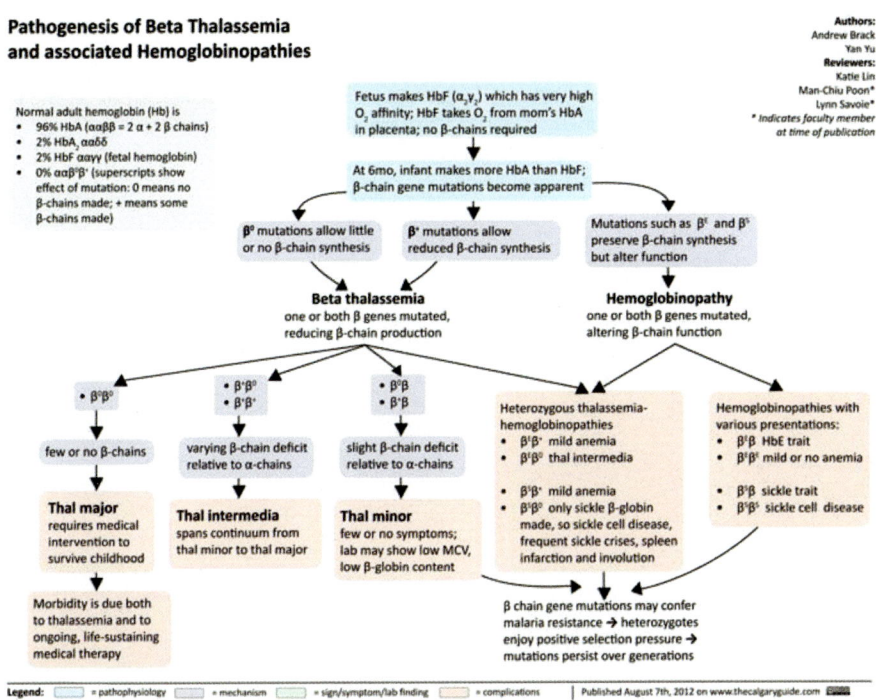

Figure 3.5. Summary of Beta Thalassemia
Source: Reproduced with permission from *The Calgary Guide to Understanding Disease*, a collaborative student/faculty project of the University of Calgary. For this, and other materials which illuminate the connection between pathophysiology and clinical symptoms and signs, visit thecalgaryguide.com.

Sickle Cell Disease

- Caused by mutations in the beta-globin gene (*HBB*).
- Carriers have an abnormal (HbS) peak on hemoglobin electrophoresis. Molecular testing can identify the causative mutation, a point mutation changing the sixth amino acid, glutamic acid, to valine (Glu6Val).
  - Partners of sickle cell carriers should be screened for beta-thalassemia and sickle cell disease; heterozygous beta-thalassemia and sickle cell mutations cause sickle-beta-thalassemia, which could be clinically severe.
- Sickle-shaped red blood cells clog arteries, causing vaso-occlusive events, which can result in pain, stroke, cardiomyopathy, bone and joint complications, etc.
- Symptoms may be exacerbated by dehydration, alcohol consumption, high altitudes, extreme temperatures, and stress.
  - Sickle cell disease carriers may become symptomatic under these conditions.

CHROMOSOME ABNORMALITIES: IN THE FETUS
Fast Facts
- The vast majority of aneuploidies are due to errors in chromosome segregation at the first meiotic division in the oocyte (thus, they are maternal in origin).
- Incidence of chromosome abnormalities:
  - 60–70% of all first trimester spontaneous abortions.
  - 6–11% of all stillbirths.
- Sex chromosome abnormalities:
  - Incidence: **1 in 400** (Nielson 1990).
    - 2.5% recurrence risk after previous sex chromosome aneuploidy (Warburton 2005).
    - No increased recurrence risk after 47,XYY or 45,XO.
- The recurrence risk of a chromosomal trisomy in a subsequent pregnancy is increased (de Souza 2009).

Table 3.8. Incidence of chromosome abnormalities by maternal age

Age at Term	Risk of Trisomy 21*	Risk of Any Chromosome Abnormality†
15‡	1:1,578	1:454
16‡	1:1,572	1:475
17‡	1:1,565	1:499
18‡	1:1,556	1:525
19‡	1:1,544	1:555
20	1:1,480	1:525
21	1:1,460	1:525
22	1:1,440	1:499
23	1:1,420	1:499
24	1:1,380	1:475
25	1:1,340	1:475
26	1:1,290	1:475
27	1:1,220	1:454
28	1:1,140	1:434
29	1:1,050	1:416
30	1:940	1:384
31	1:820	1:384
32	1:700	1:322
33	1:570	1:285
34	1:456	1:243
35	1:353	1:178
36	1:267	1:148
37	1:199	1:122
38	1:148	1:104
39	1:111	1:80
40	1:85	1:62
41	1:67	1:48
42	1:54	1:38
43	1:45	1:30
44	1:39	1:23
45	1:35	1:18
46	1:31	1:14
47	1:29	1:10
48	1:27	1:8
49	1:26	1:6
50	1:25	§

*Data from Morris JK, Wald NJ, Mutton DE, Alberman E. Comparison of models of maternal age-specific risk for Down syndrome live births. *Prenat Diagn.* 2003;23:252–8.

†Risk of any chromosomal abnormality includes the risk of trisomy 21 and trisomy 18 in addition to trisomy 13, 47,XXY, 47,XYY, Turner syndrome genotype, and other clinically significant abnormalities, 47,XXX not included. Data from Hook EB. Rates of chromosome abnormalities: at different maternal ages. *Obstet Gynecol.* 1981;58:282–5.

‡Data from Cuckle HS, Wald NJ, Thompson SG. Estimating a woman's risk of having a pregnancy associated with Down's syndrome using her age and serum alpha-fetoprotein level. *Br J Obstet Gynaecol.* 1987;94:387–402.

§Data not available.

Note: Does not include mosaicism, translocations, or marker chromosomes.

Source: Reproduced with permission from ACOG Practice Bulletin No. 163: Screening for fetal aneuploidy. *Obstet Gynecol.* 2016 May;127(5):e123-37. Copyright © 2016 The American College of Obstetricians and Gynecologists.

GENETICS

Chromosome Abnormalities: In the Fetus

Table 3.9. Chromosomal abnormalities at amniocentesis

Maternal Age (Yr)	Singleton	Down Syndrome				Singleton	All Chromosomal Abnormalities			
		White twins		African american twins			White twins		African american twins	
		One Or both	Both affected	One Or both	Both affected		One Or both	Both affected	One Or both	Both affected
25	1/885	1/481	1/5,518	1/467	1/8,300	1/1,533	1/833	1/9,583	1/809	1/14,435
26	1/826	1/447	1/5,444	1/437	1/7,553	1/1,202	1/650	1/7,939	1/636	1/11,026
27	1/769	1/415	1/5,275	1/405	1/7,659	1/943	1/509	1/6,477	1/496	1/9,413
28	1/719	1/387	1/5,126	1/379	1/6,990	1/740	1/398	1/5,277	1/390	1/7,197
29	1/680	1/364	1/5,216	1/360	1/6,242	1/580	1/310	1/4,442	1/307	1/5,313
30	1/641	1/342	1/5,039	1/339	1/5,976	1/455	1/243	1/3,561	1/240	1/4,220
31	1/610	1/324	1/5,201	1/320	1/6,560	1/357	1/190	1/3,017	1/187	1/3,796
32	1/481	1/256	1/4,028	1/255	1/4,350	1/280	1/149	1/2,319	1/148	1/2,502
33	1/389	1/206	1/3,499	1/205	1/3,948	1/219	1/116	1/1,939	1/115	1/2,183
34	1/303	1/160	1/2,727	1/159	1/3,081	1/172	1/91	1/1,518	1/91	1/1,710
35	1/237	1/125	1/2,259	1/125	1/2,305	1/135	1/71	1/1,252	1/71	1/1,278
36	1/185	1/98	1/1,721	1/97	1/1,814	1/106	1/56	1/954	1/56	1/1,003
37	1/145	1/77	1/1,374	1/77	1/1,299	1/83	1/44	1/753	1/44	1/714
38	1/113	1/60	1/992	1/59	1/1,150	1/65	1/35	1/543	1/34	1/624
39	1/89	1/47	1/812	1/47	1/813	1/51	1/27	1/435	1/27	1/436
40	1/69	1/37	1/625	1/37	1/608	1/40	1/21	1/334	1/21	1/325
41	1/55	1/29	1/434	1/31	1/247	1/31	1/17	1/222	1/18	1/133
42	1/43	1/23	1/359	1/23	1/295	1/25	1/13	1/185	1/14	1/156
43	1/33	1/18	1/203	1/18	1/257	1/19	1/10	1/105	1/10	1/128
44	1/26	1/14	1/234	1/16	1/80	1/15	1/8	1/109	1/9	1/44
45	1/21	1/11	1/210	1/11	1/168	1/12	1/6	1/90	1/7	1/76
46	1/16	1/8	1/161	1/9	1/99	1/9	1/5	1/62	1/5	1/44
47	1/13	1/7	1/128			1/7	1/4	1/42		
48	1/10	1/5	1/88			1/6	1/3	1/34		
49	1/8	1/4	1/58			1/4	1/2	1/15		

Source: Reproduced with permission from Meyers C, Adam R, Dungan J, Prenger V. Aneuploidy in twin gestations: when is maternal age advanced? *Obstet Gynecol.* 1997;89:248-51. Copyright © 1997 The American College of Obstetricians and Gynecologists.

Chromosome Abnormalities: In the Fetus — GENETICS

Table 3.10. Features of common chromosome abnormalities

Trisomy 21 Down syndrome	Incidence: 1/650 to 1,000 live births (exact risk depends on maternal age; see Table 3.9.) Clinical presentation: Short, broad hands with single palmar crease, decreased muscle tone, mental retardation, broad head with characteristic features, open mouth with large tongue, up-slanting eyes.
Trisomy 13	Incidence: 1/10,000 Clinical presentation: Multiple congenital malformations of many organs, low-set malformed ears, receding mandible, small eyes, mouth and nose with general elfin appearance, severe mental deficiency, congenital heart defects, horseshoe or double kidney, short sternum, posterior heel prominence. Typically results in fetal loss or early neonatal death.
Trisomy 18	Incidence: 1/3,000 to 8,000 Clinical presentation: Severe mental deficiency, failure to thrive, cardiac anomalies, hypertonia, clenched fists, "rocker-bottom feet" with prominent heel bone, prominent occiput, micrognathia, low-set malformed ears, short palpebral fissures. Typically results in fetal loss or early neonatal death.
47,XXY Klinefelter syndrome	Incidence: 1/500 to 1,000 newborn males Clinical presentation: Normal pregnancy, birth, childhood. Reduced testicular size, need for testosterone supplementation beginning in adolescence and through adulthood. Risk of infertility and gynecomastia. Risk of learning disabilities (reading), expressive language deficits, 50% have dyslexia.
47,XXX Trisomy X	Incidence: 1/1,000 newborn females Clinical presentation: Increased risk for early menopause and poor ovarian function. Risk of learning disability, hyperactivity, depression, and variable menses.
45,XO Turner syndrome	Incidence: 1/1,500 to 2,500 newborn females Clinical presentation: Pre/neonatal: lymphedema, risk for cardiac malformations, webbed neck, kidney malformations. Short stature, ovarian dysgenesis, hormone supplementation needed in adolescence. Additional risks include otitis media, hypertension, diabetes, thyroid disease, learning disabilities, depression. Risk of pregnancy: increased maternal cardiovascular mortality in women with XO. If there is a documented cardiac abnormality, pregnancy is an **absolute contraindication**; if no documented cardiac abnormality, pregnancy is a **relative contraindication**.
47,XYY	Incidence: 1/10,00 newborn males Clinical presentation: Appearance typically unaffected; most males have normal sexual development and are able to father children. Increased risk of learning disability, speech delay, and hyperactivity.
Triploidy 69, XXY/69, XYY/69,XXX	Incidence: 1–3% of recognized conceptions; 1/10,000 livebirths Clinical presentation: Typically results in early fetal loss; clinical presentation depends on diandric or digynic origin. If liveborn, high risk of ambiguous genitalia, rapid demise, and neonatal death.
Translocations: Exchange of segments of DNA between two chromosomes	Reciprocal translocations: 1/600 newborns. Non-homologous chromosomes exchange material and the total chromosome number remains the same. If balanced, can be phenotypically normal; however, increased risk of infertility, RPL, and chromosome abnormalities: in the fetus. Robertsonian translocations: 1/1,000 Two acrocentric chromosomes fuse, resulting in loss of the short arms. Results in balanced karyotype with 45 chromosomes. Most common is 13q14q, with frequency of 1/1,300 people. Increased risk of infertility, RPL, and chromosome abnormalities: in the fetus.

Table 3.11. Aneuploid risk of most common major anomalies

Structural Defect	Population Incidence	Aneuploidy Risk	Aneuploidy (Trisomy)
Cystic hygroma	1 in 120 (EU) at 1 in 6,000 (B)	60 at 75%	45X (80%); 21, 18, 13, XXY
Hydrops	1 in 1,500 at 1 in 4,000 (B)	30 at 80%*	13, 21, 18, 45X
Hydrocephalus	3 in 10,000 at 8 in 10,000 (LB)	3 at 8%	13, 18, triploidy
Hydranencephaly	2 in 1,000 (IA)	Minimal	Not available
Holoprosencephaly	1 in 16,000 (LB)	40 at 60%	13, 18, 18p
Cardiac defects	7 in 1,000 at 9 in 1,000 (LB)	5 at 30%	21, 18, 13, 22, 8, 9
Complete audiovisual canal		40 at 70%	21
Diaphragmatic hernia	1 in 3,500 at 1 in 4,000 (LB)	20 at 25%	13, 18, 21, 45X
Omphalocele	1 in 5,800 (LB)	30 at 40%	13, 18
Gastroschisis	1 in 10,000 at 1 in 15,000 (LB)	Minimal	Not available
Duodenal atresia	1 in 10,000 (LB)	20 at 30%	21
Bowel obstruction	1 in 2,500 at 5,000 (LB)	Minimal	Not available
Bladder outlet obstruction	1 in 1,000 at 2 in 1,000 (LB)	20 at 25%	13, 18
Prune belly syndrome	1 in 35,000 at 1 in 50,000 (LB)	Low	18, 13, 45X
Facial cleft	1 in 700 (LB)	1%	13, 18, deletions
Limb reduction	4 in 10,000 at 6 in 10,000 (LB)	8%	18
Club foot	1.2 in 1,000 (LB)	20 at 30%	18, 13, 4p-, 18q-
Single umbilical artery	1%	Minimal	Not available

B, birth; EU, early ultrasonography; IA, infant autopsy; LB, live birth.
*30% if diagnosed by 24 weeks of gestation; 80% if diagnosed by 17 weeks of gestation.

Source: Reproduced with permission from Wenstrom KD. Prenatal diagnosis of genetic disorders. In *Precis: An update in obstetrics and gynecology,* 4th Ed. Washington, DC: American College of Obstetricians and Gynecologists; 2010.

Table 3.12. Management of ultrasonographic markers for aneuploidy

Soft Marker	Imaging Criteria	Aneuploidy Association	Management
First trimester: enlarged nuchal translucency	Certified ultrasonography measurement ≥3.0 mm or above the 99th percentile for the CRL	Aneuploidy risk increases with size of NT. Also associated with Noonan syndrome, multiple pterygium syndrome, skeletal dysplasias, congenital heart disease, and other anomalies	1. Genetic counseling 2. Offer cfDNA or CVS 3. Second-trimester detailed anatomic survey and fetal cardiac ultrasonography
First trimester: cystic hygroma	Large single or multilocular fluid-filled cavities, in the nuchal region and can extend the length of the fetus	If septate, approximately 50% are aneuploidy	1. Genetic counseling 2. Offer CVS 3. Second-trimester detailed fetal anatomic survey and fetal cardiac ultrasonography
Second trimester: echogenic intracardiac foci	Echogenic tissue in one or both ventricles of the heart seen on standard four-chamber view	LR 1.4–1.8 for Down syndrome. Seen in 15–30% of Down syndrome and 4–7% euploid fetuses	1. If isolated finding, aneuploidy screening should be offered if not done previously 2. If aneuploidy screen result is negative, no further evaluation is required.
Second trimester: pyelectasis	Renal pelvis measuring ≥4 mm in anteroposterior diameter up to 20 weeks of gestation	LR 1.5–1.6 for Down syndrome	1. If isolated finding, aneuploidy screening should be offered if not performed previously 2. Repeat ultrasonography in third trimester for potential urinary tract obstruction
Second trimester: echogenic bowel	Fetal small bowel as echogenic as bone	LR 5.5–6.7 for Down syndrome. Associated with aneuploidy, intra-amniotic bleeding, cystic fibrosis, CMV	1. Further counseling 2. Offer CMV, CF, and aneuploidy screening or diagnostic testing
Second trimester: thickened nuchal fold	≥6 mm from outer edge of the occipital bone to outer skin in the midline	LR 11–18.6 with 40–50% sensitivity and >99% specificity for Down syndrome. Most powerful second-trimester marker	1. Detailed anatomic survey 2. Further detailed genetic counseling and aneuploidy screening or diagnostic testing
Second trimester: mild ventriculomegaly	Lateral ventricular atrial measurement between 10–15 mm	Associated with aneuploidy. LR 25 for Down syndrome	1. Genetic counseling 2. Second-trimester detailed anatomic ultrasound evaluation 3. Consider diagnostic testing for aneuploidy and CMV 4. Repeat ultrasound in third trimester
Second trimester: choroid plexus cysts	Discrete cyst(s) in one or both choroid plexus(es)	In isolation, no aneuploidy association	1. Second-trimester detailed anatomic survey and fetal cardiac ultrasound 2. No further follow-up if isolated 3. Consider aneuploidy screening or diagnostic testing if other markers are present

(continued)

Soft Marker	Imaging Criteria	Aneuploidy Association	Management
Second trimester: short femur length	Measurement <2.5 percentile for gestational age	LR 1.2–2.2 for Down syndrome. Can be associated with aneuploidy, IUGR, short limb dysplasia	1. Second-trimester detailed fetal anatomic evaluation for short limb dysplasia 2. Further detailed counseling 3. Consider repeat ultrasonography in third trimester for fetal growth

CF, cystic fibrosis; cfDNA, cell-free DNA; CMV, cytomegalovirus; CRL, crown-rump length; CVS, chorionic villus sampling; IUGR, intrauterine growth restriction; LR, likelihood ratio; NT, nuchal translucency.

Data from Reddy (2014), Malone (2005), Aagaard-Tillery (2009), and Nicolaides (1992).

Source: Reproduced with permission from ACOG Practice Bulletin No. 163: Screening for fetal aneuploidy. *Obstet Gynecol.* 2016 May;127(5):e123-37. Copyright © 2016 The American College of Obstetricians and Gynecologists.

GENETIC TESTING
Fast Facts
- Chromosome aberrations (e.g., aneuploidy, translocations, large deletions/duplications)
  - Detected by karyotype and/or chromosome microarray analysis
- Microdeletions (e.g., Y chromosome microdeletions)
  - Detected by PCR and/or microarray analysis
- Small mutations (i.e., single gene disorders such as cystic fibrosis)
  - Detected by DNA analysis methods such as genotyping and sequencing
    - Genotyping can cost-effectively detect the most common disease-causing mutations in a gene
    - Sequencing provides increased detection rates by detecting any disease-causing mutation within a gene (with the exception of large deletions/duplications); however, traditional applications of sequencing also detect variants of unknown significance (VUS)

Preconception
Preimplantation Genetic Diagnosis (PGD)
- Allows for genetic testing to be performed on a cell or cells from a developing embryo created through IVF.
- Biopsy/testing can take place at various stages of development: polar bodies, blastomeres, and blastocysts can be biopsied and analyzed; current trends appear to favor trophectoderm biopsy of 5–10 cells per embryo (Forman 2013).
- Healthy embryos, free of the tested disorder, are selectively transferred.
- Can be performed for all single gene disorders as long as the DNA mutations are known. Can also test embryos for HLA matching, chromosome rearrangements, aneuploidy screening. Testing for multiple indications is often possible.
- Limitations: not 100% accurate and prenatal testing is still recommended; biopsy is an invasive procedure that can damage embryos

Gamete/Embryo Donation
- Using gametes from a donor reduces the risk of passing on a genetic disorder. This is an option for dominant, X-linked, and recessive genetic disorders.
- For recessive disorders, the donor would need to undergo screening for the disorders prior to undergoing treatment.
- Egg donation can decrease the likelihood of aneuploidy due to age-related risks.
  - Limitations: donation reduces the risk but does not guarantee an embryo/pregnancy free of genetic disorders or birth defects.

During Pregnancy
Noninvasive Prenatal Testing (NIPT)
- Detects common aneuploidies (i.e., trisomies 13, 18, 21) by sequence analysis of cell-free fetal DNA in maternal serum.
- Performed as early as 10 weeks gestation.
- Limitations: positive screens currently require follow-up with diagnostic test (CVS or amniocentesis); cannot detect open neural tube defects (e.g., spina bifida).

GENETICS

Maternal Serum Screening (MSS)
- Screens for common aneuploidies by analysis of pregnancy analytes in maternal serum. May include fetal features observed on ultrasound (nuchal translucency, nasal bone).
- Performed from 10 to 18 weeks of pregnancy.
- 85–96% detection rates, for combined first/second trimester assessments (ACOG 2007).
- Limitations: high false-positive rate; positive screens require follow-up with diagnostic test (CVS or amniocentesis).

Chorionic Villus Sampling (CVS)
- Detects chromosome abnormalities: or single gene disorders by analysis of fetal cells from placental tissue.
- Performed between 10–12 weeks of gestational age.
- Risk of complication, including pregnancy loss: 1/1,000 (Caughey 2006).
- Risk of placental mosaicism: 1/100 (1%).

Amniocentesis
- Detects chromosome abnormalities: or single gene disorders by analysis of fetal cells from amniotic fluid.
- Performed between **15–20 weeks of gestation**; may be done later with increased risk of preterm labor.
- Risk of complication, including pregnancy loss: <1/1,000 (<0.1%; Eddleman 2006).

Other Options

Testing after Birth
- Newborn screening can detect children with cystic fibrosis and numerous other genetic disorders. Screening panels vary by state (http://www.cdc.gov/newbornscreening/).
- Symptomatic testing, once a child has symptoms of a disorder.

Adoption
- Can reduce the risk of having a child with a genetic disorder when reproductive partners are known carriers.

Table 3.13. Characteristics, advantages, and disadvantages of common screening tests for aneuploidy

Screening Test	Gestational Age Range for Screening (Weeks)	Detection Rate for Down Syndrome (%)	Screen Positive Rate* (%)	Advantages	Disadvantages	Method
First trimester[†]	11–14‖	82–87	5	1. Early screening 2. Single test 3. Analyte assessment of other adverse outcome	Lower DR than combined tests NT required	NT+PAPP-A and hCG
Triple screen	15–22	69	5	1. Single test 2. No specialized US required 3. Also screens for open fetal defects 4. Analyte assessment for other adverse outcomes	Lower DR than with first-trimester or quad screening Lowest accuracy of the single lab tests	hCG, AFP, uE3
Quad screen[†]	15–22	81	5	1. Single test 2. No specialized US required 3. Also screens for open fetal defects 4. Analyte assessment for other adverse outcomes	Lower DR than combined tests	hCG, AFP, uE3, DIA
Integrated[†]	11–14, then 15–22	96	5	Highest DR of combined tests Also screens for open fetal defects	Two samples needed before results are known	NT+PAPP-A, then quad screen
Sequential[‡]: Stepwise	11–14, then 15–22	95	5	First-trimester results provided; Comparable performance to integrated, but FTS results provided; also screens for open fetal defects; analyte assessment for other adverse outcomes.	Two samples needed	NT+hCG+ PAPP-A then quad screen
Contingent screening[‡]		88–94	5	First-trimester test result: Positive: diagnostic test offered Negative: no further testing Intermediate: second-trimester test offered Final: risk assessment incorporates first- and second-trimester results	Possibly two samples needed	NT+hCG+ PAPP-A, then quad screen

(continued)

GENETICS

Screening Test	Gestational Age Range for Screening (Weeks)	Detection Rate for Down Syndrome (%)	Screen Positive Rate* (%)	Advantages	Disadvantages	Method
Serum Integrated[†]	11–14; then 15–22	88	5	1. DR compares favorably with other tests 2. No need for NT	Two samples needed; no first-trimester results	PAPP-A+quad
Cell-free DNA[§]	10–term	99 (in patients who receive a result)	0.5	1. Highest DR for Down syndrome 2. Can be performed at any gestational age after 10 weeks 3. Low false-positive rate in high-risk women (or women at high risk of Down syndrome)	1. NPV and PPV not clearly reported 2. Higher false-positive rate in women at low risk of Down syndrome 3. Limited information about three trisomies and fetal sex 4. Results do not always represent a fetal DNA result	Three roughly equivalent molecular methods
Nuchal Translucency[†]	11–14[‖]	64–70	5	Allows individual fetus assessment in multifetal gestations. Provides additional screening for fetal anomalies and possibly for twin-twin transfusion syndrome	1. Poor screen in isolation 2. Ultrasound certification necessary	US only

AFP, alpha fetoprotein; DIA, dimeric inhibin-A; DR, detection rate; FTS, first-trimester screening; hCG, human chorionic gonadotropin; NPV, negative predictive value; NT, nuchal translucency; PAPP-A, pregnancy-associated plasma protein A; PPV, positive predictive value; uE3, unconjugated estriol; US, ultrasonography.

*A screen positive test result includes all positive test results: the true positives and false positives.

[†]First-trimester combined screening: 87%, 85%, and 82% for measurements performed at 11 weeks, 12 weeks, and 13 weeks, respectively (Malone 2005).

[‡]Because of variations in growth and conception timing, some fetuses at the lower and upper gestational age limits may fall outside the required crown-rump length range. Also, different laboratories use slightly different gestational age windows for their testing protocol.

[§]Cuckle (2005).

[‖]Bianchi (2012); Palomaki (2011).

Source: Reproduced with permission from ACOG Practice Bulletin No. 163: Screening for fetal aneuploidy. *Obstet Gynecol.* 2016 May;127(5):e123-37. Copyright © 2009 The American College of Obstetricians and Gynecologists.

Table 3.14. Adverse pregnancy outcomes associated with maternal serum markers for aneuploidy

	Preeclampsia	Birthweight Less Than 10th Percentile	Preterm Birth	Fetal Death at or Before 24 Wk	Fetal Death After 24 Wk
PAPP-A (<0.42 MoM)	+/++	++/+++	+(32 wk or less) ++(less than 34 wk)	++	++/+++
Free β-hCG (<0.21 MoM)	−	−/++	−	+++	−
AFP (>2.0 MoM)	−	++	−(32 wk or less) +(37 wk)	+++	−/+++
hCG (>2.0 MoM)[†]	−	−	−	−	−(greater than 24 wk) +++(greater than 500 g)
uE3 (<0.5 MoM)	−	+/++	−	+++	−
Inhibin A (>2.0 MoM)	++	+	++	−	++

PAPPA, pregnancy-associated plasma protein-A; MoM, multiples of the median; AFP, alpha-fetoprotein; uE3, unconjugated estriol.

+, adjusted odds ratio (OR) greater than 1.0; ++, adjusted OR greater than 2.0; +++ adjusted OR greater than 3.0; −, adjusted OR not significant ($P \geq .05$).

[*]The information in the table is based on the studies, which are referenced in the source article.

[†]Although an isolated human chorionic gonadotropin (hCG) was not significantly associated with the adverse outcomes, a hCG level greater than 2.0 MoM was significantly associated with preeclampsia, birth weight less than the 10th percentile for gestational age, preterm birth 32 weeks or less, and early and late fetal loss.

Source: Reproduced with permission from Dugoff L; Society for Maternal-Fetal Medicine. First- and second-trimester maternal serum markers for aneuploidy and adverse obstetric outcomes. *Obstet Gynecol.* 2010 May;115(5):1052-61. Copyright © 2010 The American College of Obstetricians and Gynecologists.

Table 3.15. Management recommendations for women with maternal serum markers for aneuploidy but without evident aneuploidy

Maternal Serum Analyte	Trimester	Cutoff*	Management Recommendations
PAPP-A	First	Less than 0.4 MoM	Patient counseling regarding anticipated fetal activity in the late second and third trimester
hCG	Second	Greater than 3.0 MoM	Patient counseling regarding the signs and symptoms suggestive of preterm labor and preeclampsia[†]
Inhibin A	Second	Greater than 2.0 MoM	Consider ultrasound assessment of fetal growth in the late second and third trimester
uE3	Second	Less than 0.5 MoM	
AFP	Second	Greater than 2.0 MoM	Patient counseling regarding anticipated fetal activity in the late second and third trimester
			Patient counseling regarding the signs and symptoms suggestive of preterm labor and preeclampsia
			Consider ultrasound assessment of fetal growth in the late second and third trimester[‡]
			If there is evidence of a low-lying placenta/placenta previa in the second or third trimester, the potential diagnosis of placenta accreta should be considered
uE3	Second	Less than 0.25 MoM	Counseling and/or further genetic evaluation for disorders such as Smith-Lemli-Opitz syndrome and steroid sulfatase deficiency

PAPPA, pregnancy-associated plasma protein-A; MoM, multiples of the median; hCG, human chorionic gonadotropin; uE3, unconjugated estriol; AFP, alpha-fetoprotein.

*The actual MoM values reported for each analyte may vary for different labs.

[†]This does not apply to women with isolated low uE3 levels.

[‡]If a diagnosis of intrauterine growth restriction is established, the patient may benefit from fetal Doppler velocimetry studies including the umbilical arteries and middle cerebral artery.

Source: Reproduced with permission from Dugoff L; Society for Maternal-Fetal Medicine. First- and second-trimester maternal serum markers for aneuploidy and adverse obstetric outcomes. *Obstet Gynecol.* 2010 May;115(5):1052-61. Copyright © 2010 The American College of Obstetricians and Gynecologists.

NEURAL TUBE DEFECTS

Table 3.16. Neural tube defect pathophysiology

Neural Tube Defect	Malformation
Cranial	
Anencephaly	Failure of fusion of cephalic portion of neural folds; absence of all or part of brain, neurocranium, and skin
Exencephaly	Failure of scalp and skull formation; exteriorization of abnormally formed brain
Encephalocele	Failure of skull formation; extrusion of brain tissue into membranous sac
Iniencephaly	Defect of cervical and upper thoracic vertebrae; abnormally formed brain tissue and extreme retroflexion of upper spine
Spinal	
Spina bifida	Failure of fusion of caudal portion of neural tube, usually of 3–5 contiguous vertebrae; spinal cord or meninges or both exposed to amniotic fluid
Meningocele	Failure of fusion of caudal portion of neural tube; meninges exposed
Meningomyelocele	Failure of fusion of caudal portion of neural tube; meninges and neural tissue exposed
Myeloschisis	Failure of fusion of caudal portion of neural tube; flattened mass of neural tissue exposed
Holorachischisis	Failure of fusion of vertebral arches; entire spinal cord exposed
Craniorachischisis	Co-existing anencephaly and rachischisis

Source: Reproduced with permission from Cheschier N; ACOG Practice Bulletin No. 44: Neural tube defects. *Int J Gynaecol Obstet.* 2003 Oct;83(1):123-33. Copyright © 2003 The American College of Obstetricians and Gynecologists.

TERATOGENICITY

Table 3.17. Safety of common over-the-counter medications during pregnancy

Medication	Drug Class	Pregnancy Risk Category*	Crosses the Placenta?	Use in Pregnancy
Diphenhydramine (Benadryl)	First-generation (nonselective) antihistamine/antiemetic	B	Yes	Possible oxytocin-like effects at high doses
Brompheniramine	First-generation (nonselective) antihistamine	C	Not known	Limited data
Chlorpheniramine	First-generation (nonselective) antihistamine	C	Not known	Drug of choice
Pheniramine	Ophthalmic antihistamine/decongestant (pheniramine 0.3%/naphazoline 0.025%)	C	Not known	Limited data; likely low risk with limited use
Cetirizine (Zyrtec)	Second-generation (selective, nonsedating) antihistamine	B	Not known	Acceptable alternative to first-generation agents
Loratadine (Claritin)	Second-generation (selective, nonsedating) antihistamine	B	Not known	Acceptable alternative to first-generation agents
Fexofenadine (Allegra)	Second-generation (selective, nonsedating) antihistamine	C	Not known	No human data, animal data suggest some risk
Phenylephrine	Sympathomimetic decongestant	C	Yes[†]	Safety not established, should be avoided in first trimester
Pseudoephedrine	Sympathomimetic decongestant	C	Not known	Behind-the-counter purchase; possible association with gastroschisis, small intestinal atresia, and hemifacial microsomia; should be avoided in first trimester
Guaifenesin	Expectorant	C	Not known	Safety not established, should be avoided in first trimester
Dextromethorphan	Nonnarcotic antitussive	C	Not known	Appears to be safe in pregnancy
Acetaminophen	Nonnarcotic analgesic/antipyretic	B	Yes	Drug of choice
Aspirin	Salicylate analgesic/antipyretic	C in the first and second trimesters, D in the third trimester	Yes	Should be avoided in pregnancy unless needed for specific indications
Naproxen	NSAID analgesic	B in the first and second trimesters, D in the third trimester	Yes	Should be avoided in the third trimester
Ibuprofen	NSAID analgesic	C in the first and second trimesters, D in the third trimester	Yes	Should be avoided in the third trimester

(continued)

Teratogenicity **GENETICS**

Medication	Drug Class	Pregnancy Risk Category*	Crosses the Placenta?	Use in Pregnancy
Cimetidine (Tagamet)	Selective histamine H2 antagonist	B	Yes	Potential weak antiandrogenic activity (only observed in animal studies)
Famotidine (Pepcid)	Selective H2 antagonist	B	Yes	Limited human data
Nizatidine (Axid)	Selective H2 antagonist	B	Yes	Limited human data
Ranitidine (Zantac)	Selective H2 antagonist	B	Yes	May be preferable to cimetidine for chronic use
Omeprazole (Prilosec)	Proton pump inhibitor	C[†]	Yes	Most human data suggest it is safe throughout pregnancy
Aluminum hydroxide	Antacid	Not available	Not known	Considered safe in pregnancy; risk of neurotoxicity with high doses
Calcium carbonate	Antacid	Not available	Yes	Drug of choice; risk of milk-alkali syndrome with high doses
Magnesium hydroxide, magnesium carbonate	Antacid	Not available	Not known	Considered safe in pregnancy; magnesium may cause tocolysis in late pregnancy, but this is not a risk with over-the-counter preparations
Simethicone (available as a single agent and contained in multiple combination antacids)	Antiflatulent	C	No	Limited data; not absorbed, so considered safe in pregnancy
Bismuth subsalicylate (Pepto-Bismol)	Antidiarrheal	C	Not known	Insufficient data; should be avoided during pregnancy, especially in the second and third trimesters because it has a salicylate portion[‡]
Loperamide (Imodium)	Antidiarrheal	C	Not known	Limited human data; questionable association with cardiovascular defects
Mineral oil	Emollient laxative	C	No (not absorbed)	Should be avoided in pregnancy, may interfere with absorption of fat-soluble vitamins[§]
Castor oil	Laxative/oxytocic	X	Not known	Should be avoided in pregnancy, potential for maternal/fetal morbidity
Polyethylene glycol 3350 (Miralax)	Osmotic laxative	C	Not known	Drug of choice for chronic constipation

FDA, Food and Drug Administration.

*Based on pregnancy risk category definitions from the FDA (Table 2) and other sources.

[†]Proton pump inhibitors as a class are rated FDA category B, including esomeprazole (Nexium), rabeprazole (Aciphex), and lansoprazole (Prevacid), based largely on animal data, which do not suggest any fetal risk; human data are limited.

[‡]Hydrolyzes into bismuth salts and sodium salicylate in the intestinal tract. Sodium salicylate is not thought to suppress platelet function like the salicylate moiety found in aspirin; however, given the concerns over potential fetal toxicity from chronic salicylate exposure, avoidance in the latter half of pregnancy may be prudent.

[§]The American Gastroenterological Association recommends avoidance presumably because of the risk of neonatal coagulopathy and hemorrhage arising from interference with maternal vitamin K absorption.

Information from references 10 through 16. Source: Reproduced with permission from Servey J, Chang J. Over-the-counter medications in pregnancy. *Am Fam Physician.* 2014 Oct 15;90(8):548-55. Copyright © 2014 American Academy of Family Physicians.

Table 3.18. Psychiatric medications during pregnancy and breastfeeding

Medication Class	Birth defects	Pregnancy	Delivery	Neonatal	Lactation	Treatment options
Benzodiazepines	Possible increased incidence of cleft lip or palate	Ultrasonography for facial morphology	Floppy infant syndrome	Withdrawal syndrome	Infant sedation reported	Clonazepam Lorazepam Alprazolam
Selective serotonin reuptake inhibitors, selective norepinephrine reuptake inhibitors, and tricyclic antidepressants	None confirmed	Decreased serum concentrations across pregnancy	None	Neonatal, withdrawal syndrome	None	Fluoxetine Sertraline Paroxetine Citalopram Nortriptyline
Lithium	Increased incidence of heart defects	Ultrasonography or fetal echocardiography for heart development or both Decreased serum concentrations across pregnancy	Intravenous fluids Increased risk for lithium toxicity in mother	Increased risk for lithium toxicity in infant	Monitor infant complete blood count, thyroid-stimulating hormone levels, and lithium levels	Sustained release lithium
Antiepileptic Drugs	Increased incidence of birth defects	Decreased serum concentrations across pregnancy Folate supplementation, vitamin K for some antiepileptic drugs	None	Neonatal symptoms, vitamin K for some antiepileptic drugs	Monitor infant complete blood count, liver enzyme levels, antiepileptic drug levels	Lamotrigine Carbamazepine
Antipsychotic Medications	None Confirmed	Avoid anticholinergic medications for side effects	None	Possible risk for neuroleptic malignant syndrome and intestinal obstruction	None	Haloperidol

Source: Reproduced with permission from ACOG Practice Bulletin No. 92: Use of psychiatric medications during pregnancy and lactation. *Obstet Gynecol.* 2008 Apr;111(4):1001-20. Copyright © 2008 The American College of Obstetricians and Gynecologists.

Teratogenicity

Table 3.19. Medications contraindicated during pregnancy

Agent	Comments
Angiotensin-converting enzyme inhibitors (antihypertensive), and angiotension II receptor blockers	May cause kidney abnormalities in fetus when used in second or third trimesters.
HMG-CoA reductase inhibitors (statins)	A range of abnormalities has been reported for exposures during the fourth through ninth week of gestation.
Androgens and testosterone derivatives	Cause masculinization of female fetus.
Carbamazepine (anticonvulsant)	Risk of fetal death, mental retardation, and malformed hearts, genitals, cleft palates, and arteries. Should be switched to another, less teratogenic agent before conception whenever possible. Use should be reserved only for cases where benefit outweighs risk.
Coumadin derivatives	Risk of bone and cartilage deformities, mental retardation, and vision problems. Should be switched to heparin before conception whenever possible.
Folic acid antagonists	Risk of spontaneous abortion and malformations.
Leflunomide, thalidomide	Risk of limb deformities. Use only with strict pregnancy prevention protocols.
Lithium (antidepressant)	Associated with increased risk of cardiovascular anomalies.
Phenytoin (anticonvulsant)	Risk of fetal hydantoin syndrome, including intrauterine growth restriction with small head circumference, dysmorphic facies, orofacial clefts, cardiac defects, and distal digital hypoplasia. Use should be reserved only for when benefit outweighs risk.
Streptomycin and kanamycin (antiinfective)	Risk of ototoxicity.
Tetracycline (antiinfective)	Risk to developing bones and teeth causing discoloration of teeth and skeletal abnormalities.
Valproic acid (anticonvulsive)	Risk of central nervous system dysfunction, spina bifida, development delay, intrauterine growth retardation, and cardiac anomalies. Should be switched to another, less teratogenic agent before conception whenever possible. If benefit of use outweighs risk, should be administered in 3–4 divided doses and should not be combined with carbamazepine and phenobarbitol.
Isotretinoin, known as Accutane (antiacne)	Elevated risk of spontaneous abortion and many anomalies.

Source: Reproduced with permission from Dunlop AL, Gardiner PM, Shellhaas CS, Menard MK, McDiarmid MA. The clinical content of preconception care: the use of medications and supplements among women of reproductive age. *Am J Obstet Gynecol.* 2008 Dec;199(6 Suppl 2):S367-72. Copyright © 2008 Elsevier.

CHAPTER 4
Ultrasound

FETAL ANATOMY SCAN

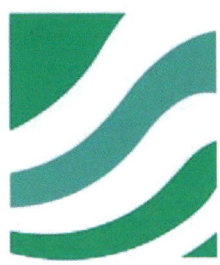
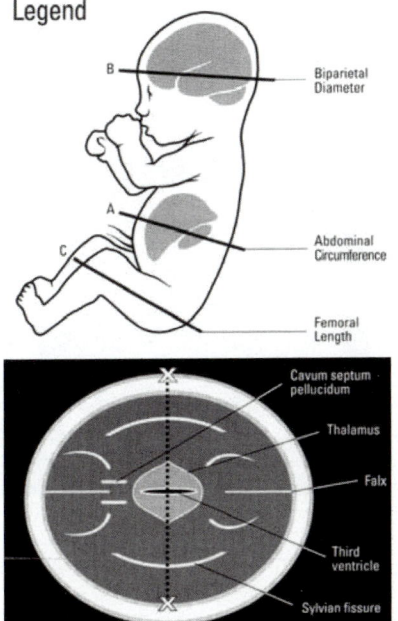
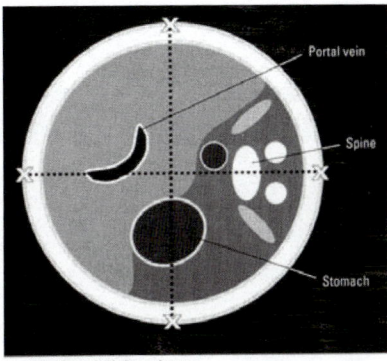
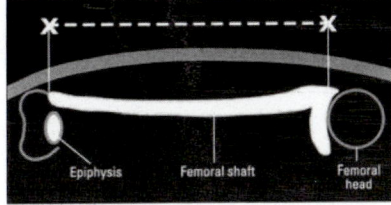

Figure 4.1. Fetal anatomic landmarks
Source: Reproduced with permission from Advanced Technology Laboratories (ATL), Bothell, Washington. *Clinical* Source: Jeanne Crowley, RDMS, and Sabrina Craigo, MD, Center for Prenatal Diagnosis, New England Medical Center, Boston, Massachusetts.

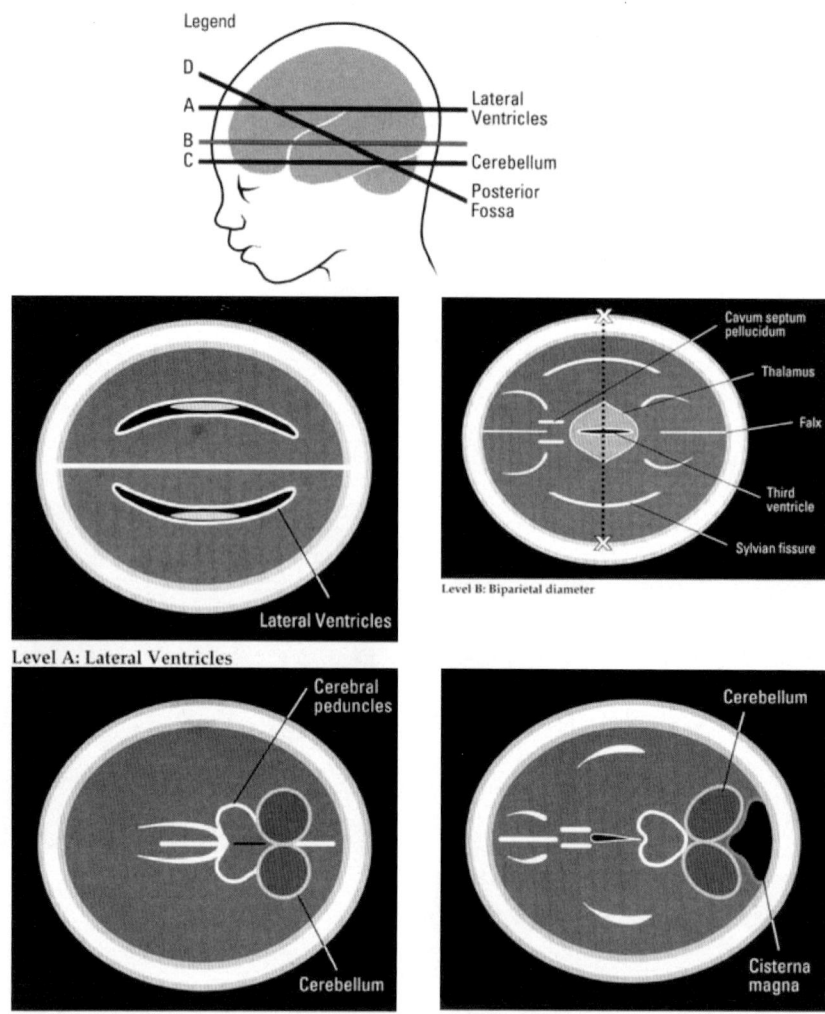

Figure 4.2. Fetal intracranial anatomy
Source: Reproduced with permission from Advanced Technology Laboratories (ATL), Bothell, Washington. *Clinical* Source: Jeanne Crowley, RDMS, and Sabrina Craigo, MD, Center for Prenatal Diagnosis, New England Medical Center, Boston, Massachusetts.

Fetal Anatomy

1. General
- First determine situs:
  - Identify fetal position
  - Locate fetal stomach and other abdominal organs
  - Verify relationship of fetal stomach to fetal heart
  - Apex of heart should be to the left

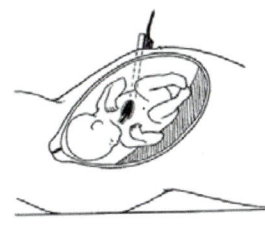

2. Four-Chamber
- Obtain a four-chamber view. Locate and verify:
  - An intact interventricular septum
  - Right and left atria approximately the same size
  - Right and left ventricles approximately equal sizes
  - Free movement of mitral and tricuspid valves
  - Foramen ovale flap in left atrium

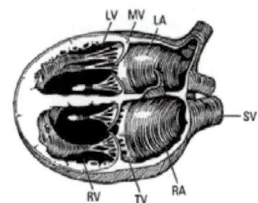

3. Long Axis Left Ventricle
- Obtain a long axis view of the left ventricle. Locate and verify:
  - Intact interventricular septum
  - Continuity of the ascending aorta with
    - Mitral valve posterior
    - Interventricular septum anterior

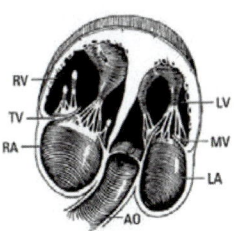

(continued)

4. Short Axis of Great Vessels
- Obtain the short axis view of the great vessels. Locate:
  - Pulmonary artery, which should exit the anterior (right) ventricle and bifurcate

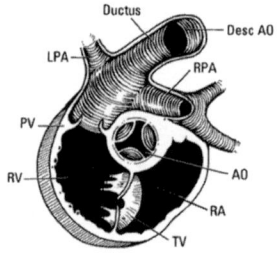

5. Aortic Arch
- Locate the aortic arch and verify that:
  - The aorta exits from the posterior (left) ventricle (not shown)
  - Three head and neck vessels should branch from the aorta

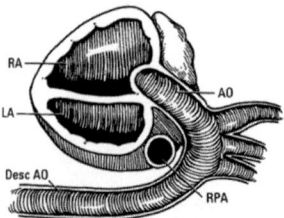

6. Pulmonary Artery-Ductus Arteriosus
- Locate the descending aorta and confirm:
  - Continuity of the ductus arteriosus with the descending aorta

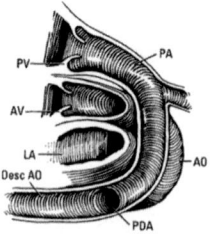

Figure 4.3. Fetal echocardiography
Source: Reproduced with permission from Advanced Technology Laboratories (ATL), Bothell, Washington. *Clinical* Source: Joshua A. Copel, MD, Director, Division of Maternal-Fetal Medicine, Department of Obstetrics and Gynecology, Yale University School of Medicine, New Haven, CT.

TRANSVAGINAL SONOGRAPHY

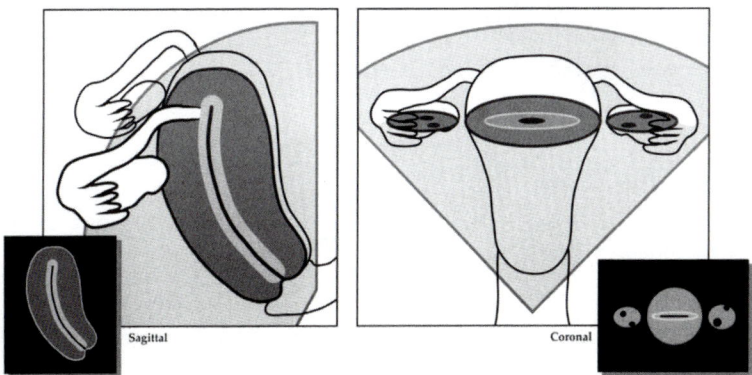

Figure 4.4. Endovaginal ultrasonography
Source: Reproduced with permission from Advanced Technology Laboratories (ATL), Bothell, Washington. *Clinical* Source: Kris M. Holoska, RDMS, Antenatal Testing Unit, Pennsylvania Hospital, Philadelphia, Pennsylvania.

Basic Principles of Scanning
- Develop a routine to systematically scan all pelvic structures.
- Each structure must be scanned in two planes perpendicular to one another.
  - Transducer's position should be monitored during insertion. Once the probe has been properly inserted, the operator should observe the screen at all times, and the position of the probe is determined by optimal visualization of the pelvic viscera. The orientation of the probe is controlled by angulation (accomplished by up and down movement of the transducer handle) and rotation:
    - The probe can be rotated 90 degrees around its axis to obtain sagittal and coronal plane images.
    - The probe can be angled in any plane to direct the plane of image.
    - Deeper insertion or withdrawal can be used to bring the area of interest within the focal zone of the transducer.
  - The scan area needs to be thought of as a pie-shaped area emanating from the transducer:

ULTRASOUND

Transvaginal Sonography

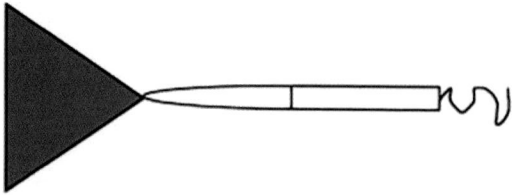

- Rotation of the transducer changes the spatial orientation of that pie between longitudinal and coronal planes:

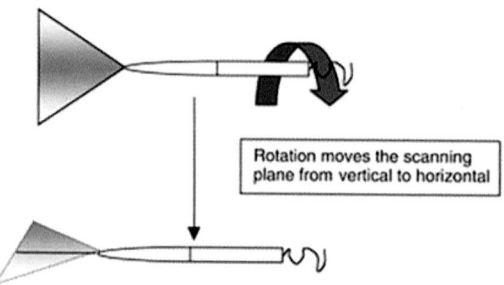

- Angling the probe (moving the probe up or down) allows for proper orientation of the probe with respect to the pelvic structures, depending on their position (e.g., anteversion, retroversion) within the pelvis:

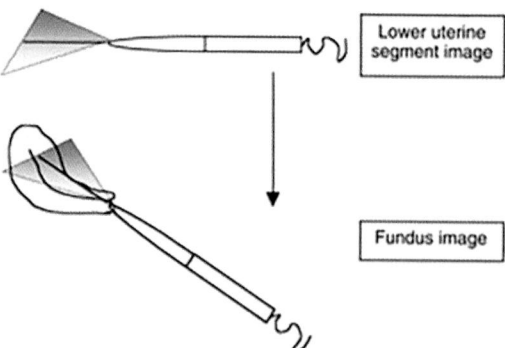

- The right to left orientation of the image in the coronal plane is controlled in two ways: (1) image direction button on the machine itself and (2) direction of rotation from the sagittal plane.
  - For example, if the image direction is set on the machine in such a way that the bladder is in the upper left corner while scanning in the sagittal plane, rotation of the probe 90 degrees clockwise will maintain the right to left orientation (patient's left will be displayed on the left of the screen). Rotation of the probe 90 degrees counterclockwise will change that orientation, and now patient's left will be displayed on the right of the screen (Callen 2000).

Figure 4.5. Basic principles of scanning

ULTRASOUND DIAGNOSIS OF PREGNANCY FAILURE

Table 4.1. Guidelines for transvaginal ultrasonographic diagnosis of pregnancy failure in a woman with an intrauterine pregnancy of uncertain viability*

Findings Diagnostic of Pregnancy Failure	Findings Suspicious for, but Not Diagnostic of, Pregnancy Failure[†]
Crown–rump length of ≥7 mm and no heartbeat	Crown–rump length of <7 mm and no heartbeat
Mean sac diameter of ≥25 mm and no embryo	Mean sac diameter of 16–24 mm and no embryo
Absence of embryo with heartbeat ≥2 wk after a scan that showed a gestational sac without a yolk sac	Absence of embryo with heartbeat 7–13 days after a scan that showed a gestational sac without a yolk sac
Absence of embryo with heartbeat ≥11 days after a scan that showed a gestational sac with a yolk sac	Absence of embryo with heartbeat 7–10 days after a scan that showed a gestational sac with a yolk sac
	Absence of embryo ≥6 wk after last menstrual period
	Empty amnion (amnion seen adjacent to yolk sac, with no visible embryo)
	Enlarged yolk sac (>7 mm)
	Small gestational sac in relation to the size of the embryo (<5 mm difference between mean sac diameter and crown-rump length)

*Criteria are from the Society of Radiologists in Ultrasound Multispecialty Consensus Conference on Early First Trimester Diagnosis of Miscarriage and Exclusion of a Viable Intrauterine Pregnancy, October 2012.

[†]When there are findings suspicious for pregnancy failure, follow-up ultrasonography at 7 to 10 days to assess the pregnancy for viability is generally appropriate.

Source: From Doublet PM, Benson CB, Bourne T, et al. Diagnostic criteria for nonviable pregnancy early in the first trimester. *N Engl J Med*. 2013 Oct 10;369(15):1443-51. Copyright © 2013 Massachusetts Medical Society. Reprinted with permission from the Massachusetts Medical Society.

Table 4.2. Diagnostic and management guidelines related to the possibility of a viable intrauterine pregnancy in a woman with a pregnancy of unknown location*

Finding	Key Points
No intrauterine fluid collection adnexa on ultrasonography[†]	A single measurement of hCG, regardless of its value, does not reliably distinguish among normal (or near-normal) between ectopic and intrauterine pregnancy (viable or nonviable).
	If a single hCG measurement is <3000 mIU/mL, presumptive treatment for ectopic pregnancy with the use of methotrexate or other pharmacologic or surgical means should not be undertaken, in order to avoid the risk of interrupting a viable intrauterine pregnancy.
	If a single hCG measurement is ≥3000 mIU/mL, a viable intrauterine pregnancy is possible but unlikely. However, the most likely diagnosis is a nonviable intrauterine pregnancy, so it is generally appropriate to obtain at least one follow-up hCG measurement and follow-up ultrasonogram before undertaking treatment for ectopic pregnancy.
Ultrasonography not yet performed	The hCG levels in women with ectopic pregnancies are highly variable, often <1000 mIU/mL, and the hCG level does not predict the likelihood of ectopic pregnancy rupture. Thus, when the clinical findings are suspicious for ectopic pregnancy, transvaginal ultrasonography is indicated even when the hCG level is low.

*Criteria are from the Society of Radiologists in Ultrasound Multispecialty Consensus Conference on Early First Trimester Diagnosis of Miscarriage and Exclusion of a Viable Intrauterine Pregnancy, October 2012.

[†]Near normal (i.e., inconsequential) adnexal findings include corpus luteum, a small amount of free pelvic fluid, and paratubal cyst.

Source: From Doublet PM, Benson CB, Bourne T, et al. Diagnostic criteria for nonviable pregnancy early in the first trimester. *N Engl J Med*. 2013 Oct 10;369(15):1443-51. Copyright © 2013 Massachusetts Medical Society. Reprinted with permission from the Massachusetts Medical Society.

TRANSVAGINAL CERVICAL LENGTH
Cervix Measurement Criteria

Using transvaginal imaging, take repeated measurements of the cervix until you get three measurements that meet all nine criteria listed below and that differ by less than 10%. Of these excellent measures, record the **SHORTEST BEST**. When submitting images for the CLEAR image review, reviewers recommend that participants not submit cervical images from a patient with an existing cerclage. Although CLEAR will accept cervical images obtained in women with a cerclage in place, sonographers should be aware that it can be more difficult to demonstrate the required landmarks in these patients.

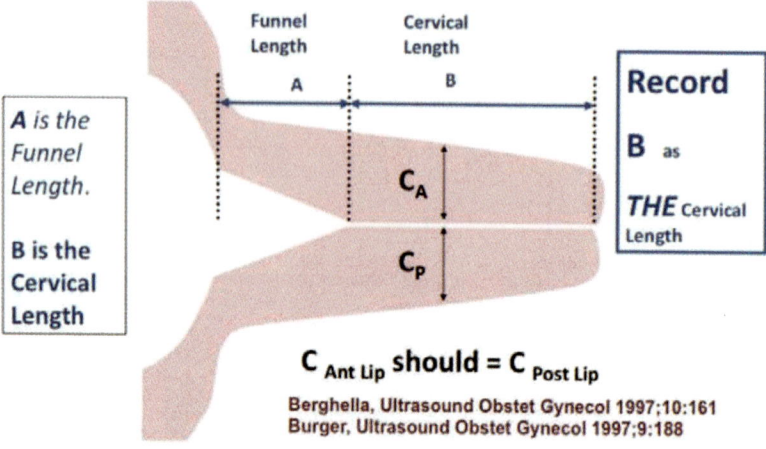

Figure 4.6. Measurement of the cervical length for preterm labor risk assessment

1. Measurement is taken on a transvaginal image:
   - Transvaginal measurements are the gold standard for ultrasound cervix measurements.
   - Short cervix can be missed on transabdominal scans.
2. The transvaginal image is filled primarily with the cervix and the field of view is optimized for measurement:
   - Approximately 75% of the image should be occupied by the cervix.
   - The bladder should be visible.
3. The anterior width of the cervix equals the posterior width:
   - The anterior cervical thickness is equal to the posterior cervical thickness.
   - The echogenicity is similar both anterior and posterior.
   - There is limited concavity created by the transducer.
4. The maternal bladder is empty:
   - The maternal bladder has a variable effect on the cervical length.
5. The internal os is seen:
   - The internal os is a small triangular area at the superior portion of the endocervical canal.
   - The internal os is adjacent to the uterine cavity.

6. The external os is seen:
   - The external os is a small triangular area at the inferior portion of the endocervical canal.
   - The anterior and posterior portions of the cervix come together at the external os.
7. The endocervical canal is visible throughout:
   - The endocervical canal is a linear echogenicity created by the interface between the anterior and posterior walls of the cervix.
   - The canal extends between the internal and external os.
8. Caliper placement is correct:
   - Calipers are placed where the anterior and posterior walls of the cervix touch at the internal and external os.
   - Calipers do not extend to the outermost edge of the cervical tissue.
   - Calipers extend along the endocervical canal.
   - If the cervix is curved two or more linear measurements are performed and the values added together to obtain the cervical length. Do not trace the cervical length.
9. Cervix mobility is considered:
   - Insert transvaginal probe to view the cervix—withdraw probe until the image blurs to reduce compression from the transducer, then reapply just enough pressure to create best image.
   - Visualize the cervix for 3–5 minutes and watch for shortening or funneling.
   - Apply mild suprapubic or fundal pressure to watch for funneling. Reduce probe pressure while fundal or suprapubic pressure applied.

Source: Reproduced with permission from The Perinatal Quality Foundation.

The Perinatal Quality Foundation (PQF) was established in 2005. The mission of PQF is to improve the quality of Maternal-Fetal Medicine medical services by providing state-of-the-art educational programs and evidence-based, statistically valid monitoring systems to evaluate current practices and facilitate the transition of emerging technologies into clinical care.

As evidence built to support a role for progesterone to prevent preterm birth in subsets of patients with short cervical length, the need to standardize the measurement of the cervix became apparent. PQF convened a task force in November 2011 with representatives and experts. Membership on the task force included representatives from the American College of Radiology (ACR), the American College of Obstetrics and Gynecology (ACOG), the American College of Osteopathic Obstetrics and Gynecology (ACOOG), the American Institute of Ultrasound in Medicine, the Society of Diagnostic Medical Sonographers (SDMS), and the Society of Maternal Fetal Medicine (SMFM). The task force developed a consensus education initiative that presented standard criteria for sonographic cervical measurement in pregnancy.

The Cervical Length Education and Review program (CLEAR) is a product of task force deliberations. The CLEAR program provides educational lectures, optional examinations, and scored image reviews. Those who complete the lectures and who pass the examination and image review receive documents verifying that they have completed the CLEAR program. They also qualify for CME provided by both SDMS and ACOG. Names of those who complete the program are listed on the CLEAR website.

The volunteers and staff involved in the development of the CLEAR program hope that the site will facilitate measurement of the cervix in a standard and accurate manner. The site is designed for education and practice.

Please contact us if you have suggestions or questions at CLEARSupport@perinatalquality.org or visit us on the internet at https://clear.perinatalquality.org.

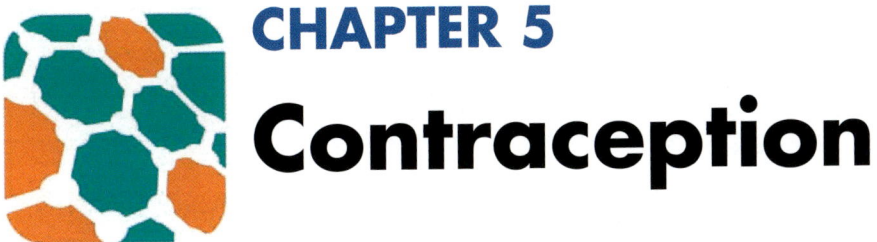

CHAPTER 5
Contraception

CONTRACEPTIVE CHOICES

Table 5.1. Percentage of women experiencing an unintended pregnancy during the first year of typical use and the first year of perfect use of contraception, and the percentage continuing use at the end of the first year

Method (1)	% of Women Experiencing an Unintended Pregnancy Within the First Year of Use		% of Women Continuing Use at 1 Year[3]
	Typical use[1] (2)	Perfect use[2] (3)	(4)
No method[4]	85	85	
Spermicides[5]	28	18	42
Fertility awareness-based methods	24		47
Standard Days method[6]		5	
TwoDay method[6]		4	
Ovulation method[6]		3	
Symptothermal method[6]		0.4	
Withdrawal	22	4	46
Sponge			36
Parous women	24	20	
Nulliparous women	12	9	
Condom[7]			
Female (fc)	21	5	41
Male	18	2	43
Diaphragm[8]	12	6	57
Combined pill and progestin-only pill	9	0.3	67
Evra patch	9	0.3	67
NuvaRing	9	0.3	67
Depo-Provera	6	0.2	56

(continued)

CONTRACEPTION

Contraceptive Choices

Method (1)	% of Women Experiencing an Unintended Pregnancy Within the First Year of Use		% of Women Continuing Use at 1 Year[3] (4)
	Typical use[1] (2)	Perfect use[2] (3)	
Intrauterine contraceptives			
ParaGard (copper T)	0.8	0.6	78
Mirena (LNg)	0.2	0.2	80
Implanon	0.05	0.05	84
Female sterilization	0.5	0.5	100
Male sterilization	0.15	0.10	100

[1] Among *typical* couples who initiate use of a method (not necessarily for the first time), the percentage who experience an accidental pregnancy during the first year if they do not stop use for any other reason. Estimates of the probability of pregnancy during the first year of typical use for spermicides, withdrawal, fertility awareness-based methods, the diaphragm, the male condom, the oral contraceptive pill, and Depo-Provera are taken from the 1995 National Survey of Family Growth corrected for underreporting of abortion; see the text for the derivation of estimates for the other methods.

[2] Among couples who initiate use of a method (not necessarily for the first time) and who use it *perfectly* (both consistently and correctly), the percentage who experience an accidental pregnancy during the first year if they do not stop use for any other reason. See the text for the derivation of the estimate for each method.

[3] Among couples attempting to avoid pregnancy, the percentage who continue to use a method for 1 year.

[4] The percentages becoming pregnant in columns (2) and (3) are based on data from populations where contraception is not used and from women who cease using contraception in order to become pregnant. Among such populations, about 89% become pregnant within 1 year. This estimate was lowered slightly (to 85%) to represent the percentage who would become pregnant within 1 year among women now relying on reversible methods of contraception if they abandoned contraception altogether.

[5] Foams, creams, gels, vaginal suppositories, and vaginal film.

[6] The Ovulation and TwoDay methods are based on evaluation of cervical mucus. The Standard Days method avoids intercourse on cycle days 8 through 19. The Symptothermal method is a double-check method based on evaluation of cervical mucus to determine the first fertile day and evaluation of cervical mucus and temperature to determine the last fertile day.

[7] Without spermicides.

[8] With spermicidal cream or jelly.

[9] ella, Plan B One-Step, and Next Choice are the only dedicated products specifically marketed for emergency contraception. The label for Plan B One-Step (1 dose is 1 white pill) says to take the pill within 72 hours after unprotected intercourse. Research has shown that all of the brands listed here are effective when used within 120 hours after unprotected sex. The label for Next Choice (1 dose is 1 peach pill) says to take 1 pill within 72 hours after unprotected intercourse and another pill 12 hours later. Research has shown that both pills can be taken at the same time with no decrease in efficacy or increase in side effects and that they are effective when used within 120 hours after unprotected sex. The Food and Drug Administration has in addition declared the following 19 brands of oral contraceptives to be safe and effective for emergency contraception: Ogestrel (1 dose is 2 white pills), Nordette (1 dose is 4 light-orange pills), Cryselle, Levora, Low-Ogestrel, Lo/Ovral or Quasence (1 dose is 4 white pills), Jolessa, Portia, Seasonale or Trivora (1 dose is 4 pink pills), Seasonique (1 dose is 4 light-blue-green pills), Enpresse (1 dose is 4 orange pills), Lessina (1 dose is 5 pink pills), Aviane or LoSeasonique (1 dose is 5 orange pills), Lutera or Sronyx (1 dose is 5 white pills), and Lybrel (1 dose is 6 yellow pills).

[10] However, to maintain effective protection against pregnancy, another method of contraception must be used as soon as menstruation resumes, the frequency or duration of breastfeeds is reduced, bottle feeds are introduced, or the baby reaches 6 months of age.

Source: Reproduced with permission from Trussell J. Contraceptive efficacy. In: Hatcher RA, Trussell J, Nelson AL, Cates W, Kowal D, Policar M. Contraceptive Technology: Twentieth Revised Edition. New York: Ardent Media; 2011.

Table 5.2. Classification of migraine

Migraine with Aura	Migraine
Visual disturbance in both eyes (i.e., homonymous hemianopsia)	Nausea ± vomiting
Flashing or moving scotoma	Photophobia
Unilateral numbness	Phonophobia
"Pins & needles" in extremities	Watery eyes
Unilateral weakness	Taste or smell sensations
Aphasia or other speech difficulties	

Source: Adapted from Hatcher R, Cwiak C. When a chronically ill patient needs contraceptives. *Cont Ob/Gyn.* 2003;Oct:70-82. *Contemporary Ob/Gyn* is a copyrighted publication of Advanstar Communications Inc. All rights reserved.

Table 5.3. Reductions in cancer risks with use of specific contraceptive methods compared with nonusers

	Use Duration	Risk Reduction
Endometrial cancer		
Combination hormonal methods	1 yr	40%
	12 yr	72%
	20 yr after discontinuation	50%
DMPA	Ever-use	79%
	Protection persists ≥8 yr after discontinuation	
IUDs	Limited data	40–60%
Ovarian cancer		
Combination hormonal methods	3–6 mo	40%
	>5 yr	50%
	Protection persists ≥30 yr after discontinuation	
Colorectal cancer		
Combination hormonal methods	Ever-use	16–18%
	96 mo	40%

DMPA, depot medroxyprogesterone acetate; IUD, intrauterine device.

Source: Reprinted with permission from Kavnitz AM, Speroff L. Contraception in the perimenopausal woman. *Dialogues in Contraception.* 2005;9(1):1–3.

MEDICAL ELIGIBILITY FOR HORMONAL CONTRACEPTIVE USE

Table 5.4. Medical eligibility criteria for contraceptive use

Condition	Sub-Condition	Cu-IUD		LNG-IUD		Implant		DMPA		POP		CHC	
		I	C	I	C	I	C	I	C	I	C	I	C
Age		Menarche to <20 yrs:2		Menarche to <20 yrs:2		Menarche to <18 yrs:1		Menarche to <18 yrs:2		Menarche to <18 yrs:1		Menarche to <40 yrs:1	
		≥20 yrs:1		≥20 yrs:1		18-45 yrs:1		18-45 yrs:1		18-45 yrs:1		≥40 yrs:2	
						>45 yrs:1		>45 yrs:2		>45 yrs:1			
Anatomical abnormalities	a) Distorted uterine cavity	4		4									
	b) Other abnormalities	2		2									
Anemias	a) Thalassemia	2		1		1		1		1		1	
	b) Sickle cell disease‡	2		1		1		1		1		2	
	c) Iron-deficiency anemia	2		1		1		1		1		1	
Benign ovarian tumors	(including cysts)	1		1		1		1		1		1	
Breast disease	a) Undiagnosed mass	1		2		2*		2*		2*		2*	
	b) Benign breast disease	1		1		1		1		1		1	
	c) Family history of cancer	1		1		1		1		1		1	
	d) Breast cancer‡												
	i) Current	1		4		4		4		4		4	
	ii) Past and no evidence of current disease for 5 years	1		3		3		3		3		3	
Breastfeeding	a) <21 days postpartum					2*		2*		2*		4*	
	b) 21 to <30 days postpartum												
	i) With other risk factors for VTE					2*		2*		2*		3*	
	ii) Without other risk factors for VTE					2*		2*		2*		3*	
	c) 30-42 days postpartum												
	i) With other risk factors for VTE					1*		1*		1*		3*	
	ii) Without other risk factors for VTE					1*		1*		1*		2*	
	d) >42 days postpartum					1*		1*		1*		2*	
Cervical cancer	Awaiting treatment	4	2	4	2	2		2		1		2	
Cervical ectropion		1		1		1		1		1		1	
Cervical intraepithelial neoplasia		1		2		2		2		1		2	
Cirrhosis	a) Mild (compensated)	1		1		1		1		1		1	
	b) Severe‡ (decompensated)	1		3		3		3		3		4	
Cystic fibrosis‡		1*		1*		1*		2*		1*		1*	
Deep venous thrombosis (DVT)/Pulmonary embolism (PE)	a) History of DVT/PE, not receiving anticoagulant therapy												
	i) Higher risk for recurrent DVT/PE	1		2		2		2		2		4	
	ii) Lower risk for recurrent DVT/PE	1		2		2		2		2		3	
	b) Acute DVT/PE	2		2		2		2		2		4	
	c) DVT/PE and established anticoagulant therapy for at least 3 months												
	i) Higher risk for recurrent DVT/PE	2		2		2		2		2		4*	
	ii) Lower risk for recurrent DVT/PE	2		2		2		2		2		3*	
	d) Family history (first-degree relatives)	1		1		1		1		1		2	
	e) Major surgery												
	i) With prolonged immobilization	1		2		2		2		2		4	
	ii) Without prolonged immobilization	1		1		1		1		1		2	
	f) Minor surgery without immobilization	1		1		1		1		1		1	
Depressive disorders		1*		1*		1*		1*		1*		1*	

Key:	
1 No restriction (method can be used)	3 Theoretical or proven risks usually outweigh the advantages
2 Advantages generally outweigh theoretical or proven risks	4 Unacceptable health risk (method not to be used)

(continued)

Medical Eligibility for Hormonal Contraceptive Use — CONTRACEPTION

Condition	Sub-Condition	Cu-IUD I	Cu-IUD C	LNG-IUD I	LNG-IUD C	Implant I	Implant C	DMPA I	DMPA C	POP I	POP C	CHC I	CHC C
Diabetes	a) History of gestational disease	1		1		1		1		1		1	
	b) Nonvascular disease												
	i) Non-insulin dependent	1		2		2		2		2		2	
	ii) Insulin dependent	1		2		2		2		2		2	
	c) Nephropathy/retinopathy/neuropathy‡	1		2		2		3		2		3/4*	
	d) Other vascular disease or diabetes of >20 years' duration‡	1		2		2		3		2		3/4*	
Dysmenorrhea	Severe	2		1		1		1		1		1	
Endometrial cancer‡		4	2	4	2	1		1		1		1	
Endometrial hyperplasia		1		1		1		1		1		1	
Endometriosis		2		1		1		1		1		1	
Epilepsy‡	(see also Drug Interactions)	1		1		1*		1*		1*		1*	
Gallbladder disease	a) Symptomatic												
	i) Treated by cholecystectomy	1		2		2		2		2		2	
	ii) Medically treated	1		2		2		2		2		3	
	iii) Current	1		2		2		2		2		3	
	b) Asymptomatic	1		2		2		2		2		2	
Gestational trophoblastic disease‡	a) Suspected GTD (immediate postevacuation)												
	i) Uterine size first trimester	1*		1*		1*		1*		1*		1*	
	ii) Uterine size second trimester	2*		2*		1*		1*		1*		1*	
	b) Confirmed GTD												
	i) Undetectable/non-pregnant ß-hCG levels	1*	1*	1*	1*	1*		1*		1*		1*	
	ii) Decreasing ß-hCG levels	2*	1*	2*	1*	1*		1*		1*		1*	
	iii) Persistently elevated ß-hCG levels or malignant disease, with no evidence or suspicion of intrauterine disease	2*	1*	2*	1*	1*		1*		1*		1*	
	iv) Persistently elevated ß-hCG levels or malignant disease, with evidence or suspicion of intrauterine disease	4*	2*	4*	2*	1*		1*		1*		1*	
Headaches	a) Nonmigraine (mild or severe)	1		1		1		1		1		1*	
	b) Migraine												
	i) Without aura (includes menstrual migraine)	1		1		1		1		1		2*	
	ii) With aura	1		1		1		1		1		4*	
History of bariatric surgery‡	a) Restrictive procedures	1		1		1		1		1		1	
	b) Malabsorptive procedures	1		1		1		1		3		COCs: 3 / P/R: 1	
History of cholestasis	a) Pregnancy related	1		1		1		1		1		2	
	b) Past COC related	1		2		2		2		2		3	
History of high blood pressure during pregnancy		1		1		1		1		1		2	
History of Pelvic surgery		1		1		1		1		1		1	
HIV	a) High risk for HIV	2	2	2	2	1		1*		1		1	
	b) HIV infection					1*		1*		1*		1*	
	i) Clinically well receiving ARV therapy	1	1	1	1	If on treatment, see Drug Interactions							
	ii) Not clinically well or not receiving ARV therapy‡	2	1	2	1	If on treatment, see Drug Interactions							

Abbreviations: C=continuation of contraceptive method; CHC=combined hormonal contraception (pill, patch, and, ring); COC=combined oral contraceptive; Cu-IUD=copper-containing intrauterine device; I=initiation of contraceptive method; LNG-IUD=levonorgestrel-releasing intrauterine device; NA=not applicable; POP=progestin-only pill; P/R=patch/ring
‡ Condition that exposes a woman to increased risk as a result of pregnancy. *Please see the complete guidance for a clarification to this classification: www.cdc.gov/reproductivehealth/unintendedpregnancy/USMEC.htm.

(continued)

CONTRACEPTION
Medical Eligibility for Hormonal Contraceptive Use

Condition	Sub-Condition	Cu-IUD		LNG-IUD		Implant		DMPA		POP		CHC	
		I	C	I	C	I	C	I	C	I	C	I	C
Hypertension	a) Adequately controlled hypertension	1*		1*		1*		2*		1*		3*	
	b) Elevated blood pressure levels (*properly taken measurements*)												
	i) Systolic 140-159 or diastolic 90-99	1*		1*		1*		2*		1*		3*	
	ii) Systolic ≥160 or diastolic ≥100‡	1*		2*		2*		3*		2*		4*	
	c) Vascular disease	1*		2*		2*		3*		2*		4*	
Inflammatory bowel disease	(*Ulcerative colitis, Crohn's disease*)	1		1		1		2		2		2/3*	
Ischemic heart disease‡	Current and history of	1		2	3	2	3	3		2	3	4	
Known thrombogenic mutations‡		1*		2*		2*		2*		2*		4*	
Liver tumors	a) Benign												
	i) Focal nodular hyperplasia	1		2		2		2		2		2	
	ii) Hepatocellular adenoma‡	1		3		3		3		3		4	
	b) Malignant‡ (hepatoma)	1		3		3		3		3		4	
Malaria		1		1		1		1		1		1	
Multiple risk factors for atherosclerotic cardiovascular disease	(e.g., older age, smoking, diabetes, hypertension, low HDL, high LDL, or high triglyceride levels)			1		2		2*		3*		2*		3/4*	
Multiple sclerosis	a) With prolonged immobility	1		1		1		2		1		3	
	b) Without prolonged immobility	1		1		1		2		1		1	
Obesity	a) Body mass index (BMI) ≥30 kg/m²	1		1		1		1		1		2	
	b) Menarche to <18 years and BMI ≥ 30 kg/m²	1		1		1		2		1		2	
Ovarian cancer‡		1		1		1		1		1		1	
Parity	a) Nulliparous	2		2		1		1		1		1	
	b) Parous	1		1		1		1		1		1	
Past ectopic pregnancy		1		1		1		1		2		1	
Pelvic inflammatory disease	a) Past												
	i) With subsequent pregnancy	1	1	1	1	1		1		1		1	
	ii) Without subsequent pregnancy	2	2	2	2	1		1		1		1	
	b) Current	4	2*	4	2*	1		1		1		1	
Peripartum cardiomyopathy‡	a) Normal or mildly impaired cardiac function												
	i) <6 months	2		2		1		1		1		4	
	ii) ≥6 months	2		2		1		1		1		3	
	b) Moderately or severely impaired cardiac function	2		2		2		2		2		4	
Postabortion	a) First trimester	1*		1*		1*		1*		1*		1*	
	b) Second trimester	2*		2*		1*		1*		1*		1*	
	c) Immediate postseptic abortion	4		4		1*		1*		1*		1*	
Postpartum (nonbreastfeeding women)	a) <21 days					1		1		1		4	
	b) 21 days to 42 days												
	i) With other risk factors for VTE					1		1		1		3*	
	ii) Without other risk factors for VTE					1		1		1		2	
	c) >42 days					1		1		1		1	
Postpartum (in breastfeeding or non-breastfeeding women, including cesarean delivery)	a) <10 minutes after delivery of the placenta												
	i) Breastfeeding	1*		2*									
	ii) Nonbreastfeeding	1*		1*									
	b) 10 minutes after delivery of the placenta to <4 weeks	2*		2*									
	c) ≥4 weeks	1*		1*									
	d) Postpartum sepsis	4		4									

(continued)

Medical Eligibility for Hormonal Contraceptive Use — CONTRACEPTION

Condition	Sub-Condition	Cu-IUD		LNG-IUD		Implant		DMPA		POP		CHC	
		I	C	I	C	I	C	I	C	I	C	I	C
Pregnancy		4*		4*		NA*		NA*		NA*		NA*	
Rheumatoid arthritis	a) On immunosuppressive therapy	2	1	2	1	1		2/3*		1		2	
	b) Not on immunosuppressive therapy	1		1		1		2		1		2	
Schistosomiasis	a) Uncomplicated	1		1		1		1		1		1	
	b) Fibrosis of the liver‡	1		1		1		1		1		1	
Sexually transmitted diseases (STDs)	a) Current purulent cervicitis or chlamydial infection or gonococcal infection	4	2*	4	2*	1		1		1		1	
	b) Vaginitis (including trichomonas vaginalis and bacterial vaginosis)	2	2	2	2	1		1		1		1	
	c) Other factors relating to STDs	2*	2	2*	2	1		1		1		1	
Smoking	a) Age <35	1		1		1		1		1		2	
	b) Age ≥35, <15 cigarettes/day	1		1		1		1		1		3	
	c) Age ≥35, ≥15 cigarettes/day	1		1		1		1		1		4	
Solid organ transplantation‡	a) Complicated	3	2	3	2	2		2		2		4	
	b) Uncomplicated	2		2		2		2		2		2*	
Stroke‡	History of cerebrovascular accident	1		2		2	3	3		2	3	4	
Superficial venous disorders	a) Varicose veins	1		1		1		1		1		1	
	b) Superficial venous thrombosis (acute or history)	1		1		1		1		1		3*	
Systemic lupus erythematosus‡	a) Positive (or unknown) antiphospholipid antibodies	1*	1*	3*		3*		3*	3*	3*		4*	
	b) Severe thrombocytopenia	3*	2*	2*		2*		3*	2*	2*		2*	
	c) Immunosuppressive therapy	2*	1*	2*		2*		2*	2*	2*		2*	
	d) None of the above	1*	1*	2*		2*		2*		2*		2*	
Thyroid disorders	Simple goiter/ hyperthyroid/hypothyroid	1		1		1		1		1		1	
Tuberculosis‡ (see also Drug Interactions)	a) Nonpelvic	1	1	1	1	1*		1*		1*		1*	
	b) Pelvic	4	3	4	3	1*		1*		1*		1*	
Unexplained vaginal bleeding	(suspicious for serious condition) before evaluation	4*	2*	4*	2*	3*		3*		2*		2*	
Uterine fibroids		2		2		1		1		1		1	
Valvular heart disease	a) Uncomplicated	1		1		1		1		1		2	
	b) Complicated‡	1		1		1		1		1		4	
Vaginal bleeding patterns	a) Irregular pattern without heavy bleeding	1		1	1	2		2		2		1	
	b) Heavy or prolonged bleeding	2*		1*	2*	2*		2*		2*		1*	
Viral hepatitis	a) Acute or flare	1		1		1		1		1		3/4*	2
	b) Carrier/Chronic	1		1		1		1		1		1	1
Antiretroviral therapy All other ARV's are 1 or 2 for all methods.	Fosamprenavir (FPV)	1/2*	1*	1/2*	1*	2*		2*		2*		3*	
Anticonvulsant therapy	a) Certain anticonvulsants (phenytoin, carbamazepine, barbiturates, primidone, topiramate, oxcarbazepine)	1		1		2*		1*		3*		3*	
	b) Lamotrigine	1		1		1		1		1		3*	
Antimicrobial therapy	a) Broad spectrum antibiotics	1		1		1		1		1		1	
	b) Antifungals	1		1		1		1		1		1	
	c) Antiparasitics	1		1		1		1		1		1	
	d) Rifampin or rifabutin therapy	1		1		2*		1*		3*		3*	
SSRIs		1		1		1		1		1		1	
St. John's wort		1		1		2		1		2		2	

Updated July 2016. This summary sheet only contains a subset of the recommendations from the U.S. MEC. For complete guidance, see: http://www.cdc.gov/reproductivehealth/unintendedpregnancy/USMEC.htm. Most contraceptive methods do not protect against sexually transmitted diseases (STDs). Consistent and correct use of the male latex condom reduces the risk of STDs and HIV.

CS266008-A

AIDS, acquired immunodeficiency syndrome; ARV, antiretroviral; BMI, body mass index; C, continuation of contraceptive method; COC, combined oral contraceptive; DM, diabetes mellitus; DVT, deep venous thrombosis; β-hCG, beta-human chorionic gonadotropin; HIV, human immunodeficiency virus; I, initiation of contraceptive method; IUD, intrauterine device; LNG-IUD, levonorgestrel-releasing IUD; NA, not applicable; P, combined hormonal contraceptive patch; PE, pulmonary embolism; R, combined hormonal vaginal ring; STI, sexually transmitted infection; VTE, venous thromboembolism.

*Condition that exposes a woman to increased risk as a result of an unintended pregnancy.

†Please see the complete guidance for a clarification to this classification, www.cdc.gov/reproductivehealth/usmec.

(continued)

CONTRACEPTION — Medical Eligibility for Hormonal Contraceptive Use

‡Please refer to the U.S. Medical Eligibility Criteria for Contraceptive Use guidance related to drug interactions at the end of this chart.

§See Tepper N, Curtis KM, Jamieson DJ, Marchbanks PA. Update to CDC's U.S. medical eligibility criteria for contraceptive use, 2010: revised recommendations for the use of contraceptive methods during the postpartum period. Centers for Disease Control and Prevention (CDC). *MMWR*. 2011;60:878–83. Available at: http://www.cdc.gov/mmwr/pdf/wk/mm6026.pdf. Retrieved July 7, 2011.

‖Clarification: For women with other risk factors for venous thromboembolism, these risk factors may increase the classification to a "4"; for example, see Smoking, DVT/PE, Thrombogenic Mutations, and Peripartum Cardiomyopathy.

Source: http://www.cdc.gov/reproductivehealth/contraception/pdf/summary-chart-us-medical-eligibility-criteria_508tagged.pdf. Accessed on July 29, 2016.

BARRIER CONTRACEPTIVES
Diaphragm
- Safe method with rare side effects.
- Urinary tract infection twice as common.
- Reduces rate of sexually transmitted infections (STIs).
- Successful fitting is crucial to efficacy.
- Insert no longer than 6 hours prior to coitus.
- Remove 6–24 hours after coitus.
- Use with spermicide.
- Assess fit annually.

Cervical Cap (Prentif)
- Safe method with rare side effects.
- Only 4 sizes and harder to place.
- Insert 20 minutes to 4 hours prior to coitus.
- Successful fitting is crucial to efficacy.
- Can leave in place for 24–36 hours.

Spermicides
- Nonoxynol-9, Octoxynol-9, Mefegol.
- Proven STI protection.
- Apply 10–30 minutes prior to coitus.
- High failure rate.

Condoms
- 6 billion used worldwide annually.
- Latex condoms 0.3–0.8 mm thick.
- Natural skin condoms do not protect against HIV and other STIs.
- Do not use with oil-based lubricants.
- Inconsistent use accounts for most failures.

ORAL CONTRACEPTIVES

Fast Facts

- Contraception but not an absolute anovulatory effect (with current lower EE doses):
  - Ovulation still occurs in approximately 3% of cycles (Teichmann 1995)
  - Turbidity of cervical mucus
  - Inhibit spinnbarkeit
  - Suppression of endometrial gland maturation → decidualized
- Efficacy of OCs at inhibiting ovulation based on when OC use was initiated (Baerwald 2006):
  - Follicle diameter of 10 mm, 0/16 ovulations
  - Follicle diameter 14 mm, 4/14
  - Follicle diameter 18 mm, 14/15

Mechanism of Action

- E and progestin are given every day for 3 of 4 weeks.
- Contraception efficacy derived from the negative feedback actions of progestins.
- Bleeding is controlled by the E component.
- P4 inhibits luteinizing hormone (LH).
- E inhibits follicle-stimulating hormone (FSH) and LH.
- E minimizes irregular shedding of endometrium and BTB.
- E potentiates the action of progestin via ↑ progestin receptors (thus allowing ↓ progestin dose).
- Multiphasic formulations.
  - The aim is to alter steroid levels to ↓ metabolic effects and ↓ BTB/amenorrhea.

Steroid Components of Oral Contraceptives

Estrogen Component

- Estradiol (E2) is the most potent natural estrogen (E) and the major E secreted by the ovaries. An ethinyl group at the C-17 position makes E2 orally active. All current oral contraceptives (OCs) use ethinyl estradiol (EE), estradiol valerate or mestranol.
- Potentiates the action of the progestogenic component by ↑ progesterone (P4) receptors.
- Stabilizes the endometrium to minimize breakthrough bleeding (BTB) and irregular shedding.

Progestin Component—Synthetic Progestins

- Potency varies depending on the target organ and endpoint being studied.
  - The biologic effect of the various progestational components in current low-dose OCs is approximately the same.

Table 5.5. Pharmacologic profiles of progesterone and various progestins

Progesterone/ Progestins	Pharmacologic Activity			
	Progestogenic	Androgenic	Antiandrogenic	Antimineralocorticoid
Progesterone	+	−	(+)	+
Drospirenone	+	−	+	+
Gestodene[a]	+	(+)	−	(+)
Norgestimate[b]	+	(+)	−	−
Levonorgestrel	+	(+)	−	−
Desogestrel[c]	+	(+)	−	−
Dienogest[a]	+	−	+	−
Cyproterone acetate[a]	+	−	+	−

+, effect; (+), negligible effect at therapeutic doses; −, no effect.

[a]Not available in the United States.

[b]Main metabolite levonorgestrel.

[c]Active metabolite 3-ketodesogestrel.

Source: Adapted from Krattenmacher R. Drospirenone: pharmacology and pharmacokinetics of a unique progestogen. *Contraception*. 2000;62:29-38.

METABOLIC EFFECTS OF ORAL CONTRACEPTIVES

Myocardial Infarction
- Second-generation OCs ↑ risk of myocardial infarction by approximately twofold among users even after controlling for cardiovascular risk factors (Tanis 2001).
- Major mortality risk in smokers >35 years of age.

Ischemic Stroke
- Risk of ischemic stroke is not significantly different in women with simple migraine (no aura) compared to those with classic migraine (with aura; Curtis 2002).
- OCs should not be used for women with visual changes or focal neurologic deficits associated with migraines.

Hemorrhagic Stroke
- <35 years old → no increased risk for OC users.
- >35 years old → 2.2-fold higher risk for users (95% confidence interval [CI], 1.5–3.3; Farley 1999).

Venous Thromboembolism
- Minimal risk of thrombosis associated with OCs (perhaps on the order of 3 out of 10,000 woman-years vs. 8 out of 10,000 woman-years in pregnancy); most VTE are asymptomatic and never diagnosed making estimates suspect at best.
- If a woman has a known inherited or acquired thrombophilia, or personal history of idiopathic VTE, she should not take an estrogen-containing OC; there is no justification to screen for prothrombotic mutations with a family history of venous thromboembolism (Grimes 2012).

Hypertension
- No ↑ incidence of clinically significant hypertension (HTN) has been reported to date.
- Hormonal contraception can safely be provided based on careful review of medical history and blood pressure (BP) measurement; for most women, no further evaluation is necessary (Stewart 2001).

Carbohydrate Metabolism
- Insulin resistance and glucose changes with low-dose monophasic and multiphasic OCs are so minimal that it is now believed that they are of no clinical significance.
- OCs do not increase risk of diabetes mellitus (DM).

Other Effects
- Minimally ↑ risk of gallbladder disease (secondary to change in composition of bile due to ↑ cholesterol from E), although low-dose OCs have yet to be tested.
- OCs contraindicated in acute or chronic cholestatic liver disease.
- Nausea and breast discomfort are most intense within first few months and usually disappear (lower incidence with low-dose pills).
- No causal association between OCs and weight gain (Gupta 2000).
- ↑ Erythrocyte sedimentation rate (ESR)/total Fe-binding capacity; ↓ prothrombin time (PT).

- Telangiectasia; melasma
- Thick cervical mucus (leukorrhea)
- Rarely → depression/↓ libido.
- Progestin-associated side effects: mood swings, depression, fatigue, ↓ libido, weight gain.

ORAL CONTRACEPTIVES AND CANCER

Breast Cancer
- After 2 years of use, there is a 40% reduction in fibrocystic disease.
- There are conflicting data, but epidemiologic studies have generally not demonstrated a strong association between OC use and breast cancer (Collaborative Group on Hormonal Factors in Breast Cancer 1996).
- Small increase in relative risk of localized breast cancer if <35 yo associated with current OC use (RR = 1.24; 95% CI, 1.15–1.33) (Collaborative Group on Hormonal Factors in Breast Cancer 1996).
- Small increase if <35 yo with past OC use within 1 to 4 years (RR = 1.16; 95% CI, 1.08–1.23) compared with controls.
- Risk declines after stopping use and disappears within 10 years.
- No difference in risk of breast cancer in ever-users and controls by age 50.
- A case-control study on a total of 4,575 women aged 35–64 years found current or former OC use was not associated with a significant ↑ risk of breast cancer: odds ratio (OR), 1.0 (0.8–1.3; Marchbanks 2002).

Cervical Cancer
- Risk for dysplasia and carcinoma in situ ↑ with use of OCs for >1 year; invasive cancer may be ↑ after 5 years of use, reaching a twofold ↑ after 10 years; ↑ risk for both adenocarcinoma and squamous cell carcinoma (Smith 2003; Green 2003).
- Risk seems to ↓ after discontinuation of OCs.
- Risk in human papillomavirus (HPV)-positive.
- OC users may be related to the 16a-hydroxyestrone metabolite of E2, which can act as a cofactor with oncogenic HPV to promote cell proliferation (Newfield 1998).
- There are many confounding variables, and the conclusions regarding cervical cancer are not definite.

Endometrial Cancer
- ↓ cancer risk (adenocarcinoma, adenosquamous carcinoma, and adenoacanthoma) by 56%, 67%, and 72% with use of combined OCs for 4, 8, and 12 years (Schlesselma 1999).
- Protection persists for up to 20 years after discontinuation (Schlesselman s 1999).
- Lower dose (30–35 mg) OCs provide comparable protection (Weiderpass 1999).

Ovarian Cancer
- ↓ cancer risk (serous, endometrioid, mucinous, and clear cell) by 41%, 54%, and 61% with use of OCs for 4, 8, and 12 years (Schlesselman 1999; Ness 2000; Royar 2001).
- Protection persists for up to 20 years after discontinuation (Schlesselman 1999).
- There may not be a protective effect for those with *BRCA1* or *BRCA2* mutation (Modan 2001), although a case-control study found a 50% ↓ in risk in past OC users with *BRCA* mutations compared with OC nonusers with the same mutations (Narod 1998).

Colorectal Cancer
- OCs may protect women from developing colorectal cancer:
  - Relative risk (RR) of colon cancer in OC users: 0.82 (95% confidence interval [CI], 0.74–0.92; Fernandez 2001).

Tumors of the Liver
- Evidence for an association between OC use and hepatic adenoma is good, while the evidence for an association with focal nodular hyperplasia and/or hepatocellular carcinoma is inconclusive.

Table 5.6. Summary of oral contraceptives and cancer

Form of Cancer	Risk with Oral Contraceptives (OCs)
Breast	Small increase in RR in women under 35 (risk goes from 1/1,000 to 1.24/1,000) but this risk declines after stopping OCs and disappears within 10 years; no increased risk in women over 35 who were current or former users of OCs. Data are inconsistent on the risk of breast cancer associated with OC use in *BRCA* mutation carriers (Cibula 2011).
Cervical	OCs used for <5 years did not increase the risk of cervical cancer but use for 5 to 9 years showed ↑ risk (OR = 2.82; 95% CI, 1.46–5.42).
Endometrial	OCs ↓ endometrial cancer by 56%, 67%, and 72% with OC use for 4, 8, and 12 years, respectively.
Ovarian	OCs ↓ ovarian cancer by 41%, 54%, and 61% with OC use for 4, 8, and 12 years, respectively. Protective effects start after just 3 to 6 months of use and continue for up to 20 years after discontinuation. There are protective benefits for women at risk for hereditary ovarian cancer (*BRCA1* and *BRCA2*).

Source: Adapted from Practice Committee of American Society for Reproductive Medicine. Hormonal contraception: recent advances and controversies. *Fertil Steril.* 2008 Nov;90(5 Suppl):S103-113.

ORAL CONTRACEPTIVES AND REPRODUCTION
Inadvertent Use While Pregnant
- Initial reports linking OCs to congenital malformations have not been substantiated.
- Risk of a significant congenital anomaly is no greater than the general rate of 2–3%.

Subsequent Fertility
- 98.9% incidence of spontaneous menses or pregnancy within 90 days; median time to return to menses = 32 days (Davis 2008).
- Spontaneous loss: Prospective case-control study revealed that use of OCs for >2 years could be associated with a higher risk of miscarriage, or 2.56 (95% CI, 1.16–5.67; Garcia-Enguidanos 2005).
- Pregnancy outcome: ↑ dizygotic twinning (1.6% vs. 1.0%) in women who conceive soon after cessation of OCs.
- Conception rates at 12 months following discontinuation of various contraceptives:

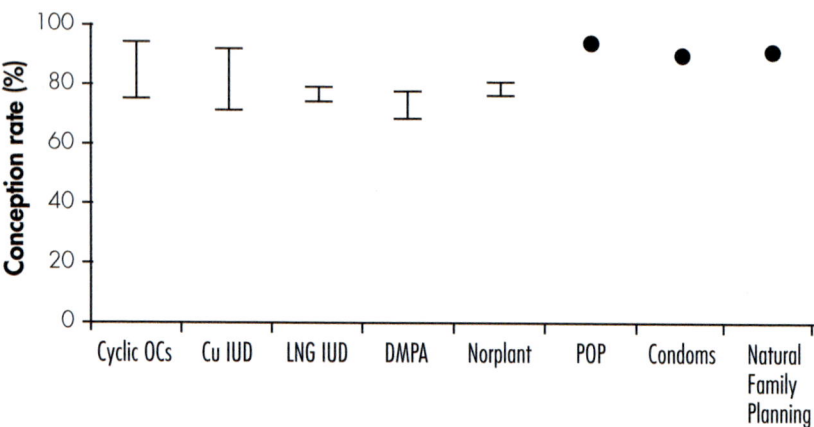

Figure 5.1. Twelve-month conception rates following discontinuation of various contraceptive methods
Source: Reproduced with permission from Barnhart KT, Schreiber CA. Return to fertility following discontinuation of oral contraceptives. *Fertil Steril.* 2009 Mar;91(3):659-63. Copyright © 2009 The American Society for Reproductive Medicine.

Oral Contraceptives and Breastfeeding
- ↓ quantity and quality of lactation (no matter the starting month), although no impairment of infant growth.
- ↓ lactation at 3.7 months vs. 4.6 months for controls.
- It has been argued that the threshold for ovulation suppression is ≥5 feedings for ≥65 minutes/day of suckling duration.
- Amenorrheic women who exclusively breastfeed at regular intervals, including nighttime, during the first 6 months have the contraceptive protection equivalent to that provided by OCs; with menstruation or after 6 months, the risk of ovulation increases.

- The progestin-only pill has no negative impact on breast milk, and some studies show ↑ milk production.

Initiation of Oral Contraceptives in Postpartum Period
- Rule of 3s for postpartum (pp) contraception:
  - Full Breastfeeding → begin OCs *3 months* pp
  - Partial or no Breastfeeding → begin in *third week* pp

Postpill Amenorrhea
- There is no evidence that OCs cause secondary amenorrhea.
  - Women who have not resumed menstrual function within 6 months should be evaluated as any other patient with secondary amenorrhea.

ORAL CONTRACEPTIVE MANAGEMENT ISSUES

Surveillance
- Monitor blood pressure yearly all other health surveillance as per health recommendations.

Proper Pill Taking
- Immediate initiation of the pill ("Quick Start" protocol) improves short-term continuation and compliance in adolescents (Lara-Torre 2002; Westhoff 2007).
- Effective contraception is present during the first cycle of pill use, provided the pills are started on the fifth day of cycle; Sunday starts usually avoid weekend bleeding.
- Postponing a period can be achieved by omitting the 7-day hormone-free interval.
- Missed pills:
  - 1 Missed pill → take 1 pill as soon as possible, then resume.
  - 2 Missed pills (in first 2 weeks) → take 2 pills × 2 days with backup × 7 days.
  - 3 Missed pills (in third week or more than 2 anytime) → backup × 7 days.

Clinical Problems
Breakthrough Bleeding
- Most frequently occurs in first few months of use (10–30% in first month, 1–10% in third month).
- Occurs due to tissue breakdown as the endometrium adjusts its architecture.
  - Take the pill at the same time every day.
  - If BTB just before end of pill cycle → stop pills, wait 7 days, and start new cycle.
- Control of BTB: estradiol valerate, 5 mg IM 3 1 dose.
- There is There is no evidence that any specific formulation is significantly superior to any other in terms of the rate of BTB; in general, pills with higher doses of E and lower doses of P4 have the lowest rates of BTB.
- Try switching from an estrane to a gonane.

Amenorrhea
- There is no harmful, permanent consequence of developing amenorrhea while taking OCs.
- Incidence: First year = 1%; several years = 5%.

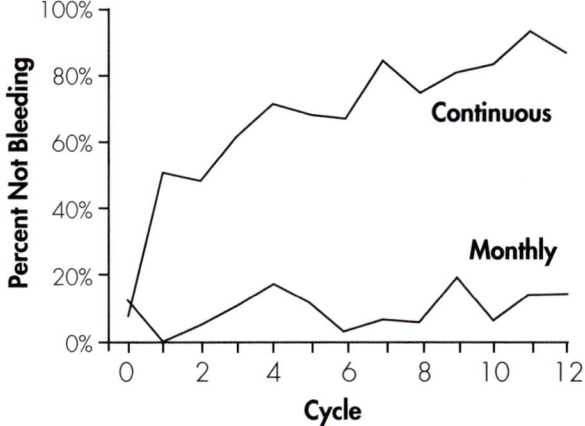

Figure 5.2. Rates of amenorrhea for continuous vs. monthly oral contraceptives
Source: Reproduced with permission from Miller L, Hughes JP. Continuous combination oral contraceptive pills to eliminate withdrawal bleeding: a randomized trial. *Obstet Gynecol.* 2003 101[4]:653. Copyright © 2003 The American College of Obstetricians and Gynecologists.

Weight Gain
- No association between OCs and weight gain.

Acne
- Improvement shown (even with 20-mg-EE OCs; Thorneycroft 1999)
  - E2 → ↓ gonadotropins + ↑ sex hormone–binding globulin (SHBG) to bind T
  - Progestins → ↓ gonadotropins + ↑ T metabolism + ↓ 5a-reductase

Ovarian Cysts
- OCs do not hasten resolution of functional ovarian cysts; surgery would be warranted if persistent beyond 2–3 cycles (Grimes 2011).
- Functional ovarian cysts occur less frequently in women taking higher-dose OCs.

CURRENTLY AVAILABLE ORAL CONTRACEPTIVES

Table 5.7. Currently available oral contraceptives

Type (Progestin/Estrogen)	Product	Progestin (mg)	Estrogen (mcg)	Active Tablets
COMBINATION BIPHASIC	Ortho-Novum 10/11	0.5	35	10 white
Norethindrone/EE		1	35	11 peach
Desogestrel/EE	Kariva	0.15	20	21 white
		—	10	5 light blue
	Mircette	0.15	20	21 white
		—	10	5 light blue
COMBINATION TRIPHASIC	Cyclessa	0.1	25	7 light orange
Desogestrel/EE		0.125	25	7 orange
		0.15	25	7 red
	Velivet	0.1	25	7 beige
		0.125	25	7 orange
		0.15	25	7 pink
Norethindrone/EE	Aranelle	0.5	35	7 light yellow
		1	35	9 white
		0.5	35	5 light yellow
	Nortrel 7/7/7	0.5	35	7 light yellow
		0.75	35	7 blue
		1	35	7 peach
	Ortho-Novum 7/7/7	0.5	35	7 white
		0.75	35	7 light peach
		1	35	7 peach
	Tri-Norinyl	0.5	35	7 blue
		1	35	9 yellow-green
		0.5	35	5 blue
Norgestimate/EE	Ortho Tri-Cyclen	0.18	35	7 white
		0.215	35	7 light blue
		0.25	35	7 blue
	Ortho Tri-Cyclen Lo	0.18	25	7 white
		0.215	25	7 light blue
		0.25	25	7 dark blue
	Ti-Previfern	0.18	35	7 white
		0.215	35	7 light blue
		0.25	35	7 blue
	Tri-Sprintec	0.18	35	7 gray
		0.215	35	7 light blue
		0.25	35	7 blue
Levonorgestrel/EE	Enpresse	0.05	30	6 pink
		0.075	40	5 white
		0.125	30	10 orange

(continued)

Currently Available Oral Contraceptives — CONTRACEPTION

Type (Progestin/Estrogen)	Product	Progestin (mg)	Estrogen (mcg)	Active Tablets
Levonorgestrel/EE (continued)	Tri-Levlen	0.05	30	6 brown
		0.075	40	5 white
		0.125	30	10 light yellow
COMBINATION MULTIPHASIC	Natazia	—	3,000	2 dark yellow
Dienogest/Estradiol valerate		2	2,000	5 medium red
		3	2,000	17 light yellow
		—	1,000	2 dark red
COMBINATION ESTROPHASIC	Estrostep Fe	1	20	5 white triangle
Norethindrone acetate/EE		1	30	7 white square
		1	35	9 white round
	Tilia Fe	1	20	5 white triangle
		1	30	7 white square
		1	35	9 white round
	Tri-Legest Fe	1	20	5 light pink round
		1	30	7 light yellow round
		1	35	9 light blue round
PROGESTIN-ONLY	Camila	0.35	none	light pink
Norethindrone	Errin	0.35	none	yellow
	Micronor	0.35	none	lime green
	Nor-QD	0.35	none	yellow
	Ovrette	0.35	none	light pink
	Jolivette	0.35	none	light green
	Nora-BE	0.35	none	white
COMBINATION EXTENDED CYCLE	Introvale	0.15	30	peach
Levonorgestrel/EE	Jolessa	0.15	30	pink
	LoSeasonique	0.1	20	84 orange
		—	10	7 yellow
	Lybrel	0.09	20	yellow
	Seasonale	0.15	30	Pink
	Seasonique	0.15	30	84 light blue-green
		—	10	7 yellow
COMBINATION MONOPHASIC	Balziva	0.4	35	light peach
Norethindrone/EE	Brevicon	0.5	35	blue
*as norethindrone acetate	Junel 21 1/20	1*	20	yellow
	Junel Fe 1/20	1*	20	yellow
	Junel 21 1.5/30	1.5*	30	pink
	Juenl Fe 1.5/30	1.5*	30	pink
	Loestrin 1/20	1*	20	white
	Loestrin Fe 1/20	1*	20	white
	Loestrin 24 Fe	1*	20	white
	Loestrin 1.5/30	1.5*	30	green
	Loestrin Fe 1.5/30	1.5*	30	green

(continued)

CONTRACEPTION

Currently Available Oral Contraceptives

Type (Progestin/Estrogen)	Product	Progestin (mg)	Estrogen (mcg)	Active Tablets
Norethindrone/EE (continued)	Lo Loestrin Fe	1*	10	24 blue
		—	10	2 white
	Norinyl 1 + 35	1	35	yellow-green
	Nortrel 0.5/35	0.5	35	light yellow
	Nortrel 1/35	1	35	yellow
	Ortho-Novum 1/35	1	35	peach
	Ovcon 35 Fe	0.4	35	peach
	Femcon Fe	0.4	35	white
	Ovcon 50	1	50	yellow
Levonorgestre/EE	Altavera	0.15	30	peach
	Aviane	0.1	20	orange
	Lessina	0.1	20	pink
	Levien	0.15	30	light orange
	Levlite	0.1	20	pink
	Nordette	0.15	30	light orange
	Portia	0.15	30	pink
Norgestrel/EE	Cryselle	0.3	30	white
	Lo/ovral	0.3	30	white
Ethynodiol diacetate/EE	Kelnor 1/35	1	35	light yellow
Norethindrone/mestranol	Norinylw 1 + 50	1	50	white
	Ortho-Novum 1/50	1	50	yellow
Desogestrel/EE	Apri	0.15	30	rose
	Desogen	0.15	30	white
	Ortho-cepi	0.15	30	orange
Drospirenone/EE	Ocella	3	30	yellow
	Yasmin	3	30	yellow
	Yaz	3	20	light pink
Norgestimate/EE	Ortho-Cyclen	0.25	35	blue
	Sprintec	0.25	35	blue
COMBINATION MONOPHASIC w. FOLATE	Beyaz	3	20	24 pink
Drospirenone/EE/levomefolate calcium (as Metafolin) 451 µg plus levomefolate calcium (as Metafolin) 451 µg only (4 light orange tabs)				
Drospirenone/EE/levomefolate calcium 451µg plus levomefolate calcium 451 µg only (7 light orange tabs)	Safyral	3	30	21 orange

(continued)

Currently Available Oral Contraceptives — CONTRACEPTION

Brand	Manufacturer	Estrogen	Progestin	Regimen	Clinical Considerations
Le-Seasonique	Duramed Pharmaceuticals (Montvale, NY)	10–20 mcg EE	0.1 mg LNG	• 84 days EE 20 mcg/LNG • 7 days EE 10 mcg	• Extended cycle • Continuous EE may improve suppression of ovulation and decrease withdrawal bleeding
Natazia	Bayer Schering Pharma AG (Leverkusen, Germany)	1–3 mg E2V	2–3 mg DNG	• Days 1–2: E2V 3 mg • Days 3–7: E2V 2 mg/DNG 2 mg • Days 8–24: E2V 2 mg/DNG 3 mg • Days 25–26: E2V 1 mg • Days 27–28: placebo	• Extended dosing • Only estradiol-based pill available in US • Effective treatment for heavy menstrual bleeding • Instructions for missed pills more complicated
Beyaz	Bayer Schering Pharma AG (Leverkusen, Germany)	20 mcg EE	3 mg DRSP	• 24 days EE/DRSP/levomefolate • 4 days levomefolate	• Extended dosing • DRSP shown to be beneficial for acne and PCOS symptoms • Provides folic acid
Lo-Loestrin Fe	Warner Chilcott (Rockaway, NJ)	10 mcg EE	1 mg NET	• 24 days EE/NET • 2 days EE • 2 days placebo	• Extended dosing • Lowest-dose EE pill • Common for patients to have no withdrawal bleeding

FDA, Food and Drug Administration; EE, ethinyl estradiol; LNG, levonorgestrel; E2V, estradiol valerate; DNG, dienogest; DRSP, drospirenone; PCOS, polycystic ovary syndrome; NET, norethindrone.

ORAL CONTRACEPTIVES—PROGESTIN ONLY

Mechanism of Action
Prevents ovulation; thickens cervical mucus; causes endometrial changes that may prevent implantation (rare); reduces activity of cilia in the fallopian tube.

Side Effects
Similar to COCs—though estrogen-related side effects (e.g., nausea, breast tenderness, bloating) are diminished; menstrual irregularity (most common); irregular bleeding; prolonged bleeding episodes; amenorrhea.

Serious Adverse Reactions
Similar to COCs with reduced risk of clotting problems; potential cardiovascular effects are controversial; ectopic pregnancy (rare).

Contraindications/Precautions
Undiagnosed genital bleeding; current CAD or cerebrovascular disease; known or suspected hormone-dependent neoplasia; history of benign or malignant liver neoplasm.

Key Counseling Points
- Does not protect against STIs or HIV infection.
- Taken daily, with no hormone-free interval.
- Take pills at the same time each day for maximum effectiveness.
- Appropriate action if:
- Pill is taken 3 hours late
  - Take pill as soon as possible. If taken the next day, take 2 pills, and complete the cycle pack.
  - Use backup contraception for 48 hours.
- ≥1 pill is missed: Stop taking pills. Discard cycle pack.
  - Use EC if necessary (see pg. 313). Menses should begin within 2–3 weeks (unless pregnant).
  - Start a new cycle pack on the day menses begins. Use backup contraception from the time the error is discovered until the third day of the new cycle pack.

Additional Considerations
- Initial Dose: Can be started on any day of the week once pregnancy is ruled out.
- Return of fertility: No delay
- One-year failure rate: Typical vs. Perfect User: 8% vs. 0.3%
- Drug interactions: Similar to COCs
- Data indicate that the cervical mucus becomes impenetrable rapidly, so backup contraception is only needed until the third consecutive pill taken at the same time each day is ingested.
- In clinical studies, failure rates have been reported as high as 13% (McCann 1994).

TRANSDERMAL CONTRACEPTIVE
- Ortho Evra (Ortho-McNeil)

Description
- Three-layer patch delivers 0.15 mg/d of norelgestromin and 20 mcg/day of EE

Mechanism of Action
- Similar to COCs

Application Issues
- Applied 1 patch/week for 3 weeks followed by a patch-free week.
- May be applied to 4 areas: lower abdomen, buttocks, upper outer arm, and upper torso, excluding breasts.
- New patch is applied to a different area of skin, on the same day of the week as previous patch.
- Initial use: Can be started on any day of the week once pregnancy is ruled out.
- If >5 days since start of menstrual bleeding, or postpartum, or postabortion, backup contraceptive method is recommended for 7 days.

Side Effects: Serious Adverse Effects
- Similar to COCs
- Skin irritation

Key Counseling Points
- Does not protect against lower genital tract STIs or HIV infection.
- Spotting or BTB may occur during the first 3 cycles of use.
- Physician should be aware if pregnancy is suspected or if any of the following occur: sudden severe headache, visual disturbances, numbness in an arm or leg, severe abdominal pain, prolonged episodes of bleeding, or amenorrhea.
  - Appropriate action if patch is detached:
    - If <24 hours, patch should be reapplied to the same body location or, if not adhering well, a new patch should be applied immediately. No backup contraception is needed.
    - If >24 hours, apply a new patch. Use backup contraception method for 7 days.

Additional Considerations
- Return of fertility: No delay
- One-year failure rate: Perfect Use: 0.3%
- Contraindications/precautions: Similar to COCs
- Drug interactions: Similar to COCs

INJECTABLE CONTRACEPTIVE

Product
- Depo-Provera (Pfizer)
- Depo-subQ Provera 104 (Pfizer)

Description
- 150 mg/1 mL suspension of DMPA (injected intramuscularly only)
- 104 mg/0.65 mL medroxyprogesterone acetate (injected subcutaneously only)

Mechanism of Action
- Prevents ovulation by inhibiting luteinizing hormone surge
- Thickens cervical mucus to block sperm entry into the upper reproductive tract
- Slows tubal motility
- Causes endometrial changes that may prevent implantation (rare)

Administration Issues
- Only use as a long-term birth control method (for example, longer than 2 years) if other birth control methods are inadequate for the patient.
  - First injection can be administered on any day, as long as pregnancy is ruled out.
  - If >5 days since start of menses, postpartum, or postabortion, backup contraceptive method is recommended for 7 days.
- Pregnancy should be ruled out if the woman returns for repeat injection more than 13 weeks after the last injection.
- Shake vial vigorously before use to ensure uniform suspension.

Duration of Efficacy
- 3 months

Side Effects/Serious Adverse Effects
- Irregular bleeding, weight gain, breast tenderness, headaches
- Prolonged use may result in significant loss of bone density with greater loss the longer the drug is administered; may not be completely reversible after discontinuation

Contraindications
- Undiagnosed abnormal genital bleeding
- Known or suspected pregnancy
- Acute liver disease
- Benign or malignant liver tumors
- Known or suspected malignancy of the breast

Key Counseling Points
- Does not protect against lower genital tract STIs or HIV infection.
- Most women experience irregular unpredictable bleeding during the first year.
- Return every 3 months for repeat injection.

- Physician should be aware if pregnancy is suspected or if any of the following occur: sudden severe headache, visual disturbances, numbness in an arm or leg, severe abdominal pain, prolonged episodes of bleeding, or amenorrhea.

Additional Considerations
- Return of fertility: Delayed; as many as 30% of women may not conceive within 12 months; delay may be >2 years.
- One-year failure rate: Typical vs. Perfect Use: 0.3% vs. 6%.
- Drug interactions: Aminoglutethimide may significantly depress MPA levels and reduce efficacy; contraceptive efficacy is not reduced with antiepileptic (phenobarbital and carbamazepine) use.

   Source: Kaunitz A. Injectable long-acting contraceptives. *Clin Obstet Gynecol.* 2001;44:82–84; Speroff L. Bone mineral density and hormonal contraception. *Dialogues in Contraception.* 2002;7:2–3.

VAGINAL CONTRACEPTIVE RING

Device
- NuvaRing (Organon)

Description
- Flexible, ethylene vinylacetate ring approximately 54 mm in diameter
- Releases 0.12 mg etonogestrel and 15 mcg EE daily

Mechanism of Action
- Similar to COCs

Use Issues
- Initial use: Can be inserted on any day of the week once pregnancy is ruled out.
- If >5 days since start of menstrual bleeding, or postpartum, or postabortion, backup contraceptive method is recommended for 7 days.
- Self-inserted ring is left in place for 3 weeks, then removed for 1 week.
- Menses is expected during the ring-free week.

Side Effects/Serious Adverse Effects
- Similar to COCs

Key Counseling Points
- Does not protect against lower genital tract STIs or HIV infection.
- Spotting or BTB may occur during the first 3 cycles of use.
- Physician needs to be aware if pregnancy is suspected or if any of the following occur: sudden severe headache, visual disturbances, numbness in an arm or leg, severe abdominal pain, prolonged episodes of bleeding, or amenorrhea.

Appropriate Action If Ring Is Removed
- >3 hours: Backup contraceptive method must be used until the ring has been used continuously for 7 days.

Additional Considerations
- Return of fertility: No delay
- One-year failure rate: Perfect Use: 0.3%, Typical Use: 9%
- Contraindications/precautions: Similar to COCs
- Drug interactions: Similar to COCs

PROGESTIN IMPLANT (NEXPLANON)
Fast Facts
- Nexplanon is an implantable single, nonbiodegradable, subdermal rod containing 68 mg etonorgestrel.
  - The release rate decreases with time from approximately 60–70 µg/day in weeks 5–6 to approximately 25–30 µg/day at the end of the third year.
- Nexplanon is approved for up to 3 years of use.
- Each implant Nexplanon and Implanon are very similar but barium sulphate has been added to Nexplanon to enable detection by X-ray and the applicator has also been modified to reduce the risk of deep insertion and to facilitate one-handed insertion.
- Nexplanon may improve dysmenorrhea.
- There is little or no increased risk of thromboembolic phenomenon with Nexplanon.
- Nexplanon does not have an adverse impact on bone mineral density.

Mechanism of Action
- Prevents ovulation by inhibiting luteinizing hormone surge; thickens cervical mucus to block sperm entry into the upper reproductive tract; causes endometrial changes that may prevent implantation (rare).

Irregular Bleeding
- Fewer than 25% of women using Nexplanon will have regular bleeds.
- Infrequent bleeding is the most common pattern (approximately one-third).
- 20% of women experience amenorrhea.
- 25% of women have prolonged or frequent bleeding.

Other Issues
- Nexplanon does not offer protection against viral STIs.
- A woman with an impalpable implant should be advised to use additional precautions or avoid intercourse until the presence of an implant is confirmed.
- Combined oral contraceptive pills (cyclically or continuously for 3 months) may be helpful in cases of irregular bleeding.
- The progestogen-only implant is not known to be harmful in pregnancy, but women with a continuing pregnancy should be advised to have the implant removed. Women may retain the implant if they wish to continue the method after a noncontinuing pregnancy.

Table 5.8. Timing of initiation of Nexplanon

Situation	Starting Implant	Requirements for Additional Contraception
Women having menstrual cycles	Day 1–5 of menstrual cycle	Not required
	Any other time; consider pregnancy	7 days
Women who are amenorrhoeic	At any time if it is reasonably certain she is not pregnant	7 days
Postpartum (includes any delivery from 24 weeks' gestation)	On or before Day 21 postpartum[a]	Not required
	After Day 21 postpartum	7 days (unless menstruation recommended and Days 1–5)
Post first- or second-trimester abortion	Up to and including Day 6 postabortion[b]	Not required
	At any other time if it is reasonably certain she is not pregnant or at risk of pregnancy	7 days
Following emergency oral contraception	Implant insertion should be delayed for 5 days	7 days after levonorgestrel, 7 days after ulipristal acetate
Other situations in which pregnancy cannot be excluded	Consider quick starting implant or bridging method[c]	7 days

[a]The Summary of Product Characteristics advises insertion between Days 21 and 28. Ovulations have been noted around Day 30. FSRH advises Day 21 for postpartum contraceptive starting in line with the World Health Organization as highly unlikely women will have ovulated by Day 21 and to ensure contraceptive effect is established before ovulation.

[b]The Clinical Effectiveness Unit advises that women ideally start on the day or day after a first- or second-trimester abortion.

[c]A pregnancy test is advised no sooner that 3 weeks after unprotected sexual intercourse.

Source: Reproduced with permission from the Clinical Effectiveness Unit of the UK Faculty of Sexual & Reproductive Healthcare. Faculty of Sexual and Reproductive Healthcare. Clinical Guidance. *Combined Hormonal Contraception.* Copyright © Faculty of Sexual and Reproductive Healthcare 2012.

EMERGENCY POSTCOITAL ORAL CONTRACEPTION

Fast Facts
- Safety confirmed in several large multicenter trials.
- Appropriate candidate is reproductive-age women within 72 hours of unprotected coitus.
- Often associated with failure of barrier contraception.
- Treatment reduces pregnancy rate by 75% (range 55%–94%) based on published studies.
- Effective pregnancy rate ~2%.
- Other option: midcycle IUD placement; failure rate 0.1%.
- 98% of patients will menstruate by 21 days after treatment (mean 7–9 days).

Table 5.9. Options for emergency contraception

Regimen	Formulation	Timing of Use After Unprotected Sexual Intercourse*	Access	FDA Labeled for Use as Emergency Contraception
Selective progesterone receptor modulator	1 tablet, containing 30 mg of ulipristal acetate	Up to 5 days	Requires a prescription	Yes
Progestin only	1 tablet, containing 1.5 mg of levonorgestrel	Up to 3 days	Available over the counter without age restriction	Yes
	2 tablets, each containing 0.75 mg of levonorgestrel	Up to 3 days	Available over the counter to those 17 years and older with photo identification	Yes
Combined progestin–estrogen pills	A variety of formulations can be used[†]	Up to 5 days	Requires a prescription	No[‡]
Copper IUD[§]	N/A	Up to 5 days	Requires office visit and insertion by a clinician	No[‡]

FDA, Food and Drug Administration; IUD, intrauterine device; N/A, not applicable.

*Emergency contraception is best used as soon as possible after unprotected sex.

[†]A variety of formulations of combined oral contraceptives can be used for emergency contraception. For a list of appropriate formulations, see http://ec.princeton.edu/questions/dose.html#dose.

[‡]Although these methods are not FDA labeled for use as emergency contraception, they have been found to be safe and effective when used for emergency contraception and can be used off-label for this indication.

[§]The copper IUD is the most effective method of emergency contraception.

Source: Reprinted with permission from ACOG Practice Bulletin No. 152: Emergency contraception. *Obstet Gynecol.* 2015 Sep;126(3):e1-e11. Copyright © 2015 The American College of Obstetricians and Gynecologists.

Table 5.10. Oral contraceptives that can be used for emergency contraception in the United States

Brand	Company	First Dose[b]	Second Dose[b] (12 Hours Later)	Ulipristal Acetate Per Dose (mg)	Ethinyl Estradiol Per Dose (mcg)	Levonorgestrel Per Dose (mg)[c]
Ulipristal acetate (dedicated EC pills)						
ella	Afaxys	1 white pill	None	30	-	-
Progestin-only (dedicated EC pills)						
Aftera[c]	Teva	1 white pill	None	-	-	1.5
AfterPill[d]	Syzygy	1 white pill	None	-	-	1.5
EContra Ez[e]	Afaxys	1 white pill	None	-	-	1.5
Levonorgestrel Tablets	Perrigo	2 white pills	None[b]	-	-	1.5
My Way	Gavis	1 white pill	None	-	-	1.5
Next Choice One Dose	Actavis	1 peach pill	None	-	-	1.5
Plan B One-Step	Teva	1 white pill	None	-	-	1.5
Take Action	Teva	1 white pill	None	-	-	1.5
Combined progestin and estrogen pills (regular oral contraceptive pills)						
Altavera	Sandoz	4 peach pills	4 peach pills	-	120	0.60
Amethia	Watson	4 white pills	4 white pills	-	120	0.60
Amethia Lo	Watson	5 white pills	5 white pills	-	100	0.50
Amethyst	Watson	6 white pills	6 white pills	-	120	0.54
Aviane	Teva	5 orange pills	5 orange pills	-	100	0.50
Camrese	Teva	4 light blue-green pills	4 light blue-green pills	-	120	0.60
CamreseLo	Teva	5 orange pills	5 orange pills	-	100	0.50
Cryselle[f]	Teva	4 white pills	4 white pills	-	120	0.60
Enpresse	Teva	4 orange pills	4 orange pills	-	120	0.60
Introvale	Sandoz	4 peach pills	4 peach pills	-	120	0.60
Jolessa	Teva	4 pink pills	4 pink pills	-	120	0.60
Lessina	Teva	5 pink pills	5 pink pills	-	100	0.50
Levora	Watson	4 white pills	4 white pills	-	120	0.60
Lo/Ovral[f]	Akrimax	4 white pills	4 white pills	-	120	0.60
LoSeasonique	Teva	5 orange pills	5 orange pills	-	100	0.50
Low-Ogestrel[f]	Watson	4 white pills	4 white pills	-	120	0.60
Lutera	Watson	5 white pills	5 white pills	-	100	0.50
Lybrel	Wyeth	6 yellow pills	6 yellow pills	-	120	0.54
Nordette	Teva	4 light-orange pills	4 light-orange pills	-	120	0.60
Ogestrel[f]	Watson	2 white pills	2 white pills	-	100	0.50
Portia	Teva	4 pink pills	4 pink pills	-	120	0.60
Quasense	Watson	4 white pills	4 white pills	-	120	0.60
Seasonale	Teva	4 pink pills	4 pink pills	-	120	0.60

(continued)

Brand	Company	First Dose[b]	Second Dose[b] (12 Hours Later)	Ulipristal Acetate Per Dose (mg)	Ethinyl Estradiol Per Dose (mcg)	Levonorgestrel Per Dose (mg)[c]
Seasonique	Teva	4 light-blue-green pills	4 light-blue-green pills	-	120	0.60
Sronyx	Watson	5 white pills	5 white pills	-	100	0.50
Trivora	Watson	4 pink pills	4 pink pills	-	120	0.50

Source: Reprinted with permission from website of the Office of Population Research, Princeton University. http://ec.princeton.edu/questions/dose.html#dose. Accessed on February 10, 2016.

INTRAUTERINE DEVICE
Fast Facts
- Most widely used reversible contraceptive in the world.
- <1% of U.S. couples use this excellent method of contraception.
- Two IUD choices now available in the United States: copper IUD, levonorgestrel IUS (20 micrograms levonorgestrel released per day).

Contraindications
- PID currently or within the past 3 months
- History of recurrent PID
- Postabortion or postpartum endometritis or septic abortion within the past 3 months
- Known or suspected untreated endocervical gonorrhea, chlamydia, or mucopurulent cervicitis
- Undiagnosed abnormal vaginal bleeding
- Pregnancy or suspicion of pregnancy
- Severely distorted uterine cavity
- Suspected or known uterine perforation occurring with placement of a uterine sound during the current insertion procedure
- History of symptomatic actinomycosis confirmed by culture, but not asymptomatic colonization
- Known cervical cancer that has yet to be treated
- Known endometrial cancer
- Known pelvic tuberculosis
- Acute liver disease or liver tumor (benign or malignant)
- Known or suspected breast cancer

Table 5.11. Five-year cumulative pregnancy rates and side effects leading to discontinuation of IUD

Side Effect	Levonorgestrel IUD	Copper IUD
Pregnancy	0.5%	5.9%
Bleeding problems	13.7%	20.9%
Amenorrhea	6.0%	0%
Hormonal side effects	12.1%	2.0%
Pelvic inflammatory disease	0.8%	2.2%

Source: Leonhardt KK. 2001 guide to contraceptive management. *Ob/Gyn Special Edition.* 2001;4:17-22. Reproduced with permission of McMahon Publishing Group.

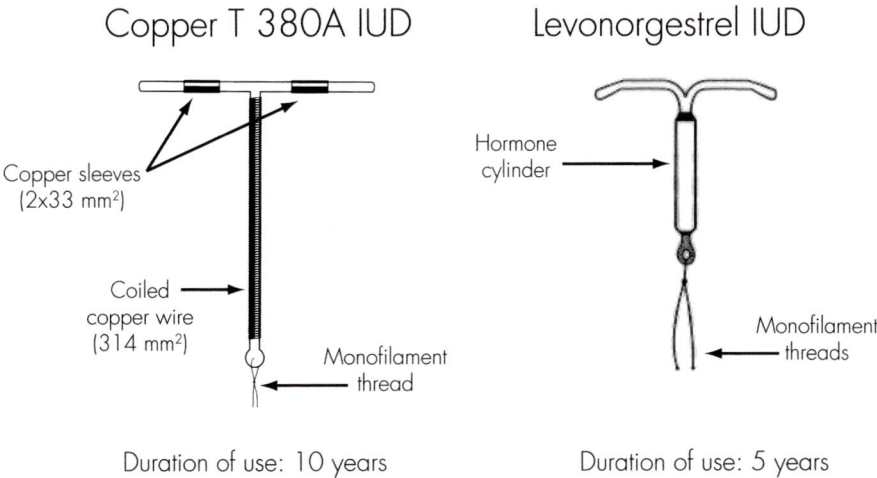

Figure 5.3. Available IUDs

Levonorgestrel Intrauterine System (Mirena/Skyla)
- Levonorgestrel, 52 mg (initial release rate of 20 mg/day); approved for up to 5 years of use.
- Effective treatment for heavy menstrual bleeding.
- Intrauterine systems (IUS) do not increase the risk of infertility, STI, or ectopic pregnancy.
- Women with no current STI and if not engaged in risky sexual behaviors are appropriate candidates for IUS, regardless of age, parity, or history of ectopic pregnancy.
- ~90% decreased menstrual blood loss by 1 year.
- Five-year pregnancy rate: 0.71/100 women; ectopic rate: 0.02/100 women years.
- Immediate insertion following first-trimester uterine aspiration resulted in higher rates of IUS use at 6 months without increased risk of complications (Bednarek 2011).
- A low-dose (13.5 mg) levonorgestrel-releasing intrauterine device (Skyla) became available in 2013. It is smaller in size than the Mirena and may be easier to insert in nulliparous.

CONTRACEPTION — Intrauterine Device

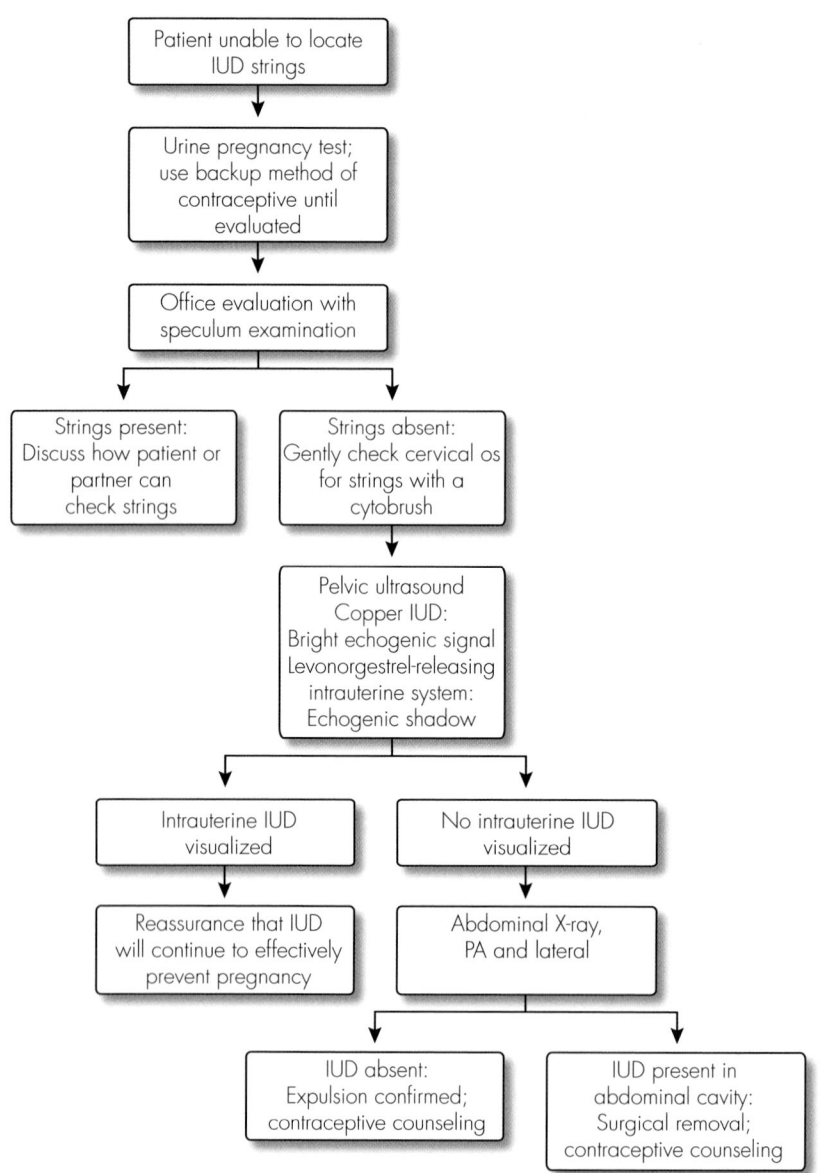

Figure 5.4. Algorithm for locating lost IUD strings
Source: Reproduced with permission from Blumenthal PD, Edelman A. Hormonal contraception. *Obstet Gynecol.* 2008 Sep;112(3):670-84. Copyright © 2008 The American College of Obstetricians and Gynecologists.

FEMALE STERILIZATION
Fast Facts
- Most frequent indication for laparoscopy in United States.
- Preoperative counseling is essential (including failure rate).
- Reversal of sterilization dependent on procedure performed.
    - Clips/bands have highest reversal success rates (>70%).
    - Incurs increased risk of ectopic pregnancy.

Laparoscopic Tubal Ligation
- Performed as an interval procedure.
- Must clearly identify fimbria/tube.
    - Falope rings applied to the round ligament do not prevent pregnancies.
- Perform prior to ovulation to prevent conception around the time of surgery.
- Most popular techniques.
    - Fulguration (with or without division), thermocautery, Falope rings, clips.

Postpartum Tubal Ligation
- Either at time of cesarean section or after vaginal delivery.
- Patient selection important.
    - No history of pelvic adhesions
    - No history of significant PID
    - Body habitus
- If patient is ambivalent, then defer to interval procedure.
- Empty bladder prior to performing procedure.
- Informed consent should always be documented.
- Be sure to follow up on path report to ensure the tubes were indeed excised.
- Uchida/Irving have lowest failure rates.

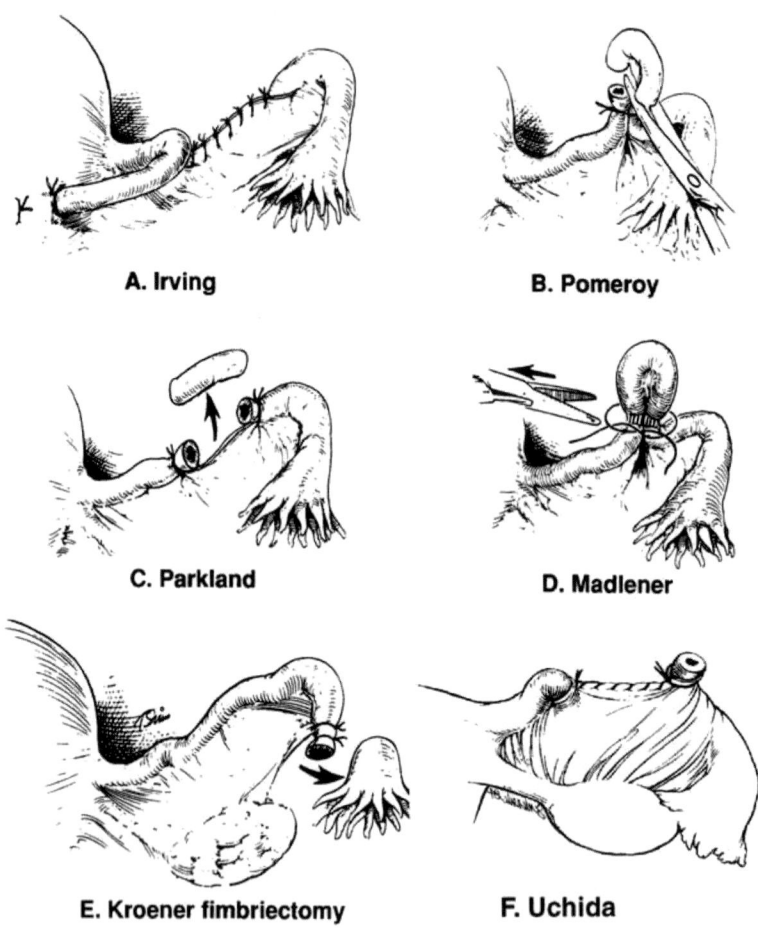

Figure 5.5. Types of tubal ligation
Source: Cunningham FG, MacDonald PC, Gant NF, et al. Family planning. In: *Williams Obstetrics.* 20th Ed. Stamford, CT. Appleton & Lange; 1997; and Depp R. Cesarean delivery and other surgical procedures. In: Gabbe SG, Niebyl JR, Simpson JL, ed. *Obstetrics: Normal and Problem Pregnancies, 2nd Ed.* New York: Churchill Livingstone; 1991. Reproduced with the permission of McGraw-Hill Education.

Hysteroscopic Sterilization (Essure Adiana Procedure)
- Hysteroscopic tubal occlusion represents an extremely effective sterilization technique.
- In the Essure procedure, a 4 mm by 1 mm polyester/nickel/titanium/steel microinsert is placed into the interstitial portion of each fallopian tube under hysteroscopic guidance.
  - Benign tissue ingrowth around the device results in complete tubal occlusion
- Adiana sterilization relies upon a combination of controlled thermal damage to the lining of the fallopian tube followed by insertion of a nonabsorbable biocompatible silicone elastomer matrix within the tubal lumen. Occlusion is achieved by fibroblast ingrowth into the matrix.
- Essure's bilateral placement rate is 94.6%. Adiana's bilateral placement rate is 94%; after a second procedure, 95% achieve bilateral placement.
- Both Essure and Adiana reduced procedural discomfort and increased patient satisfaction when compared with laparoscopic tubal ligation.
- Transcervical female sterilization has a very favorable cost profile.
- Adiana will be similarly or slightly less economically efficient than Essure given equipment cost.
- Both systems are well tolerated with low rates of adverse events.
- Effectiveness depends upon proper placement and confirmation of tubal occlusion:
  - Confirming proper device placement during the procedure
  - Confirming tubal occlusion at 90 days
  - Understanding the risk of pregnancy for women who do not follow-up
- Both procedures are usually done under local anesthesia and take 5–30 minutes.
- Both methods should result in minimal menstrual changes and no hormonal changes.

Table 5.12. Some characteristics of essure and adiana

	Essure	Adiana
Method	A microinsert comprising (1) an inner coil of stainless steel and polyethylene terephthalate fibers and (2) an outer coil of nickel titanium is placed in the interstitial portion of each fallopian tube by means of hysterectomy.	A delivery catheter is placed in the tubal ostium. The tip of the catheter contains an electrode array that can deliver thermal injury when activated. After the thermal event, a silicon implant is released into the tube.
Follow-up	Hysterosalpingography is used to assess successful tubal occlusion approximately 3 months after the procedure. Before successful occlusion is demonstrated, the patient should use another form of contraception.	
Additional equipment	None.	Requires a device-specific radiofrequency generator to induce thermal damage.

Source: Adapted from Palmer SN, Greenberg JA. Transcervical sterilization: a comparison of Essure permanent birth control system and Adiana permanent contraception system. *Rev Obstet Gynecol.* 2009 Spring;2(2):84-92.

Table 5.13. Pregnancy rates by sterilization methods

Method	5-year (Per 1,000 Procedures)	10-year (Per 1,000 Procedures)	Ectopic (Per 1,000 Procedures)
Postpartum partial salpingectomy	6.3	7.5	1.5
Bipolar coagulation*	16.5	24.8	17.1
Silicone band methods	10.0	17.7	7.3
Spring clip	31.7	36.5	8.5
Hysteroscopy (Essure)[†]	1.64	—	—
Vasectomy	11.3		No association

*Secondary analysis of 5-year failure rates with bipolar coagulation performed in different decades found that failure was significantly lower in later periods, reflecting improved technique with the method: 19.5 per 1,000 procedures for 1978–1982 versus 6.3 per 1,000 procedures for 1985–1987 (Peterson 1999).

[†]Food and Drug Administration recommended projections based on Bayesian statistical analysis (Baskinski 2010).

Data from Basinski CM. A review of clinical data for currently approved hysteroscopic sterilization procedures. *Rev Obstet Gynecol.* 2010;3:101–10; Jamieson DJ, Costello C, Trussell J, Hillis SD, Marchbanks PA, Peterson HB. The risk of pregnancy after vasectomy. US Collaborative Review of Sterilization Working Group (published erratum appears in *Obstet Gynecol.* 2004;104:200). *Obstet Gynecol.* 2004;103:848–50; Peterson HB, Xia Z, Hughes JM, Wilcox LS, Tylor LR, Trussell J. The risk of pregnancy after tubal sterilization: findings from the U.S. Collaborative Review of Sterilization. *Am J Obstet Gynecol.* 1996;174:1161–8, discussion 1168–70; Peterson HB, Xia Z, Hughes JM, Wilcox LS, Tylor LR, Trussell J. The risk of ectopic pregnancy after tubal sterilization. U.S. Collaborative Review of Sterilization Working Group. *N Engl J Med.* 1997;336:762–7; and Peterson HB, Xia Z, Wilcox LS, Tylor LR, Trussell J. Pregnancy after tubal sterilization with bipolar electrocoagulation. U.S. Collaborative Review of Sterilization Working Group. *Obstet Gynecol.* 1999;94:163–7.

Source: Reproduced with permission from American College of Obstetricians and Gynecologists. ACOG Practice bulletin No. 133: Benefits and risks of sterilization. *Obstet Gynecol.* 2013 Feb;121(2 Pt 1):392-404. Copyright © 2013 The American College of Obstetricians and Gynecologists.

CHAPTER 6
Gynecology

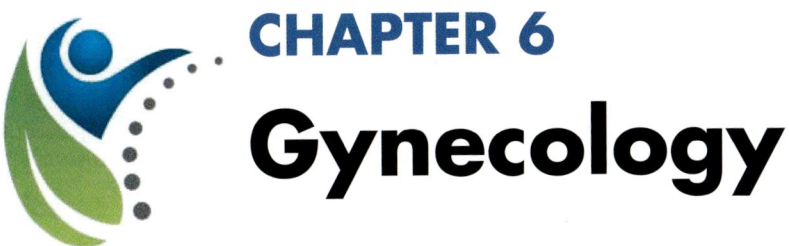

ABNORMAL UTERINE BLEEDING
Definition
- Abnormal menstrual volume, duration, regularity, or frequency

Table 6.1. Suggested "normal" limits for menstrual parameters in the midreproductive years

Clinical Dimensions of Menstruation and Menstrual Cycle	Descriptive Terms	Normal Limits (5th to 95th Percentiles)
Frequency of menses (d)	Frequent	<24
Normal		24–38
Infrequent		>38
Regularity of menses, cycle-to-cycle variation over 12 mo (d)	Absent	—
	Regular	Variation ± 2–20 days
	Irregular	Variation >20 days
Duration of flow (d)	Prolonged	>8.0
	Normal	4.5–8.0
	Shortened	<4.5
Volume of monthly blood loss (mL)	Heavy	>80
	Normal	5–80
	Light	<5

Source: Reproduced with permission from Fraser IS, Critchley HO, Munro MG, Broder M; Writing Group for this Menstrual Agreement Process. A process designed to lead to international agreement on terminologies and definitions used to describe abnormalities of menstrual bleeding. *Fertil Steril.* 2007 Mar;87(3):466-76. Copyright © 2007 The American Society for Reproductive Medicine.

Newer Terminology

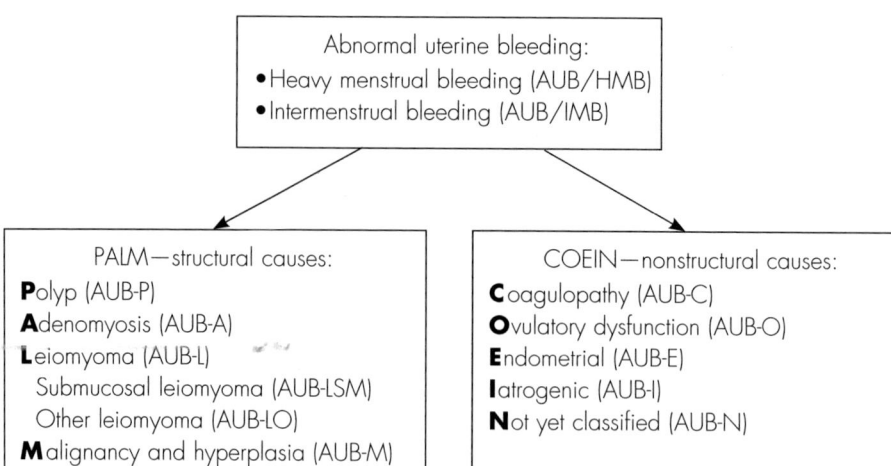

Figure 6.1. PALM-COEIN classification of abnormal uterine bleeding
Source: Reproduced with permission from Munro MG. *Abnormal Uterine Bleeding*. Cambridge: Cambridge University Press; Copyright © 2010.

Table 6.2. Systemic etiologies for abnormal uterine bleeding

Coagulation disorders
    von Willebrand's disease
    Thrombocytopenia
    Acute leukemia
    Advanced liver disease
Endocrinopathies
    Thyroid disease, hyperprolactinemia
    Polycystic ovary syndrome or elevated circulating androgens
    Cushing syndrome
Anovulation or oligoovulation
    Idiopathic
    Stress, exercise, obesity, rapid weight changes
    Polycystic ovary syndrome or endocrinopathies as above
Drugs
    Contraception: oral/transdermal/vaginal contraceptive, intrauterine device, medroxyprogesterone acetate (Depo-Provera)
    Anticoagulants
    Antipsychotics
    Chemotherapy
    Drugs related to dopamine metabolism: tricyclic antidepressants, phenothiazines, antipsychotic drugs
Trauma
    Sexual intercourse
    Sexual abuse
    Foreign bodies
    Pelvic trauma
Other
    Urinary system disorders: urethritis, cystitis, bladder cancer
    Inflammatory bowel disease, hemorrhoids

Table 6.3. Genital tract disorders leading to abnormal uterine bleeding

	Uterus	Cervix	Vagina	Vulva
Infection	Endometritis	Cervicitis	Bacterial vaginosis, STDs, atrophic vaginitis	STD
Benign	Polyps, endometrial hyperplasia, adenomyosis, leiomyo-mas	Polyps, ectropion, endometriosis	Gartner's duct cysts, polyps, adenomyosis	Skin tags, condylomata, angiokeratoma
Cancer	Adenocarcinoma, sarcoma	Invasive or metastatic cancer	Vaginal cancer	Vulvar cancer

STD, sexually transmitted disease.

Table 6.4. Causes of abnormal uterine bleeding by age group

- Neonates
    - Estrogen withdrawal
- Premenarchal
    - Foreign body
    - Adenomyosis
    - Trauma, abuse
    - Vulvovaginitis
    - Cancer (i.e., sarcoma botryoides)
    - Precocious puberty
- Early postmenarche
    - Anovulation: hypothalamic immaturity (>90% of cases)
    - Stress: exercise induced
    - Pregnancy
    - Infection
    - Coagulation disorder
- Reproductive age
    - Anovulation
    - Pregnancy
    - Endocrine disorder
    - Polyps/fibroids/adenomyosis
    - Medication related (oral contraceptives)
    - Infection
    - Sarcoma, ovarian
    - Coagulation disorder
- Perimenopausal
    - Anovulation leading to unopposed estrogen and hyperplasia
    - Polyp/fibroid/adenomyosis
    - Cancer
- Postmenopausal
    - Atrophy
    - Cancer/polyp
    - Estrogen therapy
    - Selective estrogen receptor modulators

Source: Reproduced with permission from APGO Educational Series on Women's Health. *Abnormal Uterine Bleeding.* Copyright © 2002.

Abnormal Uterine Bleeding — GYNECOLOGY

Initial Evaluation

History
- Timing: frequency, temporal pattern, last menstrual period
- Nature of bleeding: duration, postcoital, quantity, temporal pattern
- Associated symptoms: pain, fever, vaginal discharge, changes in bowel/bladder function
- Pertinent medical history, history of bleeding disorders (family history as well), and medication history
- Changes in weight, excessive exercise, chronic illness, stress

Physical Examination
- General: signs of systemic illness, ecchymosis, thyromegaly, evidence of hyperandrogenism (hirsutism, acne, male pattern balding), acanthosis nigricans
- Pelvic: determine site of bleeding; assess contour, size, and tenderness of the uterus; any suspicious lesions or tumors

Laboratory Testing
- Urine pregnancy test to rule out pregnancy-related bleeding
  - Serum β-human chorionic gonadotropin (β-hCG) if there has been a recent pregnancy (rule out trophoblastic disease)
- Pap smear
- Complete blood count (CBC) and platelets
- Thyroid-stimulating hormone to exclude hypothyroidism
- Liver function tests in those with chronic liver or renal disease
- Determine ovulatory status
- Menstrual cycle charting: >10 days of variance from one cycle to the next suggests anovulatory cycles.
- Normal menstrual cycle length: 24–35 days
- Luteinizing hormone (LH) urine predictor kit: False positives include premature ovarian failure, menopause, and polycystic ovary syndrome (on occasion)
- Screening for disorders of hemostasis (see Table 6.5 below)

Table 6.5. Clinical screening for an underlying disorder of hemostasis in the patient with excessive bleeding

Initial screening for an underlying disorder of hemostasis in patients with excessive menstrual bleeding should be structured by medical history (positive screen comprises any of the following):*

1. **Heavy Menstrual bleeding since menarche**
2. **One of the following:**
    Postpartum hemorrhage
    Surgery-related bleeding
    Bleeding associated with dental work
3. **Two or more of the following symptoms:**
    Bruising one to two times per month
    Epistaxis one to two times per month
    Frequent gum bleeding
    Family history of bleeding symptoms

*Patients with a positive screen should be considered for further evaluation, including consultation with a hematologist and testing of von Willebrand factor and ristocetin cofactor.

Source: Reproduced with permission from Management of acute abnormal uterine bleeding in nonpregnant reproductive-aged women. Committee Opinion No. 557. American College of Obstetricians and Gynecologists. *Obstet Gynecol.* 121:891-96, 2013. Copyright © 2013 The American College of Obstetricians and Gynecologists.

Endometrial Biopsy

- Consider performing in all women >35 years of age with abnormal uterine bleeding
- Consider in women with a history of unopposed estrogen exposure and abnormal uterine bleeding
- Consider in women with risk factors for endometrial hyperplasia:
    - Obesity, chronic anovulation, history of breast cancer, selective estrogen receptor modulator (tamoxifen) use
    - Family history of endometrial, ovarian, breast, or colon cancer (Farquhar 1999)

Table 6.6. Summary of initial evaluation of the patient with abnormal uterine bleeding

History and physical
Pregnancy tests: exclude pregnancy or trophoblastic disease
Pap smear
CBC/PLTs
TSH
LFTs (those with chronic liver or renal disease)
PT/PTT, factor VIII, von Willebrand's factor antigen (if suspicious history)
Ovulatory status
Menstrual charting
Luteal phase length (24–35 days)
LH urine predictor kits
Endometrial biopsy
Transvaginal ultrasound (possible sonohysterogram or hysteroscopy)

CBC, complete blood count; LFT, liver function tests; PLT, platelet; PT/PTT, prothrombin time and partial thromboplastin time; TSH, thyroid-stimulating hormone.

Secondary Evaluation
Transvaginal Ultrasound (TVS)
- Evaluates for structural lesions in the setting of abnormal pelvic examination or normal endometrial biopsy.
- Can demonstrate a thickened endometrial lining; cannot reliably distinguish between submucous fibroids, polyps, adenomyosis, and neoplastic change.
- Utility of TVS in excluding endometrial abnormalities is more reliable in postmenopausal women.
- In premenopausal women, TVS should be performed on cycle days 4–6; if returns with an endometrial stripe >5 mm → obtain sonohysterogram.
  - In 200 premenopausal women with AUB, 16 of 80 women (20%!) with an endometrial stripe <5 mm had an endometrial polyp or submucosal fibroid seen on sonohysterogram (Breitkopf 2004).

Sonohysterography
- Allows for careful evaluation of cavity by infusing sterile saline into the endometrial cavity and monitoring by TVS.
- Can better detect smaller lesions such as polyps or small submucosal fibroids.
- Advantage: higher sensitivity in detecting polyps than TVS alone (94% vs. 75%, respectively; Kamel 2000).
- Disadvantage: no tissue for histologic diagnosis.

Hysteroscopy
- Direct visualization of the endometrial cavity.
- Considered the gold standard for the diagnosis of abnormal uterine bleeding.
- Can biopsy or excise lesions identified.

Treatment
Acute Heavy Abnormal Uterine Bleeding
- Stabilize the hemodynamically compromised patient.
- IV access, fluids, blood products as needed.
- Management depends upon the cause of AUB.
- If AUB is the result of break-through bleeding on OCPs or other progestin form of contraception, then treatment will require estrogen if ultrasound confirms a thin endometrium.
- If AUB is the result of chronic anovulation in PCOS or obese patient with a thickened endometrium, then treatment will require progestins or D&C.

Table 6.7. Medical options to treat acute abnormal uterine bleeding

Drug	Source	Suggested Dose	Dose Schedule	Potential Contraindications and Precautions According to FDA Labeling*
Conjugated equine estrogen	DeVore GR, Owens O, Kane N. Use of intravenous Premarin in the treatment of dysfunctional uterine bleeding—a double-blind randomized control study. *Obstet Gynecol.* 1982;59:285–91.	25 mg IV	Every 4–6 hours for 24 hours	Contraindications include, but are not limited to, breast cancer, active or past venous thrombosis or arterial thromboembolic disease, and liver dysfunction or disease. The agent should be used with caution in patients with cardiovascular or thromboembolic risk factors.
Combined oral contraceptives[1]	Munro MG, Mainor N, Basu R, Brisinger M, Barreda L. Oral medroxyprogesterone acetate and combined oral contraceptives for acute uterine bleeding: a randomized controlled trial. *Obstet Gynecol.* 2006;108:924–9.	Monophasic combined oral contraceptive that contains 35 micrograms of ethinyl estradiol	Three times per day for 7 days	Contraindications include, but are not limited to, cigarette smoking (in women aged 35 years or older), hypertension, history of deep vein thrombosis or pulmonary embolism, known thromboembolic disorders, cerebrovascular disease, ischemic heart disease, migraine with aura, current or past breast cancer, severe liver disease, diabetes with vascular involvement, valvular heart disease with complications, and major surgery with prolonged immobilization.
Medroxyprogesterone acetate[2]	Munro MG, Mainor N, Basu R, Brisinger M, Barreda L. Oral medroxyprogesterone acetate and combination oral contraceptives for acute uterine bleeding: a randomized controlled trial. *Obstet Gynecol.* 2006;108:924–9.	20 mg orally	Three times per day for 7 days	Contraindications include, but are not limited to, active or past deep vein thrombosis or pulmonary embolism, active or recent arterial thromboembolic disease, current or past breast cancer, and impaired liver function or liver disease.
Tranexamic acid	James AH, Kouides PA, Abdul-Kadir R, Dietrich JE, Edlund M, Federici AB, et al. Evaluation and management of acute menorrhagia in women with and without underlying bleeding disorders: consensus from an international expert panel. *Eur J Obstet Gynecol Reprod Biol.* 2011;158:124–34.	1.3 g orally[3] or 10 mg/kg IV (maximum 600 mg/dose)	Three times per day for 5 days (every 8 hours)	Contraindications include, but are not limited to, acquired impaired color vision and current thrombotic or thromboembolic disease. The agent should be used with caution in patients with a history of thrombosis (because of uncertain thrombotic risks), and concomitant administration of combine oral contraceptives needs to be carefully considered.

FDA indicates Food and Drug Administration; IV, intravenously.

*The US Food and Drug Administration's labeling contains exhaustive lists of contraindications for each of these therapies. In treating women with acute abnormal uterine bleeding, physicians often must weigh the relative risks of treatment against the risk of continued bleeding in the context of the patient's medical history and risk factors.

[1]Other combined oral contraceptive formulations, dosages, and schedules may also be effective.

[2]Other progestins (such as norethindrone acetate), dosages, and schedules may also be effective.

[3]Other dosages and schedules may also be effective.

Source: Reproduced with permission from American College of Obstetricians and Gynecologists. Committee Opinion No. 557: Management of acute abnormal uterine bleeding in nonpregnant reproductive-aged women. *Obstet Gynecol.* 2013;121:891-96. Copyright © 2013 The American College of Obstetricians and Gynecologists.

Abnormal Uterine Bleeding   GYNECOLOGY

Chronic Heavy Abnormal Uterine Bleeding

Table 6.8. Medical options to treat abnormal uterine bleeding

	↓ Blood Flow (%)	Comments
Oral contraceptives	50	Continuous or cyclic[a]
Levonorgestrel intrauterine device	80–90	May induce amenorrhea
Nonsteroidal antiinflammatory drugs	20–50	Effective in ovulatory women
Cyclic progestin	—	Particularly in anovulatory bleeding
Antifibrinolytics (tranexamic acid, 650 mg, 2 tablets PO t.i.d. during menses, maximum × 5 days	50	Side effects: nausea, leg cramps, potential deep venous thrombosis risk
Gonadotropin-releasing hormone agonists and antagonists	—	Hypoestrogenemia side effects: hot flashes, osteopenia; limit use to 6 months

[a]May need an oral contraceptive with a more estrogenic progestin, such as ethynodiol diacetate; if the endometrium is thick on oral contraceptives, then a higher dose of progestin (1 mg norethindrone) may be necessary. Could use such an oral contraceptive 3 times a day for a week followed by one pill for the next 3 weeks.

Failed Medical Therapy or Known Surgical Indication

- Hysteroscopy/dilatation and curettage.
- Endometrial ablation.
- Approximately 20% of patients require further surgery, with 10% needing hysterectomy.
- Hysterectomy: definitive surgery.

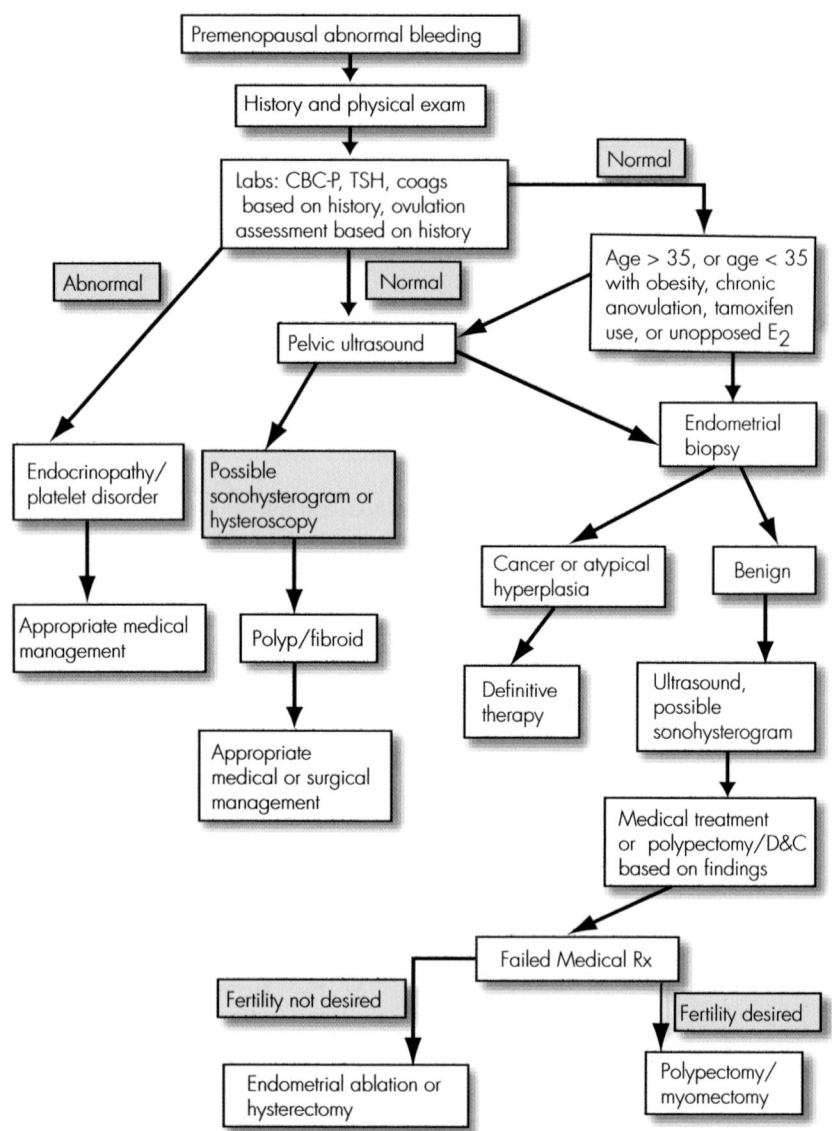

Figure 6.2. Evaluation of premenopausal abnormal bleeding
CBC-P, complete blood count/platelets; coags, coagulation disorders; D&C, dilatation and curettage; E2, estradiol; Rx, treatment; TSH, thyroid-stimulating hormone.

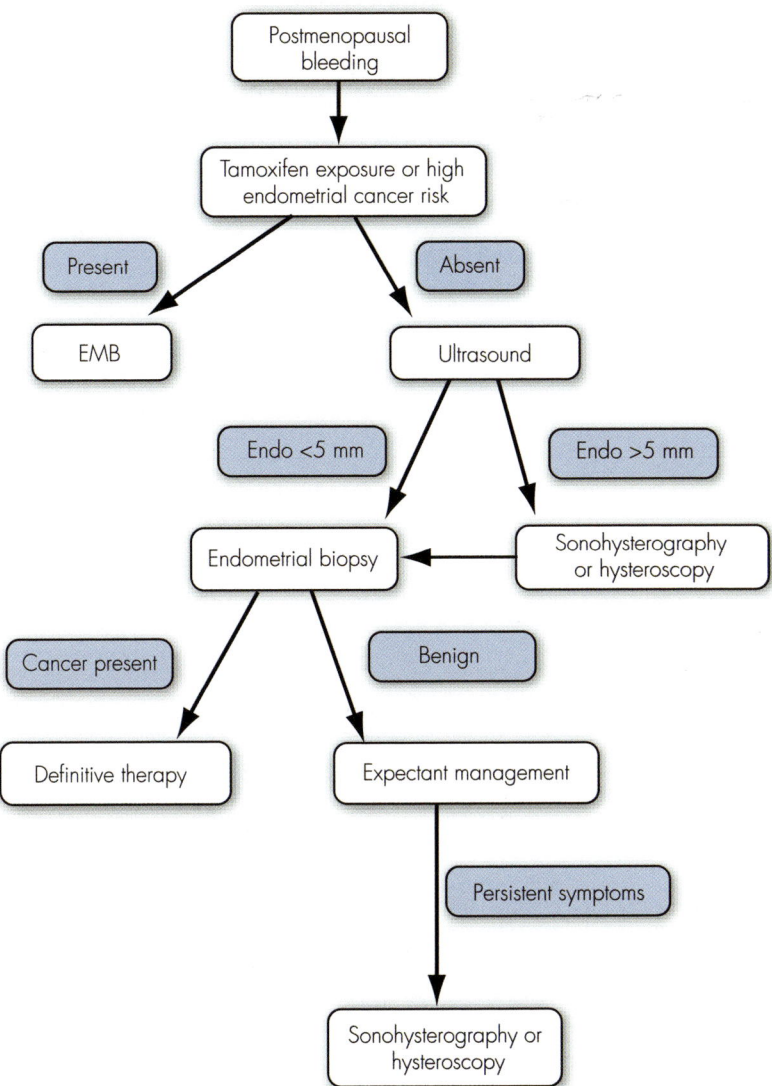

Figure 6.3. Evaluation of postmenopausal abnormal bleeding
EMB, endometrial biopsy; Endo, endometrium.

ENDOMETRIAL ABLATION

Table 6.9. Outcomes of endometrial ablation

Device	Global Endometrial Ablation/Rollerball Ablation (%)		
	Satisfaction Rate	Amenorrhea Rate*	Diary Success (Score: 75 or Less)
ThermaChoice (thermal balloon)	96/99[†]	13.9/24.4	80.2/84.3
Hydro ThermAblator (circulated hot fluid)	— [‡]	35.3/47.1	68.4/76.4
Her Option (cryotherapy)	86/88[§]	22.2/46.5	67.4/73.3
NovaSure (RF electrosurgery)	92/93[†]	36.0/32.2	77.7/74.4
MEA (microwave energy)	99/99[†]	55.3/45.8	87.0/83.2

RF, radiofrequency; MEA, Microsulis Endometrial Ablation.
*Based on intent to treat.
[†]Patients reported being satisfied or very satisfied.
[‡]Quality-of-life scores compared with baseline only.
[§]Patients reported being very or extremely satisfied.
Source: Reproduced with permission from Sharp HT. Assessment of new technology in the treatment of idiopathic menorrhagia and uterine leiomyomata. *Obstet Gynecol.* 2006 Oct;108(4):990-1003. Copyright © 2006 The American College of Obstetricians and Gynecologists.

Table 6.10. Contraindications to global endometrial ablation

Pregnancy or desire to be pregnant in the future
Known or suspected endometrial carcinoma
Premalignant change of the endometrium[a]
Active pelvic inflammatory disease or hydrosalpinx[a]
Prior classic cesarean delivery or transmural myomectomy
Uterine anomaly (e.g., septate uterus, bicornuate uterus, or unicornuate uterus)
Intrauterine device in place
Active urinary tract infection at the time of treatment[a]

[a]Relative contraindications.

Table 6.11. Recommended preoperative checklist for global endometrial ablation

Document failure, refusal, or intolerance to medical management.
Confirm that patient does not desire future pregnancy.
Establish a plan for contraception.
Exclude endometrial hyperplasia or malignancy with a tissue sample.
Perform adequate endometrial imaging to exclude a lesion that would preclude the use of global endometrial ablation.
Exclude pregnancy.

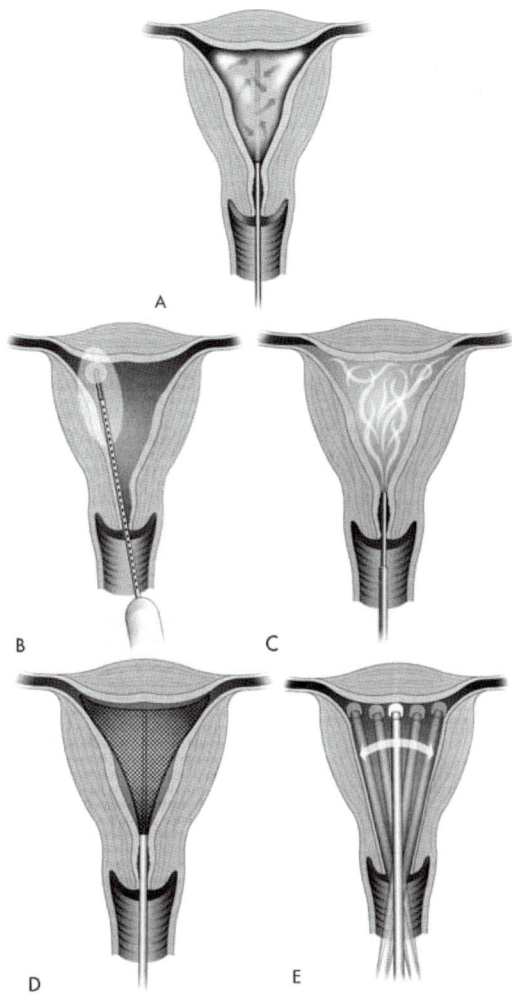

Figure 6.4. Options for global endometrial ablation
(A) ThermaChoice uterine balloon therapy. Heated fluid circulates within the ThermaChoice uterine balloon.
(B) Her Option cryoablation. A cryoprobe is placed within the uterine cavity near the cornu, resulting in ice ball formation. **(C)** Hydro Thermablation. A hysteroscope and the hydrothermablation sheath are inserted into the uterine cavity to allow heated fluid to circulate within the uterine cavity. **(D)** NovaSure radiofrequency ablation. The electrode fans out to fit within the uterine cavity. **(E)** Microwave Endometrial Ablation. The Microsulis Endometrial Ablation wand is inserted into the uterine fundus and moved back and forth while it is being withdrawn.

Source: Reproduced with permission from Sharp HT. Assessment of new technology in the treatment of idiopathic menorrhagia and uterine leiomyomata. *Obstet Gynecol.* 2006 Oct;108(4):990-1003. Copyright © 2006 The American College of Obstetricians and Gynecologists. Illustrations: John Yanson.

ECTOPIC PREGNANCY
Fast Facts
- Ectopic pregnancies represent 9% of all maternal deaths.
- Prior pelvic inflammatory disease, especially related to *C. trachomatis*, is the major risk factor.

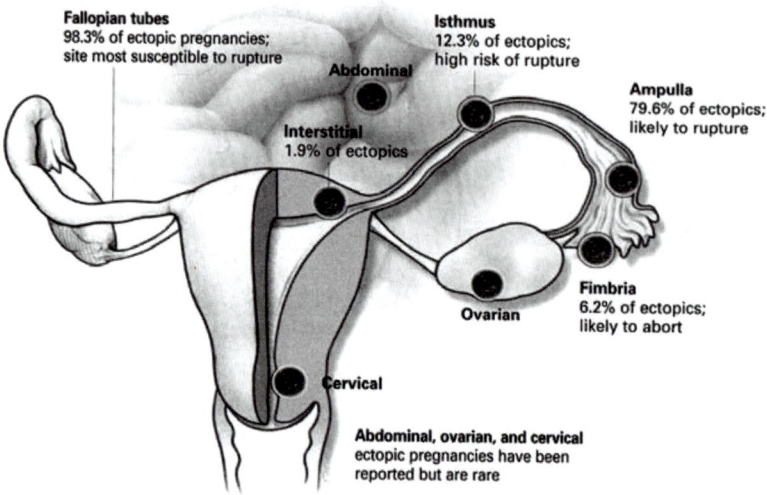

Figure 6.5. Locations of ectopic pregnancy
Source: Reprinted with permission from Buster JE, Barnhart K. Ectopic pregnancy: a 5-step plan for medical management. *OBG Management*. 2004;74-86. Copyright © Frontline Medical Communications. All rights reserved. Artist: Scott Bodell.

Diagnosis
- Serum β-hCG positive 8–9 days after ovulation, produced from cytotrophoblasts.
- β-hCG rises >53% in 48 hours with normal intrauterine pregnancy.
- Rule of 10s for normal pregnancies:
  - β-hCG = 100 mIU/mL at time of missed menses
  - β-hCG = 100,000 mIU/mL at 10 weeks (peak)
  - β-hCG = 10,000 mIU/mL at term
- β-hCG elimination half-life = approximately 1 day.
- 90% of ectopics have β-hCG <6500 mIU/mL.

Table 6.12. Useful ultrasonographic findings in the evaluation of women at risk for an ectopic pregnancy

Pregnancy and Gestational Age	Ultrasonographic Findings	Comments
Normal intrauterine pregnancy		
Gestational age, 4 to <5 wk from last menstrual period	Eccentrically placed small gestational sac, 0.2 to 0.5 cm in diameter, may be visible within one layer of endometrium	
Gestational age, 5 wk from last menstrual period	Double decidua sign: two echogenic rings surrounded by intrauterine fluid collection	Needs to be differentiated from a pseudo-sac; sometimes associated with an ectopic pregnancy
Gestational age, 5.5 wk from last menstrual period	Yolk sac visualized within the gestational sac	Considered to be definitive confirmation of an intrauterine pregnancy
Gestational age, 6 wk from last menstrual period	An embryonic pole should be visualized	
Gestational age, 6.5 wk from last menstrual period	Fetal cardiac activity apparent	
Nonviable intrauterine pregnancy		
Anembryonic gestation	Gestational sac with a mean diameter of >2 cm, without evidence of a fetal pole	The gestational sac is often asymmetric
Embryonic or fetal death	Crown-rump length of >0.5 cm without fetal cardiac activity	
Ectopic (tubal) pregnancy		
Viable extrauterine pregnancy	Extrauterine gestational sac with fetal pole and cardiac activity	Presence of a yolk sac or fetal pole has positive predictive value of almost 100% for identifying ectopic pregnancy
Nonviable extrauterine gestation	Extrauterine gestational sac with a fetal pole, without cardiac activity	Fetal pole with or without cardiac activity seen in 13% of ectopic pregnancies diagnosed by ultrasonography
Ring sign	Adnexal mass with a hyperechoic ring around a gestational sac	Seen in 20% of ectopic pregnancies diagnosed by ultrasonography
Nonhomogeneous mass	Adnexal mass separate from the ovary	Seen in 60% of ectopic pregnancies diagnosed by ultrasonography; positive predictive value ranges from 80 to 90%

*Bipolar radiofrequency, microwave, circulating hot water, thermal balloon, cryotherapy.
¶Laser or roller ball ablation, wire loop resection.
□Difference between types of ablation is statistically significant

Source: Reproduced with permission from Barnhart KT. Clinical practice. Ectopic pregnancy. *N Engl J Med.* 2009 Jul 23;361(4):379-87. Copyright © 2009 Massachusetts Medical Society. Reproduced with permission of the Massachusetts Medical Society.

Table 6.13. Treatment outcomes for ectopic pregnancy

Method	Number of Studies	Number of Patients	Number with Successful Resolution
Conservative laparoscopic surgery	32	1626	1516 (93%)
Variable-dose methotrexate	12	338	314 (93%)
Single-dose methotrexate	7	393	340 (87%)
Direct-injection methotrexate	21	660	502 (76%)
Expectant management	14	628	425 (68%)

		Subsequent Fertility Rate	
Method	Tubal Patency Rate	Intrauterine Pregnancy	Ectopic
Conservative laparoscopic surgery	170/223 (76%)	366/647 (57%)	87/647 (13%)
Variable-dose methotrexate	136/182 (75%)	55/95 (58%)	7/95 (7%)
Single-dose methotrexate	61/75 (81%)	39/64 (61%)	5/64 (8%)
Direct-injection methotrexate	130/162 (80%)	87/152 (57%)	9/152 (6%)
Expectant management	60/79 (76%)	12/14 (86%)	1/14 (7%)

Source: Reproduced with permission from Pisarska MD, Carson SA, Buster JE. Ectopic pregnancy. *Lancet.* 1998;351:1115-20. Copyright © 1998 Elsevier.

Consider Total or Partial Salpingectomy in Situations Noted Below

- Childbearing complete
- Second ectopic in the same tube
- Uncontrolled bleeding
- Severely damaged tube
- Normal appearing contralateral tube
- Isthmic or interstitial ectopic
- Ectopic occurring after prior BTL
- All ectopic pregnancies

Methotrexate Therapy for Ectopic Pregnancy

- Reported success rates of 67–100% in selected patients.
- Average time to resolution (β-hCG <15 mIU/mL) for those successfully treated with MTX = approximately 35 days, although it can take up to 109 days (Lipscomb 1998).
- Longest interval between initial treatment and rupture = 42 days (Lipscomb 2000).
- Pretreatment β-hCG level is the only significant prognosticator of failure (Lipscomb 1999).
- Previous EP appears to be an independent risk factor for MTX failure (failure rate of 18.6% in those with a prior EP compared to a 6.8% failure rate for first-time EP; Lipscomb 2004).
- If the initial β-hCG <1000 mIU/mL, 88% resolve without MTX (this is equivalent to MTX efficiency; Trio 1995).

Ectopic Pregnancy GYNECOLOGY

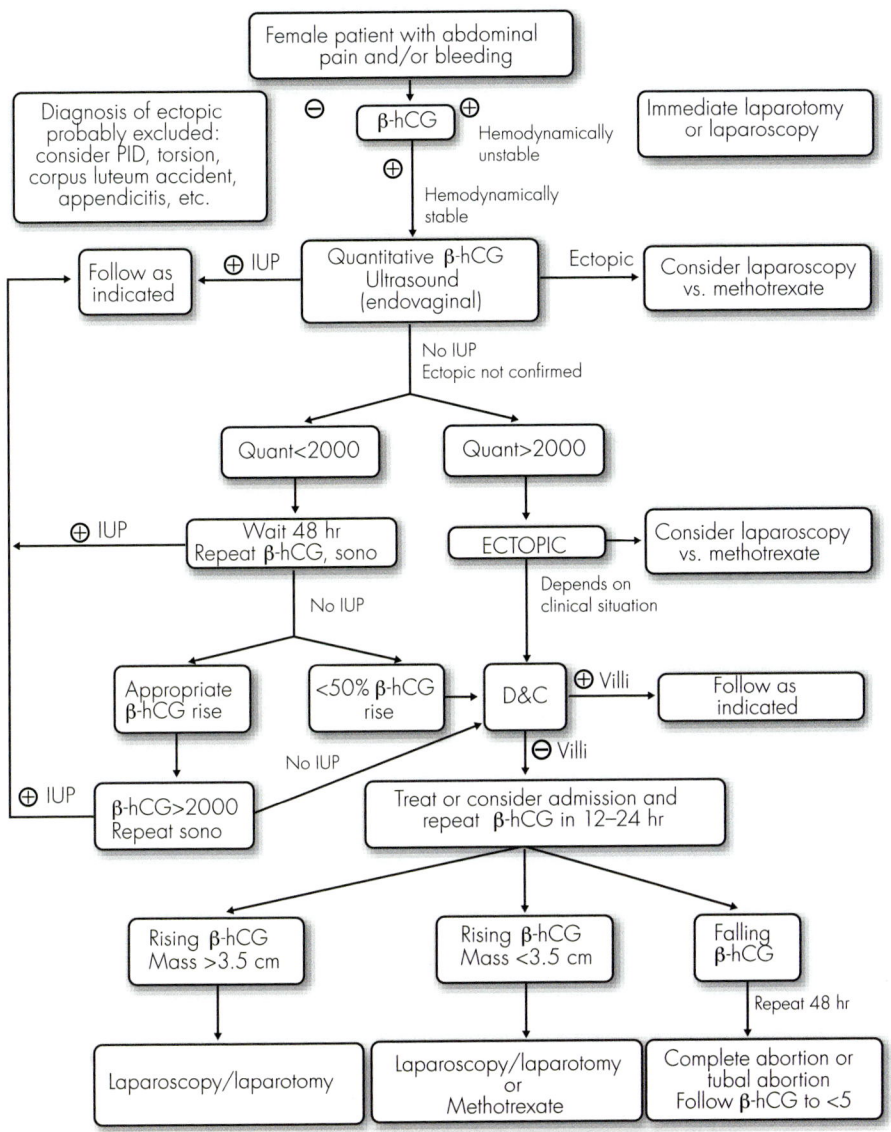

Figure 6.6. Algorithm for the management of ectopic pregnancy
Source: Adapted from Carson SA, Buster JE. Ectopic pregnancy. *N Engl J Med.* 1993; 329(16):1174-81; and Stovall TG, Ling FW. Ectopic pregnancy. Diagnostic and therapeutic algorithms minimizing surgical intervention. *J Reprod Med.* 1993;38(10):807-812.

Table 6.14. Contraindications to MTX therapy of ectopic pregnancy

Contraindication	ACOG	ASRM
Absolute contraindications	Breastfeeding; laboratory evidence of immunodeficiency; preexisting blood dyscrasias (bone marrow hypoplasia, leukopenia, thrombocytopenia, or clinically significant anemia); known sensitivity to methotrexate; active pulmonary disease; peptic ulcer disease; hepatic, renal, or hematologic dysfunction; alcoholism; alcoholic or other chronic liver disease	Breastfeeding; evidence of immunodeficiency; moderate-to-severe anemia, leukopenia, or thrombocytopenia; sensitivity to methotrexate; active pulmonary or peptic ulcer disease; clinically important hepatic or renal dysfunction; intrauterine pregnancy
Relative contraindications	Ectopic mass >3.5 cm; embryonic cardiac motion	Ectopic mass >4 cm detected by transvaginal ultrasonography; embryonic cardiac activity detected by transvaginal ultrasonography; patient declines blood transfusion; patient is not able to participate in follow-up; high initial hCG level (>5000 mIU/mL)
Choice of regimen based on hCG level	Multidose regimen of methotrexate may be appropriate if presenting hCG value >5000 mIU/mL	Single-dose regimen of methotrexate better in patients with a low initial hCG level

Source: Reproduced with permission from Barnhart KT. Clinical practice. Ectopic pregnancy. *N Engl J Med.* 2009 Jul 23;361(4):379-87. Copyright © 2009 Massachusetts Medical Society. Reproduced with permission of the Massachusetts Medical Society.

Table 6.15. Single-dose MTX treatment protocol for ectopic pregnancy

Treatment Day	Laboratory Evaluation	Intervention
Pretreatment	hCG, CBC with differential, liver function tests, creatinine, blood type, and antibody screen	Rule out spontaneous abortion RHOgam if Rh negative
1	hCG	MTX 50 mg/m² IM
4	hCG	
7	hCG	MTX 50 mg/m² IM if β-hCG decreased <15% between days 4 and 7

CBC, complete blood count; MTX, methotrexate; IM, intramuscularly.

Source: Reproduced with permission from Practice Committee of the American Society for Reproductive Medicine. Medical treatment of ectopic pregnancy: a committee opinion. *Fertil Steril.* 2013;100:638-44. Copyright © 2013 The American Society for Reproductive Medicine.

Table 6.16. Two-dose MTX treatment protocol for ectopic pregnancy

Day 0: MTX, 50 mg/m^2 IM	β-hCG, ALT, Cr, CBC, type and screen	Rho(D) immune globulin (RhoGAM; 300 mcg IM) if Rh negative
Day 4: MTX, 50 mg/m^2 IM	β-hCG	
Day 7	β-hCG, ALT, Cr, CBC	If not ↓ by 15% from day 4, administer third and fourth doses of MTX, 50 mg/m^2 IM on day 7 and 11.
		If >15% decline from day 4, check hCG weekly until <5 mIU/mL
Day 11	β-hCG	If not ↓ by 15% from day 7, consider surgical treatment.
		If >15% decline from day 7, check hCG weekly until <5 mIU/mL

ALT, alanine aminotransferase; β-hCG, β-human chorionic gonadotropin; CBC, complete blood count; Cr, creatinine; MTX, methotrexate.

If follow-up hCG value plateau or rise, consider surgical intervention.

Source: Reproduced with permission from Barnhart K, Hummel AC, Sammel MD, Menon S, Jain J, Chakhtoura N. Use of "2-dose" regimen of methotrexate to treat ectopic pregnancy. *Fertil Steril.* 2007; 87:250-56. Copyright © 2007 The American Society for Reproductive Medicine.

Table 6.17. Multi-dose MTX treatment protocol for ectopic pregnancy

Treatment Day	Laboratory Evaluation	Intervention
Pretreatment	hCG, CBC with differential, liver function tests, creatinine, blood type, and antibody screen	Rule out spontaneous abortion
		RhoGAM if Rh negative
1	hCG	MTX 1.0 mg/kg IM
2		LEU 0.1 mg/kg IM
3	hCG	MTX 1.0 mg/kg IM if <15% decline day 1–day 3
		If >15%, stop treatment and start surveillance
4		LEU 0.1 mg/kg IM
5	hCG	MTX 1.0 mg/kg IM if <15% decline day 3–day 5
		If >15%, stop treatment and start surveillance
6		LEU 0.1 mg/kg IM
7	hCG	MTX 1.0 mg/kg IM if <15% decline day 5–day 7
		If >15%, stop treatment and start surveillance
8		LEU 0.1 mg/kg IM

CBC, complete blood count; MTX, methotrexate; IM, intramuscularly; LEU, leucovorin.

Note: Surveillance every 7 days (until hCG <5 mIU/mL). Screening laboratory studies should be repeated every week after the last dose of MTX.

Source: Reproduced with permission from Practice Committee of the American Society for Reproductive Medicine. Medical treatment of ectopic pregnancy: a committee opinion. *Fertil Steril.* 2013;100:638-44. Copyright © 2013 The American Society for Reproductive Medicine.

Table 6.18. Caveats for physicians and patients regarding the use of MTX

- Avoid intercourse until hCG is undetectable.
- Avoid pelvic examinations and ultrasound during surveillance of MTX therapy.
- Avoid sun exposure to limit risk of MTX dermatitis.
- Avoid foods and vitamins containing folic acid.
- Avoid gas-forming foods because they produce pain.
- Avoid new conception until hCG is undetectable.

MTX, methotrexate; *hCG*, human chorionic gonadotropin.

Source: Reproduced with permission from Practice Committee of the American Society for Reproductive Medicine. Medical treatment of ectopic pregnancy: a committee opinion. *Fertil Steril.* 2013;100:638-44. Copyright © 2013 The American Society for Reproductive Medicine.

Table 6.19. Predictors of failure of methotrexate treatment for ectopic pregnancy

- Adnexal fetal cardiac activity
- Size and volume of the gestational mass (>4 cm)
- High initial hCG concentration (>5,000 mIU/mL)
- Presence of free peritoneal blood
- Rapidly increasing hCG concentrations (>50%/48 hr) before MTX

Continued rapid rise in hCG concentrations during MTX.

Source: Reproduced with permission from Practice Committee of the American Society for Reproductive Medicine. Medical treatment of ectopic pregnancy: a committee opinion. *Fertil Steril.* 2013;100:638-44. Copyright © 2013 The American Society for Reproductive Medicine.

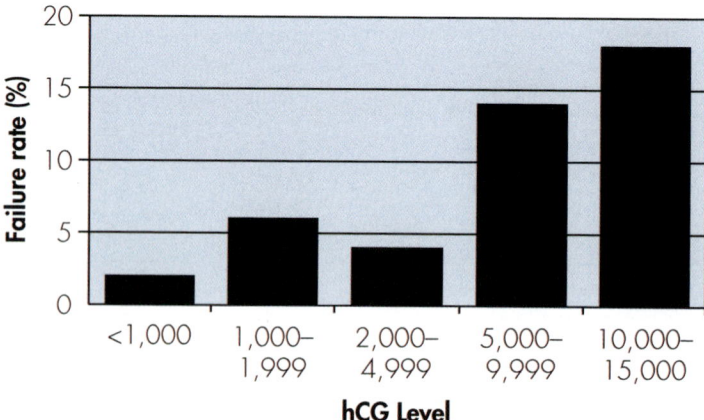

Figure 6.7. Single-dose MTX treatment failure based on β-hCG levels

Source: Reproduced with permission from Practice Committee of the American Society for Reproductive Medicine. Medical treatment of ectopic pregnancy: a committee opinion. *Fertil Steril.* 2013;100:638-44. Copyright © 2013 The American Society for Reproductive Medicine.

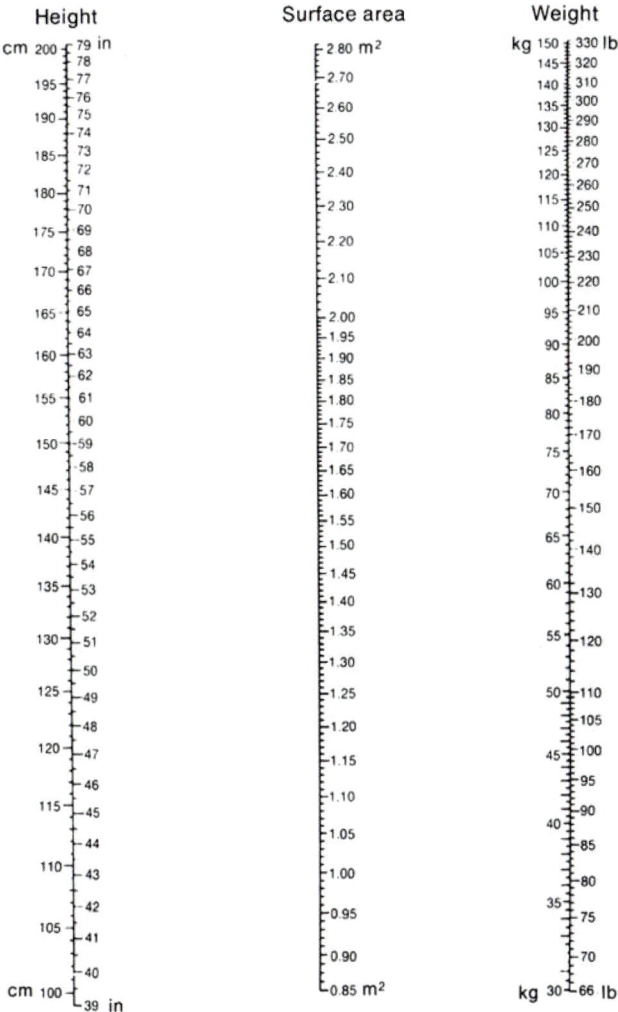

Figure 6.8. Body surface nomogram
Source: Chu CS, Rubin SC. Basic Principles of Chemotherapy. In *Clinical Gynecologic Oncology*, 8th Ed. DiSaia PJ and Creasman WT eds. Copyright © 2012. Elsevier. Philadelphia. Reproduced with permission of the publisher.

PREGNANCY OF UNKNOWN LOCATION
Fast Facts
- Pregnancy of unknown location (PUL) is a descriptive term used to classify a pregnancy when a TVS has shown no signs of either an intrauterine or extrauterine pregnancy or retained products of conception.
- PUL is not a diagnosis.
- PUL is a term used to classify a pregnancy until the final clinical outcome is known.
- Any woman classified as having a PUL needs follow-up to determine the final clinical outcome, which may be an ongoing viable IUP, a failed pregnancy, an EP, or, rarely, a persisting PUL.

Categorization System for Initial Ultrasound Findings:
- Definite EP: extrauterine gestational sac with yolk sac and/or embryo (with or without cardiac activity).
- PUL-probable EP: inhomogeneous adnexal mass or extrauterine sac-like structure.
- "True" PUL: no signs of either an intrauterine or extrauterine pregnancy on TVS.
- PUL-probable IUP: intrauterine gestational sac-like structure.
- Definite IUP: intrauterine gestational sac with yolk sac and/or embryo (with or without cardiac activity).

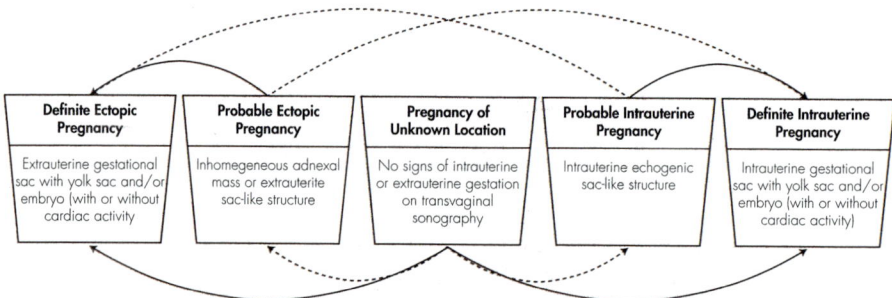

Figure 6.9. Classification of ultrasound findings for a woman with a positive pregnancy test
Source: Reproduced with permission from Barnhart K, van Mello NM, Bourne T, et al. Pregnancy of unknown location: a consensus statement of nomenclature, definitions, and outcome. *Fertil Steril.* 2011 Mar 1;95(3):857-66. Copyright © 2011 The American Society for Reproductive Medicine.

PUL or Early IUP?
- A small intrauterine gestational sac-like structure may not be a true gestation sac but a collection of fluid in the endometrial cavity ("pseudosac").
- Some sonographers will classify such a finding as a PUL.

PUL or Miscarriage?
- A pregnant woman with no definitive IUP and with a history of heavy bleeding could represent a complete miscarriage or an ectopic.
- In a study of 152 women with such a history, 5.9% were subsequently found to have an underlying EP (Condous 2005).

- A slightly thickened or irregular endometrium could represent retained products of conception.
- Where no definitive retained products of conception are seen, it would seem appropriate to adopt the safer approach and manage these cases as PUL, thus also avoiding the possibility of curettage in the presence of a potentially viable early IUP.

PUL or EP?
- Definitive diagnosis of an EP requires an extrauterine gestational sac with a yolk sac or embryo to be visualized (Barnhart 2011).
- An inhomogeneous adnexal mass more accurately should be referred to as "probable EP" (Barnhart 2011).
- The stricter criteria for making a definitive diagnosis of EP become particularly relevant when treatment with methotrexate is being considered.

GYNECOLOGY — Ectopic Pregnancy

Management of PUL

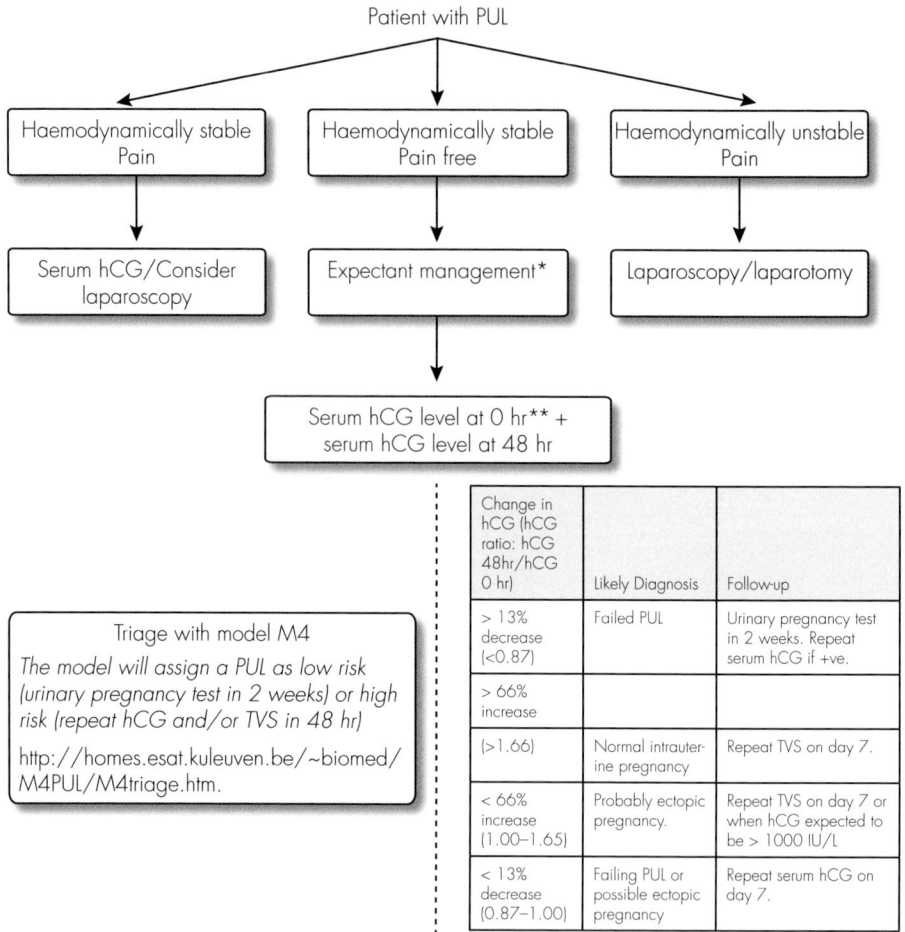

Figure 6.10. Algorithm for the management of pregnancy of unknown location (PUL)
Source: Reproduced with permission from Kirk E, Bottomley C, Bourne T. Diagnosing ectopic pregnancy and current concepts in the management of pregnancy of unknown location. *Hum Reprod Update*. 2014 Mar-Apr;20(2):250-61. Reproduced with permission of Oxford University Press on behalf of the European Society of Human Reproduction and Embryology (ESHRE).

FALSE-POSITIVE BETA-HCG

- The frequency of false-positive β-hCG is between 1 in 10,000 and 1 in 100,000 tests.
- A false-positive β-hCG is usually <150 mIU/mL.
- Most false positives are due to interference by non-hCG substances (i.e., anti-animal immunoglobulin antibodies).
- Characteristically, the serum is positive but the urine is negative because the heterophilic antibodies are usually immunoglobulins G with a molecular weight of ~160,000 diopter and are not easily filtered through the renal glomeruli. In addition, serial dilutions of serum are not parallel to the hCG standard.

Table 6.20. Causes of false-positive serum hCG

Interference by non-hCG substances
Anti-animal heterophilic immunoglobulin antibodies
hLH or hLH β-subunit
Rheumatoid factor
Nonspecific serum factors
Injection of exogenous hCG
Pituitary hCG-like substance
Assay contaminants

HCG, human chorionic gonadotropin; hLH, human luteinizing hormone.

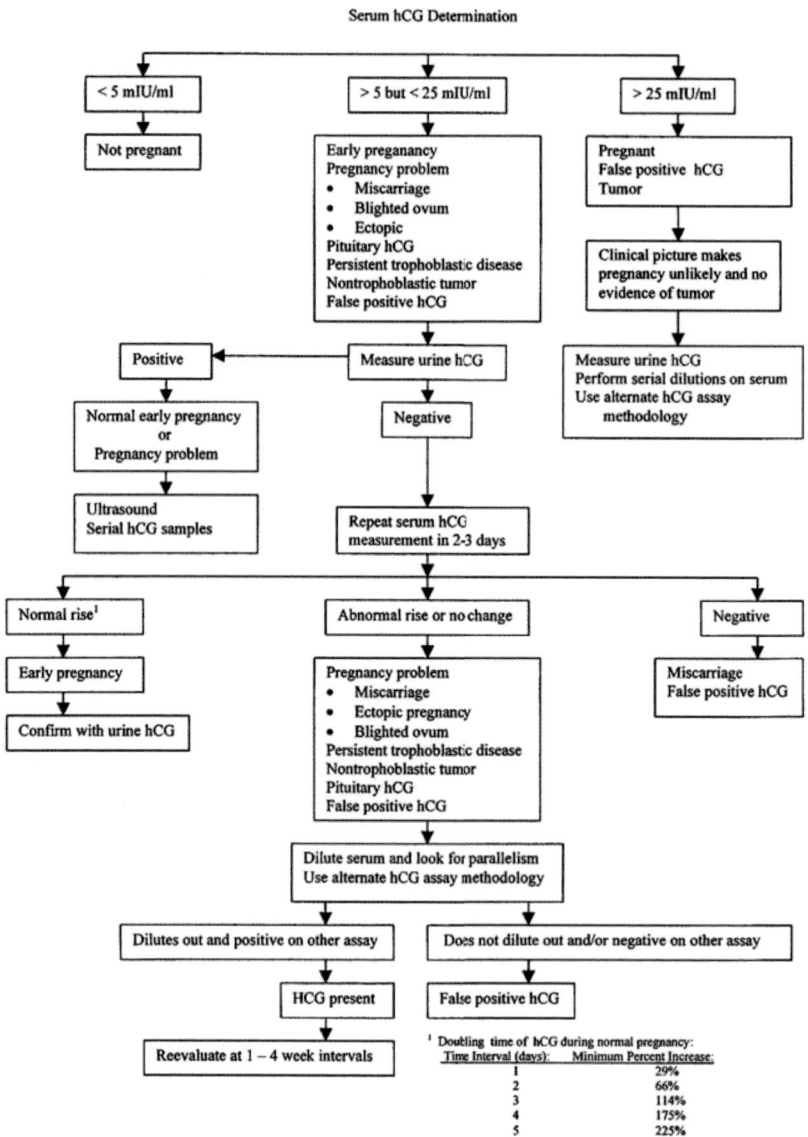

Figure 6.11. Algorithm for the evaluation of false positive beta-hCG
Source: Reproduced with permission from Braunstein, GD. False-positive serum human chorionic gonadotropin results: causes, characteristics, and recognition. *Am J Obstet Gynecol.* 2002;187[1]:217. Copyright © 2002 Elsevier.

MANAGEMENT OF FIRST-TRIMESTER PREGNANCY FAILURE

Table 6.21. Management of spontaneous abortion

	Advantages	Disadvantages	Success	Contraindications	Follow-up/Other
Expectant management No intervention. Awaiting natural passage of tissue.	Possible avoidance of: • Surgery, anesthesia, medicine. Perception of more: • Natural, privacy, control. Safe option for most.	Time until resolution is unpredictable, which may cause anxiety. No tissue for karyotyping. Highest chance of: • Unscheduled surgery. • More bleeding. POCs may be recognizable if >10 weeks.	Depends on type of abortion (i.e., incomplete vs. anembryonic) and length of follow-up. By day 7: 25–50% success By day 14: 50–80% success	Hemodynamically or medically unstable patients. Pelvic infection or sepsis. Pregnancy of unknown location, ectopic, or molar pregnancy. Caution if Hb ≤9.5 g/dL. History of coagulopathy or current anticoagulants.	Transvaginal ultrasound in 1 week. Look for expulsion of gestational sac (GS). Endometrial thickness is not predictive of success or need for surgery. β-hCG follow-up **not** needed if GS expulsed.
Medical management Use of medications to expel uterine tissue. Misoprostol 800 mcg vaginally, with repeat dose on day 3 if needed, is the most well-studied regimen.	Possible avoidance of: • Surgery, anesthesia. Perception of more: • Natural, privacy, control. Safe option for most.	Increased rates of: • Nausea, vomiting, diarrhea, cramping (compared with surgical). No tissue for karyotyping. POCs may be recognizable if >10 weeks.	Highest for women with symptoms (cramping and bleeding). Differs by type: • Incomplete/inevitable: 93% • Embryonic/fetal demise: 88% • Anembryonic gestation: 81%	Same as above, plus: Allergy or contraindication to prostaglandins.	Same as above. Counseling: average of 12 days bleeding after misoprostal.
Surgical management Mechanical removal of tissue from uterus.	Predictable start and finish. Anesthesia available. Standard of care for septic abortion, hemorrhage, molar pregnancy.	Patient may have delay until surgery can occur. Risk of anesthesia. Surgical risk.	>97% Does not vary by gestational age.	None May be challenging in patients with morbid obesity or uterine anomalies.	If chorionic villi or gestational sac obtained, β-hCG follow-up **not** needed. Can be performed in office or OR.

No difference in complications after medical versus surgical management for:		
Hemorrhage requiring hospitalization with or without blood transfusion (1%)	Fever (3–4%)	Decrease in hemoglobin ≥2 g/dL (4–9%)
	ED visit to hospital within 24 hr of treatment (2–3%)	
Hospitalization for endometritis (<1%)	Unscheduled hospital visits (17–23%)	Decrease in hemoglobin ≥3 g/dL (1–5%)

BhCG, beta human chorionic gonadotropin; ED, emergency department; EPF, early pregnancy failure; GS, gestational sac; Hb, hemoglobin; Ig, immunoglobulin; OR, operating room; POC, products of conception.

All options are medically safe, so patient preference should be guiding force deciding EPF management.

All patients need blood type documented and Rh Ig if Rh negative.

Source: Reproduced with permission from Gariepy AM and Stanwood NL. Medical management of early pregnancy failure. *Cont Ob/Gyn.* May 2013:26-33. Copyrighted 2016 Advanstar. 121944:0216DS.

Table 6.22. Absolute contraindications to mifepristone/misoprostol for medical abortion

Contraindication	Explanation
Confirmed or suspected ectopic pregnancy or undiagnosed adnexal mass	Mifepristone/misoprostol will not treat an ectopic pregnancy resulting from a reduced numbers of progestin receptors as compared to a normal intrauterine pregnancy.
Intrauterine device (IUD) in place	Remove any IUD before treatment with mifepristone/misoprostol.
Chronic adrenal failure or current long-term corticosteroid therapy	Mifepristone can bind to glucocorticoid receptors and possibly potentiate adrenal insufficiency.
History of allergy to mifepristone, misoprostol, or other prostaglandin	
Severe anemia, known coagulopathy, or anticoagulant therapy	The lack of supervision with the blood loss may be problematic, even if the blood loss with medical abortion is similar to that with surgical abortion.

Source: Reproduced with permission from Isley MM and Blumenthal P. Medical abortion what's old, what's new? Cont Ob/Gyn. April 2008:30-38. Copyrighted 2016 Advanstar. 121944:0216DS.

Table 6.23. Comparison of common medical abortion regimens

Common Regimens	Overall Success Rate (%)	Advantages and Disadvantages	Gestational Age
Mifepristone 600 mg orally, followed by misoprostol 400 micrograms orally 48 hours later (regimen approved by the Food and Drug Administration)	92[1]	Must return to office or clinic for misoprostol administration; can be used only up to 49 days of gestation	Up to 49 days
Mifepristone 200 mg orally, followed by misoprostol 800 micrograms vaginally, buccally, or sublingually 24–48 hours later (alternative evidence-based regimens; with vaginal administration, misoprostol may be administered 6 hours or less after mifepristone)	95–99[2-7]	Compared with the regimen approved by the Food and Drug Administration: • More effective • Less time to expulsion • Fewer adverse effects • Lower cost • More convenient because allows home administration of isoprostol	Up to 63 days
Methotrexate, 50 mg/m² intramuscularly or 50 mg vaginally plus misoprostol, 800 micrograms vaginally 3–7 days later	92–96[8-10]	Compared with mifepristone-misoprostol regimen: • Takes longer for expulsion in 20–30% of women • Readily available medications • Low drug cost	Up to 49 days
Misoprostol only, 800 micrograms vaginally or sublingually administered every 3 hours for three doses (with vaginal administration, dosing interval may be as long as 12 hours)	84–85[11]	• Significantly higher incidence of adverse effects than other regimens • Readily available medication • Low drug cost	Up to 63 days

[1] Spitz (1998).
[2] Schaff (2001).
[4] el-Refaey (1995).
[5] von Hertzen (2003).
[6] Creinin (2004).
[7] von Hertzen (2010).
[8] Creinin (1999).
[10] Wiebe (2002).
[11] von Hertzen (2007).

Source: Reproduced with permission from American College of Obstetricians and Gynecologists. Practice Bulletin No. 143: Medical management of first-trimester abortion. *Obstet Gynecol.* 2014 Mar;123(3):676-92. Copyright © 2014 The American College of Obstetricians and Gynecologists.

EVALUATION OF THE SEXUAL ASSAULT PATIENT
Fast Facts
- Sexual assault is the most underreported crime in the United States.
- 50% of assaults occur in the victim's home.
- Ob/Gyn physicians are often required to provide ER evaluation of rape victims.
- Use of special consent forms and rape victim evaluation kit can be helpful.

Rape Tray Contents
- Sealed package of microscope slides with frosted tips
- Eye dropper bottle with 0.9% normal saline
- Six to twelve packages of sterile cotton swabs
- Eight to twelve sterile tubes
- Urine container
- Sterile, unused, and packaged comb
- Sterile scissors
- Two to four Papanicolaou smear mailers
- Package of gummed labels
- Nail scraper
- An outline for conducting the examination

GYNECOLOGY

Evaluation

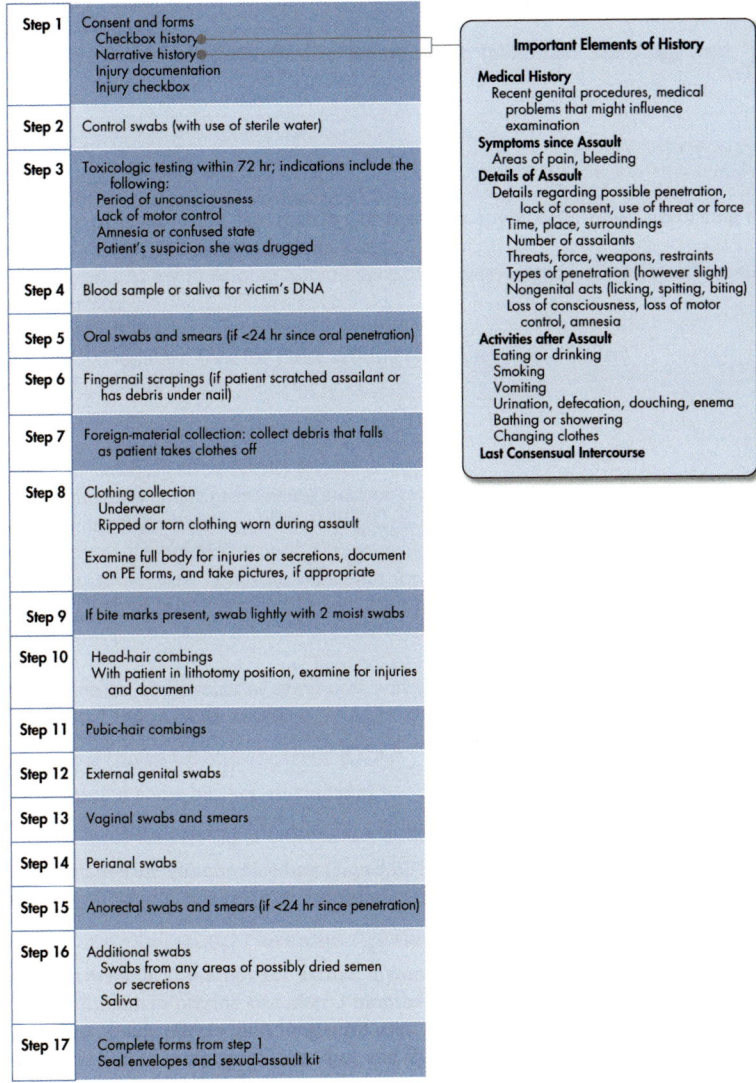

Figure 6.12. Steps in obtaining samples for a sexual assault evidence collection kit and medical-history taking

Source: Reproduced with permission from Linden JA. Clinical practice. Care of the adult patient after sexual assault. *N Engl J Med.* 2011 Sep 1;365(9):834-41. Copyright © 2011 Massachusetts Medical Society. Reproduced with permission of the Massachusetts Medical Society.

Options for Sexually Transmitted Disease Prophylaxis

Table 6.24. Drug therapies for the prevention of sexually transmitted infections and pregnancy after sexual assault

Infection or Condition	Recommended Treatment	Comments
Gonorrhea	Ceftriaxone (250 mg intramuscularly) or cefixime (400 mg orally in a single dose); azithromycin (2 g orally in a single dose) in patients with penicillin allergy	Avoid the use of ceftriaxone and cefixime in patients with severe anaphylactic reactions to penicillin and avoid the use of azithromycin in patients with erythromycin allergy; drugs may cause diarrhea and nausea
Chlamydia	Azithromycin (1 g orally in a single dose) or doxycycline (100 mg orally twice a day for 7 days)	Avoid the use of doxycycline in pregnant women or in children <8 yr of age
Trichomoniasis	Metronidazole (2 g orally in a single dose)	Avoid use with alcohol; drug may cause nausea and vomiting
Hepatitis B	Hepatitis B vaccination if not already immunized, with first dose given in the emergency department	Administer the second dose at 1–2 mo and the third dose at 4–6 mo
HIV*	Combination therapy with tenofovir plus emtricitabine (Truvada) (1 tab orally once a day for 28 days) or combination therapy with lamivudine plus zidovudine (Combivir) (1 tab orally twice a day for 28 days); if higher risk, consider adding combination therapy with lopinavir plus ritonavir (Kaletra) (400 mg of lopinavir and 100 mg of ritonavir [two tabs] orally twice a day for 28 days)	Treat if assailant is HIV-positive and there was significant exposure; consider risk according to type of assault, preferably in consultation with local specialist, who should also be consulted if the patient is pregnant. Side effects are as follows—Truvada: headache, diarrhea, nausea and vomiting, renal toxicity, lactic acidosis; Combivir: headache, fatigue, insomnia, nausea and vomiting, pancreatitis, elevated liver enzymes, neutropenia, anemia, lactic acidosis; Kaletra: rash, nausea, vomiting, abdominal pain, taste changes, elevated liver enzymes
Tetanus	Tetanus booster (if indicated)	
Pregnancy	Levonorgestrel, or Plan B (1.5 mg orally in a single dose)	Drug may cause nausea, vomiting, vaginal bleeding, abdominal cramping, early or late menses

*Most experts recommend treatment if the assailant is known or suspected to be positive for the human immunodeficiency virus (HIV). Multiple regimens are available, and other regimens may be advised by specialists in HIV prophylaxis, depending on the preference of the patient, resistance pattern to antiretroviral medications in the area, and the availability of medication. An antiemetic (e.g., ondansetron or prochlorperazine) should be prescribed, since the medications administered may cause nausea.

Source: Reproduced with permission from Linden JA. Clinical practice. Care of the adult patient after sexual assault. N Engl J Med. 2011 Sep 1;365(9):834-41. Copyright © 2011 Massachusetts Medical Society. Reproduced with permission of the Massachusetts Medical Society.

Follow-up

- Only 20–30% of patients will return for follow-up.
- Consider arranging for patient to be seen by same MD in follow-up.

Follow-up Testing

- 2 weeks: Gonorrhea/chlamydia
- 4 weeks: Hepatitis B
- 6 weeks: Pregnancy, trichomonas, human papillomavirus, vaginosis
- 3 months: Gonorrhea/chlamydia, HIV
- 6 months: Hepatitis B, HIV, rapid plasma reagin

PELVIC PAIN

Fast Facts
- Frustrating disease for patient and physician
- Many possible etiologies
- Excessive use of narcotics can lead to drug dependency

Etiology

Gynecologic
- Extrauterine
  - Adhesions
  - Chronic ectopic pregnancy
  - Chronic pelvic infection
  - Endometriosis
  - Residual ovary syndrome
- Uterine
  - Adenomyosis
  - Chronic endometritis
  - Leiomyomata
  - Intrauterine contraceptive device
  - Pelvic congestion
  - Pelvic support defects
  - Polyps

Urologic
- Chronic urinary tract infection
- Detrusor overactivity
- Interstitial cystitis
- Stone
- Suburethral diverticulitis
- Urethral syndrome

Gastrointestinal
- Cholelithiasis
- Chronic appendicitis
- Constipation
- Diverticular disease
- Enterocolitis
- Gastric/duodenal ulcer
- Inflammatory bowel disease (Crohn's disease, ulcerative colitis)
- Irritable bowel syndrome
- Neoplasia

Musculoskeletal
- Coccydynia
- Disk problems

- Degenerative joint disease
- Fibromyositis
- Hernias
- Herpes zoster (shingles)
- Low back pain
- Levator ani syndrome (spasm of pelvic floor)
- Myofascial pain (trigger points, spasms)
- Nerve entrapment syndromes
- Osteoporosis (fractures)
- Pain posture
- Scoliosis/lordosis/kyphosis
- Strains/sprains

Other

- Abuse (physical or sexual, prior or current)
- Heavy metal poisoning (lead, mercury)
- Hyperparathyroidism
- Porphyria
- Psychiatric disorders (depression, bipolar disorders, inadequate personality disorder)
- Psychosocial stress (marital discord, work stress)
- Sickle cell disease
- Sleep disturbances
- Somatoform disorders
- Substance use (especially cocaine)
- Sympathetic dystrophy
- Tabes dorsalis (third degree syphilis)

Table 6.25. Medical treatment of chronic pelvic pain

Class/Medication	Dosing	Side Effects	Considerations
Tricyclic antidepressants (TCAs)		Sedation, dry mouth, constipation, weight gain, tachycardia, hyperglycemia	Urinary retention
Amitriptyline	• 10–25 mg qhs • Titrate 10–25 mg/week to 75–150 qhs	Pelvic exam/Pelvic U/S/Pelvic MRI to evaluate anatomy	
Nortriptyline	• 10 mg qhs • Titrate 10 mg/week to 50–100 mg qhs		
Desipramine	• 20 mg daily • Titrate 10–25 mg/week to 75–100 mg daily		
Selective norepinephrine reuptake inhibitors (SNRIs)		Sedation, headache, dizziness	Hepatic dysfunction, caution with serotonergic drugs (risk for serotonin syndrome), rapid-cycling bipolar. Taper off required.
Duloxetine	• 20 mg daily • Titrate 20 mg/week to 60–90 mg daily		
Desvenlofaxine	• 37.5 mg twice daily • Titrate 37.5 mg/week until maximum dose of 150–225 mg daily		
Gamma-aminobutyric acid analogues		Sedation, dizziness, anxiety	Taper off required
Gabapentin	**First month:** • 100 mg qhs × 1 week • 200 mg qhs × 1 week • 300 mg qhs × 1 week • 100 mg q am/300 mg qhs **Second month:** • 300 mg tid • If some relief, can continue to increase incrementally to 600 mg po tid. Max dose 3600 mg/24 hr		

(continued)

Class/Medication	Dosing	Side Effects	Considerations
Pregabalin	**First month:** • 25 mg qhs × 1 week • 25 mg bid × 1 week • 25 mg q am, 50 mg qhs × 1 week • 50 mg bid × 1 week **Second month:** • 50 mg tid • If some relief, can continue to increase to 150 mg tid. Max dose 600 mg daily		
Anxiolytics		Sedation	Dependency. Taper off required. Do not use with additional benzodiazepines.
Clonazepam	0.5 mg qhs		
Muscle relaxants		Sedation	Avoid in patients with myasthenia gravis, liver disease, narrow-angle glaucoma, sleep apnea.
Flexeril	10 mg q 8 hr pm for spasm		
Valium	10 mg per vagina q 8 hr pm for pain		

Source: Carey E, Findley, A. Caring for patients with chronic pelvic pain. *Cont Ob/Gyn*. January 6, 2015. Copyrighted 2016. Advanstar. 121944:0216DS

Table 6.26. Strategies for treating primary dysmenorrhea

Strategy	Route/Dose	Advantages	Disadvantages
Ovulation suppression			
Hormonal contraceptives	Oral, transdermal, intravaginal	Provides contraception, regular bleeding, lighter flow	21 days of medication for 2–4 days of relief, prescription required
Prostaglandin suppression			
Ibuprofen	Oral (800 mg to 1200 mg initial, 800 mg every 6 hr)	Widely available, proven effective	Risk of gastrointestinal upset, prescription required
Mefenamic acid (Ponstel)	Oral (250 mg to 500 mg initial, 250 mg, every 6 hr)	Proven effective in reducing uterine activity and subjective pain	Risk of gastrointestinal upset, prescription required
Naproxen sodium (Anaprox, Naprosyn)	Oral (250 mg to 500 mg initial, 250 mg twice daily)	Widely available, proven effective in reducing uterine activity and subjective pain, twice daily dosing	Risk of gastrointestinal upset, prescription required
Continuous low-level topical heat			
ThermaCare	Topical (low abdomen or back)	Non-prescription, no systemic side effects, proven effective in reducing uterine activity and subjective pain (comparable to prescription therapy), individual heat patches effective for 8–10 hr	Effectiveness reduced if heat patch is deprived of oxygen

Source: Reprinted with permission from Smith RP. Finding the best approach to dysmenorrhea. *Cont Ob/Gyn.* 2006;Nov:54-60. *Cont Ob/Gyn* is a copyrighted publication of Advanstar Communications Inc. All rights reserved.

ENDOMETRIOSIS

Fast Facts
- Found in 5–15% of reproductive age women undergoing laparoscopy
- 1/3 of these have infertility concerns

Symptoms
- None (!)
- Cyclic pre- and peri-menstrual pain
- Dyspareunia (vaginal hyperalgesia)
- Chronic pelvic pain
- Dyschezia and/or dysuria
- Infertility

Etiology
- Sampson: retrograde flow (monkey studies)
- Halban: lymphatic-vascular spreading (lung, brain, pericardium)
- Meyer: coelomic (found in males and infants)
- Dmowski: decrease in cellular immunity

Pathology
- Ectopic endometrial glands
- Ectopic endometrial stroma
- Adjacent hemorrhage
- Common locations: uterosacral ligament, ovary, cul-de-sac

Treatment

Medical
- Primary therapy for pain-related symptoms but not for infertility patients
- Gonadotropin-releasing hormone (GnRH) agonists
  - Buserelin
  - Triptorelin
  - Decapeptyl
  - Goserelin (Zoladex)
  - Leuprolide (Lupron)
  - Nafarelin (Synarel)
- Consider hormonal treatment of hypoestrogenic side effects ("add-back" therapy; see page 67)

Alternatives (Side Effects, Costs, Duration of Treatment >6 Months)
- Continuous oral contraceptives for 6–12 months
- Norethindrone acetate 5 mg PO q day
- Depot medroxyprogesterone acetate subcutaneous-104 × 3 months or longer
- Danazol 200–800 mg PO q day × 6 months
- Aromatase inhibitors (letrozole 2.5 mg PO q day with continuous progestins)

Table 6.27. Progestins in the medical management of endometriosis

Type	Dose	Duration	Expected Pain Reduction
Oral medroxyprogesterone acetate	10 mg three times a day, maximum total dose 100 mg daily	6 months	Improvement of symptoms in 80% of patients
Norethindrone acetate	5 mg daily and maximum total dose 15 mg daily	6 months	Significantly less than GnRH agonists
Depot medroxyprogesterone acetate (DMPA)	150 mg every 12–14 weeks		As effective as leuprolide and danazol in randomized trials
Subcutaneous medroxyprogesterone acetate	104 mg every 12–14 weeks	Up to 18 months	Comparable to GnRH agonists
Levonorgestrel-releasing intrauterine system (LNG-IUS)	52 mg levonorgestrel covered by silicone that releases 20 μg/day for 5 years	Up to 36 months	Significant improvement in pain scores
Etonogestrel subdermal implant	68 mg of etonogestrel, which is released over a 3-year period	Up to 36 months	4/5 were satisfied with pain relief

Source: Reproduced from Bedaiwy MA and Liu J. Long-term management of endometriosis: medical therapy and treatment of infertility. *SRM*. 2010 Aug:10-14. Copyright © 2010 The American Society for Reproductive Medicine.

GYNECOLOGY

Endometriosis

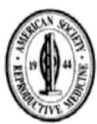

**AMERICAN SOCIETY FOR REPRODUCTIVE MEDICINE
REVISED CLASSIFICATION OF ENDOMETRIOSIS**

Patient's Name _____ Date _____

Stage I (Minimal) - 1-5
Stage II (Mild) - 6-15
Stage III (Moderate) - 16-40
Stage IV (Severe) - >40
Total _____

Laparoscopy _____ Laparotomy _____ Photography _____
Recommended Treatment _____
_____
Prognosis _____

	ENDOMETRIOSIS	<1cm	1-3cm	>3cm
PERITONEUM	Superficial	1	2	4
	Deep	2	4	6
OVARY	R Superficial	1	2	4
	Deep	4	16	20
	L Superficial	1	2	4
	Deep	4	16	20
	POSTERIOR CULDESAC OBLITERATION	Partial		Complete
		4		40
	ADHESIONS	<1/3 Enclosure	1/3-2/3 Enclosure	>2/3 Enclosure
OVARY	R Filmy	1	2	4
	Dense	4	8	16
	L Filmy	1	2	4
	Dense	4	8	16
TUBE	R Filmy	1	2	4
	Dense	4*	8*	16
	L Filmy	1	2	4
	Dense	4*	8*	16

*If the fimbriated end of the fallopian tube is completely enclosed, change the point assignment to 16.

Denote appearance of superficial implant types as red [(R), red, red-pink, flamelike, vesicular blobs, clear vesicles], white [(W), opacifications, peritoneal defects, yellow-brown], or black [(B) black, hemosiderin deposits, blue]. Denote percent of total described as R___%, W___% and B___%. Total should equal 100%.

Additional Endometriosis: _____ Associated Pathology: _____

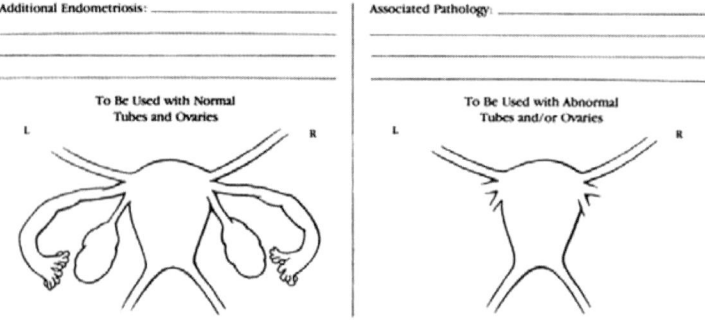

Figure 6.14. American Society for Reproductive Medicine revised classification of endometriosis

Source: Reproduced with permission from Revised American Society for Reproductive Medicine. Classification of endometriosis: 1996. *Fertil Steril.* 1997;(67):817-21. Copyright © 1996 The American Society for Reproductive Medicine.

(continued)

Endometriosis

GYNECOLOGY

EXAMPLES & GUIDELINES

STAGE I (MINIMAL)

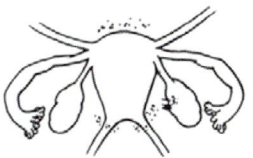

PERITONEUM
  Superficial Endo — 1-3cm - 2
R. OVARY
  Superficial Endo — < 1cm - 1
  Filmy Adhesions — < 1/3 - 1
    TOTAL POINTS   4

STAGE II (MILD)

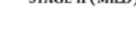
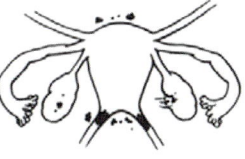

PERITONEUM
  Deep Endo — > 3cm - 6
R. OVARY
  Superficial Endo — < 1cm - 1
  Filmy Adhesions — < 1/3 - 1
L. OVARY
  Superficial Endo — < 1cm - 1
    TOTAL POINTS   9

STAGE III (MODERATE)

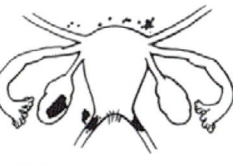

PERITONEUM
  Deep Endo — > 3cm - 6
CULDESAC
  Partial Obliteration - 4
L. OVARY
  Deep Endo — 1-3cm - 16
    TOTAL POINTS   26

STAGE III (MODERATE)

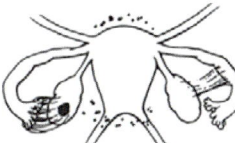

PERITONEUM
  Superficial Endo — > 3cm -4
R. TUBE
  Filmy Adhesions — < 1/3 - 1
R. OVARY
  Filmy Adhesions — < 1/3 - 1
L. TUBE
  Dense Adhesions — < 1/3 - 16*
L. OVARY
  Deep Endo — < 1 cm -4
  Dense Adhesions — < 1/3 -4
    TOTAL POINTS   30

STAGE IV (SEVERE)

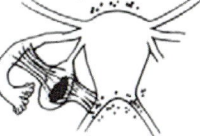

PERITONEUM
  Superficial Endo — > 3cm -4
L. OVARY
  Deep Endo — 1-3cm - 32**
  Dense Adhesions — < 1/3 - 8**
L. TUBE
  Dense Adhesions — < 1/3 - 8**
    TOTAL POINTS   52

*Point assignment changed to 16
**Point assignment doubled

STAGE IV (SEVERE)

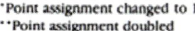
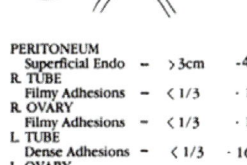

PERITONEUM
  Deep Endo — > 3cm - 6
CULDESAC
  Complete Obliteration - 40
R. OVARY
  Deep Endo — 1-3cm - 16
  Dense Adhesions — < 1/3 - 4
L. TUBE
  Dense Adhesions — > 2/3 - 16
L. OVARY
  Deep Endo — 1-3cm - 16
  Dense Adhesions — > 2/3 - 16
    TOTAL POINTS   114

Determination of the stage or degree of endometrial involvement is based on a weighted point system. Distribution of points has been arbitrarily determined and may require further revision or refinement as knowledge of the disease increases.

To ensure complete evaluation, inspection of the pelvis in a clockwise or counterclockwise fashion is encouraged. Number, size and location of endometrial implants, plaques, endometriomas and/or adhesions are noted. For example, five separate 0.5cm superficial implants on the peritoneum (2.5 cm total) would be assigned 2 points. (The surface of the uterus should be considered peritoneum.) The severity of the endometriosis or adhesions should be assigned the highest score only for peritoneum, ovary, tube or culdesac. For example, a 4cm superficial and a 2cm deep implant of the peritoneum should be given a score of 6 (not 8). A 4cm deep endometrioma of the ovary associated with more than 3cm of superficial disease should be scored 20 (not 24).

In those patients with only one adenexa, points applied to disease of the remaining tube and ovary should be multiplied by two. **Points assigned may be circled and totaled. Aggregation of points indicates stage of disease (minimal, mild, moderate, or severe).

The presence of endometriosis of the bowel, urinary tract, fallopian tube, vagina, cervix, skin etc., should be documented under "additional endometriosis." Other pathology such as tubal occlusion, leiomyomata, uterine anomaly, etc., should be documented under "associated pathology." All pathology should be depicted as specifically as possible on the sketch of pelvic organs, and means of observation (laparoscopy or laparotomy) should be noted.

Property of the American Society for Reproductive Medicine 1996

For additional supply write to: American Society for Reproductive Medicine,
1209 Montgomery Highway, Birmingham, Alabama 35216

ENDOMETRIOSIS FERTILITY INDEX
Fast Facts
- Previous scoring systems such as ASRM (see pages 362–363) have been criticized for their inability to predict non-IVF conception rates.
- EFI was created using a different approach:
  - Data was collected prospectively, then infertility outcomes were assessed, and comprehensive statistical analysis was used to derive a new staging system from the data.
  - The new staging system has been externally validated in five additional studies.

Least Function Score
- The functional score measures the ability of the tube and ovary to work together and grades the following:
  - The ability of the fimbria to move over the ovary and to pick up an egg.
  - The ability of the ovary to house eggs, develop follicles, ovulate eggs, and allow them to be picked up by the fimbria.
- Because pregnancy requires the functioning of all three—tube, fimbria, and ovary—the lowest score of those three structures determines the ability of that side to function effectively.
- The total least function score is obtained by adding the lowest score from the right side to the lowest score from the left side to give a combined total of potential for reproductive function in the pelvis.
  - A completely normal pelvis would have a score of 4 + 4 = 8 and have excellent reproductive potential.
  - A completely nonfunctional pelvis with no chance of reproductive potential would have a score of 0 + 0 = 0.

Table 6.28. Descriptions of least function terms for Endometriosis Fertility Index scoring

Structure	Dysfunction	Description
Tube	Mild	Slight injury to serosa of the fallopian tube
	Moderate	Moderate injury to serosa or muscularis of the fallopian tube; moderate limitation in mobility
	Severe	Fallopian tube fibrosis or mild/moderate salpingitis isthmica nodosa; severe limitation in mobility
	Nonfunctional	Complete tubal obstruction, extensive fibrosis or salpingitis isthmica nodosa
Fimbria	Mild	Slight injury to fimbria with minimal scarring
	Moderate	Moderate injury to fimbria, with moderate scarring, moderate loss of fimbrial architecture and minimal intrafimbrial fibrosis
	Severe	Severe injury to fimbria, with severe scarring, severe loss of fimbrial architecture and moderate intrafimbrial fibrosis
	Nonfunctional	Severe injury to fimbria, with extensive scarring, complete loss of fimbrial architecture, complete tubal occlusion or hydrosalpinx
Ovary	Mild	Normal or almost normal ovarian size; minimal or mild injury to ovarian serosa
	Moderate	Ovarian size reduced by one-third or more; moderate injury to ovarian surface
	Severe	Ovarian size reduced by two-thirds or more; severe injury to ovarian surface
	Nonfunctional	Ovary absent or completely encased in adhesions

Source: Reproduced with permission from Adamson GD, Pasta DJ. Endometriosis fertility index: the new, validated endometriosis staging system. *Fertil Steril.* 2010. 94(5):1609-15. Copyright © 2010 The American Society for Reproductive Medicine

ENDOMETRIOSIS FERTILITY INDEX (EFI) SURGERY FORM

LEAST FUNCTION (LF) SCORE AT CONCLUSION OF SURGERY

Score	Description
4 =	Normal
3 =	Mild Dysfunction
2 =	Moderate Dysfunction
1 =	Severe Dysfunction
0 =	Absent or Nonfunctional

Fallopian Tube: Left [ ] Right [ ]
Fimbria: Left [ ] Right [ ]
Ovary: Left [ ] Right [ ]

To calculate the LF score, add together the lowest score for the left side and the lowest score for the right side. If an ovary is absent on one side, the LF score is obtained by doubling the lowest score on the side with the ovary.

Lowest Score: Left [ ] + Right [ ] = LF Score [ ]

ENDOMETRIOSIS FERTILITY INDEX (EFI)

Historical Factors

Factor	Description	Points
Age		
	If age is ≤ 35 years	2
	If age is 36 to 39 years	1
	If age is ≥ 40 years	0
Years Infertile		
	If years infertile is ≤ 3	2
	If years infertile is > 3	0
Prior Pregnancy		
	If there is a history of a prior pregnancy	1
	If there is no history of prior pregnancy	0
Total Historical Factors		

Surgical Factors

Factor	Description	Points
LF Score		
	If LF Score = 7 to 8 (high score)	3
	If LF Score = 4 to 6 (moderate score)	2
	If LF Score = 1 to 3 (low score)	0
AFS Endometriosis Score		
	If AFS Endometriosis Lesion Score is < 16	1
	If AFS Endometriosis Lesion Score is ≥ 16	0
AFS Total Score		
	If AFS total score is < 71	1
	If AFS total score is ≥ 71	0
Total Surgical Factors		

EFI = TOTAL HISTORICAL FACTORS + TOTAL SURGICAL FACTORS: Historical [ ] + Surgical [ ] = EFI Score [ ]

ESTIMATED PERCENT PREGNANT BY EFI SCORE

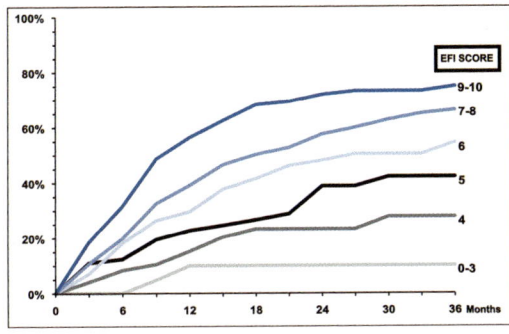

Figure 6.15. Endometriosis fertility index surgery form
Source: Reproduced with permission from Adamson GD, Pasta DJ. Endometriosis fertility index: the new, validated endometriosis staging system. *Fertil Steril.* 2010. 94(5):1609-15. Copyright © 2010 The American Society for Reproductive Medicine.

GONADOTROPIN-RELEASING HORMONE ANALOGS

Fast Facts
- Native GnRH is a decapeptide
- Substitutions at position 6 produce various agonists
- Native LH-releasing hormone isolated 1971 by Schally and Guillemin
- Secreted in pulsatile fashion by hypothalamus
- Serum half-life 2–8 minutes
- Initiates synthesis and release of LH and follicle-stimulating hormone

Analogs
- Most agonists substitution of D amino acid at position 6
- Most antagonists substitutions and modification at position 2
- Use of agonists results in transient upregulation of GnRH receptors followed by reversible downregulation and desensitization

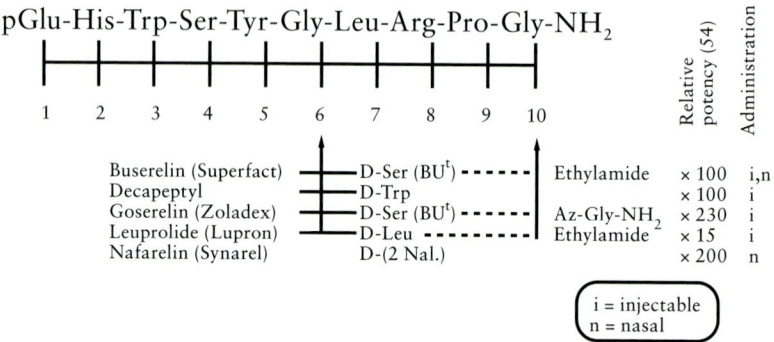

Figure 6.16. Amino acid sequence of GnRH and GnRH-agonists

Indications
- Endometriosis
- Leiomyomata (preoperative shrinkage)
- In vitro fertilization and other assisted reproductive technologies
- Precocious puberty
- Prostate carcinoma
- Breast carcinoma (many trials)

Adverse Effects
- Hypoestrogenic state (hot flashes, decreased libido, vaginal dryness, decreased bone mass)
- Androgenic (acne, myalgias, edema, weight gain)

Table 6.29. Add-back therapy for patients treated with GnRH-agonists

Author (Reference)	No. of Patients	Add-back Therapy	Symptoms	Vasomotor Symptoms	Bone Mineral Density
Surrey, et al.	19	a) NEt (10 mg/day)	↓	↓	No change
		b) NEt (2.5 mg/day) + cyclic etidronate disodium (400 mg/day)	↓	↓	No change (DXA spine)
Hornstein, et al.	201	a) NEt Ac (5 mg/day)	↓	↓	No change
		b) NEt Ac (5 mg/day) + CEE (0.625 mg/day)	↓	↓	No change
		c) NEt Ac (5 mg/day) + CEE (1.25 mg/day)	↓	↓	No change (DXA spine)
					(All less than GnRH-a alone)

CEE, conjugated equine estrogens; DXA, dual energy X-ray absorptiometry; GnRH-a, gonadotropin-releasing hormone agonist; NEt, norethindrone; NEt Ac, norethindrone acetate.

Source: Data from Surrey, et al. Prolonged gonadotropin-releasing hormone agonist treatment of symptomatic endometriosis: the role of cyclic sodium etidronate and low-dose norethindrone "add-back" therapy. *Fertil Steril.* 1995;63:747-55; and Hornstein, et al. Leuprolide acetate depot and hormonal add-back in endometriosis: a 12-month study. Lupron Add-Back Study Group. *Obstet Gynecol.* 1998;91:16-24.

Table 6.30. Use of add-back therapy for patients on long-term GnRH-agonists

GnRH-agonist Use	Add-back	Bone Density Scan	Recommended Agent
6 mo	Optional	High-risk patients only	a) Norethindrone acetate 2.5 mg daily
			b) Conjugated equine estrogens 0.3–0.625 mg (or equivalent) + medroxyprogesterone acetate 5 mg daily
6–12 mo	Required	Every 6–12 mo	Norethindrone acetate 5 mg daily
Retreatment	Required	Prior to retreatment	Norethindrone acetate 5 mg daily

Source: Data from Surrey, et al. Prolonged gonadotropin-releasing hormone agonist treatment of symptomatic endometriosis: the role of cyclic sodium etidronate and low-dose norethindrone "add-back" therapy. *Fertil Steril.* 1995;63:747-55; and Hornstein, et al. Leuprolide acetate depot and hormonal add-back in endometriosis: a 12-month study. Lupron Add-Back Study Group. *Obstet Gynecol.* 1998;91:16-24.

LAPAROSCOPY
Fast Facts
- 1805: Bozzanie examines urethra with light reflector.
- 1910: Jocobaeus in Sweden creates pneumoperitoneum in humans and uses endoscope.
- 1968: Cohen and Fear write first American article in 30 years.
- 1970s: Semm in Germany describes techniques for adhesion lysis, adnexectomy, and myomectomy.
- 1972: American Association of Gynecologic Laparoscopists founded.
- 1973: Shapiro and Adler describe laparoscopic removal of ectopic pregnancy.

Indications
Diagnosis
- Evaluation of benign pelvic mass
- Pelvic pain
- Acute (torsion, pelvic inflammatory disease, ectopic, appendicitis, etc.)
- Infertility
- Evaluation of uterine perforation
- Evaluation of pelvis prior to vaginal hysterectomy

Therapy
- Sterilization
- Fulguration of endometriosis
- Ectopic pregnancy
- Gamete intrafallopian transfer
- Ovarian cystectomy
- Oophorectomy
- Lysis of adhesions
- Appendectomy
- Hysterectomy, myomectomy, incontinence surgery

Preop Evaluation
- Patients must be well informed about all risks of planned procedure
- Routine history and physical
- Laboratory studies as indicated (β-hCG, CBC, etc.)
- Bowel prep where appropriate (GoLytely or Fleet's enema)
- Antibiotics at discretion of surgeon

Critical Analysis
- Fair evidence to suggest superiority of laparoscopy in treatment of:
  - Ectopic pregnancy
  - Endometriosis
  - Polycystic ovary syndrome resistant to clomiphene
- Superiority of laparoscopy over laparotomy in more advanced procedures requires further evaluation and is more surgeon-specific.

HYSTEROSCOPY

Fast Facts
- 1895: Bumm reports on uterine endoscope
- 1914: Heineberg introduces improved uteroscope
- 1925: Rubin describes using CO_2 as distention media
- 1968: Menken uses high viscosity media

Indications

Abnormal Uterine Bleeding
- Diagnosis and therapy
  - Ablation of endometrium
  - Excision of endometrial polyps
  - Excision of submucous fibroids

Intrauterine Foreign Bodies
- Diagnosis and therapy
  - Location of displaced intrauterine device with visually directed removal of intrauterine device
  - Location of foreign bodies with visually directed removal of foreign bodies

Infertility or Recurrent Pregnancy Wastage
- Diagnosis and therapy
  - Resection of Müllerian fusion defects
  - Division of endometrial adhesions

Table 6.31. Options for evaluation of the uterus

Anatomic Abnormality	Hysteroscopy	D&C	HSG	Ultrasound	MRI
Fibroids					
Intramural	+	−	+	+++	+++
Submucous	+++	+	++	++	+++
Intrauterine synechiae	+++	−	++	−	−
Bicornuate/septate uterus	+++	+	+++	+	+++
Endometrial polyps	++	+	+	+	++
Endometrial hyperplasia	+++	+++	−	+	−
Endometrial cancer	++	+++	+	+	−
Assessing tubal patency	+/−	−	+++	−	−

−, not helpful; +, occasionally helpful; ++, often helpful; +++, very helpful; D&C, dilatation and curettage; HSG, hysterosalpingogram.

Source: Adapted from Corfman RS. Indications for hysteroscopy. *Obstet Gynecol Clin NA*. 1988;15(1):41-49; Lavy G. Hysteroscopy as a diagnostic aid. *Obstet Gynecol Clin NA*. 1988;15(1):61-72.

Table 6.32. Comparison of hysteroscopic distension media

Type	Advantages	Disadvantages and Safety Precautions
Carbon dioxide gas	Ease of cleaning and maintaining equipment Clear view of cavity	To minimize the risk of gas embolization, the flow of carbon dioxide should be limited to 100 mL/min with intrauterine pressure of less than 100 mm Hg and used with a hysteroscopic insufflator. Insufflators designed for use in laparoscopy must not be used for hysteroscopy.
Electrolyte-poor fluid (e.g., glycine, 1.5%; sorbitol, 3%; and mannitol, 5%)	Compatible with radiofrequency energy Monopolar devices require electrolyte-poor fluids.	Excessive absorption of these fluids can cause hyponatremia, hyperammonemia, and decreased serum osmolality with the potential for seizures, cerebral edema, and death.
Electrolyte-containing fluid	Readily available Isotonic Media of choice during diagnostic hysteroscopy and in operative cases where mechanical, laser, or bipolar energy is used	Although the risk of hyponatremia and decreased serum osmolality can be reduced by using these media, pulmonary edema and congestive heart failure can still occur. Careful attention should be paid to fluid input and output, with particular attention to the fluid deficit.

Source: Reproduced with permission from American College of Obstetricians and Gynecologists. Technology Assessment No. 7: Hysteroscopy. *Obstet Gynecol.* 2011;117:1486-91. Copyright © 2011 The American College of Obstetricians and Gynecologists.

POSTOPERATIVE MANAGEMENT
Postoperative Orders
1. Admit
2. Because . . . Diagnosis
3. Condition
4. Diet
5. Exercise . . . Activity
6. Fluids (IV)
7. Graphics (vitals, weights, urine output, etc.)
8. Hypersensitivities . . . Allergies
9. Input/Output
10. Junk (Foley, nasogastric tube, stereotactic catheter drainage, spirometry, drains)
11. Call house officer for . . .
12. Labs
13. Meds
14. Narcotics (see patient controlled analgesia [PCA] orders)
15. Oxygen
16. Position (semi-Fowler's, knee chest, etc.)
17. Respiratory therapy
18. X-rays

Table 6.33. Patient-controlled analgesia

Drug	Bolus Dose (mg)	Lockout Interval (Min)	Continuous Infusion (mg/Hr)
Agonists			
Fentanyl	0.015–0.05	3–10	0.02–0.1
Hydromorphone	0.1–0.5	5–15	0.2–0.5
Meperidine	5–15	5–15	5–40
Methadone	0.5–3	10–20	
Morphine	0.5–3	5–20	1–10
Sufentanil	0.003–0.015	3–10	0.004–0.03
Agonists-antagonists			
Buprenorphine	0.03–0.2	10–20	
Pentazocine	5–30	5–15	6–40

Source: Reproduced with permission from Barash PG, Cullen BF, Stoeling RK, eds. *Handbook of Clinical Anesthesia,* 2nd Ed. Philadelphia: J.B. Lippincott; 1993.

Table 6.34. Post-operative pain management

Drug	Route	Maximum Daily Dose (mg)	Analgesic Effect		
			Onset (hr)	Peak (hr)	Duration (hr)
Nonopioids					
Salicylates					
Aspirin	PO	3600	0.5–1	0.5–2	2–4
Diflunisal	PO	2000	1–2	2–3	8–12
Propionic acids					
Fenoprofen	PO	3200	1	1–2	4–6
Ibuprofen	PO	3200	0.5	1–2	4–6
Naproxen	PO	1500	1	2–4	4–7
Indoles					
Indomethacin	PO	200	0.5	1–2	4–6
Sulindac	PO	400		2–4	
Ketorolac	IM	120	0.5–1	1	4–6
Oxicams					
Piroxicam	PO	20	1	3–5	48–72
P-ampinophenols					
Acetaminophen	PO	1200	0.5	0.5–1	2–4
Phenacetin	PO	2400		1	
Opioids					
Morphine	IV	2.5	Rapid	0.125	
Codeine	IM	15–60	0.25–0.5	1–5	4–6
	PO	15–60	0.25–1	0.5–2	3–4
Hydromorphone	IM	1–4	0.3–0.5	1	2–3
Oxycodone	PO	5	0.5	1–2	3–6
Methadone	PO	2.5–10	0.5–1	1.5–2	4–8
Propoxyphene	PO	32–65	0.25–1	1–2	3–6
Meperidine	IM	0.3–0.6	0.12–0.5	1	2–4
Buprenorphine	IM	0.3–0.6	0.12	1	6–8
Butorphanol	IM	2–4	0.1–0.2	0.5–1	3–4
Nalbuphine	IM	10–20	0.25	1	3–6
	IV	1–5			
Pentazocine	IM	30–60	0.12–0.5	1–3	3–6
	PO	50			4–7

Source: Reproduced with permission from Barash PG, Cullen BF, Stoeling RK, eds. *Handbook of Clinical Anesthesia*, 2nd Ed. Philadelphia: J.B. Lippincott; 1993.

UROGYNECOLOGY

Table 6.35. Common findings for the different types of urinary incontinence

Finding	Stress Incontinence	Detrusor Instability	Intrinsic Sphincter Deficiency	Overflow Incontinence	Functional Incontinence
Loss with Valsalva	+	–	+	+	–
Difficulty starting stream	–	–	–	+	–
Urge incontinence	–	+	–	+	+
Constant wetness	–	–	+	+	–
Hypermobile Valsalva	+	+/–	+/–	+/–	+/–
Elevated postvoid residual	–	–	–	+	–
Neurologic disease	–	+/–	+/–	+/–	+/–
Severe genital prolapse	+/–	+/–	+/–	+/–	+/–

Table 6.36. Differential diagnosis of urinary incontinence in women

Genitourinary Etiology

Filling and storage disorders
- Urodynamic stress incontinence
- Detrusor overactivity (idiopathic)
- Detrusor overactivity (neurogenic)
- Mixed types

Fistula
- Vesical
- Ureteral
- Urethral

Congenital
- Ectopic ureter
- Epispadias

Nongenitourinary Etiology

Functional
- Neurologic
- Cognitive
- Psychologic
- Physical impairment

Environmental

Pharmacologic

Metabolic

Source: Reproduced with permission from ACOG Practice Bulletin No. 155: Urinary incontinence in women. *Obstet Gynecol*. 2015;126(5):e66-e81. Copyright © 2015 The American College of Obstetricians and Gynecologists.

Table 6.37. Common causes of transient urinary incontinence

Urinary tract infection or urethritis
Atrophic urethritis or vaginitis
Drug side effects
Pregnancy
Increased urine production
• Metabolic (hyperglycemia, hypercalcemia)
• Excess fluid intake
• Volume overload
Delirium
Restricted mobility
Stool impaction
Psychologic

Source: Reproduced with permission from APGO Educational Series on Women's Health Issues. Clinical management of urinary incontinence. 2004:8-21.

Table 6.38. DIAPPERS mnemonic for transient causes of urinary incontinence

D	Delirium or acute confusion
I	Infection (symptomatic urinary tract infection)
A	Atrophic vaginitis or urethritis
P	Pharmaceutical agents
P	Psychological disorder (depression, behavioral disturbance)
E	Excess urine output (due to excess fluid intake, diuretics, congestive heart failure, etc.)
R	Restricted mobility
S	Stool impaction

Source: Reproduced with permission from APGO Educational Series on Women's Health Issues. Clinical management of urinary incontinence. 2004:8-21.

Table 6.39. Common medications used to treat urinary incontinence

Drug	Dosage
Stress incontinence	
Pseudoephedrine (Sudafed)	15–30 mg, 3 times daily
Vaginal estrogen ring (Estring)	Insert into vagina once every 3 mo
Vaginal estrogen cream	0.5–1 g, apply in vagina every night
Overactive bladder	
Oxybutynin ER (Ditropan XL)	5–15 mg, every morning
Generic oxybutynin	2.5–10 mg, 2–4 times daily
Tolterodine (Detrol)	1–2 mg, 2 times daily
Imipramine (Tofranil)	10–75 mg, every night
Dicyclomine (Bentyl)	10–20 mg, 4 times daily
Hyoscyamine (Cystospaz)	0.375 mg, 2 times daily

Source: Reproduced with permission from APGO Educational Series on Women's Health Issues. Clinical management of urinary incontinence. 2004:8-21.

Table 6.40. Therapy to facilitate urine storage/bladder filling

Bladder Related (Inhibiting Bladder Contractility, Decreasing Sensory Input, or Increasing Bladder Capacity)	Outlet Related (Increasing Outlet Resistance)
Behavioral therapy	**Behavioral therapy**
Education	**Electrical stimulation**
Fluid restriction	**Pharmacologic therapy**
Bladder training	Alpha-adrenergic agonists
Timed bladder emptying or scheduled voiding	Tricyclic antidepressants; 5-hydroxy-tryptamine and norepinephrine uptake inhibitors
Pelvic floor physiotherapy with or without biofeedback	
Pharmacologic therapy	Beta-adrenergic antagonists, agonists
Anticholinergic agents	Estrogens
Drugs with mixed actions	**Vaginal and perineal occlusive or supportive devices; urethral plugs**
Calcium antagonists	
Prostaglandin inhibitors	**Nonsurgical periurethral compression**
Beta-adrenergic agonists	**Periurethral bulking agents (polytef, collagen, or pyrolytic carbon-coated beads)**
Alpha-adrenergic antagonists	
Tricyclic antidepressants: 5-hydroxy-tryptamine and norepinephrine reuptake inhibitors	**Vesicourethral suspension with or without prolapse repair (female)**
Dimethyl sulfoxide	**Sling procedures with or without prolapse repair (female)**
Capsaicin, resiniferatoxin, and like agents	**Closure of the bladder outlet**
Electrical stimulation and neuromodulation	**Artificial urinary sphincter**
Acupuncture and electroacupuncture	**Bladder outlet reconstruction**
Interruption of innervation	**Myoplasty**
Less central (sacral rhizotomy, elective sacral rhizotomy)	*Circumventing the problem*
Peripheral motor and sensory block	**Antidiuretic hormone-like agents**
Augmentation cystoplasty (bowel, auto, tissue engineering)	**Short-acting diuretics**
	Intermittent catheterization
	External collecting devices
	Absorbent products
	Continuous catheterization
	Urinary diversion

Source: Reproduced with permission from APGO Educational Series on Women's Health Issues. Clinical management of urinary incontinence. 2004:8-21.

Urogynecology GYNECOLOGY

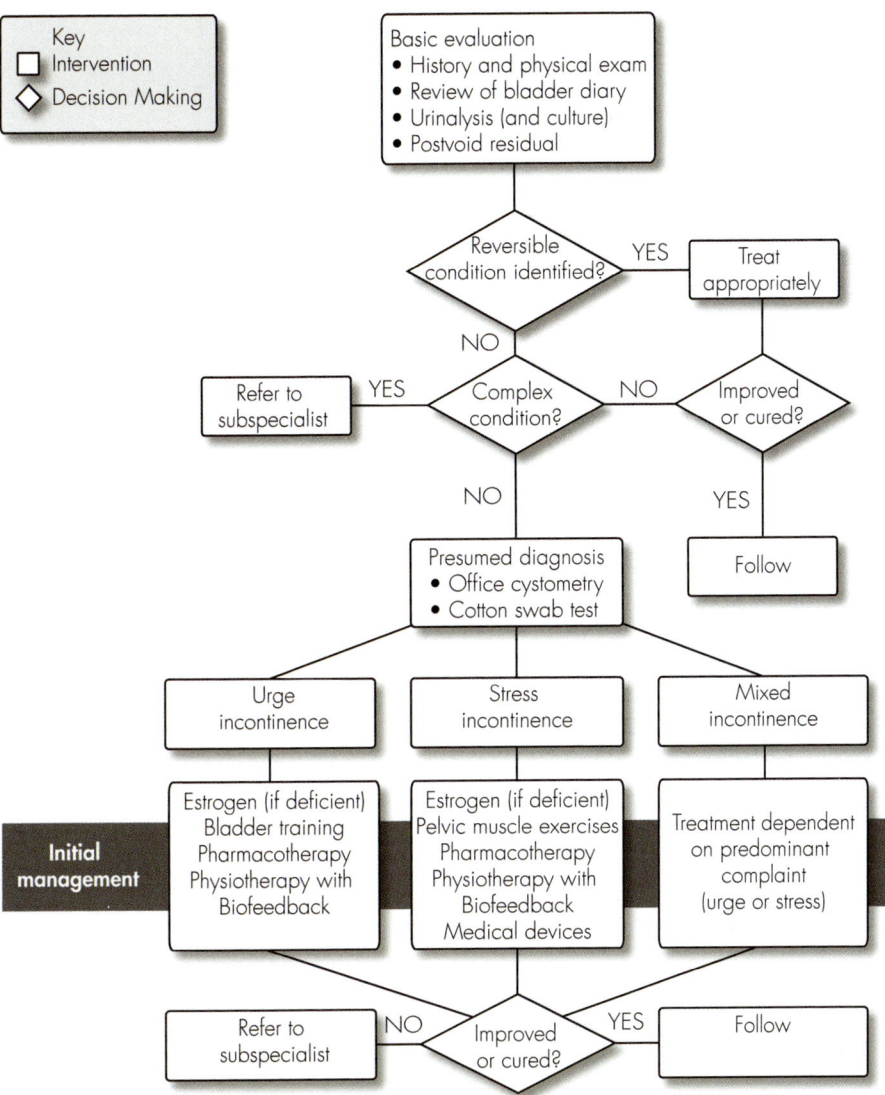

Figure 6.17. Diagnosis and treatment algorithm for urinary incontinence
Source: Reproduced with permission from APGO Educational Series on Women's Health Issues. Clinical management of urinary incontinence. 2004:8-21.

GYNECOLOGY — Urogynecology

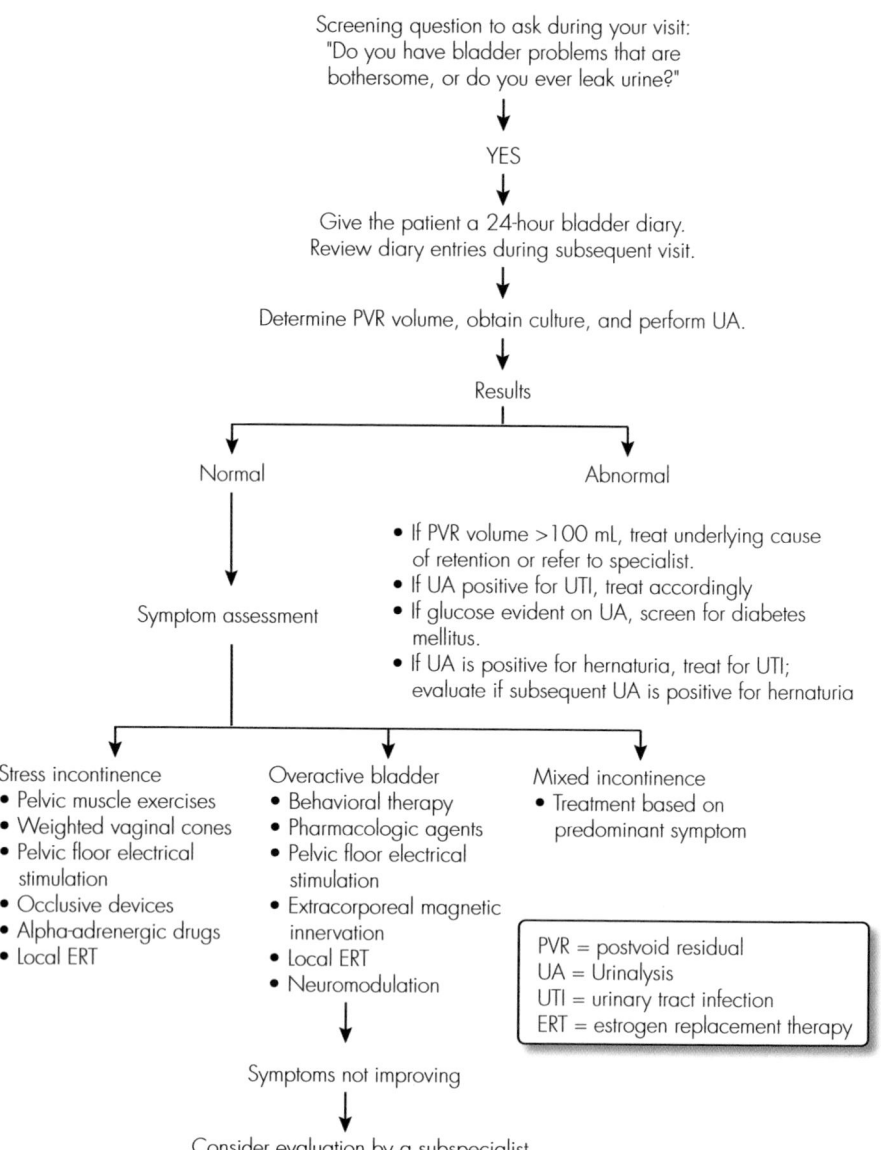

Figure 6.18. Evaluation and treatment algorithm for urinary incontinence
Source: Reproduced with permission from APGO Educational Series on Women's Health Issues. Clinical management of urinary incontinence. 2004:8-21.

VULVAR DYSTROPHIES
Nonneoplastic Epithelial Disorders
- New classification based on gross and histopathologic findings
- Squamous cell hyperplasia (formerly hyperplastic dystrophy)
- Lichen sclerosus
- Other dermatoses

Squamous Cell Hyperplasia
- Most represent lichen simplex chronicus
- Gross appearance variable
- Microscopic evaluation
  - Hyperkeratosis
  - Acanthosis
  - Parakeratosis

Lichen Sclerosus
- Classic lesion—crinkled (cigarette paper), parchment-like
- Biopsy
  - Hyperkeratosis
  - Epithelial thinning
- Often associated with foci of hyperplastic and thinning epithelium ("mixed dystrophy")
  - Squamous cell hyperplasia found in 27–35%
  - Intraepithelial neoplasia found in 5%

Therapy
- First step before therapy: biopsy, biopsy, biopsy

Squamous Cell Hyperplasia
- Topical steroids (bid to tid)
- 0.025–0.01% triamcinolone acetonide
- 0.1% β-methasone valerate and crotamiton (Eurax) in 7:3 mix

Lichen Sclerosus
- Topical testosterone no longer recommended
- Clobetasol (Temovate 0.05%) cream very effective
  - Use bid × 1 month, then qHS × 2 months, then 2×/week for 3 months
    - Complete regression can occur with this treatment
- Crotamiton (Eurax) 10% cream for pruritus

VULVODYNIA

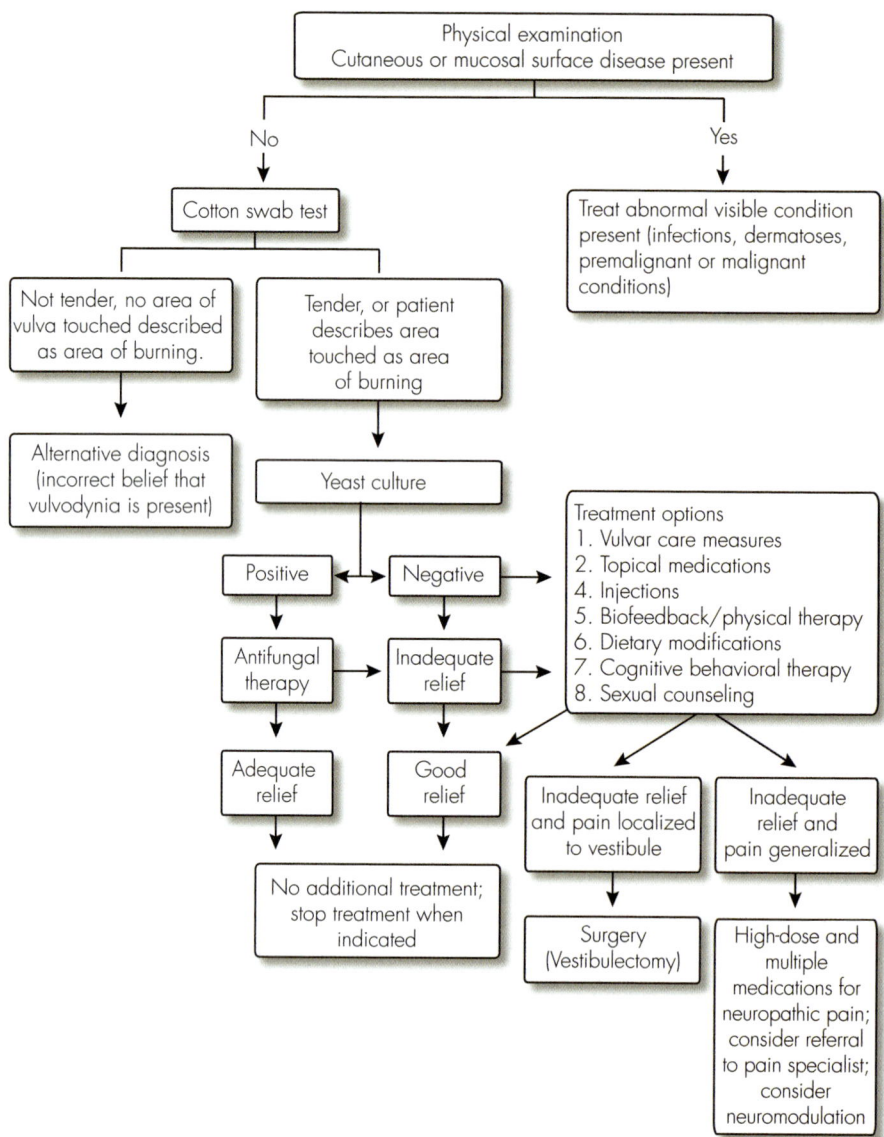

Figure 6.19. Vulvodynia treatment algorithm
Source: Modified from Haefner HK, Collins ME, Davis GD, et al. The vulvodynia guideline. *J Low Genit Tract Dis.* 2005 Jan;9(1):40-51.Reprinted with permission from ACOG Committee Opinion. Vulvodynia. *Obstet Gynecol.* 2006;108(4):1049-1052. Copyright © 2006 The American College of Obstetricians and Gynecologists.

Treatment Options for Vulvodynia

Table 6.41. Treatment options for vulvodynia[a]

Treatment	Dosage/Regimen	Side Effects
Topical		
Avoidance of topical irritants and allergens	Use mild soap or water for cleansing area, wear cotton underwear, and use fragrance-free sanitary products.	None
Estrogen (if estrogen-deficiency is indicated by parabasal cells on normal saline preparation)	Vaginal cream used daily for 3 wk, then 2–3 times/wk as needed.	Local: infrequent burning. Systemic: unclear
Topical lidocaine, 5% gel or cream	Topically to area of tenderness prior to intercourse, or nightly, applying lidocaine gel to a cotton ball that is then placed in the introitus and used overnight. Treatment duration is undetermined.	Occasional sensitivity/irritation
Cromolyn cream, 4%	Apply three times/day to area of tenderness.	Sensitivity to the agent or vehicle
Oral agents (commonly started at first visit)		
Tricyclic antidepressants	Amitriptyline, starting at 25 mg/day at bedtime for 10 days, increasing by 25-mg increments as tolerated to typical dosage of 50–100 mg/day (maximum dosage, 250 mg/day). Desipramine or imipramine at similar dosage. Nortriptyline at similar dosage, but to maximum of 100 mg/day.	Oral dryness, constipation, fatigue, weight gain (less common). Occasional neurologic symptoms, cardiac arrhythmias, or urinary retention require discontinuation
Paroxetine	10–20 mg/day, increasing as needed and tolerated to a maximum of 60 mg/day.	Occasional restlessness, weight gain, fatigue, anorgasmia
Venlafaxine	37.5 mg/day for 10 days, increasing to 75 mg/day; may increase to maximum of 225 mg/day.	Anorgasmia, gastrointestinal problems, anxiety
Gabapentin	300 mg/day, increasing every 4 days by 300 mg/day (divided into three doses) to a maximum of 900 mg three times/day.	Headache, nausea, vomiting, fatigue, dizziness
Calcium citrate (due to the citrate component)	Two tablets twice per day, increasing to 3–4 tablets twice/day.	Tablets are large and difficult for some to swallow. Not indicated for women with a history of calcium-based renal stones
Other therapeutic regimes		
Pelvic-floor physical therapy and/or biofeedback	Performed by physical therapist who has undergone appropriate training.	Discomfort, numerous visits, compliance with home exercises, possible high cost
Cognitive behavioral therapy	Sessions with a therapist; study included eight 2-hr group meetings over 12 wk, but may need ongoing treatment.	Time/commitment for full course of sessions
Low-oxalate diet	Ranges from highly restrictive diet to avoidance of a small number of high-risk foods.	Poor compliance

(continued)

GYNECOLOGY — Vulvodynia

Treatment	Dosage/Regimen	Side Effects
Surgery (rarely used)		
Perineoplasty/vestibulectomy (hypersensitive tissue is removed and replaced with vaginal mucosa advancement).	Surgical procedure confined to the posterior introitus; for women who have not responded to other treatments.	Discomfort, recovery time; rare reports of bleeding, infection, hematoma, wound separation, vaginismus, vaginal stenosis

[a]None of these options has been approved by the Food and Drug Administration specifically for the indication of vulvodynia.

Source: Reprinted with permission from Reed BD. Vulvodynia. *The Female Patient.* 2005;30:48-54.

FIBROIDS

Prevalence
- Cumulative incidence of fibroids by age 50 of 70–80% (Baird 2003)
- Prevalence of uterine myomas in the first trimester of pregnancy (prospective cohort study; Laughlin 2009)
  - 18% in African American women
  - 10% in Hispanic women
  - 8% in white women

Classification

Leiomyoma Subclassification System

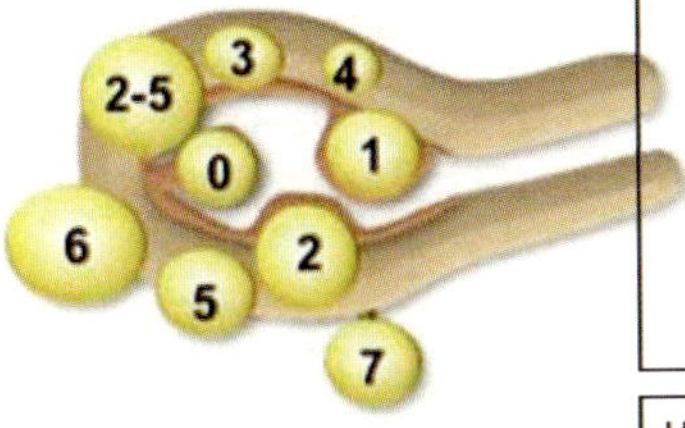

SM—Submucosal	0	Pedunculated intracavitary
	1	< 50% Intramural
	2	≥ 50% Intramural
O—Other	3	Contacts endometrium; 100% Intramural
	4	Intramural
	5	Subserosal ≥ 50% Intramural
	6	Subserosal < 50% Intramural
	7	Subserosal Pedunculated
	8	Other (specify; e.g., cervical, parasitic)

Hybrid Leiomyomas (impact both endometrium and serosal)		Two numbers are listed separated by a hyphen. By convention, the first refers to the relationship with the endometrium while the second refers to the relationship with to the serosa. One example is below.
	2–5	Submucosal and subserosal, each with less than half the diameter in the endometrial and peritoneal cavities, respectively.

Figure 6.20. FIGO classification of system for leiomyomas
Source: Adapted with permission from Munro MG. *Abnormal Uterine Bleeding*. Cambridge: Cambridge University Press; 2010.

Fibroids and Bleeding

- Most common symptom is menorrhagia or hypermenorrhea
- Obstructive effect on uterine vasculature may lead to endometrial venule extasia → proximal congestion in the myometrium/endometrium → hypermenorrhea
- ↑ size of uterine cavity (sometimes appreciated on hysterosalpingogram) leads to greater surface area for endometrial sloughing

Fibroids and Infertility

- Sole factor for infertility in <10% of infertility cases (Wallach 1995)
- Submucosal is most likely to cause infertility, then intramural, then subserosal (Farhi 1995)
- Prospective study of small (≤5 cm) intramural fibroids on the cumulative outcome of up to 3 attempts of IVF/ICSI (Khalaf 2006):
  - ↓ 40% pregnancy rate with each cycle
  - ↓ 45% cumulative ongoing pregnancy rate
  - ↓ 49% cumulative live birth rate
    - Still unclear if this negative impact can be ameliorated by a myomectomy
- Submucosal mechanism of infertility:
  - Dysfunctional uterine contractility (Vollenhoven 1990)
  - Focal endometrial vascular disturbance
  - Endometrial inflammation; endometritis
  - Secretion of vasoactive substances
  - Enhanced androgen environment (Buttram 1981)
    - Patients advised to wait 4–6 months after myomectomy before attempting to conceive
    - Uterine artery embolization not recommended in patients considering future fertility

Table 6.42. Complications of uterine fibroids during pregnancy

	Qidwai GI, et al.[2]			Stout MJ, et al.[1]		
	Fibroid (n = 401)	No fibroids (n = 14,703)	P	Fibroid (n = 2,058)	No fibroids (n = 61,989)	P
Preterm delivery <37 weeks	19%	13%	0.001	15%	10%	<0.01
Preterm premature rupture of membranes	7%	6%	0.630	3%	2%	0.03
Placental abruption	2%	2%	0.623	1%	0.7%	<0.01
Placenta previa	4%	2%	0.028	1%	0.5%	<0.01
Malpresentation	13%	8%	0.003	5%	3%	<0.01
Cesarean delivery	49%	21%	<0.001	33%	24%	<0.01
Postpartum hemorrhage[*]	8%	3%	<0.001	—	—	—

[*] Defined as estimated blood loss of >1000 mL (vaginal birth) and >1,500 mL (cesarean delivery).

Source: Reproduced with permission from Kase BA and Blackwell SC. SMFM Consult. Fibroids in pregnancy: meaning and management. *Cont Ob/Gyn.* 2014 Dec. Copyright © 2016 Advanstar. 121944:0216DS.

Fibroid Treatment Options
- Asymptomatic fibroids can be followed without intervention (perhaps yearly imaging and symptom assessment).
- Relief of symptoms warrants further management (abnormal bleeding, pain, pressure, infertility).

Surgical Options
- Mainstay of fibroid management (Falcone 2013)
  - Myomectomy
    - Choice of laparotomy, laparoscopy, or hysteroscopy is determined according to fibroid size, location, and surgeon's skills.
    - Key aspect of myomectomy is avoidance of damage to endometrium and repair of uterine defects.
  - Hysterectomy
  - Endometrial ablation (not for those seeking pregnancy in the future)
  - Myolysis (Stewart 2006)

Nonsurgical Options
- Uterine artery embolization (UAE)
  - UAE performed under radiologic guidance results in a significant reduction of uterine volume and improvement in quality of life (Goodwin 2008).
- Magnetic resonance-guided focused-ultrasound surgery (MRgFUS)
  - Results in short-term symptom reduction for women with symptomatic uterine leiomyomas with a good safety profile (Stewart 2006).

Medical Treatment Options
~75% of women get some relief of symptoms within a year, but there is a high long-term failure rate (Carlson 1994; ACOG 2008).

1. Combination Oral Contraceptives (COC)
- Can be helpful in some but not all patients.

2. Levonorgestrel-Releasing Intrauterine System (IUS)
- Reduction in uterine volume/bleeding (Sayed 2011).
- Intracavitary fibroid(s) is a relative contraindication for an IUS.

3. Gonadotropin-Releasing Hormone Agonists (GnRHa)
- Most effective medical therapy for uterine myomas.
- 35–60% reduction in uterine size after 3 months of treatment.
- Hypoestrogenic side effects limit long-term use.
  - Add-back (0.625 conjugated estradiol and 2.5 mg MPA or 5 mg norethindrone acetate) should be used after initial phase of down-regulation accomplished.
- Primarily used as preoperative therapy (× 3 months).

4. Ulipristal Acetate—Progesterone Receptor Modulator
- Not available in the US except as a 30-mg dose in ella (emergency contraceptive).
- Significantly high rate of menorrhagia resolution and fibroid volume reduction (Donnez 2014).

5. Tranexamic Acid — Antifibrinolytic Agent
- Useful in the treatment of heavy menstrual bleeding but not to be taken along with COCs

6. Mifepristone
- Progesterone antagonist
- Administered orally or vaginally
- Effective in reducing uterine fibroid volume and improve quality of life (Steinauer 2004; Yerushalmi 2014)

CHAPTER 7
Infectious Diseases

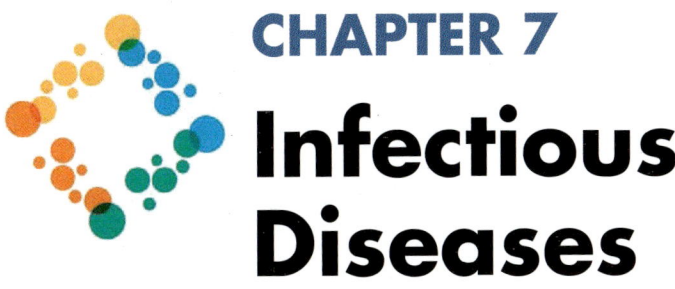

GROUP B *STREPTOCOCCUS*
Fast Facts
- A leading cause of life-threatening perinatal infections in United States.
- 15–30% of women are asymptomatic carriers.
- Infection rate has decreased from 1.8/1000 in 1990 to 0.34/1000 live births in 2004.
- Early onset infection (80% within 6 hours of delivery)—4% neonatal mortality of term infants and 23% mortality in preterm infants.

Table 7.1. Procedures for collecting clinical specimens for culture of group B *Streptococcus* (GBS) at 35–37 weeks' gestation

- Swab the lower vagina (vaginal introitus), followed by the rectum (i.e., insert swab through the anal sphincter) using the same swab or two different swabs. Cultures should be collected in the outpatient setting by the health care provider or, with appropriate instruction, by the patient herself. Cervical, perianal, perirectal, or perineal specimens are not acceptable, and a speculum should not be used for culture collection.
- Place the swab(s) into a nonnutritive transport medium. Appropriate transport systems (e.g., Stuart's or Amies with or without charcoal) are commercially available. GBS isolates can remain viable in transport media for several days at room temperature; however, the recovery of isolates declines over one to four days, especially at elevated temperatures, which can lead to false-negative results. When feasible, specimens should be refrigerated before processing.
- Specimen requisitions should indicate clearly that specimens are for group B streptococcal testing. Patients who state that they are allergic to penicillin should be evaluated for risk for anaphylaxis. If a woman is determined to be at high risk for anaphylaxis,* susceptibility testing for clindamycin and erythromycin should be ordered.

*Patients with a history of any of the following after receiving penicillin or a cephalosporin are considered to be at high risk for anaphylaxis: anaphylaxis, angioedema, respiratory distress, or urticaria.

Source: Reproduced from Verani JR, McGee L, Schrag SJ; Division of Bacterial Diseases, National Center for Immunization and Respiratory Diseases, Centers for Disease Control and Prevention (CDC). Prevention of perinatal group B streptococcal disease—revised guidelines from CDC, 2010. *MMWR Recomm Rep*. 2010 Nov 19;59(RR-10):1-36.

Table 7.2. Comparison of key points in the 2002 and 2010 centers for disease control and prevention guidelines for the prevention of perinatal group B streptococcal disease

Topic in the Guidelines	Key Points Unchanged from 2002	Key Points Changed from 2002
Universal screening for GBS acid amplification tests for intrapartum testing for GBS	Universal screening at 35–37 weeks of gestation remains the sole strategy for IAP.	Permissive statement for limited role of nucleic
Preterm delivery		New and separate algorithms for preterm labor and for PPROM (see Fig. 7.1 and Fig. 7.2)
GBS specimen collection and processing	Rectovaginal swab specimens collected at 35–37 weeks of gestation remains the recommendation.	Transport options clarified Identification options expanded to include use of chromogenic media and nucleic acid amplification tests Laboratories to report GBS in concentrations of greater than or equal to 10^4 CFU in urine culture specimens (previously, it was GBS "in any concentration")
Intrapartum antibiotic prophylaxis	Penicillin remains drug of choice with ampicillin as an alternative. Cefazolin remains the drug of choice for penicillin allergy without anaphylaxis, angioedema, respiratory distress, or urticaria. GBS isolates from women at high risk of anaphylaxis should be tested for susceptibility to clindamycin and erythromycin. Vancomycin use is recommended if isolate is resistant to either clindamycin or erythromycin.	Definition of high risk for anaphylaxis is clarified Minor change in penicillin dose permitted Erythromycin is no longer recommended under any circumstances D-test recommended to detect inducible resistance in isolates tested for susceptibility to clindamycin and erythromycin
Other obstetric management issues		Data are not sufficient to make recommendations regarding the timing of procedures intended to facilitate progression of labor, such as amniotomy, in GBS-colonized women. Intrapartum antibiotic prophylaxis is optimal if administered at least 4 hours before delivery; therefore, such procedures should be timed accordingly, if possible. No medically necessary obstetric procedure should be delayed in order to achieve 4 hours of GBS prophylaxis before delivery.
Newborn management		Algorithm now applies to all newborns, whether or not from GBS-positive mothers. Clarification of "adequate" IAP. See full CDC guidelines for details.

CDC, Centers for Disease Control and Prevention; CFU, colony-forming units; GBS, group B streptococci; IAP, intrapartum antibiotic prophylaxis; PROM, premature rupture of membranes.

Source: Reproduced with permission from American College of Obstetricians and Gynecologists Committee on Obstetric Practice. ACOG Committee Opinion No. 485: Prevention of early-onset group B streptococcal disease in newborns. *Obstet Gynecol.* 2011 Apr;117(4):1019-27. Copyright © 2011 The American College of Obstetricians and Gynecologists.

Table 7.3. Indications and nonindications for intrapartum antibiotic prophylaxis to prevent early-onset group B streptococcal (GBS) disease

Intrapartum GBS Prophylaxis Indicated	Intrapartum GBS Prophylaxis Not Indicated
• Previous infant with invasive GBS disease	• Colonization with GBS during a previous pregnancy (unless an indication for GBS prophylaxis is present for current pregnancy)
• GBS bacteriuria during any trimester of the current pregnancy*	• GBS bacteriuria during previous pregnancy (unless an indication for GBS prophylaxis is present for current pregnancy)
• Positive GBS vaginal-rectal screening culture in late gestation† during current pregnancy*	• Negative vaginal and rectal GBS screening culture in late gestation† during the current pregnancy, regardless of intrapartum risk factors

• Unknown GBS status at the onset of labor (culture not done, incomplete, or results unknown) and any of the following:
  ○ Delivery at <37 weeks' gestation§
  ○ Amniotic membrane rupture ≥18 hours
  ○ Intrapartum temperature ≥100.4°F (≥38.0°C)¶
  ○ Intrapartum NAAT** positive for GBS
	• Cesarean delivery performed before onset of labor on a woman with intact amniotic membranes, regardless of GBS colonization status or gestational age

NAAT, Nucleic acid amplification tests

*Intrapartum antibiotic prophylaxis is not indicated in this circumstance if a cesarean delivery is performed before onset of labor on a woman with intact amniotic membranes.

†Optimal timing for prenatal GBS screening is at 35–37 weeks' gestation.

§Recommendations for the use of intrapartum antibiotics for prevention of early-onset GBS disease in the setting of threatened preterm delivery are presented in Figures 7.1 and 7.2.

¶If amnionitis is suspected, broad-spectrum antibiotic therapy that includes an agent known to be active against GBS should replace GBS prophylaxis.

**NAAT testing for GBS is optional and might not be available in all settings. If intrapartum NAAT is negative for GBS but any other intrapartum risk factor (delivery at <37 weeks' gestation, amniotic membrane rupture at ≥18 hours, or temperature ≥100.4°F [≥38.0°C]) is present, then intrapartum antibiotic prophylaxis is indicated.

Source: Reproduced from Verani JR, McGee L, Schrag SJ; Division of Bacterial Diseases, National Center for Immunization and Respiratory Diseases, Centers for Disease Control and Prevention (CDC). Prevention of perinatal group B streptococcal disease—revised guidelines from CDC, 2010. *MMWR Recomm Rep.* 2010 Nov 19;59(RR-10):1-36.

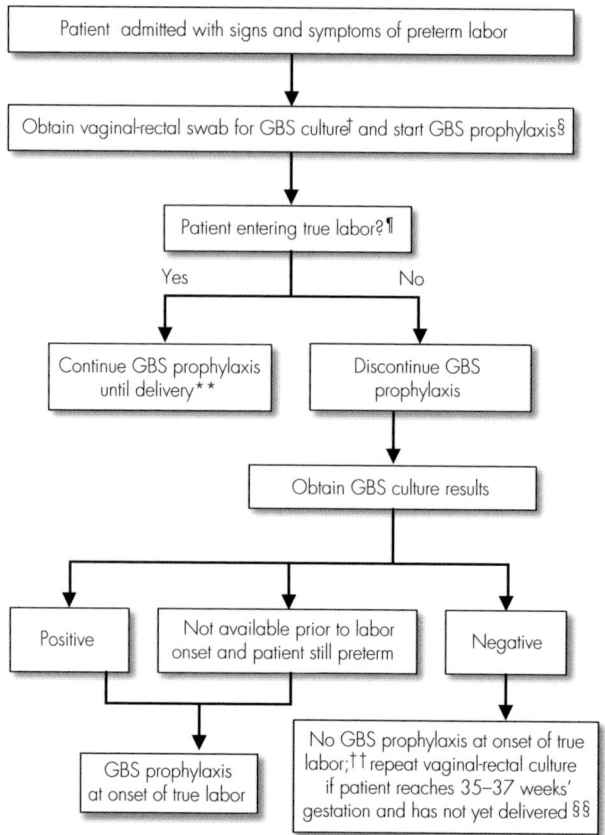

Figure 7.1. Algorithm for screening for group B streptococcal (GBS) colonization and use of intrapartum prophylaxis for women with preterm* labor (PTL)

* At <37 weeks and 0 days' gestation.

† If patient has undergone vaginal-rectal GBS culture within the preceding 5 weeks, the results of that culture should guide management. GBS-colonized women should receive intrapartum antibiotic prophylaxis. No antibiotics are indicated for GBS prophylaxis if a vaginal-rectal screen within 5 weeks was negative.

§ See Figure 7.4 for recommended antibiotic regimens.

¶ Patient should be regularly assessed for progression to true labor; if the patient is considered not to be in true labor, discontinue GBS prophylaxis.

** If GBS culture results become available prior to delivery and are negative, then discontinue GBS prophylaxis.

†† Unless subsequent GBS culture prior to delivery is positive.

§§ A negative GBS screen is considered valid for 5 weeks. If a patient with a history of PTL is readmitted with signs and symptoms of PTL and had a negative GBS screen >5 weeks prior, she should be rescreened and managed according to this algorithm at that time.

Source: Reproduced from Verani JR, McGee L, Schrag SJ; Division of Bacterial Diseases, National Center for Immunization and Respiratory Diseases, Centers for Disease Control and Prevention (CDC). Prevention of perinatal group B streptococcal disease—revised guidelines from CDC, 2010. *MMWR Recomm Rep.* 2010 Nov 19;59(RR-10):1-36.

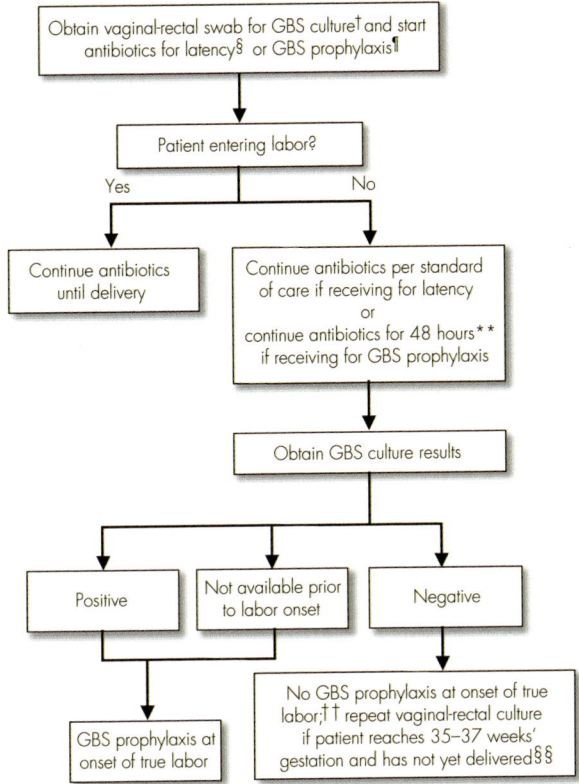

Figure 7.2. Algorithm for screening for group B streptococcal (GBS) colonization and use of intrapartum prophylaxis for women with preterm* premature rupture of membranes (PPROM)

* At <37 weeks and 0 days' gestation.

† If patient has undergone vaginal-rectal GBS culture within the preceding 5 weeks, the results of that culture should guide management. GBS-colonized women should receive intrapartum antibiotic prophylaxis. No antibiotics are indicated for GBS prophylaxis if a vaginal-rectal screen within 5 weeks was negative.

§ Antibiotics given for latency in the setting of PPROM that include ampicillin 2 g intravenously (IV) once, followed by 1 g IV every 6 hours for at least 48 hours are adequate for GBS prophylaxis. If other regimens are used, GBS prophylaxis should be initiated in addition.

¶ See Figure 7.4 for recommended antibiotic regimens.

** GBS prophylaxis should be discontinued at 48 hours for women with PPROM who are not in labor. If results from a GBS screen performed on admission become available during the 48-hour period and are negative, GBS prophylaxis should be discontinued at that time.

†† Unless subsequent GBS culture prior to delivery is positive.

§§ A negative GBS screen is considered valid for 5 weeks. If a patient with PPROM is entering labor and had a negative GBS screen >5 weeks prior, she should be rescreened and managed according to this algorithm at that time.

Source: Reproduced from Verani JR, McGee L, Schrag SJ; Division of Bacterial Diseases, National Center for Immunization and Respiratory Diseases, Centers for Disease Control and Prevention (CDC). Prevention of perinatal group B streptococcal disease—revised guidelines from CDC, 2010. *MMWR Recomm Rep.* 2010 Nov 19;59(RR-10):1-36.

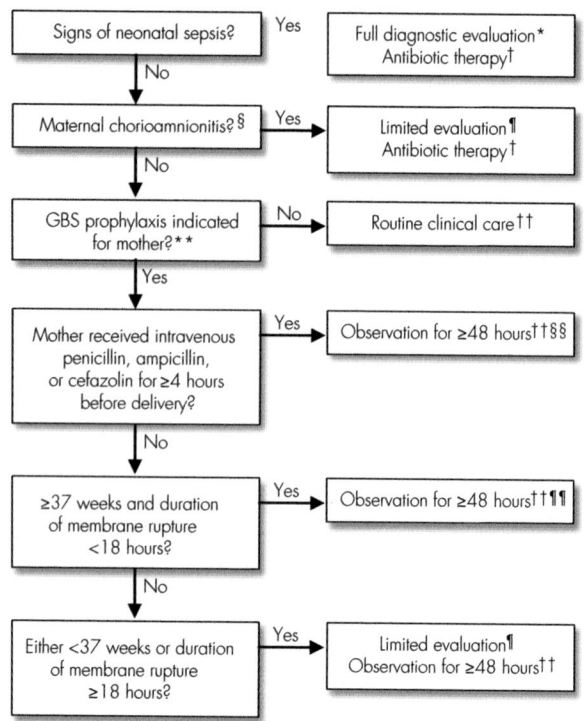

Figure 7.3. Algorithm for secondary prevention of early-onset group B streptococcal (GBS) disease among newborns

* Full diagnostic evaluation includes a blood culture, a complete blood count (CBC) including white blood cell differential and platelet counts, chest radiograph (if respiratory abnormalities are present), and lumbar puncture (if patient is stable enough to tolerate procedure and sepsis is suspected).

† Antibiotic therapy should be directed toward the most common causes of neonatal sepsis, including intravenous ampicillin for GBS and coverage for other organisms (including *Escherichia coli* and other gram-negative pathogens) and should take into account local antibiotic resistance patterns.

§ Consultation with obstetric providers is important to determine the level of clinical suspicion for chorioamnionitis. Chorioamnionitis is diagnosed clinically and some of the signs are nonspecific.

¶ Limited evaluation includes blood culture (at birth) and CBC with differential and platelets (at birth and/or at 6–12 hours of life).

** See Table 7.3 for indications for intrapartum GBS prophylaxis.

†† If signs of sepsis develop, a full diagnostic evaluation should be conducted and antibiotic therapy initiated.

§§ If ≥37 weeks' gestation, observation may occur at home after 24 hours if other discharge criteria have been met, access to medical care is readily available, and a person who is able to comply fully with instructions for home observation will be present. If any of these conditions is not met, the infant should be observed in the hospital for at least 48 hours and until discharge criteria are achieved.

¶¶ Some experts recommend a CBC with differential and platelets at age 6–12 hours.

Source: Reproduced from Verani JR, McGee L, Schrag SJ; Division of Bacterial Diseases, National Center for Immunization and Respiratory Diseases, Centers for Disease Control and Prevention (CDC). Prevention of perinatal group B streptococcal disease—revised guidelines from CDC, 2010. *MMWR Recomm Rep.* 2010 Nov 19;59(RR-10):1-36.

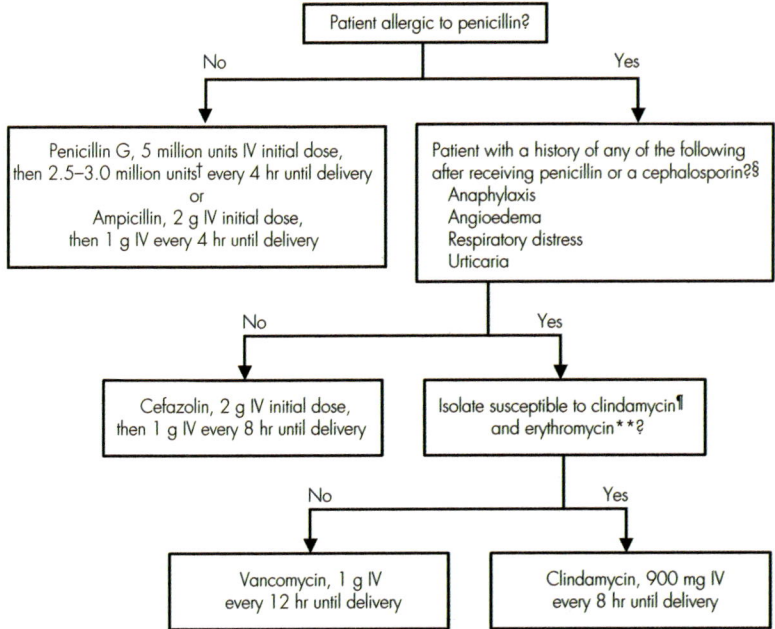

Figure 7.4. Recommended regimens for intrapartum antibiotic prophylaxis for prevention of early-onset group B streptococcal (GBS) disease*

IV, intravenously.

* Broader spectrum agents, including an agent active against GBS, might be necessary for treatment of chorioamnionitis.

† Doses ranging from 2.5 to 3.0 million units are acceptable for the doses administered every 4 hours following the initial dose. The choice of dose within that range should be guided by which formulations of penicillin G are readily available to reduce the need for pharmacies to specially prepare doses.

§ Penicillin-allergic patients with a history of anaphylaxis, angioedema, respiratory distress, or urticaria following administration of penicillin or a cephalosporin are considered to be at high risk for anaphylaxis and should not receive penicillin, ampicillin, or cefazolin for GBS intrapartum prophylaxis. For penicillin-allergic patients who do not have a history of those reactions, cefazolin is the preferred agent because pharmacologic data suggest it achieves effective intraamniotic concentrations. Vancomycin and clindamycin should be reserved for penicillin-allergic women at high risk for anaphylaxis.

¶ If laboratory facilities are adequate, clindamycin and erythromycin susceptibility testing should be performed on prenatal GBS isolates from penicillin-allergic women at high risk for anaphylaxis. If no susceptibility testing is performed, or the results are not available at the time of labor, vancomycin is the preferred agent for GBS intrapartum prophylaxis for penicillin-allergic women at high risk for anaphylaxis.

** Resistance to erythromycin is often but not always associated with clindamycin resistance. If an isolate is resistant to erythromycin, it might have inducible resistance to clindamycin, even if it appears susceptible to clindamycin. If a GBS isolate is susceptible to clindamycin, resistant to erythromycin, and testing for inducible clindamycin resistance has been performed and is negative (no inducible resistance), then clindamycin can be used for GBS intrapartum prophylaxis instead of vancomycin.

Source: Reproduced from Verani JR, McGee L, Schrag SJ; Division of Bacterial Diseases, National Center for Immunization and Respiratory Diseases, Centers for Disease Control and Prevention (CDC). Prevention of perinatal group B streptococcal disease—revised guidelines from CDC, 2010. *MMWR Recomm Rep.* 2010 Nov 19;59(RR-10):1-36.

INTRA-AMNIOTIC INFECTION

Definition
- A bacterial infection of the chorion, amnion, and amniotic fluid often diagnosed during a prolonged labor.

Diagnosis
- Maternal temperature 100.4° F/38.0° C with no other obvious source and one of the following additional findings:
  - Fetal tachycardia
  - Maternal tachycardia
  - Abdominal tenderness
  - Foul-smelling amniotic fluid
  - Leukocytosis
  - Positive amniotic fluid culture

Risk Factors
- Prolonged rupture of membranes
- Multiple vaginal exams in labor and internal monitoring

Antibiotics
- Mezlocillin 4 g IV q4–6hrs or piperacillin 3–4 g IV q4hrs
- Ticarcillin/clavulanic acid 3.1 g IV q6hrs
- Ampicillin/sulbactam 3 g IV q4–6hrs
- Ampicillin 2 g IV q6hrs and gentamicin 1.5 mg/kg load then 1.0 mg/kg q8hrs (if delivery by cesarean section, add clindamycin 900 mg IV q6hrs)

Comments
- Some clinicians continue antibiotics for 24–48 hours afebrile following delivery.
- Chorioamnionitis is not an indication for cesarean delivery.
- Fetal outcome is improved by maternal antibiotic therapy and ↓ temperature. Give IV fluids and acetaminophen for maternal and fetal resuscitation.
- Always consider other sources of maternal fever (pyelonephritis, pneumonia, appendicitis).
- Watch for postpartum hemorrhage and dystocia secondary to inadequate uterine action.
- Chorioamnionitis may represent a risk factor for cerebral palsy.

Table 7.4. Clinical diagnosis of chorioamnionitis

Test	Result Suggesting Chorioamnionitis	Comments
Clinical parameters		Generally nonspecific[4]
Fever	Temperature >100.4 twice or >101 once	95–100 sensitive[4]
Maternal tachycardia	>100/min	50–80% sensitive
Fetal tachycardia	>160/min	40–70% sensitive
Fundal tenderness	tenderness on palpation	4–25% sensitive
Vaginal discharge	Foul-smelling discharge	5–22% sensitive
Amniotic fluid parameters		
Culture	Microbial growth	Diagnostic gold-standard
Gram stain	Bacteria or white blood cells (>6/HPF)	24% sensitive, 99% specific [31]
Glucose level	<15 mg/dL	Affected by maternal hyperglycemia 57% sensitive, 74% specific[31]
Interleukin 6	>7.9 ng/mL	81% sensitive, 75% specific[31]
Matrix Metalloproteinase	Positive result	90% sensitive and 80% specific[30]
White blood cell count	>30/cubic mm	57% sensitive, 78% specific[31]
Leukocyte esterase	Positive (dipsticks)	85–91% sensitive, 95–100% specific[26,32]

[4]Newton (1993).
[31]Romero (1993).
[30]Kim (2007).
[26]Riggs (1998).
[32]Hoskins (1990).

Source: Reproduced with permission from Tita AT, Andrews WW. Diagnosis and management of clinical chorioamnionitis. *Clin Perinatol.* 2010 Jun;37(2):339-54. Copyright © 2010 Elsevier.

FEBRILE MORBIDITY AND ENDOMYOMETRITIS

Definition
- Two temperature elevations to >38° C (100.4° F; outside the first 24 hours after delivery) or
- A temperature of >38.7° C (101.5° F) at any time

Etiology
- Seven Ws of febrile morbidity
    - Womb (endomyometritis)
    - Wind (atelectasis, pneumonia)
    - Water (urinary tract infection or pyelonephritis)
    - Walk (deep vein thrombosis or pulmonary embolism)
    - Wound (wound infection, episiotomy infection)
    - Weaning (breast engorgement, mastitis, breast abscess)
    - Wonder (drug fever—wonder drugs)

Evaluation
- Physical examination including pelvic exam to rule out hematoma or retained membranes
- Complete blood count with differential, urinalysis, urine, and blood cultures as indicated
- Chest X-ray, ultrasound as indicated

Treatment
- Cefotetan 1–2 g IV q12hrs
- Mezlocillin 4 g IV q4–6hr or piperacillin 3–4 g IV q4hrs
- Ticarcillin/clavulanate 3.1 g IV q6hrs
- Ampicillin/sulbactam 3 g IV q4–6hrs
- Gentamicin 1.5 mg/kg load then 1.0 mg/kg q8hrs (or 5 mg/kg q24hrs) and clindamycin 900 mg IV q6hrs (plus ampicillin 2 g IV q6hrs as needed to cover enterococcus)

Comments
- Continue IV antibiotics until 24–48 hours afebrile and improved physical exam.
- Oral antibiotics following IV antibiotics have not been shown to be of proven value.
- If unresponsive following 48–72 hours of IV antibiotics, reexamine the patient.
    - Consider broadening antibiotic coverage to cover enterococcus if using gentamicin and clindamycin.
    - Consider pelvic abscess.
    - Consider septic pelvic thrombophlebitis.
    - Consider drug fever.

MASTITIS AND BREAST ABSCESS
Fast Facts
- Affects 2–3% of nursing mothers.
- Most frequently seen as a nonepidemic mammary cellulitis.
- Usually *Staphylococcus aureus* and must consider MRSA.
- Other pathogens: *b-hemolytic streptococci, H. influenzae, H. parainfluenzae,* Escherichia coli, *Klebsiella pneumoniae.*
- Must distinguish between simple engorgement and infectious process.
- Outpatient antibiotic therapy usually successful but consider IV antibiotics if unresponsive or patient compliance/tolerance uncertain or patient appears septic.
- Breast abscess can form even on antibiotics; surgical drainage may be necessary or ultrasound guided needle aspiration could be considered.

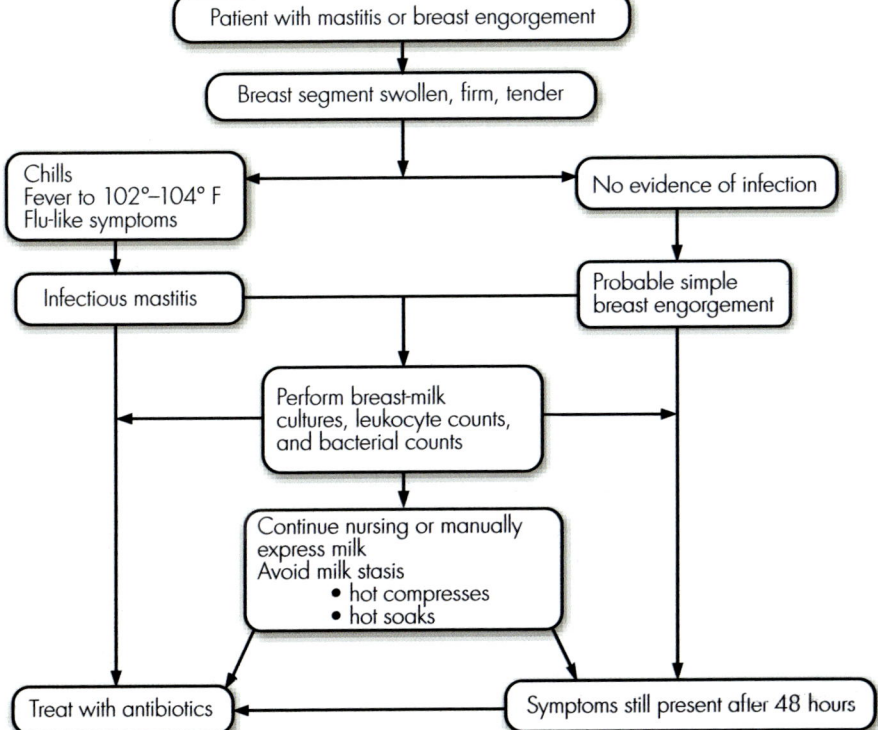

Figure 7.5. Evaluation of the patient with mastitis
Source: Reproduced with permission from Hager, W. David. Managing mastitis. *Cont Ob/Gyn.* 2004:Jan;33-47. *Cont Ob/Gyn* is a copyrighted publication of Advanstar Communications Inc. All rights reserved.

Drug Regimens

Table 7.5. Drug regimens for the treatment of mastitis

Cephalexin (Keflex) 500 mg orally every 6 hr for 7 days
Amoxicillin/Clavulante potassium (Augmentin) 875 mg orally every 12 hr for 7 days
Azithromycin (Zithromax) 500 mg initially, then 250 mg orally daily for 5–7 days
Dicloxacillin 250–500 mg orally every 8 hr for 7 days
Clindamycin 300 mg orally every 8 hr for 7 days

Source: Reproduced with permission from Hager, W. David. Managing mastitis. *Cont Ob/Gyn*. 2004:Jan;33-47. *Cont Ob/Gyn* is a copyrighted publication of Advanstar Communications Inc. All rights reserved.

Prevention

- Avoid cracked or fissured nipples.
- Use plain water to clean nipple area (No. soap or alcohol).
- Increase duration of nursing gradually to avoid soreness.
- Use breast shield or topical cream to help healing of cracked nipples.
- Place finger in corner of baby's mouth during feeding to break sucking force.
- Treat recurrent mastitis promptly but continue breastfeeding.

Patient Information: What to Do If You Develop Mastitis?

Table 7.6. Patient information: what to do if you develop mastitis

If you have symptoms that suggest you have mastitis, you'll need to heed the following advice:

- Continue breastfeeding, starting on the affected side.
- If your baby doesn't feed well or will not feed on the affected breast, empty the breast using a piston-type, hospital breast pump.
- If possible, remain in bed for the first 48 hr.
- Drink more fluids.
- Reduce your salt intake.
- Take acetaminophen or ibuprofen to reduce fever and discomfort so milk letdown will occur and the breast can be emptied.
- Apply moist heat to speed up milk letdown and ease soreness; cool packs may be used initially to decrease swelling.
- Apply gentle massage to move the milk forward and increase drainage from the infected area.
- Avoid breast shells and tight-fitting bras.
- Avoid tight clothing and underwire bras.
- Wash your hands before handling the infected breast.
- Lanolin creams may be used to treat nipples. Your physician may prescribe medication if you develop a fungal infection of the nipple.
- Make sure your baby is in a comfortable nursing position that does not pull excessively on your nipple; if necessary, talk to a lactation consultant to evaluate your nursing technique.
- If you have a fever, the doctor may prescribe antibiotics for 7–10 days. Schedule a follow-up appointment in 7 days so that the doctor can check for an abscess. If your symptoms don't respond within 48 hr of antibiotic treatment, notify the physician.

Source: Reproduced with permission from Hager, W. David. Managing mastitis. *Cont Ob/Gyn*. 2004:Jan;33-47. *Cont Ob/Gyn* is a copyrighted publication of Advanstar Communications Inc. All rights reserved.

HEPATITIS

Table 7.7. Overview of viral hepatitis

	A	B	C	D	E
Virus Family	Picornaviridae	Hepadnaviridae	Flaviviridae	N/A	Appears to be member of Caliciviridae
Transmission	Fecal-oral, permucosal	Percutaneous, permucosal	Percutaneous, permucosal	Percutaneous, permucosal	Fecal-oral (especially contaminated water)
Chronicity	None	6–10% of adults	75–85%	Average 6%	Unknown 25–50% of children (1–5 years of age) 70–90% of infants
Onset	Usually abrupt	Usually insidious	Insidious	Usually abrupt	Usually abrupt average 40 days; range 15–60 days
Incubation	Average 28 days; range 15–45 days; ~0.3%	Average 60–90 days; range 45–180 days	Average 6–7 wk; range 2–26 wk	21–90 days	
Mortality		0.5–1.0%	0.2%–0.4%	2–20% with coinfection, up to 30% with superinfection	About 1–2%; 15–20% in pregnant women

Source: Reprinted with permission from APGO Educational Series on Women's Health Issues. *Sexually transmitted infections hepatitis B and C: the Ob/Gyn's role.* 2002:1–17.

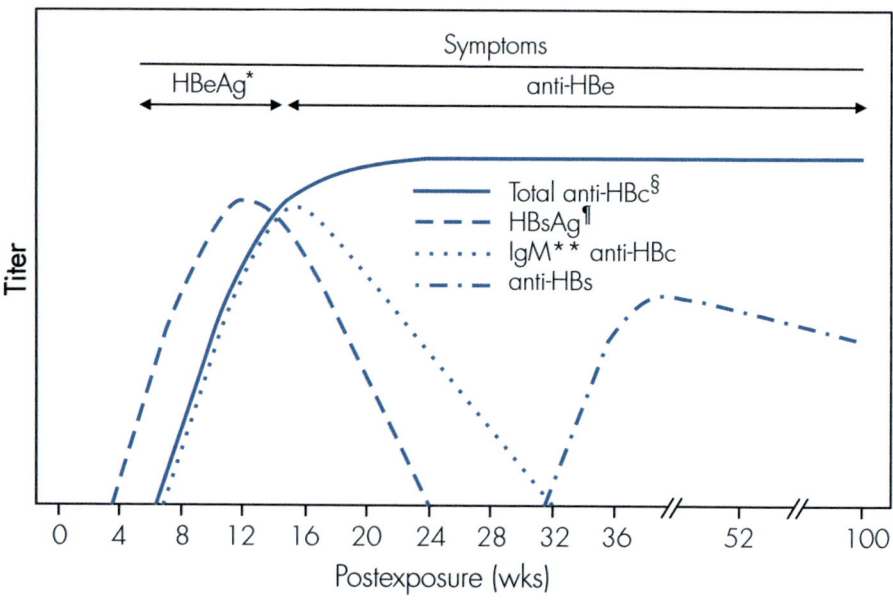

Figure 7.6. Typical serologic course of acute hepatitis B

* Hepatitis B e antigen.
† Antibody to HBeAg.
§ Antibody to hepatitis B core antigen.
¶ Hepatitis B surface antigen.
** Immunoglobulin M.
†† Antibody to HBsAg.
Source: Reproduced from Weinbaum CM, Williams I, Mast EE, Wang SA, Finelli L, Wasley A, Neitzel SM, Ward JW; Centers for Disease Control and Prevention (CDC). Recommendations for identification and public health management of persons with chronic hepatitis B virus infection. *MMWR Recomm Rep.* 2008 Sep 19;57(RR-8):1-20.

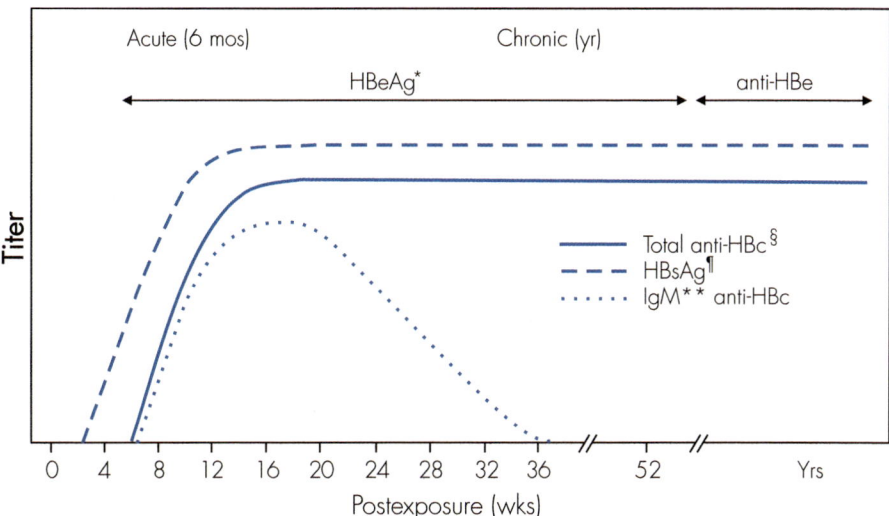

Figure 7.7. Progression to chronic hepatitis B

 * Hepatitis B e antigen.
 † Antibody to HBeAg.
 § Antibody to hepatitis B core antigen.
 ¶ Hepatitis B surface antigen.
 ** Immunoglobulin M.
 Source: Reproduced from Weinbaum CM, Williams I, Mast EE, Wang SA, Finelli L, Wasley A, Neitzel SM, Ward JW; Centers for Disease Control and Prevention (CDC). Recommendations for identification and public health management of persons with chronic hepatitis B virus infection. *MMWR Recomm Rep.* 2008 Sep 19;57(RR-8):1-20.

Table 7.8. Interpretation of serologic test results* for hepatitis B

HBsag	Total anti-HBc	Igm anti-HBc	Anti-HBs	Interpretation
−	−	−	−	Never infected
+†	−	−	−	Early acute infection; transient (up to 18 days) after vaccination
+	+	+	−	Acute infection
−	+	+	−	Acute resolving infection
−	+	−	+	Recovered from past infection and immune
+	+	−	−	Chronic infection
−	+	−	−	False positive (i.e., susceptible); past infection; "low-level" chronic infection§; passive transfer to infant born to HBsAg-positive mother
−	−	−	+	Immune if concentration is >10 mIU/mL, passive transfer after HBIG administration

Anti-HBc, antibody to hepatitis B core antigen; anti-HBs, antibody to hepatitis B surface antigen; HBsAg, hepatitis B surface antigen; IgM, immunoglobulin M; mIU/mL, Milli-international units per milliliter.

*Symbol for negative test result, "−"; symbol for positive test result, "+."

†To ensure that an HBsAg-positive test result is not false-positive, samples with repeatedly reactive HBsAg results should be tested with an FDA-cleared neutralizing confirmatory test.

§Persons positive for only anti-HBc are unlikely to be infectious except under unusual circumstances involving direct percutaneous exposure to large quantities of blood (e.g., blood transfusion and organ transplantation).

Source: Reproduced from Workowski KA, Bolan GA. Sexually transmitted diseases treatment guidelines, 2015. *MMWR Recomm Rep.* 2015 Jun 5;64(RR-03):1-137.

Table 7.9. Interpretation of serologic test results for hepatitis B

HBsAg	negative	Susceptible
anti-HBc	negative	
anti-HBs	negative	
HBsAg	negative	Immune due to natural infection
anti-HBc	positive	
anti-HBs	positive	
HBsAg	negative	Immune due to hepatitis B vaccination
anti-HBc	negative	
anti-HBs	positive	
HBsAg	positive	Acutely infected
anti-HBc	positive	
IgM anti-HBc	positive	
anti-HBs	negative	
HBsAg	positive	Chronically infected
anti-HBc	positive	
IgM anti-HBc	negative	
anti-HBs	negative	
HBsAg	negative	Interpretation unclear; four possibilities:
anti-HBc	positive	1. Resolved infection (most common)
anti-HBs	negative	2. False-positive anti-HBc, thus susceptible
		3. "Low-level" chronic infection
		4. Resolving acute infection

Source: Adapted from Mast EE, Margolis HS, Fiore AE, et al; Advisory Committee on Immunization Practices (ACIP). A comprehensive immunization strategy to eliminate transmission of hepatitis B virus infection in the United States: recommendations of the Advisory Committee on Immunization Practices (ACIP) part 1: immunization of infants, children, and adolescents. *MMWR Recomm Rep.* 2005 Dec 23;54(RR-16):1-31. Erratum in: *MMWR.* 2006 Feb 17;55(6):158-59.

Available Hepatitis B Vaccines

Two single-antigen vaccines and three combination vaccines are currently licensed in the United States.

Single-Antigen Hepatitis B Vaccines
- ENGERIX-B®
- RECOMBIVAX HB®

Combination Vaccines
- COMVAX®: Combined hepatitis B–*Haemophilus influenzae* type b (Hib) conjugate vaccine. Cannot be administered before age 6 weeks or after age 71 months.
- PEDIARIX®: Combined hepatitis B, diphtheria, tetanus, acellular pertussis (DTaP), and inactivated poliovirus (IPV) vaccine. Cannot be administered before age 6 weeks or after age 7 years.
- TWINRIX®: Combined hepatitis A and hepatitis B vaccine. recommended for persons aged ≥18 years who are at increased risk for both hepatitis A virus and HBV infections.

Table 7.10. Recommended doses of currently licensed formulation for hepatitis B vaccine

Recommended Doses of Currently Licensed Formulations of Hepatitis B Vaccine, By Age Group and Vaccine Type

Age Group		Single-antigen Vaccine				Combination Vaccine					
		Recombivax HB		Engerix-B		Comvax*		Pediarix[†]		Twinrix[§]	
		Dose (μg)[¶]	Vol (mL)	Dose (μg)[¶]	Vol (mL)	Dose (μg)[¶]	Vol (mL)	Dose (μg)[¶]	Vol (mL)	Dose (μg)[¶]	Vol (mL)
Infants (<1 yr)		5	0.5	10	0.5	5	0.5	10	0.5	NA**	NA
Children (1–10 yr)		5	0.5	10	0.5	5*	0.5	10[†]	0.5	NA	NA
Adolescents	11–15 yr	10[††]	1.0	NA	NA	NA	NA	NA	NA	NA	NA
	11–19 yr	5	0.5	10	0.5	NA	NA	NA	NA	NA	NA
Adults (≥20 yr)		10	1.0	20	1.0	NA	NA	NA	NA	20[§]	1.0
Hemodialysis patients and other immunocompromised persons	<20 yr[§§]	5	0.5	10	0.5	NA	NA	NA	NA	NA	NA
	≥20 yr	40[¶¶]	1.0	40***	2.0	NA	NA	NA	NA	NA	NA

*Combined hepatitis B–*Haemophilus influenzae* type b conjugate vaccine. This vaccine cannot be administered at birth, before age 6 weeks, or after age 71 months.

[†]Combined hepatitis B, diphtheria, tetanus, acellular pertussis adsorbed, inactivated poliovirus vaccine. This vaccine cannot be administered at birth, before age 6 weeks, or at age >7 years.

[§]Combined hepatitis A and hepatitis B vaccine. This vaccine is recommended for persons aged ≥18 years who are at increased risk for both hepatitis B virus and hepatitis A virus infections.

[¶]Recombinant hepatitis B surface antigen protein dose.

**Not applicable.

[††]Adult formulation administered on a 2-dose schedule.

[§§] Higher doses might be more immunogenic, but no specific recommendations have been made.

[¶¶]Dialysis formulation administered on a 3-dose schedule at 0, 1, and 6 months.

***Two 1.0-mL doses administered at one site, on a 4-dose schedule at 0, 1, 2, and 6 months.

Source: From http://www.cdc.gov/hepatitis/hbv/hbvfaq.htm#vaccFAQ. Accessed on June 2, 2015.

HEPATITIS C
Fast Facts
- Hepatitis C is now the leading indication for liver transplantation in many U.S. medical centers.
- Approximately 50% of hepatitis C cases result from IV drug use.
- Risk of sexual transmission in a discordant monogamous couple is 5% over 10–20 years.
- 85–90% of infected patients are unable to clear the virus and are chronically infected.
- No guidelines for hepatitis C and pregnancy exist.
- Perinatal transmission accounts for probably 2–8% of cases, but it is higher in human immunodeficiency virus (HIV)–positive women.
- Breastfeeding is not an established risk factor. Recommend breastfeeding but discuss nipple care and avoiding breastfeeding temporarily if nipples are cracked and actively bleeding.
- Pregnant women cannot be treated with alpha interferon or ribavirin. There is currently no data on the use of novel antiviral drugs in pregnancy.
- No evidence that cesarean delivery reduces risk of transmission. Cesarean delivery only for standard obstetrical indications.
- Risk of transmission is increased by higher maternal viral load, use of internal fetal monitors, and prolonged rupture of membranes (≥6hr) in labor.

Table 7.11. Interpretation of results of tests for hepatitis C virus (HCV) infection and further actions

Test Outcome	Interpretation	Further Action
HCV antibody nonreactive	No HCV antibody detected	Sample can be reported as nonreactive for HCV antibody. No further action required.
		If recent HCV exposure in person tested is suspected, test for HCV RNA.*
HCV antibody reactive	Presumptive HCV infection	A repeatedly reactive result is consistent with current HCV infection, or past HCV infection that has resolved, or biologic false positively for HCV antibody. Test for HCV RNA to identify current infection.
HCV antibody reactive, HCV RNA detected	Current HCV infection	Provide person tested with appropriate counseling and link person tested to medical care and treatment.†
HCV antibody reactive, HCV RNA not detected	No current HCV infection	No further action required in most cases.
		If distinction between true positivity and biologic false positivity for HCV antibody is desired, and if sample is repeatedly reactive in the initial test, test with another HCV antibody assay.
		In certain situations§ follow up with HCV RNA testing and appropriate counseling.

*If HCV RNA testing is not feasible and person tested is not immunocompromised, do follow-up testing for HCV antibody to demonstrate seroconversion. If the person tested is immunocompromised, consider testing for HCV RNA.

†It is recommended before initiating antiviral therapy to retest for HCV RNA in a subsequent blood sample to confirm HCV RNA positivity.

§If the person tested is suspected of having HCV exposure within the past 6 months, or has clinical evidence of HCV disease, or if there is concern regarding the handling or storage of the test specimen.

Source: Reproduced from Centers for Disease Control and Prevention (CDC). Testing for HCV infection: an update of guidance for clinicians and laboratorians. *MMWR.* 2013 May 10;62(18):362-65.

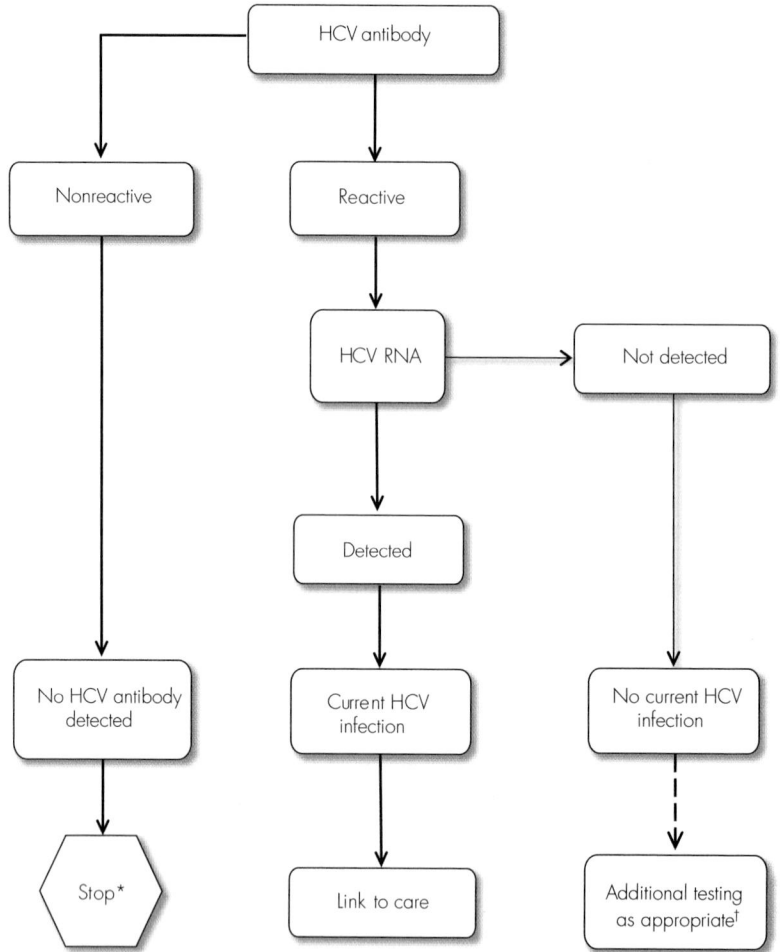

Figure 7.8. Recommended testing sequence for identifying current hepatitis C virus (HCV) infection

* For persons who might have been exposed to HCV within the past 6 months, testing for HCV RNA or follow-up testing for HCV antibody is recommended. For persons who are immunocompromised, testing for HCV RNA can be considered.

† To differentiate past, resolved HCV infection from biologic false positivity for HCV antibody, testing with another HCV antibody assay can be considered. Repeat HCV RNA testing if the person tested is suspected to have had HCV exposure within the past 6 months or has clinical evidence of HCV disease, or if there is concern regarding the handling or storage of the test specimen.

Source: Reproduced from Centers for Disease Control and Prevention (CDC). Testing for HCV infection: an update of guidance for clinicians and laboratorians. *MMWR*. 2013 May 10;62(18):362-65.

MANAGEMENT OF TUBERCULOSIS IN PREGNANCY

Fast Facts
- Untreated tuberculosis (TB) disease represents a greater hazard to a pregnant woman and her fetus than does its treatment.
- Treatment of pregnant women should be initiated whenever the probability of TB is moderate to high.
- Infants born to women with untreated TB may be of lower birth weight than those born to women without TB and, in rare circumstances, the infant may be born with TB.
- Although the drugs used in the initial treatment regimen for TB cross the placenta, they do not appear to have harmful effects on the fetus.

Treatment

Latent TB Infection (LTBI)
- Isoniazid (INH) administered either daily or twice weekly for 9 months is the standard regimen for the treatment of LTBI in pregnant women.
  - Women taking INH should also take pyridoxine (vitamin B6) supplementation.
  - The 12-dose regimen of INH and Rifapentine (RPT) is not recommended for pregnant women or women expecting to be pregnant within the next 3 months.

TB Disease
- Pregnant women should start treatment as soon as TB is suspected.
- The preferred initial treatment regimen is INH, rifampin (RIF), and ethambutol (EMB) daily for 2 months followed by INH and RIF daily, or twice weekly for 7 months (for a total of 9 months of treatment).
- Streptomycin should not be used because it has been shown to have harmful effects on the fetus. In most cases, pyrazinamide (PZA) is not recommended to be used because its effect on fetus is unknown.

HIV Infection
- HIV-infected pregnant women who are suspected of having TB disease should be treated without delay.
- TB treatment regimens for HIV-infected pregnant women should include a rifamycin.
  - Although the routine use of PZA during pregnancy is not recommended in the United States, the benefits of a TB treatment regimen that includes PZA for HIV-infected pregnant women may outweigh the undetermined potential risks to the fetus.

Antituberculosis Drugs Are Contraindicated in Pregnant Women
- Streptomycin
- Kanamycin
- Amikacin
- Capreomycin
- Fluoroquinolones
  - Women who are being treated for drug-resistant TB should receive counseling concerning the risk to the fetus because of the known and unknown risks of second-line antituberculosis drugs.

Breastfeeding

- Breastfeeding should not be discouraged for women being treated with the first-line antituberculosis drugs because the concentrations of these drugs in breast milk are too small to produce toxicity in the nursing newborn.
- For the same reason, drugs in breast milk are not an effective treatment for TB disease or LTBI in a nursing infant.
- Breastfeeding women taking INH should also take pyridoxine (vitamin B6) supplementation.

   Source: National Center for HIV/AIDS, Viral hepatitis, STD, and TB Prevention, Division of Tuberculosis Elimination. TB elimination, tuberculosis and pregnancy. November 2011. http://www.cdc.gov/tb/publications/factsheets/specpop/pregnancy.pdf. Accessed on April 4, 2016.

For More Information

1. CDC. Treatment of tuberculosis. *MMWR*. 2003;52(RR-11). http://www.cdc.gov/mmwr/preview/mmwrhtml/rr5211a1.htm.
2. American Thoracic Society/CDC. Targeted tuberculin testing and treatment of latent TB infection. *MMWR*. 2000:49(RR 6). http://www.cdc.gov/MMWR/PDF/rr/rr4906.pdf.
3. CDC. Guidelines for using the QuantiFERON®-TB Gold test for detecting Mycobacterium tuberculosis infection, United States. *MMWR*. 2005;54(RR-15). http://www.cdc.gov/mmwr/pdf/rr/rr5415.pdf.
4. CDC. Recommendations for use of an Isoniazid–Rifapentine regimen with direct observation to treat latent Mycobacterium tuberculosis infection. *MMWR*. 2011;60:1650–1653. http://www.cdc.gov/mmwr/preview/mmwrhtml/mm6048a3.htm?s_cid=mm6048a3_w.
5. Targeted tuberculosis (TB) testing and treatment of latent TB infection (slide set). http://www.cdc.gov/tb/publications/slidesets/LTBI/default.htm; http://www.cdc.gov/tb.

Management of Tuberculosis in Pregnancy — INFECTIOUS DISEASES

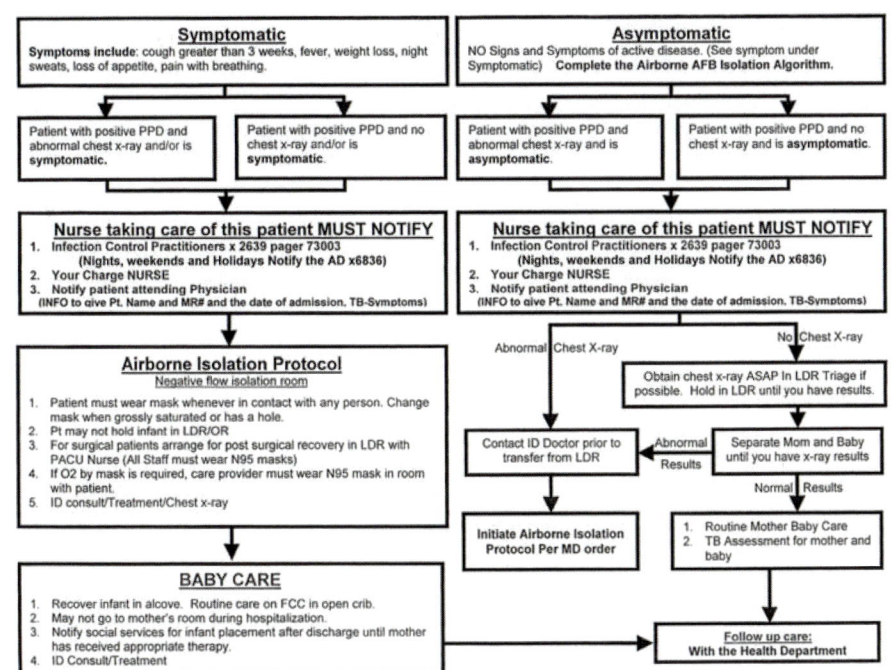

Figure 7.9. Pulmonary tuberculosis control plan
Source: Pulmonary tuberculosis control plan. Inova Fairfax Hospital, Fairfax, VA.

HUMAN IMMUNODEFICIENCY VIRUS
General Principles

Table 7.12. Use of antiretroviral drugs during pregnancy

Panel's Recommendations

- Initial evaluation of HIV-infected pregnant women should include assessment of HIV disease status and recommendations regarding initiation of combination antiretroviral therapy (cART) or the need for any modification if currently receiving cART **(AIII)**. The National Perinatal HIV Hotline (888-448-8765) provides free clinical consultation on all aspects of perinatal HIV care.

- All pregnant HIV-infected women should receive cART to prevent perinatal transmission regardless of plasma HIV RNA copy number or CD4 T lymphocyte count **(AI)**. The goal of cART is to maintain a viral load below the limit of detection throughout pregnancy.

- Combined antepartum, intrapartum, and infant antiretroviral prophylaxis is recommended because antiretroviral drugs reduce perinatal transmission by several mechanisms, including lowering maternal antepartum viral load and providing infant pre- and post-exposure prophylaxis **(AI)**.

- The known benefits and potential risks of all medication use, including antiretroviral use, during pregnancy should be discussed with all HIV-infected women **(AIII)**.

- The importance of adherence to antiretroviral regimens should be emphasized in patient counseling **(AII)**.

- Antiretroviral drug-resistance studies should be performed before starting or modifying ARV drug regimens in women whose HIV RNA levels are above the threshold for resistance testing (i.e., >500 to 1,000 copies/mL) (see Antiretroviral Drug Resistance and Resistance Testing in Pregnancy) **(AIII)**. In pregnant women not already receiving cART, consideration should be given to initiating cART before results of drug-resistance testing are available because earlier viral suppression has been associated with lower risk of transmission. If cART is initiated before results are available, the regimen should be modified, if necessary, based on resistance assay results **(BIII)**.

- Coordination of services among prenatal care providers, primary care and HIV specialty care providers, and when appropriate, mental health and drug abuse treatment services, and public assistance programs, is essential to ensure that infected women adhere to their antiretroviral drug regimens **(AIII)**.

Rating of Recommendations: A = Strong; B = Moderate; C = Optional

Rating of Evidence: I = One or more randomized trials with clinical outcomes and/or validated laboratory endpoints; II = One or more well-designed, nonrandomized trials or observational cohort studies with long-term clinical outcomes; III = Expert opinion

Source: Reproduced from Panel on Treatment of HIV-Infected Pregnant Women and Prevention of Perinatal Transmission. Recommendations for use of antiretroviral drugs in pregnant HIV-1-infected women for maternal health and interventions to reduce perinatal HIV transmission in the United States. Available at http://aidsinfo.nih.gov/contentfiles/lvguidelines/PerinatalGL.pdf. Accessed April 4, 2016. All items were last updated August 6, 2015; last reviewed August 6, 2015.

Human Immunodeficiency Virus — INFECTIOUS DISEASES

Table 7.13. What to start: initial combination regimens for antiretroviral-naive pregnant women

These recommendations are for pregnant women who have never received antiretroviral therapy (ART) previously (i.e., antiretroviral-naive) and are predicated on lack of evidence of resistance to regimen components. See Table for more information on specific drugs and dosing in pregnancy. Within each drug class, regimens are listed alphabetically, and the order does not indicate a ranking of preference. It is recommended that women who become pregnant while on a stable ARV regimen with viral suppression remain on that same regimen.

Drug	Comments
Preferred Regimens	
Regimens with clinical trial data in adults demonstrating optimal efficacy and durability with acceptable toxicity and ease of use, PK data available in pregnancy, and no evidence to date of teratogenic effects or established adverse outcomes for mother/fetus/newborn. To minimize the risk of resistance, a PI regimen is preferred for women who may stop ART during the postpartum period.	
Preferred Two-NRTI Backbone	
ABC/3TC	Available as FDC. Can be administered once daily. ABC **should not be used** in patients who test positive for HLA-B*5701 because of risk of hypersensitivity reaction. ABC/3TC with ATV/r or with EFV is not recommended if pretreatment HIV RNA >100,000 copies/mL.
TDF/FTC or 3TC	TDF/FTC available as FDC. Either TDF/FTC or TDF and 3TC can be administered once daily. TDF has potential renal toxicity, thus TDF-based dual NRTI combinations should be used with caution in patients with renal insufficiency.
ZDV/3TC	Available as FDC. NRTI combination with most experience for use in pregnancy but has disadvantages of requirement for twice-daily administration and increased potential for hematologic toxicities.
Preferred PI Regimens	
ATV/r plus a Preferred Two-NRTI Backbone	Once-daily administration. Extensive experience in pregnancy. Maternal hyperbilirubinemia
DRV/r plus a Preferred Two-NRTI Backbone	Better tolerated than LPV/r. PK data available. Increasing experience with use in pregnancy. Must be used twice daily in pregnancy.
Preferred NNRTI Regimen	
EFV plus a Preferred Two-NRTI Backbone Note: May be initiated after the first 8 weeks of pregnancy	Concern because of birth defects seen in primate study; risk in humans is unclear (see Teratogenicity and Table 7). Postpartum contraception must be ensured. Preferred regimen in women who require co-administration of drugs with significant interactions with PIs or the convenience of co-formulated, single-tablet, once-daily regimen.
Preferred Integrase Inhibitor Regimen	
RAL plus a Preferred Two-NRTI Backbone	PK data available and increasing experience in pregnancy. Rapid viral load reduction. Useful when drug interactions with PI regimens are a concern. Twice-daily dosing required.
Alternative Regimens	
Regimens with clinical trial data demonstrating efficacy in adults but one or more of the following apply: experience in pregnancy is limited, data are lacking or incomplete on teratogenicity, or regimen is associated with dosing, formulation, toxicity, or interaction issues	
PI Regimens	
LPV/r plus a Preferred Two-NRTI Backbone	Abundant experience and established PK in pregnancy. More nausea than preferred agents. Twice-daily administration. Once-daily LPV/r is not recommended for use in pregnant women.
NNRTI Regimen	
RPV/TDF/FTC (or RPV plus a Preferred Two-NRTI Backbone)	RPV not recommended with pretreatment HIV RNA >100,000 copies/mL or CD4 cell count <200 cells/mm^3. Do not use with PPIs. PK data available in pregnancy but relatively little experience with use in pregnancy. Available in co-formulated single-pill once daily regimen.

INFECTIOUS DISEASES — Human Immunodeficiency Virus

Drug	Comments
Insufficient Data in Pregnancy to Recommend Routine Use in ART-Naive Women	
Drugs that are approved for use in adults but lack adequate pregnancy-specific PK or safety data	
DTG	No data on use of DTG in pregnancy
EVG/COBI/TDF/FTC Fixed Drug Combination	No data on use of EVG/COBI component in pregnancy.
FPV	Limited data on use in pregnancy.
MVC	MVC requires tropism testing before use. Few case reports of use in pregnancy.
COBI	No data on use of COBI (including co-formulations with ATV or DRV) in pregnancy.
Not Recommended	
Drugs whose use is not recommended because of toxicity, lower rate of viral suppression or because not recommended in ART-naive populations	
ABC/3TC/ZDV	Generally not recommended due to inferior virologic efficacy.
d4T	Not recommended due to toxicity.
ddI	Not recommended due to toxicity.
IDV/r	Nephrolithiasis, maternal hyperbilirubinemia.
NFV	Lower rate of viral suppression with NFV compared to LPV/r or EFV in adult trials.
RTV	RTV as a single PI is not recommended because of inferior efficacy and increased toxicity.
SQV/r	Not recommended based on potential toxicity and dosing disadvantages. Baseline ECG is recommended before initiation of SQV/r because of potential PR and QT prolongation; contraindicated with pre-existing cardiac conduction system disease. Limited data in pregnancy. Large pill burden. Twice daily dosing required.
ETR	Not recommended in ART-naive populations
NVP	Not recommended because of greater potential for adverse events, complex lead-in dosing, and low barrier to resistance. NVP should be used with caution when initiating ART in women with CD4 cell count >250 cells/mm^3. Use NVP and ABC together with caution; both can cause hypersensitivity reactions within the first few weeks after initiation.
T20	Not recommended in ART-naive populations
TPV/r	Not recommended in ART-naive populations

Key to Acronyms: 3TC = lamivudine; ABC = abacavir; ART = antiretroviral therapy; ARV = antiretroviral; ATV/r = atazanavir/ritonavir; CD4 = CD4 T lymphocyte cell; COBI = cobicistat; d4T = stavudine; ddI = didanosine; DTG = dolutegravir; DRV/r = darunavir/ritonavir; ECG = electrocardiogram; EFV = efavirenz; ETR = etravirine; EVG = elvitegravir; FDC = fixed-dose combination; FPV = fosamprenavir; FTC = emtricitabine; IDV/r = indinavir/ritonavir; LPV/r = lopinavir/ritonavir; MVC = maraviroc; NFV = nelfinavir; NRTI = nucleoside reverse transcriptase inhibitor; NNRTI = non-nucleoside reverse transcriptase inhibitor; NVP = nevirapine; PI = protease inhibitor; PPI = proton pump inhibitor; PK = pharmacokinetic; RAL = raltegravir; RPV = rilpivirine; RTV = ritonavir; SQV/r = saquinavir/ritonavir; T20 = enfuvirtide; TDF = tenofovir disoproxil fumarate; TPV = tipranavir; ZDV = zidovudine

Source: Reproduced from Panel on Treatment of HIV-Infected Pregnant Women and Prevention of Perinatal Transmission. Recommendations for use of antiretroviral drugs in pregnant HIV-1-infected women for maternal health and interventions to reduce perinatal HIV transmission in the United States. Available at http://aidsinfo.nih.gov/contentfiles/lvguidelines/PerinatalGL.pdf. Accessed April 4, 2016. All items were last updated August 6, 2015; last reviewed August 6, 2015.

Table 7.14. HIV-infected pregnant women who have never received antiretroviral drugs (antiretroviral naive)

Panel's Recommendations
• All HIV-infected pregnant women should receive combination antiretroviral therapy (cART) to reduce the risk of perinatal transmission of HIV **(AI)**. The choice of regimen should take into account current adult treatment guidelines, what is known about the use of specific drugs in pregnancy, and the risk of teratogenicity (see Table 6 and Table 7).
• Consideration should be given to initiating cART as soon as HIV is diagnosed during pregnancy; earlier viral suppression is associated with lower risk of transmission. This decision may be influenced by CD4 T lymphocyte count, HIV RNA levels, and maternal conditions (e.g., nausea and vomiting) **(AIII)**. The benefits of early cART must be weighed against potential fetal effects of drug exposure.
• Antiretroviral drug-resistance studies should be performed to guide selection of antiretroviral regimens in women whose HIV RNA levels are above the threshold for resistance testing (i.e., >500 to 1,000 copies/mL) unless drug-resistance studies have already been performed (see Antiretroviral Drug Resistance and Resistance Testing in Pregnancy) **(AI)**. If cART is initiated before the results of the drug-resistance assays are available, the antiretroviral regimen should be modified, if necessary, based on the resistance assay results **(BIII)**.
• If there is no evidence of resistance, cART regimens that are preferred for the treatment of antiretroviral-naive HIV-infected pregnant women include: a dual nucleoside reverse transcriptase inhibitor combination (abacavir/lamivudine, tenofovir disoproxil fumarate/emtricitabine or lamivudine, or zidovudine/lamivudine) and either a ritonavir-boosted protease inhibitor (atazanavir/ritonavir or darunavir/ritonavir), a non-nucleoside reverse transcriptase inhibitor (efavirenz initiated after 8 weeks of pregnancy), or an integrase inhibitor (raltegravir) (see Table 6) **(AIII)**.

Rating of Recommendations: A = Strong; B = Moderate; C = Optional

Rating of Evidence: I = One or more randomized trials with clinical outcomes and/or validated laboratory endpoints; II = One or more well-designed, nonrandomized trials or observational cohort studies with long-term clinical outcomes; III = Expert opinion

Source: Reproduced from Panel on Treatment of HIV-Infected Pregnant Women and Prevention of Perinatal Transmission. Recommendations for use of antiretroviral drugs in pregnant HIV-1-infected women for maternal health and interventions to reduce perinatal HIV transmission in the United States. Available at http://aidsinfo.nih.gov/contentfiles/lvguidelines/PerinatalGL.pdf. Accessed April 4, 2016. All items were last updated August 6, 2015; last reviewed August 6, 2015.

Table 7.15. HIV-infected pregnant women who are currently receiving antiretroviral therapy

Panel's Recommendations
• In general, HIV-infected pregnant women receiving combination antiretroviral therapy (cART) who present for care during the first trimester should continue treatment during pregnancy, assuming the regimen is tolerated and effective in suppressing viral replication (HIV-1 viral load less than lower limits of detection of the assay) **(AII)**.
• The Panel recommends that efavirenz be continued in pregnant women receiving efavirenz-based cART who present for antenatal care in the first trimester, provided the regimen is achieving virologic suppression **(CIII)**.
• HIV antiretroviral drug-resistance testing should be performed to assist in the selection of active drugs when changing antiretroviral regimens in pregnant women on therapy with virologic failure and HIV RNA levels >1,000 copies/mL **(AI)**. In individuals with HIV RNA levels >500 but <1,000 copies/mL, testing may be unsuccessful but should still be considered **(BII)** (see Lack of Viral Suppression).

Rating of Recommendations: A = Strong; B = Moderate; C = Optional

Rating of Evidence: I = One or more randomized trials with clinical outcomes and/or validated laboratory endpoints; II = One or more well-designed, nonrandomized trials or observational cohort studies with long-term clinical outcomes; III = Expert opinion

Source: Reproduced from Panel on Treatment of HIV-Infected Pregnant Women and Prevention of Perinatal Transmission. Recommendations for use of antiretroviral drugs in pregnant HIV-1-infected women for maternal health and interventions to reduce perinatal HIV transmission in the United States. Available at http://aidsinfo.nih.gov/contentfiles/lvguidelines/PerinatalGL.pdf. Accessed April 4, 2016. All items were last updated August 6, 2015; last reviewed August 6, 2015.

Table 7.16. HIV-infected pregnant women who have previously received antiretroviral treatment or prophylaxis but are not currently receiving any antiretroviral medications

Panel's Recommendations
• Obtain an accurate history of all prior antiretroviral regimens used for treatment of HIV disease or prevention of transmission, including virologic efficacy, tolerance to the medications, results of prior resistance testing, and any adherence issues **(AIII)**.
• If HIV RNA is above the threshold for resistance testing (i.e., >500 copies/mL), antiretroviral drug-resistance studies should be performed before starting an antiretroviral drug regimen (see Antiretroviral Drug Resistance and Resistance Testing in Pregnancy) **(AI)**.
• Consideration should be given to initiating combination antiretroviral therapy (cART) prior to receiving results of antiretroviral drug-resistance studies in light of data demonstrating an association between earlier viral suppression and lower risk of HIV transmission. The antiretroviral regimen should be modified based on the results of the resistance assay, if necessary **(BIII)**.
• Choose and initiate a cART regimen based on results of resistance testing if available and prior history of cART while avoiding drugs with known adverse potential for the mother or fetus/infant **(AII)**.
• Consider obtaining a consultation with specialists in treatment of HIV infection about the choice of a cART regimen in women who previously received antiretroviral drugs **(BIII)**.
• Perform repeat antiretroviral drug-resistance testing **(AI)**, assess adherence, and consult with an HIV treatment specialist to guide changes in ARV drugs in women who do not achieve virologic suppression on their antiretroviral regimens **(AIII)** (see Monitoring of the Woman and Fetus During Pregnancy).
Rating of Recommendations: A = Strong; B = Moderate; C = Optional
Rating of Evidence: I = One or more randomized trials with clinical outcomes and/or validated laboratory endpoints; II = One or more well-designed, nonrandomized trials or observational cohort studies with long-term clinical outcomes; III = Expert opinion

Source: Reproduced from Panel on Treatment of HIV-Infected Pregnant Women and Prevention of Perinatal Transmission. Recommendations for use of antiretroviral drugs in pregnant HIV-1-infected women for maternal health and interventions to reduce perinatal HIV transmission in the United States. Available at http://aidsinfo.nih.gov/contentfiles/lvguidelines/PerinatalGL.pdf. Accessed April 4, 2016. All items were last updated August 6, 2015; last reviewed August 6, 2015.

Antepartum Care

Table 7.17. Monitoring of the woman and fetus during pregnancy

Panel's Recommendations
• Plasma HIV RNA levels should be monitored at the initial visit **(AI)**; 2 to 4 weeks after initiating (or changing) antiretroviral drug regimens **(BI)**; monthly until RNA levels are undetectable **(BIII)**; and then at least every 3 months during pregnancy **(BIII)**. HIV RNA levels also should be assessed at approximately 34 to 36 weeks' gestation to inform decisions about mode of delivery (see Transmission and Mode of Delivery) and to inform decisions about optimal treatment of the newborn (see Infant ARV Prophylaxis) **(AIII)**.
• CD4 T lymphocyte (CD4) cell count should be monitored at the initial antenatal visit **(AI)** and at least every 3 months during pregnancy **(BIII)**. Monitoring of CD4 cell count can be performed every 6 months in patients on combination antiretroviral therapy (cART) with consistently suppressed viral load who have CD4 counts well above the threshold for opportunistic infection risk) **(CIII)**.
• Genotypic antiretroviral drug-resistance testing should be performed at baseline in all HIV-infected pregnant women with HIV RNA levels >1,000 copies/mL **(AI)**. In individuals with HIV RNA levels >500 but <1,000 copies/mL, testing may be unsuccessful but should still be considered **(BII)**. Tests should be performed whether the women are antiretroviral-naive or currently on therapy **(AIII)**.
• HIV drug-resistance studies should be performed before modifying antiretroviral regimens for those entering pregnancy with detectable HIV RNA levels that are above the threshold for resistance testing (i.e., >500 to 1,000 copies/mL) while receiving antiretroviral drugs. They should also be performed on women who have suboptimal viral suppression after starting ARV drugs during pregnancy **(AII)**.
• Monitoring for complications of antiretroviral drugs during pregnancy should be based on what is known about the adverse effects of the drugs a woman is receiving **(AIII)**.
• HIV-infected women taking cART during pregnancy should undergo standard glucose screening at 24 to 28 weeks' gestation **(AIII)**. Some experts would perform earlier glucose screening in women receiving ongoing protease inhibitor-based regimens initiated before pregnancy, similar to recommendations for women with risk factors for glucose intolerance **(BIII)**. For further information on protease inhibitors see Combination Antiretroviral Drug Regimens and Pregnancy Outcome.
• Early ultrasound is recommended to confirm gestational age and, if scheduled cesarean delivery is necessary, to guide timing of the procedure (see Transmission and Mode of Delivery) **(AII)**.
• In women on effective cART, no perinatal transmissions have been reported after amniocentesis, but a small risk of transmission cannot be ruled out. Amniocentesis should be performed on HIV-infected women only after initiation of an effective cART regimen and, ideally, when HIV RNA levels are undetectable **(BIII)**. In women with detectable HIV RNA levels in whom amniocentesis is deemed necessary, consultation with an expert should be considered **(BIII)**.

Rating of Recommendations: A = Strong; B = Moderate; C = Optional

Rating of Evidence: I = One or more randomized trials with clinical outcomes and/or validated laboratory endpoints; II = One or more well-designed, nonrandomized trials or observational cohort studies with long-term clinical outcomes; III = Expert opinion

Source: Reproduced from Panel on Treatment of HIV-Infected Pregnant Women and Prevention of Perinatal Transmission. Recommendations for use of antiretroviral drugs in pregnant HIV-1-infected women for maternal health and interventions to reduce perinatal HIV transmission in the United States. Available at http://aidsinfo.nih.gov/contentfiles/lvguidelines/PerinatalGL.pdf. Accessed April 4, 2016. All items were last updated August 6, 2015; last reviewed August 6, 2015.

INFECTIOUS DISEASES — Human Immunodeficiency Virus

Table 7.18. Antiretroviral drug resistance and resistance testing in pregnancy

Panel's Recommendations

- HIV drug-resistance studies should be performed before starting antiretroviral (ARV) regimens in all ARV-naive pregnant women whose HIV RNA levels are above the threshold for resistance testing (i.e., >500 to 1,000 copies/mL) unless they have already been tested for ARV resistance **(AIII)**.
- HIV drug-resistance studies should be performed before modifying ARV regimens for those entering pregnancy with detectable HIV RNA levels that are above the threshold for resistance testing (i.e., >500 to 1,000 copies/mL) while receiving ARV drugs or who have suboptimal virologic response to ARV drugs started during pregnancy **(AIII)**.
- Combination antiretroviral therapy (cART) should be initiated in pregnant women prior to receiving results of ARV-resistance studies. The ARV regimen should be modified, if necessary, based on the results of the resistance assay **(BIII)**.
- Documented zidovudine resistance does not affect the indications for use of intrapartum zidovudine **(BIII)**.
- The optimal prophylactic regimen for newborns of women with ARV resistance is unknown. Therefore, ARV prophylaxis for an infant born to a woman with known or suspected drug resistance should be determined in consultation with a pediatric HIV specialist, preferably before delivery (see Infant Antiretroviral Prophylaxis) **(AIII)**.
- HIV-infected pregnant women should be given cART to maximally suppress viral replication, which is the most effective strategy for preventing development of resistance and minimizing risk of perinatal transmission **(AII)**.
- All pregnant and postpartum women should be counseled about the importance of adherence to prescribed ARV medications to reduce the potential for development of resistance **(AII)**.
- To minimize development of resistance, pregnant women who receive a non-nucleoside reverse transcriptase inhibitor (NNRTI)-based cART regimen that is discontinued after delivery should receive either dual nucleoside analogue reverse transcriptase inhibitor agents alone **(AI)** or with a protease inhibitor **(BII)** for 7 to 30 days **(AII)** after stopping the NNRTI drug. The optimal interval between stopping an NNRTI and the other ARV drugs is unknown (see Stopping Antiretroviral Drugs During Pregnancy and Postpartum Follow-Up of HIV-Infected Women).

Rating of Recommendations: A = Strong; B = Moderate; C = Optional

Rating of Evidence: I = One or more randomized trials with clinical outcomes and/or validated laboratory endpoints; II = One or more well-designed, nonrandomized trials or observational cohort studies with long-term clinical outcomes; III = Expert opinion

Source: Reproduced from Panel on Treatment of HIV-Infected Pregnant Women and Prevention of Perinatal Transmission. Recommendations for use of antiretroviral drugs in pregnant HIV-1-infected women for maternal health and interventions to reduce perinatal HIV transmission in the United States. Available at http://aidsinfo.nih.gov/contentfiles/lvguidelines/PerinatalGL.pdf. Accessed April 4, 2016. All items were last updated August 6, 2015; last reviewed August 6, 2015.

Human Immunodeficiency Virus   INFECTIOUS DISEASES

Table 7.19. Lack of viral suppression

Panel's Recommendations
• Because maternal antenatal viral load correlates with risk of perinatal transmission of HIV, suppression of HIV RNA to undetectable levels should be achieved as rapidly as possible **(AII)**.

• If an ultrasensitive HIV RNA assay indicates failure of viral suppression (after an adequate period of treatment):
    ○ Assess adherence and resistance (if HIV RNA level is high enough for resistance testing) **(AII)**.
    ○ Consult an HIV treatment expert and consider possible antiretroviral regimen modification **(AIII)**.

• Scheduled cesarean delivery is recommended for HIV-infected pregnant women who have HIV RNA levels >1,000 copies/mL near the time of delivery **(AII)**.
Rating of Recommendations: A = Strong; B = Moderate; C = Optional
Rating of Evidence: I = One or more randomized trials with clinical outcomes and/or validated laboratory endpoints; II = One or more well-designed, nonrandomized trials or observational cohort studies with long-term clinical outcomes; III = Expert opinion

Source: Reproduced from Panel on Treatment of HIV-Infected Pregnant Women and Prevention of Perinatal Transmission. Recommendations for use of antiretroviral drugs in pregnant HIV-1-infected women for maternal health and interventions to reduce perinatal HIV transmission in the United States. Available at http://aidsinfo.nih.gov/contentfiles/lvguidelines/PerinatalGL.pdf. Accessed April 4, 2016. All items were last updated August 6, 2015; last reviewed August 6, 2015.

Table 7.20. Stopping antiretroviral drugs during pregnancy

Panel's Recommendations
• HIV-infected women receiving combination antiretroviral therapy who present for care during the first trimester should continue treatment during pregnancy **(AII)**.
• If an antiretroviral drug regimen is stopped acutely for severe or life-threatening toxicity, severe pregnancy-induced hyperemesis unresponsive to antiemetics, or other acute illnesses that preclude oral intake, all antiretroviral drugs should be stopped simultaneously and ARV therapy should be reinitiated as soon as possible **(AIII)**.
Rating of Recommendations: A = Strong; B = Moderate; C = Optional
Rating of Evidence: I = One or more randomized trials with clinical outcomes and/or validated laboratory endpoints; II = One or more well-designed, nonrandomized trials or observational cohort studies with long-term clinical outcomes; III = Expert opinion

Source: Reproduced from Panel on Treatment of HIV-Infected Pregnant Women and Prevention of Perinatal Transmission. Recommendations for use of antiretroviral drugs in pregnant HIV-1-infected women for maternal health and interventions to reduce perinatal HIV transmission in the United States. Available at http://aidsinfo.nih.gov/contentfiles/lvguidelines/PerinatalGL.pdf. Accessed April 4, 2016. All items were last updated August 6, 2015; last reviewed August 6, 2015.

INFECTIOUS DISEASES — Human Immunodeficiency Virus

Intrapartum Care

Table 7.21. Intrapartum antiretroviral therapy/prophylaxis

Panel's Recommendations

- Women should continue their antepartum combination antiretroviral therapy (cART) drug regimen on schedule as much as possible during labor and before scheduled cesarean delivery **(AIII)**.
- Intravenous (IV) zidovudine should be administered to HIV-infected women with HIV RNA >1,000 copies/mL (or unknown HIV RNA) near delivery **(AI)**, but is not required for HIV-infected women receiving cART regimens who have HIV RNA ≤1,000 copies/mL during late pregnancy and near delivery and no concerns regarding adherence to the cART regimen **(BII)**. Scheduled cesarean delivery at 38 weeks' gestation (compared to 39 weeks for most indications) is recommended for women who have HIV RNA >1,000 copies/mL near delivery (see Transmission and Mode of Delivery) **(AI)**.
- Women who present in labor with unknown HIV status should undergo expedited HIV testing **(AII)**. If the results are positive, a confirmatory HIV test should be done as soon as possible and maternal (IV zidovudine)/infant (combination antiretroviral [ARV] prophylaxis) ARV drugs should be initiated pending results of the confirmatory test **(AII)**. If the maternal confirmatory HIV test is positive, infant ARV drugs should be managed as discussed in the Infant Antiretroviral Prophylaxis section **(AI)**; if the maternal confirmatory HIV test is negative, the maternal and infant ARV drugs should be stopped.

Rating of Recommendations: A = Strong; B = Moderate; C = Optional

Rating of Evidence: I = One or more randomized trials with clinical outcomes and/or validated laboratory endpoints; II = One or more well-designed, nonrandomized trials or observational cohort studies with long-term clinical outcomes; III = Expert opinion

Source: Reproduced from Panel on Treatment of HIV-Infected Pregnant Women and Prevention of Perinatal Transmission. Recommendations for use of antiretroviral drugs in pregnant HIV-1-infected women for maternal health and interventions to reduce perinatal HIV transmission in the United States. Available at http://aidsinfo.nih.gov/contentfiles/lvguidelines/PerinatalGL.pdf. Accessed April 4, 2016. All items were last updated August 6, 2015; last reviewed August 6, 2015.

Human Immunodeficiency Virus — INFECTIOUS DISEASES

Table 7.22. Transmission and mode of delivery

Panel's Recommendations
• Scheduled cesarean delivery at 38 weeks' gestation to minimize perinatal transmission of HIV is recommended for women with HIV RNA levels >1000 copies/mL or unknown HIV levels near the time of delivery, irrespective of administration of antepartum antiretroviral drugs **(AII)**. Scheduled cesarean delivery performed solely for prevention of perinatal transmission in women receiving combination antiretroviral therapy with HIV RNA ≤1000 copies/mL is not routinely recommended due to the low rate of perinatal transmission in this group and the potential for increased complications following cesarean delivery in HIV-infected women **(AII)**. In women with HIV RNA levels ≤1000 copies/mL, cesarean delivery performed for standard obstetrical indications should be scheduled at 39 weeks' gestation **(AII)**.
• Because there is insufficient evidence to determine whether cesarean delivery after rupture of membranes or onset of labor reduces the risk of perinatal HIV transmission, management of women originally scheduled for cesarean delivery who present with ruptured membranes or in labor must be individualized at the time of presentation **(BII)**. In these circumstances, consultation with an expert in perinatal HIV (e.g., telephone consultation with the National Perinatal HIV/AIDS Clinical Consultation Center at (888) 448-8765) may be helpful in rapidly developing an individualized plan.
• Women with HIV infection should be counseled that HIV infection may put them at higher risk of surgical complications of cesarean delivery **(AII)**.
Rating of Recommendations: A = Strong; B = Moderate; C = Optional
Rating of Evidence: I = One or more randomized trials with clinical outcomes and/or validated laboratory endpoints; II = One or more well-designed, nonrandomized trials or observational cohort studies with long-term clinical outcomes; III = Expert opinion

Source: Reproduced from Panel on Treatment of HIV-Infected Pregnant Women and Prevention of Perinatal Transmission. Recommendations for use of antiretroviral drugs in pregnant HIV-1-infected women for maternal health and interventions to reduce perinatal HIV transmission in the United States. Available at http://aidsinfo.nih.gov/contentfiles/lvguidelines/PerinatalGL.pdf. Accessed April 4, 2016. All items were last updated August 6, 2015; last reviewed August 6, 2015.

Table 7.23. Other intrapartum management considerations

Panel's Recommendations

• The following should generally be avoided because of a potential increased risk of transmission, unless there are clear obstetric indications:
  • Artificial rupture of membranes **(BIII)**
  • Routine use of fetal scalp electrodes for fetal monitoring **(BIII)**
  • Operative delivery with forceps or a vacuum extractor and/or episiotomy **(BIII)**

• The antiretroviral drug regimen a woman is receiving should be taken into consideration when treating excessive postpartum bleeding resulting from uterine atony:
  • In women who are receiving a cytochrome P450 (CYP) 3A4 enzyme inhibitor such as a protease inhibitor, methergine should be used only if no alternative treatments for postpartum hemorrhage are available and the need for pharmacologic treatment outweighs the risks. If methergine is used, it should be administered in the lowest effective dose for the shortest possible duration **(BIII)**.
  • In women who are receiving a CYP3A4 enzyme inducer such as nevirapine, efavirenz, or etravirine, additional uterotonic agents may be needed because of the potential for decreased methergine levels and inadequate treatment effect **(BIII)**.

Rating of Recommendations: A = Strong; B = Moderate; C = Optional
Rating of Evidence: I = One or more randomized trials with clinical outcomes and/or validated laboratory endpoints; II = One or more well-designed, nonrandomized trials or observational cohort studies with long-term clinical outcomes; III = Expert opinion

Source: Reproduced from Panel on Treatment of HIV-Infected Pregnant Women and Prevention of Perinatal Transmission. Recommendations for use of antiretroviral drugs in pregnant HIV-1-infected women for maternal health and interventions to reduce perinatal HIV transmission in the United States. Available at http://aidsinfo.nih.gov/contentfiles/lvguidelines/PerinatalGL.pdf. Accessed April 4, 2016. All items were last updated August 6, 2015; last reviewed August 6, 2015.

Postpartum Care

Table 7.24. Postpartum management

Panel's Recommendations

- Decisions regarding continuing combination antiretroviral therapy (cART) after delivery should be made in consultation with the woman and her HIV provider, ideally before delivery **(AIII)**. cART is currently recommended for all HIV-infected individuals to reduce the risk of disease progression and to prevent HIV sexual transmission **(AI)**. Decisions should take into account current recommendations for initiation of cART in adults, HIV RNA levels, adherence issues, whether a woman has an HIV-uninfected sexual partner, and patient preferences.
- Because the immediate postpartum period poses unique challenges to antiretroviral adherence, arrangements for new or continued supportive services should be made before hospital discharge for women continuing cART **(AII)**.
- Contraceptive counseling should be a critical aspect of postpartum care **(AIII)**.
- Women with a positive rapid HIV antibody test during labor require immediate linkage to HIV care and comprehensive follow-up, including confirmation of HIV infection. If infection is confirmed, a full health assessment is warranted, including evaluation for associated medical conditions, counseling related to newly diagnosed HIV infection, and assessment of need for cART and opportunistic infection prophylaxis **(AII)**.
- Breastfeeding is not recommended for HIV-infected women in the United States **(AII)**.

Rating of Recommendations: A = Strong; B = Moderate; C = Optional

Rating of Evidence: I = One or more randomized trials with clinical outcomes and/or validated laboratory endpoints; II = One or more well-designed, nonrandomized trials or observational cohort studies with long-term clinical outcomes; III = Expert opinion

Source: Reproduced from Panel on Treatment of HIV-Infected Pregnant Women and Prevention of Perinatal Transmission. Recommendations for use of antiretroviral drugs in pregnant HIV-1-infected women for maternal health and interventions to reduce perinatal HIV transmission in the United States. Available at http://aidsinfo.nih.gov/contentfiles/lvguidelines/PerinatalGL.pdf. Accessed April 4, 2016. All items were last updated August 6, 2015; last reviewed August 6, 2015.

VARICELLA
Fast Facts
- Assess varicella immunity at the beginning of pregnancy either by maternal history or laboratory confirmation of varicella IgG.
- Prior to the introduction of VZV vaccines, 0.4–0.7/1,000 pregnancies are complicated by maternal chickenpox. The rate is likely lower given the routine use of vaccination that began in 1995.
- Congenital varicella syndrome development is rare. The risk is 0.4% after first trimester exposure, 2% after second trimester exposure, and 0% with third trimester exposure.
  - Manifestations of congenital varicella include skin scarring, limb hypoplasia, chorioretinitis, and microcephaly.
  - Ultrasound findings of congenital varicella include hydrops, hyperechogenic foci in the liver and bowel, cardiac malformations, limb deformities, microcephaly, and fetal growth restriction.
- Risk of neonatal varicella is highest if the infant is delivered 2 days before onset of maternal rash through 5 days after onset of rash.
  - Neonatal varicella infection confers a high risk of death.
  - Avoid delivery during this time period if possible.
- Oral or IV acyclovir can be used to reduce the duration and severity of symptoms and may reduce morbidity and mortality.
- 10–20% of pregnant varicella patients develop varicella pneumonia, which is associated with a 40% mortality rate.
  - Maternal acyclovir does not appear to alter the risk of congenital varicella syndrome.
- There is no fetal risk in cases of maternal herpes zoster (shingles).
- Immunize if nonimmune prior to conception if possible or postpartum.
- Defer pregnancy for 1 month following second of the two immunizations (given 1 month apart).
- Breastfeeding should be avoided and the woman should be isolated from her infant with a new varicella infection.
- Breastfeeding is okay if an immunocompetent woman develops zoster as long as the lesion is not on the breast and does not contact the infant.

Source: ACOG Education Bulletin No. 258: Breastfeeding: maternal and infant aspects. *Obstet Gynecol.* 2000;96:1–16; ACOG Practice Bulletin No. 151: Cytomegalovirus, parvovirus B19, varicella zoster, and toxoplasmosis in pregnancy. *Obstet Gynecol.* 2015 Jun;125(6):1510-25.

INFECTIOUS DISEASES

RUBELLA
Fast Facts
- Infection can be communicated 7 days before and 4 days after appearance of rash.
- Rash occurs 2–3 weeks following exposure.
  - Usually lasts 3 days: "3-day measles"
- Congenital rubella syndrome can include:
  - Miscarriage or fetal death
  - Eye anomalies including cataracts, pigmentary retinopathy, micropthalmos, or congenital glaucoma
  - Cardiac anomalies include patent ductus arteriosus or peripheral pulmonary artery stenosis
  - Hearing loss
  - Neurologic manifestations including behavioral disorders, meningoencephalitis, or mental disability
- Rate of fetal infection depends on stage of gestation.
  - <11 weeks, 90% risk of congenital infection
  - 11–12 weeks, 33%
  - 13–14 weeks, 11%
  - 15–16 weeks, 24%
  - >16 weeks, 0%
- The risk of fetal anomalies is also dependent on gestational age.
  - First trimester,
    - 25%; first month → 50%; second month → 25%; third month → 10%
  - Second trimester, <1%;
  - 16–20 weeks: sensory only; >20 weeks: no reported cases

Management

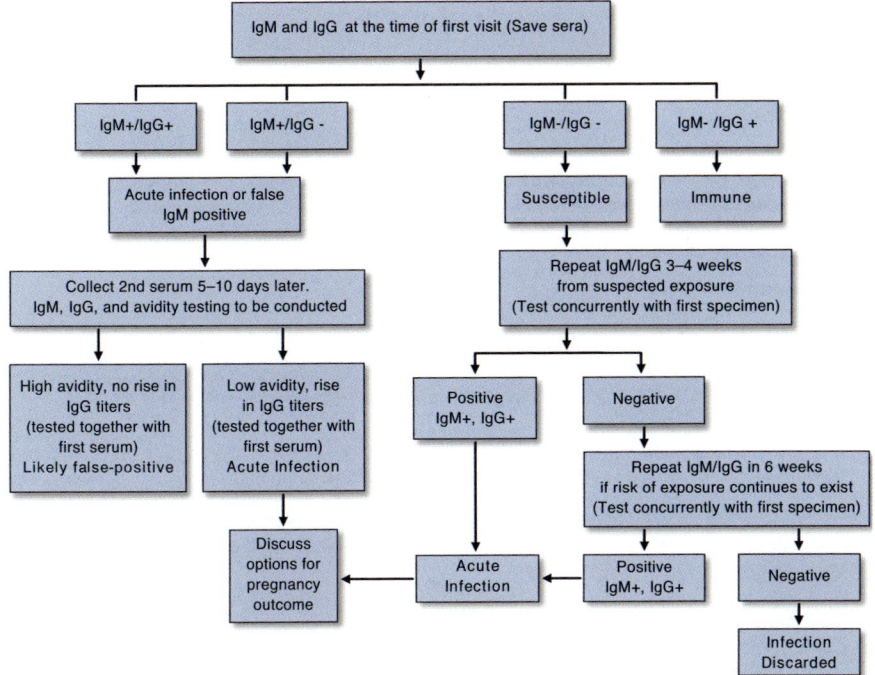

Figure 7.10. Algorithm for the management of pregnant patient exposed to rubella
Source: Reproduced from McLean H, Redd S, Abernathy MS et al. Centers for Disease Control and Prevention. *Manual for the surveillance of vaccine-preventable diseases*. Centers for Disease Control and Prevention, Atlanta, GA, September 2012. http://www.cdc.gov/vaccines/pubs/surv-manual/chpt14-rubella.html. Accessed on April 4, 2016.

TOXOPLASMOSIS
Fast Facts
- Routine screening is not recommended given that >1/3 of pregnant women will demonstrate serologic evidence of prior infection probably through ingestion of undercooked meat and contact with cat feces.
- HIV-positive pregnant women or pregnant women who are immunocompromised should be screened.
- Presence of IgG indicates immunity; IgM appears within 1 week and can last for years.
- Increasing gestational age increases fetal infection rate but diminishes severity.
- Rate of fetal infection resulting from acute maternal infection:
  - First trimester: 10–15%
  - Second trimester: 25%
  - Third trimester: 60%
- 90% of infected infants will develop sequelae, including:
  - IUGR, microcephaly, chorioretinitis and subsequent severe visual impairment, hearing loss, severe neurodevelopmental delay, rash, hepatosplenomegaly, ascites, fever, periventricular calcifications, ventriculomegaly, and seizures
- Pregnant women who suffer acute infection should be treated with spiramycin, whereas fetal infection is best treated with a combination of pyrimethamine, sulfadiazine, and folinic acid.

Source: American College of Obstetricians and Gynecologists. Practice Bulletin No. 151: Cytomegalovirus, parvovirus B19, varicella zoster, and toxoplasmosis in pregnancy. *Obstet Gynecol.* 2015 Jun;125(6):1510-25.

Diagnosis

Table 7.25. Serological criteria for the determination of the *Toxoplasma gondii* infection stage in acquired toxoplasmosis

Diagnostic Criteria			
IgG	IgG avidity	IgM	*Toxoplasma Gondii* Infection Stage
Neg	/	Neg	Seronegative
Pos	Low	Pos	Acute
Pos	Border/high	Pos	Subacute
Pos	Low	Neg	Subacute
Pos	Border/high	Border	Subacute
Pos	High	Neg	Chronic

Border, borderline; IgG avidity, TXGA-VIDAS result for specific IgG avidity; IgG, TXG-VIDAS result for specific IgG; IgM, TXMVIDAS result for specific IgM; Neg, negative; Pos, positive.

Source: Reproduced with permission from Stajner T, Bobic B, Klun I, et al. Prenatal and early postnatal diagnosis of congenital toxoplasmosis in a setting with no systematic screening in pregnancy. *Medicine.* 2016 Mar;95(9):e2979.

Toxoplasmosis

Table 7.26. Criteria for the timing of *Toxoplasma gondii* infection versus conception in pregnant women and after childbirth

First Tested	IgM	IgG Avidity	Infection Stage	Time of Infection Versus Conception
First trimester	Neg	High	Chronic	>2 mo before conception
	Pos/border	High/border	Subacute	Periconceptual cannot be excluded
	Pos	Low (0.100–0.200)	Acute	Periconceptual
	Pos	Low (<0.100)	Acute	First trimester
Second trimester	Neg	High	Chronic	>2 mo before conception
	Pos/border	High	Subacute	Periconceptual cannot be excluded
	Pos	Border	Subacute	Periconceptual
	Pos	Low (0.100–0.200)	Acute	First trimester
	Pos	Low (<0.100)	Acute	Second trimester
Third trimester	Neg	High	Chronic	>2 mo before conception
	Pos/border	High	Subacute	Periconceptual
	Border	Border	Subacute	First trimester
	Pos	Border	Subacute	Second trimester
	Pos	Low (0.100–0.200)	Acute	Second trimester
	Pos	Low (<0.100)	Acute	Third trimester
After delivery	Neg	High (>0.600)	Chronic	>2 mo before conception; considered of no risk in pregnancy
	Neg	High (0.300–0.500)	Chronic	>6 mo before delivery but periconceptual cannot be excluded
	Border	High/border	Subacute	First trimester
	Pos	High/border	Subacute	Second trimester
	Pos	Low	Acute	Third trimester

Border, borderline; m, months; Neg, negative; Pos, positive.

Source: Reproduced with permission from Stajner T, Bobic B, Klun I, et al. Prenatal and early postnatal diagnosis of congenital toxoplasmosis in a setting with no systematic screening in pregnancy. *Medicine.* 2016 Mar;95(9):e2979.

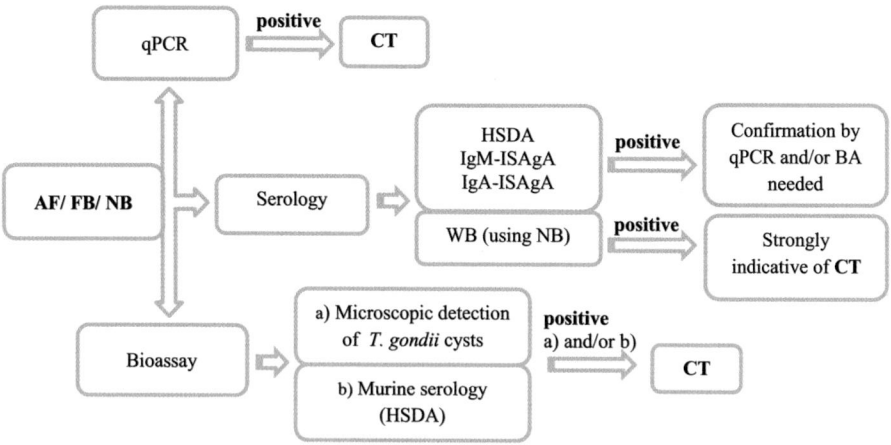

Figure 7.11. Algorithm for the diagnosis of congenital toxoplasmosis
AF, amniotic fluid; BA, bioassay; CT, congenital toxoplasmosis; FB, fetal blood; HSDA, high sensitivity direct agglutination assay; IgM-ISAgA, ISAgA test for detection of specific IgM; IgA-ISA-gA, ISAgA test for detection of specific IgA; NB, neonatal blood; qPCR, quantitative PCR; WB, Western blot.
Source: Reproduced with permission from Stajner T, Bobic B, Klun I, et al. Prenatal and early postnatal diagnosis of congenital toxoplasmosis in a setting with no systematic screening in pregnancy. *Medicine*. 2016 Mar;95(9):e2979.

CYTOMEGALOVIRUS
Fast Facts
- 0.7–4% of pregnancies are complicated by primary infections, up to 13.5% complicated by recurrent infections
- Usually asymptomatic
- Infection is transmitted through sexual contact or contact with infected blood, urine, or saliva
- Forty-day (28–60 day range) incubation period prior to development of maternal antibodies
- Cytomegalovirus (CMV) is the most common congenital infection, occurring in 0.2–2.2% of all neonates
- Risk of transmission of primary CMV increases with advancing gestational age (30% first trimester, 34–38% second trimester, and 40–72% third trimester)
  - Severity of infection, however, is increased with transmission earlier in gestation
  - CMV tetrad: mental retardation, microcephaly, chorioretinitis, cerebral calcifications. Other complications include jaundice, petechiae, thrombocytopenia, hepatosplenomeglay, growth restriction, and nonimmune hydrops, hearing loss
- Primary CMV infection: 30–40% risk of transmission, 10% with clinical signs of infection, 30% of severe infections die, and 65–80% of survivors have severe neurologic morbidity
- Recurrent CMV infection: 0.15–2% risk of transmission; infants are usually symptomatic
  - Most common sequelae is isolated hearing loss
- Transmission via cervical secretions and breast milk is usually asymptomatic
- Ultrasound findings are nonspecific for CMV infection but include: abdominal/liver calcifications, hepatosplenomegaly, echogenic bowel or kidneys, ascites, cerebral ventriculomegaly, intracranial calcifications, microcephaly, hydrops fetalis, and fetal growth restriction
- Diagnosis of fetal infection is based on amniocentesis; more reliable if done after 21 weeks of pregnancy
- Universal screening is not currently recommended as there are no proven interventions that can reduce the sequelae of fetal infection
- Inconclusive studies have suggested that antiviral medications and CMV-specific hyperimmune globulin may be beneficial; however, these treatments should be done under a research protocol and consultation with maternal-fetal medicine and or infectious disease specialist should occur

Source: American College of Obstetricians and Gynecologists. Practice Bulletin No. 151: Cytomegalovirus, parvovirus B19, varicella zoster, and toxoplasmosis in pregnancy. *Obstet Gynecol*. 2015 Jun;125(6):1510-25.

CMV Prevention
Here Are Some Simple Steps for Pregnant Women to Prevent Exposure to Saliva and Urine That Might Contain CMV
- Wash your hands often with soap and water for 15–20 seconds, especially after changing diapers, feeding a young child, wiping a young child's nose or drool, and handling children's toys.
- Do not share food, drinks, or eating utensils with young children.
- Do not put a child's pacifier in your mouth.
- Do not share a toothbrush with a young child.
- Avoid contact with saliva when kissing a child.
- Clean toys, countertops, and other surfaces that come into contact with children's urine or saliva.

Source: From the National CMV Foundation. Facts about CMV. Https://www.nationalcmv.org/NCMVF/media/ncmvf/hero/Facts_About_CMV.pdf?ext=.pdf. Accessed on April 4, 2016.

ZIKA VIRUS INFECTION
Fast Facts
- Zika virus is primarily transmitted through the bite of infected Aedes species mosquitoes.
- Zika virus can also be sexually transmitted.
- Most persons infected with Zika virus are asymptomatic.
  - Signs and symptoms, when present, are typically mild, with the most common being acute onset of fever, macular or papular rash, arthralgia, and conjunctivitis.
- There is no evidence that Zika virus will cause congenital infection in pregnancies conceived after the resolution of maternal Zika viremia.
- Data on the incubation period for Zika virus disease and the duration of Zika viremia are limited. Evidence from case reports and experience from related flavivirus infections indicate that the incubation period for Zika virus disease is likely 3–14 days.
- After symptom onset, the duration of Zika viremia may range from a few days to 1 week.
- Maternal infection during pregnancy has been linked to fetal microcephaly, intracranial calcifications, and brain and eye abnormalities.

Zika Recommendations
The Centers for Disease Control and Prevention (CDC) has updated its interim guidance for US health care providers caring for pregnant women with possible Zika virus exposure to include emerging data indicating that Zika virus RNA can be detected for prolonged periods in some pregnant women. In order to increase the proportion of pregnant women with Zika virus infection who receive a definitive diagnosis, CDC recommends expanding real-time reverse transcription-polymerase chain-reaction (rRT-PCR) testing. Other recommendations include the following:

- Women who have Zika virus disease* should wait at least 8 weeks after symptom onset to attempt conception.
- Men with Zika virus disease should wait at least 6 months after symptom onset to attempt conception.
- Women and men with possible exposure to Zika virus but without clinical illness consistent with Zika virus disease should wait at least 8 weeks after exposure to attempt conception.
- Zika virus disease is defined as having at least one of the following signs or symptoms: acute onset of fever, rash, arthralgia, conjunctivitis and laboratory confirmation of Zika virus infection. Persons who had possible Zika virus exposure and display one or more signs or symptoms consistent with Zika virus disease (acute onset of fever, rash, arthralgia, conjunctivitis) but did not have testing performed should follow recommendations for persons with Zika virus disease.
- Symptomatic pregnant women who are evaluated <2 weeks after symptom onset should receive serum and urine Zika virus rRT-PCR testing.
- Symptomatic pregnant women who are evaluated 2 to 12 weeks after symptom onset should first receive a Zika virus immunoglobulin (IgM) antibody test; if result is positive or equivocal, serum and urine rRT-PCR testing should be performed.
- For asymptomatic pregnant women who live in areas without active Zika virus transmission and who are evaluated <2 weeks after last possible exposure, rRT-PCR testing should be performed; if result is negative, a Zika virus IgM antibody test should be performed 2 to 12 weeks after the exposure.

- Asymptomatic pregnant women who do not live in an area with active Zika virus transmission, who are first evaluated 2 to 12 weeks after their last possible exposure, should first receive a Zika virus IgM antibody test; if result is positive or equivocal, serum and urine rRT-PCR should be performed.
- For symptomatic and asymptomatic pregnant women with possible Zika virus exposure who seek care >12 weeks after symptom onset or possible exposure, IgM antibody testing may be considered.
- Asymptomatic pregnant women with ongoing risk for exposure to Zika virus should receive Zika virus IgM antibody testing as part of routine obstetric care during the first and second trimesters.

Source: From Oduyebo T, Igbinosa I, Petersen EE, et al. Update: interim guidance for health care providers caring for pregnant women with possible Zika virus exposure—United States, July 2016. [Published online ahead of print July 25, 2016]. *MMWR*. doi:10.15585/mmwr.mm6529e1.

INFECTIOUS DISEASES — Zika Virus Infection

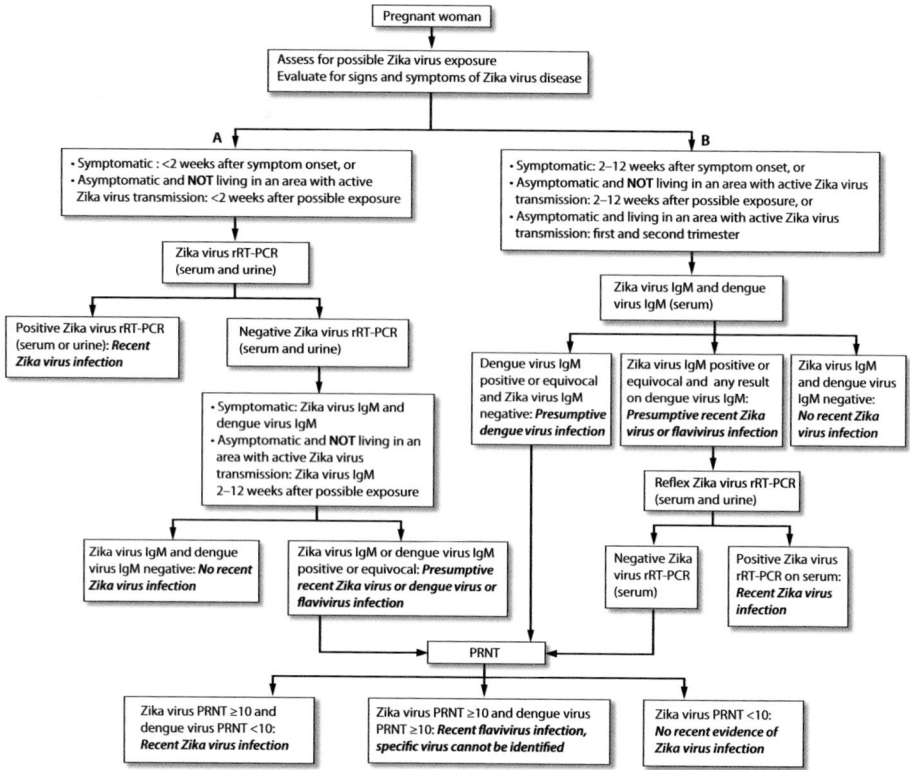

Figure 7.12. Updated interim guidance: testing algorithm*,†,§,¶ for a pregnant woman with possible Zika virus exposure** not residing in an area with active Zika virus transmission

IgM, immunoglobulin M; PRNT, plaque reduction neutralization test; rRT-PCR, real-time reverse transcription–polymerase chain reaction.

* A pregnant woman is considered symptomatic if one or more signs or symptoms (acute onset of fever, rash, arthralgia, or conjunctivitis) consistent with Zika virus disease is reported. A pregnant woman is considered asymptomatic if these symptoms are not reported.

† Testing includes Zika virus rRT-PCR on serum and urine samples, Zika virus and dengue virus IgM, and PRNT on serum samples. PRNT results that indicate recent flavivirus infection should be interpreted in the context of the currently circulating flaviviruses. Refer to the laboratory guidance for updated testing recommendations (http://www.cdc.gov/zika/laboratories/lab-guidance.html). Because of the overlap of symptoms in areas where other viral illness are endemic, evaluate for possible dengue or chikungunya virus infection.

§ Dengue virus IgM antibody testing is recommended only for symptomatic pregnant women.

¶ If Zika virus rRT-PCR testing is requested from laboratories without IgM antibody testing capacity or a process to forward specimens to another testing laboratory, storing of additional serum samples is recommended for IgM antibody testing in the event of an rRT-PCR negative result.

** Possible exposure to Zika virus includes travel to or residence in an area with active Zika virus transmission (http://wwwnc.cdc.gov/travel/notices/), or sex (vaginal sex [penis-to-vagina], anal sex [penis-to-anus], oral sex [mouth-to-penis or mouth-to-vagina], and the sharing of sex toys) without a barrier method to prevent infection (male or female condoms for vaginal or anal sex, male condoms for oral sex [mouth-to-penis], and male condoms cut to create a flat barrier or dental dams for oral sex [mouth-to-vagina]) with a partner who traveled to, or lives in, an area with active Zika virus transmission.

Source: From Oduyebo T, Igbinosa I, Petersen EE, et al. Update: interim guidance for health care providers caring for pregnant women with possible Zika virus exposure—United States, July 2016. [Published online ahead of print July 25, 2016]. *MMWR.* doi:10.15585/mmwr.mm6529e1.

Table 7.27. Clinical management of a pregnant woman with suspected Zika virus infection

Interpretation of Laboratory Results*	Prenatal Management	Postnatal Management
Recent Zika virus infection	Consider serial ultrasounds every 3–4 weeks to assess fetal anatomy and growth.† Decisions regarding amniocentesis should be individualized for each clinical circumstance.§	*Live births:* Cord blood and infant serum should be tested for Zika virus by rRT-PCR, and for Zika IgM and dengue virus IgM antibodies. If CSF is obtained for other reasons, it can also be tested. Zika virus rRT-PCR and IHC staining of umbilical cord and placenta are recommended.¶ *Fetal losses:* Zika virus rRT-PCR and IHC staining of fetal tissues is recommended.¶
Recent flavivirus infection; specific virus cannot be identified		
Presumptive recent Zika virus infection**	Consider serial ultrasounds every 3–4 weeks to assess fetal anatomy and growth.† Amniocentesis might be considered; decisions should be individualized for each clinical circumstance.	*Live births:* Cord blood and infant serum should be tested for Zika virus by rRT-PCR, and for Zika virus IgM and dengue virus IgM antibodies. If CSF is obtained for other reasons, it can also be tested. Zika virus rRT-PCR and IHC staining of umbilical cord and placenta should be considered.¶ *Fetal losses:* Zika virus rRT-PCR and IHC staining of fetal tissues should be considered.¶
Presumptive recent flavivirus infection**		
Recent dengue virus infection	Clinical management in accordance with existing guidelines.††	
No evidence of Zika virus or dengue virus infection	Prenatal ultrasound to evaluate for fetal abnormalities consistent with congenital Zika virus syndrome.† *Fetal abnormalities present:* repeat Zika virus rRT-PCR and IgM test; base clinical management on corresponding laboratory results. *Fetal abnormalities absent:* base obstetric care on the ongoing risk for Zika virus exposure risk to the pregnant woman.	

CSF, cerebrospinal fluid; IgM, immunoglobulin M; IHC, immunohistochemical; PRNT, plaque reduction neutralization test; rRT-PCR, real-time reverse transcription–polymerase chain reaction.

*Refer to the previously published guidance for testing interpretation (http://www.cdc.gov/mmwr/volumes/65/wr/mm6521e1.htm).

†Fetal abnormalities consistent with congenital Zika virus syndrome include microcephaly, intracranial calcifications, and brain and eye abnormalities.

§Health care providers should discuss risks and benefits of amniocentesis with their patients. It is not known how sensitive or specific rRT-PCR testing of amniotic fluid is for congenital Zika virus infection, whether a positive result is predictive of a subsequent fetal abnormality, and if it is predictive, what proportion of infants born after infection will have abnormalities.

¶Refer to pathology guidance for collection and submission of fetal tissues for Zika virus testing for detailed information on recommended specimen types (http://www.cdc.gov/zika/laboratories/test-specimens-tissues.html).

**rRT-PCR or PRNT should be performed for positive or equivocal IgM results as indicated. PRNT results that indicate recent flavivirus infection should be interpreted in the context of the currently circulating flaviviruses. Refer to the laboratory guidance for updated testing recommendations (http://www.cdc.gov/zika/laboratories/lab-guidance.html). Because of the overlap of symptoms and areas where other viral illnesses are endemic, evaluate for possible dengue or chikungunya virus infection.

††http://apps.who.int/iris/bitstream/10665/44188/1/9789241547871_eng.pdf.

Source: From Oduyebo T, Igbinosa I, Petersen EE, et al. Update: interim guidance for health care providers caring for pregnant women with possible Zika virus exposure—United States, July 2016. [Published online ahead of print July 25, 2016]. *MMWR.* doi:10.15585/mmwr.mm6529e1.

IMMUNIZATION DURING PREGNANCY

Table 7.28. Immunization during pregnancy

Routine	Hepatitis A	Recommended if otherwise indicated	See hepatitis A text
	Hepatitis B	Recommended in some circumstances	See hepatitis B text
	Human Papillomavirus (HPV)	Not recommended	See HPV text
	Influenza (Inactivated)	Recommended	See Influenza text
	Influenza (LAIV)	Contraindicated	See Influenza (LAIV) text
	MMR	Contraindicated	See MMR text
	Meningococcal	May be used if otherwise indicated	See Meningococcal text
	PCV13	Inadequate data for specific recommendation	See Pneumococcal Conjugate text
	PPSV23	Inadequate data for specific recommendation	See Pneumococcal Polysaccharide text
	Polio	May be used if needed	See Polio text
	Td	Should be used if otherwise indicated	See Tetanus and Diphtheria text
	Tdap	Recommended	See Tetanus, Diphtheria, and Pertussis text
	Varicella	Contraindicated	See Varicella text
	Zoster	Contraindicated	See Zoster text
Travel & Other	Anthrax	Low risk of exposure—not recommended. High risk of exposure—may be used	See Anthrax text
	BCG	Contraindicated	See BCG text
	Japanese Encephalitis	Inadequate data for specific recommendation	See Japanese Encephalitis text
	Rabies	May be used if otherwise indicated	See Rabies text
	Typhoid	Inadequate data for specific recommendation	See Typhoid text
	Smallpox	Pre-exposure—contraindicated Post-exposure—recommended	See Smallpox text
	Yellow fever	May be used if benefit outweighs risk	See Yellow Fever text

Source: Reproduced from http://www.cdc.gov/vaccines/pubs/preg-guide.htm. Accessed on February 25, 2016.

Routine Vaccinations

Hepatitis A
- Hepatitis A is an inactivated vaccine, and similar to hepatitis B vaccines, **is recommended if another high risk condition or other indication is present.**[1]

Hepatitis B
- **Pregnancy is not a contraindication to vaccination.** Limited data suggest that developing fetuses are not at risk for adverse events when hepatitis B vaccine is administered to pregnant women. Available vaccines contain noninfectious HBsAg and should cause no risk of infection to the fetus.[2]
- **Pregnant women who are identified as being at risk for HBV infection** during pregnancy (e.g., having more than one sex partner during the previous 6 months, been evaluated or treated for an STD, recent or current injection drug use, or having had an HBsAg-positive sex partner) **should be vaccinated.**[3]

Human Papillomavirus (HPV)
- **HPV vaccines are not recommended for use in pregnant women.** If a woman is found to be pregnant after initiating the vaccination series, the remainder of the 3-dose series should be delayed until completion of pregnancy. Pregnancy testing is not needed before vaccination. If a vaccine dose has been administered during pregnancy, no intervention is needed.[4]
- Patients and health care providers should report any exposure to HPV4 (Gardasil) during pregnancy to Merck at telephone, 1–877–888–4231, and any exposure to HPV2 (Cervarix) during pregnancy to GlaxoSmithKline at telephone, 888–452–9622.[4]

Influenza (Inactivated)
- Women in the second and third trimesters of pregnancy are at increased risk for hospitalization from influenza. Because vaccinating against influenza before the season begins is critical, and because predicting exactly when the season will begin is impossible, **routine influenza vaccination is recommended for all women who are or will be pregnant (in any trimester) during influenza season,** which in the United States is usually early October through late March.[5]

Influenza (LAIV)
- **Do not administer LAIV to pregnant women.**[6]

Measles, Mumps, Rubella (MMR)
- Measles-mumps-rubella (MMR) vaccine and its component vaccines **should not be administered to women known to be pregnant.** Because a risk to the fetus from administration of these live virus vaccines cannot be excluded for theoretical reasons, women should be counseled to avoid becoming pregnant for 28 days after vaccination with measles or mumps vaccines or MMR or other rubella-containing vaccines.[7]
- Because of the importance of protecting women of childbearing age against rubella and varicella, reasonable practices in any vaccination program include asking women if they are pregnant or might become pregnant in the next 4 weeks; not vaccinating women who state that they are or plan to become pregnant; explaining the theoretical risk for the fetus of MMR, varicella, or MMRV vaccine were administered to a woman who is pregnant; and counseling women who are vaccinated not to become pregnant during the 4 weeks after MMR, varicella, or MMRV vaccination.

- Routine pregnancy testing of women of childbearing age before administering a live-virus vaccine is not recommended. If a pregnant woman is inadvertently vaccinated or becomes pregnant within 4 weeks after MMR or varicella vaccination, she should be counseled about the theoretical basis of concern for the fetus; however, MMR or varicella vaccination during pregnancy should not be considered a reason to terminate pregnancy.[5]
- Rubella-susceptible women who are not vaccinated because they state they are or may be pregnant should be counseled about the potential risk for CRS and the importance of being vaccinated as soon as they are no longer pregnant.[8]
- A registry of susceptible women vaccinated with rubella vaccine between 3 months before and 3 months after conception—the "Vaccine in Pregnancy (VIP) Registry"—was kept between 1971 and 1989. No evidence of CRS occurred in the offspring of the 226 women who received the current RA 27/3 rubella vaccine and continued their pregnancy to term.[8]

Meningococcal (MenACWY Or MPSV4)
- **Pregnancy should not preclude vaccination with MenACWY or MPSV4, if indicated.** Women of childbearing age who become aware that they were pregnant at the time of MenACWY vaccination should contact their health care provider or the vaccine manufacturer so that their experience might be captured in the vaccine manufacturer's registry of vaccination during pregnancy. Any adverse event following receipt of MenACWY, MPSV4, or Hib-MenCY-TT vaccine should be reported to VAERS at telephone 1–800–822–7967 or at http://vaers.hhs.gov/index.[9]

Pneumococcal Conjugate (PCV13)
- ACIP has not published pregnancy recommendations for PCV13 at this time. (Use of PCV13 is limited among women of childbearing age.)

Pneumococcal Polysaccharide (PPSV23)
- **The safety of the PPSV23 vaccine during the first trimester of pregnancy has not been evaluated,** although no adverse consequences have been reported among newborns whose mothers were inadvertently vaccinated during pregnancy.[10]

Polio (IPV)
- Although no adverse effects of IPV have been documented among pregnant women or their fetuses, **vaccination of pregnant women should be avoided on theoretical grounds.** However, if a pregnant woman is at increased risk for infection and requires immediate protection against polio, IPV can be administered in accordance with the recommended schedules for adults.[11]

Tetanus, Diphtheria, and Pertussis (TDAP); and Tetanus and Diphtheria (TD)
- Health care personnel should **administer a dose of Tdap during each pregnancy** irrespective of the patient's prior history of receiving Tdap. To maximize the maternal antibody response and passive antibody transfer to the infant, **optimal timing for Tdap administration is between 27 and 36 weeks of gestation,** although Tdap may be given at any time during pregnancy.[12]
- For women not previously vaccinated with Tdap, if Tdap is not administered during pregnancy, Tdap should be administered immediately postpartum.[12]
- Available data from . . . studies do not suggest any elevated frequency or unusual patterns of adverse events in pregnant women who received Tdap, and the few serious adverse events reported were unlikely to have been caused by the vaccine.[13]

- *Wound Management:* If a Td booster is indicated for a pregnant woman, health care providers should administer Tdap.[12]
- *Unknown or Incomplete Tetanus Vaccination:* To ensure protection against maternal and neonatal tetanus, pregnant women who never have been vaccinated against tetanus should receive three vaccinations containing tetanus and reduced diphtheria toxoids. The recommended schedule is 0, 4 weeks and 6 through 12 months. Tdap should replace 1 dose of Td, preferably between 27 and 36 weeks gestation.[12]
- Providers are encouraged to report administration of Tdap to a pregnant woman, regardless of trimester, to the appropriate manufacturer's pregnancy registry: for Adacel® to sanofi pasteur, telephone 1–800–822–2463 and for Boostrix® to GlaxoSmithKline Biologicals, telephone 1–888–825–5249.[14]

Varicella

- Because the effects of the varicella virus on the fetus are unknown, **pregnant women should not be vaccinated.** Nonpregnant women who are vaccinated should avoid becoming pregnant for 1 month after each injection. For persons without evidence of immunity, having a pregnant household member is not a contraindication for vaccination.[15]
- Wild-type varicella poses a low risk to the fetus. Because the virulence of the attenuated virus used in the vaccine is less than that of the wild-type virus, the risk to the fetus, if any, should be even lower.[15]
- Because of the importance of protecting women of childbearing age against rubella and varicella, reasonable practices in any vaccination program include asking women if they are pregnant or might become pregnant in the next 4 weeks; not vaccinating women who state that they are or plan to become pregnant; explaining the theoretical risk for the fetus of MMR, varicella, or MMRV vaccine were administered to a woman who is pregnant; and counseling women who are vaccinated not to become pregnant during the 4 weeks after MMR, varicella, or MMRV vaccination.
- Routine pregnancy testing of women of childbearing age before administering a live-virus vaccine is not recommended. If a pregnant woman is inadvertently vaccinated or becomes pregnant within 4 weeks after MMR or varicella vaccination, she should be counseled about the theoretical basis of concern for the fetus; however, MMR or varicella vaccination during pregnancy should not be considered a reason to terminate pregnancy.[5]
- In 1995, Merck and Co., Inc., in collaboration with CDC, established a Pregnancy Registry to monitor the fetal and pregnancy outcomes of women who inadvertently received varicella vaccine 3 months before or at any time during pregnancy. In 2006, the registry was expanded to include exposures to ProQuad® and Zostavax®. After 17 years of monitoring, no cases of congenital varicella syndrome or increased risk for other birth defects have been identified. However, the theoretical risk to the fetus for congenital varicella syndrome, although small, cannot be completely ruled out. In 2013, FDA approved the closure of the registry and new patient enrollment was discontinued in October 2013. Merck will continue to monitor exposures to the VZV-containing vaccines (Varivax®, ProQuad®, and Zostavax®) during pregnancy or within 3 months prior to conception. To report administration of VZV-containing vaccines to a pregnant woman, call 1–877–888–4231. See Merck's website for more information. The annual reports of registry data are available to health care providers in the U.S. from the manufacturer upon request (1–877–888–4231; updated February 2014).

Zoster

- Zoster vaccine (Zostavax®) should not be administered to pregnant women. Additionally, Zostavax is not licensed for the age groups that include women of traditional childbearing ages. To report administration of VZV-containing vaccines to a pregnant woman, call 1–877–888–4231. See *Guidelines for Vaccinating Pregnant Women: Varicella* and *Merck's Pregnancy Registries* website for more information (updated March 2014).
- In most circumstances, the decision to terminate a pregnancy should not be based on whether zoster vaccine was administered during pregnancy. Merck & Co., Inc., in collaboration with CDC, has established a pregnancy registry to monitor the maternal-fetal outcomes of pregnant women who are inadvertently administered live-attenuated VZV-based vaccines within 1 month of pregnancy (telephone 1–877–888–4231).[16]

Travel and Other Vaccines

Anthrax

- In a **pre-event** setting, in which the risk for exposure to aerosolized *B. anthracis* spores is presumably low, **vaccination of pregnant women is not recommended** and should be deferred until after pregnancy.[17]
- In a **postevent** setting that poses a high risk for exposure to aerosolized *B. anthracis* spores, pregnancy is neither a precaution nor a contraindication to PEP. **Pregnant women at risk for inhalation anthrax should receive AVA** and 60 days of antimicrobial therapy as described.[17]

BCG

- **BCG vaccination should not be given during pregnancy.** Even though no harmful effects of BCG vaccination on the fetus have been observed, further studies are needed to prove its safety.[18]

Japanese Encephalitis (JE)

- No controlled studies have assessed the safety, immunogenicity, or efficacy of [Ixiaro] in pregnant women. Preclinical studies of [Ixiaro] in pregnant rats did not show evidence of harm to the mother or fetus.[19]

Rabies

- Because of the potential consequences of inadequately managed rabies exposure, pregnancy is not considered a contraindication to postexposure prophylaxis. Certain studies have indicated no increased incidence of abortion, premature births, or fetal abnormalities associated with rabies vaccination. If the risk of exposure to rabies is substantial, **pre-exposure prophylaxis also might be indicated during pregnancy.** Rabies exposure or the diagnosis of rabies in the mother should not be regarded as reasons to terminate the pregnancy.[20]

Typhoid

- No data have been reported on the use of any of the typhoid vaccines among pregnant women.[21]

Vaccinia (Smallpox)

- Because of the limited risk but severe consequences of fetal infection, **smallpox vaccine should not be administered in a pre-event setting to pregnant women or to women who are trying to become pregnant.**[22]

- Before vaccination, women of childbearing age should be asked if they are pregnant or intend to become pregnant in the next 4 weeks; women who respond positively should not be vaccinated.[22]
- If a pregnant woman is inadvertently vaccinated or if she becomes pregnant within 4 weeks after smallpox vaccination, she should be counseled regarding concern for the fetus. Smallpox vaccination during pregnancy should not ordinarily be a reason to terminate pregnancy. CDC has established a pregnancy registry to prospectively follow the outcome of such pregnancies and facilitate the investigation of any adverse pregnancy outcome among pregnant women who were inadvertently vaccinated. For enrollment in the registry, contact CDC at 404–639–8253.[22]
- Pregnant women **who have had a definite exposure to smallpox virus** (i.e., face-to-face, household, or close-proximity contact with a smallpox patient) and are, therefore, at high risk for contracting the disease, should be vaccinated. Smallpox infection among pregnant women has been reported to result in a more severe infection than among nonpregnant women. Therefore the risks to the mother and fetus from experiencing clinical smallpox substantially outweigh any potential risks regarding vaccination. In addition, vaccinia virus has not been documented to be teratogenic, and the incidence of fetal vaccinia is low.[22]
- **When the level of exposure risk is undetermined,** the decision to vaccinate should be made after assessment by the clinician and the patient of the potential risks versus the benefits of smallpox vaccination.[23]

Yellow Fever

- **Pregnancy is a precaution for Yellow Fever vaccine (YFV) administration,** compared with most other live vaccines, which are contraindicated in pregnancy. If travel is unavoidable, and the risks for YFV exposure are felt to outweigh the vaccination risks, a pregnant woman should be vaccinated. If the risks for vaccination are felt to outweigh the risks for YFV exposure, pregnant women should be issued a medical waiver to fulfill health regulations.[24]
- Because pregnancy might affect immunologic function, serologic testing to document an immune response to the vaccine should be considered.[24]
- Although no specific data are available, a woman should wait 4 weeks after receiving YFV before conceiving.[24]

References

1. CDC. Advisory Committee on Immunization Practices (ACIP) recommended immunization schedules for persons aged 0 through 18 years and adults aged 19 years and older—United States, 2013. *MMWR.* 2013;62(Suppl 1):11.
2. CDC. A comprehensive immunization strategy to eliminate transmission of hepatitis B virus infection in the United States: recommendations of the Advisory Committee on Immunization Practices (ACIP) part 2: immunization of adults. *MMWR.* 2006;55(No. RR-16):13.
3. CDC. A comprehensive immunization strategy to eliminate transmission of hepatitis B virus infection in the United States: recommendations of the Advisory Committee on Immunization Practices (ACIP) part 1: immunization of infants, children, and adolescents. *MMWR.* 2005;54(No. RR-16):14.
4. CDC. FDA licensure of bivalent human papillomavirus vaccine (HPV2, Cervarix) for use in females and updated HPV vaccination recommendations from the Advisory Committee on Immunization Practices (ACIP). *MMWR.* 2010;59(No. 20):629.
5. CDC. General recommendations on immunization: recommendations of the Advisory Committee on Immunization Practices (ACIP). *MMWR.* 2011;60(No. 2):26-27.

6. CDC. Prevention and control of influenza with vaccines: recommendations of the Advisory Committee on Immunization Practices (ACIP), 2010. *MMWR*. 2010;59(No. RR-8):39.
7. CDC. Notice to readers: revised ACIP recommendation for avoiding pregnancy after receiving a rubella-containing vaccine. *MMWR*. 2001;50(No. 49):1117.
8. CDC. Measles, mumps, and rubella—vaccine use and strategies for elimination of measles, rubella, and congenital rubella syndrome and control of mumps: recommendations of the Advisory Committee on Immunization Practices (ACIP). *MMWR*. 1998;47(No. RR-8):18, 32-33.
9. CDC. Prevention and control of meningococcal disease: recommendations of the Advisory Committee on Immunization Practices (ACIP). *MMWR*. 2013;62(No. RR-2):18.
10. CDC. Prevention of pneumococcal disease: recommendations of the Advisory Committee on Immunization Practices (ACIP). *MMWR*. 1997;46(No. RR-8):6.
11. CDC. Poliomyelitis prevention in the United States: recommendations of the Advisory Committee on Immunization Practices (ACIP). *MMWR*. 2000;49(No. RR-5):14.
12. CDC. Updated recommendations for use of tetanus toxoid, reduced diphtheria toxoid, and acellular pertussis vaccine (Tdap) in pregnant women—Advisory Committee on Immunization Practices (ACIP), 2012. *MMWR*. 2013;62(No. 07):131-5.
13. CDC. Updated recommendations for use of tetanus toxoid, reduced diphtheria toxoid and acellular pertussis vaccine (Tdap) in pregnant women and persons who have or anticipate having close contact with an infant aged <12 months – Advisory Committee on Immunization Practices (ACIP), 2011. *MMWR*. 2011;60(No. 41):1426.
14. CDC. Prevention of pertussis, tetanus, and diphtheria among pregnant and postpartum women and their infants: recommendations of the Advisory Committee on Immunization Practices (ACIP). *MMWR*. 2008;57(No. RR-4):49.
15. CDC. Prevention of varicella: recommendations of the Advisory Committee on Immunization Practices (ACIP). *MMWR*. 2007;56(No. RR-4):28, 31.
16. CDC. Prevention of herpes zoster: recommendations of the Advisory Committee on Immunization Practices (ACIP). *MMWR*. 2008;57(No. RR-5):21.
17. CDC. Use of anthrax vaccine in the United States: recommendations of the Advisory Committee on Immunization Practices (ACIP). *MMWR*. 2010;59(No. RR-6):19-21.
18. CDC's Fact Sheet on BCG (http://www.cdc.gov/tb/publications/factsheets/prevention/BCG.htm)
19. CDC. Japanese encephalitis vaccines: recommendations of the Advisory Committee on Immunization Practices (ACIP). *MMWR*. 2010;49(No. RR-1):12-15.
20. CDC. Human rabies prevention—United States, 2008: recommendations of the Advisory Committee on Immunization Practices (ACIP). *MMWR*. 2008;57(No. RR-3):20-21.
21. CDC. Typhoid immunization: recommendations of the Advisory Committee on Immunization Practices (ACIP). *MMWR*. 1994;43(No. RR-14):7.
22. CDC. Recommendations for using smallpox vaccine in a pre-event vaccination program: supplemental recommendations of the Advisory Committee on Immunization Practices (ACIP) and the Healthcare Infection Control Practices Advisory Committee (HICPAC). *MMWR*. 2003;52(No. RR-7):9-11.
23. CDC. Vaccinia (smallpox) vaccine: recommendations of the Advisory Committee on Immunization Practices (ACIP). *MMWR*. 2001;50(No. RR-10):12 & 19.
24. CDC. Yellow fever vaccine: recommendations of the Advisory Committee on Immunization Practices (ACIP). *MMWR*. 2010;59(No. RR-7):13 & 21.

HPV VACCINATION

Table 7.29. Key information regarding currently available human papillomavirus vaccines

	Cervarix	Gardasil	Gardasil 9
Gender	Females Only	Females and Males in the US; Females only in the UK	Females and Males in the US
Age	9–25	9–26	Females 9–26 and Males 9–21
Recommended Age at Vaccination	11–12 in the US; 12–13 in the UK	11–12 in the US; 12–13 in the UK	11–12 in the US
HPV Strains the Vaccine Covers	HPV-16 and HPV-18	HPV-6, 11, 16 and 18	HPV-6, 11, 16, 18, 31, 33, 45, 52, and 58
Protects Against	Cervical Cancer	Anal, Cervical, Vulvar, and Vaginal Cancer; Anogenital Warts; Vaginal, Vulvar, Cervical and Anal Intraepithelial Neoplasia	Anal, Cervical, Vulvar, and Vaginal Cancer; Anogenital Warts; Vaginal, Vulvar, Cervical and Anal Intraepithelial Neoplasia
Dosage	3 over 6-month period	3 over 6-month period	3 over 6-month period

INFECTIOUS DISEASES — Urinary Tract Infections in Pregnancy

URINARY TRACT INFECTIONS IN PREGNANCY
Fast Facts
- 5% of patients develop urinary tract infection or asymptomatic bacteriuria.
- 1/3 untreated patients develop pyelonephritis.
- Pyelonephritis in pregnancy is treated as an inpatient.
- Check serum potassium level on admission (may be hypokalemic).
- Initiate renal evaluation for multiple admissions or left-sided pyelonephritis.
- Hydronephrosis usually occurs on the right because of uterine displacement.
- Consider antibiotic suppressive therapy for high-risk patients.

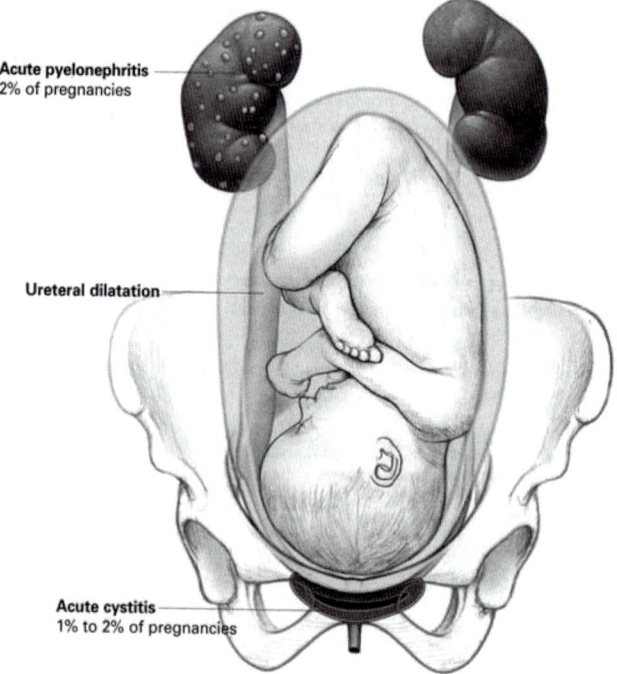

Figure 7.13. Risk factors that contribute to increased incidence of UTI in pregnancy
Mechanical changes lead to urinary stasis and ureterovesical reflux. Beginning in the 6th week of gestation and peaking at 22–24 weeks, approximately 90% of pregnant women develop **ureteral dilation,** which remains until delivery. **Increased bladder volume** and **decreased bladder and ureteral tone** contribute to increased urinary stasis and ureterovesical reflux.
Hormonal changes lead to increased bacterial growth in the urine and possibly lowered resistance to bacteria. Up to 70% of pregnant women develop **glycosuria,** which encourages bacterial growth in the urine. **Increases in urinary progestins and estrogens** may lead to decreased ability of the lower urinary tract to resist invading bacteria.
Source: Reproduced with permission from Chen KT. UTI in pregnancy: 6 questions to guide therapy. *OBG Management.* 2004;Nov:36-53. Artist: Scott Bodell.

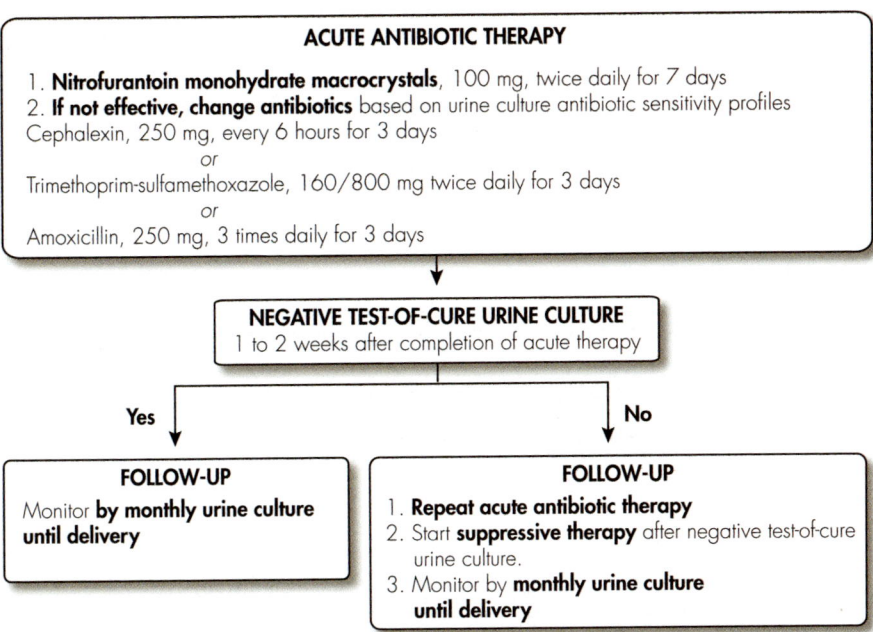

Figure 7.14. Algorithm for the management of asymptomatic bacteriuria or acute cystitis in pregnancy
Source: Reproduced with permission from Chen KT. UTI in pregnancy: 6 questions to guide therapy. *OBG Management*. 2004;Nov:36-53.

INFECTIOUS DISEASES — Urinary Tract Infections in Pregnancy

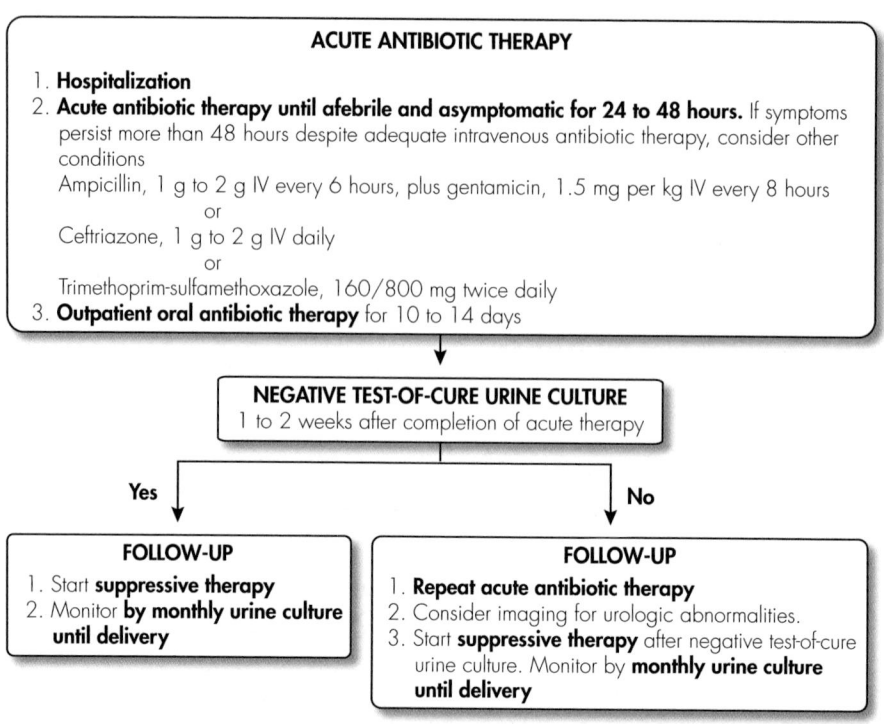

Figure 7.15. Algorithm for the management of acute pyelonephritis in pregnancy
Source: Reproduced with permission from Chen KT. UTI in pregnancy: 6 questions to guide therapy. *OBG Management*. 2004;Nov:36-53. Copyright © Frontline Medical Communications. All rights reserved. Artist: Scott Bodell.

Table 7.30. Treatment regimens for uncomplicated acute bacterial cystitis

Antimicrobial Agent	Dose	Adverse Events
Trimethoprim-sulfamethoxazole	One tablet (160 mg trimethoprim–800 mg sulfamethoxazole), twice daily for 3 days	Fever, rash, photosensitivity, neutropenia, thrombocytopenia, anorexia, nausea and vomiting, pruritus, headache, urticaria, Stevens-Johnson syndrome, and toxic epidermal necrosis
Trimethoprim	100 mg, twice daily for 3 days	Rash, pruritus, photosensitivity, exfoliative dermatitis, Stevens-Johnson syndrome, toxic epidermal necrosis, and aseptic meningitis
Ciprofloxacin	250 mg, twice daily for 3 days	Rash, confusion, seizures, restlessness, headache, severe hypersensitivity, hypoglycemia, hyperglycemia, and Achilles tendon rupture (in patients older than 60 years)
Levofloxacin	250 mg, once daily for 3 days	Same as for ciprofloxacin
Norfloxacin	400 mg, twice daily for 3 days	Same as for ciprofloxacin
Gatifloxacin	200 mg, once daily for 3 days	Same as for ciprofloxacin
Nitrofurantoin macrocrystals	50–100 mg, four times daily for 7 days	Anorexia, nausea, vomiting, hypersensitivity, peripheral neuropathy, hepatitis, hemolytic anemia, and pulmonary reactions
Nitrofurantoin monohydrate macrocrystals	100 mg, twice daily for 7 days	Same as for nitrofurantoin macrocrystals
Fosfomycin tromethamine	3 g dose (powder) single dose	Diarrhea, nausea, vomiting, rash, and hypersensitivity

Source: Reproduced with permission from American College of Obstetricians and Gynecologists. ACOG Practice Bulletin No. 91: Treatment of urinary tract infections in nonpregnant women. *Obstet Gynecol.* 2008 Mar;111(3):785-94. Copyright © 2008 The American College of Obstetricians and Gynecologists.

ACOG Practice Advisory August 4, 2016

The Food and Drug Administration (FDA) recently issued a Drug Safety Communication advising that oral and injectable fluoroquinolones should be reserved for use in patients who have no other treatment options for serious bacterial infections, including uncomplicated urinary tract infections, because the risks of serious adverse effects generally outweigh the benefits. The FDA has revised the current "Boxed Warning" on the labels of systemic fluoroquinolone antibacterial drugs to indicate that these medications are associated with disabling and potentially permanent adverse effects to the tendons, muscles, joints, nerves, and central nervous system that can occur together in the same patient. The FDA is continuing to assess safety issues with fluoroquinolones as part of its ongoing review of drugs and will provide updates if additional actions are needed.

For more information on the updated fluoroquinolone warning, see the complete FDA Drug Safety Communication. For information and clinical guidance on the management of urinary tract infections, see the American College of Obstetricians and Gynecologists' Practice Bulletin #91, "Treatment of Urinary Tract Infections in Nonpregnant Women."

VAGINITIS

Table 7.31. Diagnostic tests available for vaginitis

Test	Sensitivity %	Specificity	Comment
Bacterial vaginosis*			
pH >4.5	97	64	
Amsel's criteria	92	77	Must meet 3 of 4 clinical criteria (pH >4.5, thin watery discharge, >20% clue cells, positive "whiff" test [amine odor present with addition of base]), but similar results achieved if 2 of 4 criteria met
Nugent criteria			Gram's stain morphology score (0–10) based on lactobacilli and other morphotypes; a score of 0–3 indicates normal flora, a score of 4–6 intermediate flora, and a score of 7–10 bacterial vaginosis; high interobserver reproducibility
Papanicolaou smear	49	93	
Point-of-care tests			
QuickVue Advance pH+ amines	89	96	Positive if pH >4.7
QuickVue Advance G. vaginalis[†]	91	>95	Tests for proline iminopeptidase activity in vaginal fluid; if used when pH >4.5, sensitivity is 95% and specificity is 99%
OSOM BV Blue[†]	90	>95	Test for vaginal sialidase activity
Candida[‡]			
Wet mount			
Overall	50	97	
Growth of 3–4+ on culture	85		C. albicans a commensal agent in 10–25% of women
Growth of 1+ on culture	23		
pH ≤4.5			pH may be elevated if mixed infection with bacterial vaginosis or T. vaginalis present
Papanicolaou smear	25	72	
T. Vaginalis[§]			
Wet mount	45–60	95	Increased visibility of microorganisms with a higher burden of infection
Culture	85–90	>95	
pH >4.5	56	50	
Papanicolaou smear	92	61	False positive rate, 8% for standard Pap test and 4% for liquid-based cytologic test
Point-of-care test			
OSOM	83	98.8	Requires 10 min to perform; tests for T. vaginalis antigens

*For details, see Eschenbach, et al. and the guidelines of the American College of Obstetricians and Gynecologists (ACOG).

[†]Proline iminopeptidase and sialidase are enzymes produced by many bacteria associated with bacterial vaginosis.

[‡]For details, see Eckert, et al. and Shurbaji, et al.

[§]For details, see Soper, the ACOG guidelines, and Krieger, et al.

Source: Reprinted with permission from Eckert LO. Acute vulvovaginitis: clinical practice. *N Engl J Med.* 2006;355(12):1244-52. Copyright © 2006 Massachusetts Medical Society. All rights reserved.

Vulvovaginal Candidiasis

Table 7.32. 2015 CDC guidelines for treatment of vulvovaginal candidiasis

Over the Counter Intravaginal Agents
Clotrimazole 1% cream 5 g intravaginally daily for 7–14 days
Clotrimazole 2% cream 5 g intravaginally daily for 3 days
Miconazole 2% cream 5 g intravaginally daily for 7 days
Miconazole 4% cream 5 g intravaginally daily for 3 days
Miconazole 100 mg vaginal suppository, one suppository daily for 7 days
Miconazole 200 mg vaginal suppository, one suppository for 3 days
Miconazole 1,200 mg vaginal suppository, one suppository for 1 day
Tioconazole 6.5% ointment 5 g intravaginally in a single application
Prescription Intravaginal Agents:
Butoconazole 2% cream (single dose bioadhesive product), 5 g intravaginally in a single application
Terconazole 0.4% cream 5 g intravaginally daily for 7 days
Terconazole 0.8% cream 5 g intravaginally daily for 3 days
Terconazole 80 mg vaginal suppository, one suppository daily for 3 days
Prescription Oral Agent:
Fluconazole 150 mg orally in a single dose

Source: Reproduced from Workowski KA, Bolan GA. Sexually transmitted diseases treatment guidelines, 2015. *MMWR Recomm Rep.* 2015 Jun 5;64(RR-03):1-137.

SEXUALLY TRANSMITTED INFECTIONS

Table 7.33. Diagnostic testing for STIs

Infection	Diagnostic
Bacterial vaginosis	• Clinical criteria (3 of 4): vaginal pH >4.5, gray discharge, clue cells on wet mount, positive amine test (whiff test) • Gram's stain of vaginal discharge
Chlamydia trachomatis	• Cervical swab: nucleic acid amplification (PCR), nucleic acid hybridization, enzyme immunoassay, direct fluorescent antibody, culture • Urine: nucleic acid amplification (LCR)
Genital warts	• Clinical: raised papular, keratotic, or cauliform lesions; may also be flat • Biopsy, if there is doubt • Vesicular fluid or swab from ulcer: culture • Type-specific serology
Neisseria gonorrhoeae	• Cervical swab: nucleic acid amplification (PCR), nucleic acid hybridization, enzyme immunoassay, culture, Gram's stain • Urine: nucleic acid amplification (LCR)
Trichomonas	• Wet mount with motile trichomonads • Vaginal swab: culture, polymerase chain reaction, antigen-based point of care test
Pubic lice	• Visual identification of lice or nits; magnifying glass may help
Syphilis	• Primary and secondary: darkfield microscopy of swab from lesions, serologic tests (nontreponemal[a] and treponemal[b])

LCR, ligase chain reaction; PCR, polymerase chain reaction.

[a]Nontreponemal tests: rapid plasma reagin (RPR) test, Venereal Disease Research Laboratory (VDRL).

[b]Treponemal tests: fluorescent treponemal antibody absorbed (FTA-ABS), microhemagglutination-*Treponema pallidum* (MHA-TP).

Source: Reprinted with permission from Gunter J. Sexually transmitted infections update. *OB/GYN Special Edition.* 2005:19-24.

2015 CDC GUIDELINES
Chlamydia

Table 7.34. 2015 CDC guidelines for treatment of chlamydia

Non-pregnant Patient Recommended Regimens
Azithromycin 1 g orally in a single dose
Doxycycline 100 mg orally twice a day for 7 days
Alternative Regimens:
Erythromycin base 500 mg orally four times a day for 7 days
Erythromycin ethylsuccinate 800 mg orally four times a day for 7 days
Levofloxacin 500 mg orally once daily for 7 days
Ofloxacin 300 mg orally twice a day for 7 days
Pregnant Patient Recommended Regimens
Azithromycin 1 g orally in a single dose
Alternative Regimens:
Amoxicillin 500 mg orally three times a day for 7 days
Erythromycin base 500 mg orally four times a day for 7 days
Erythromycin base 250 mg orally four times a day for 14 days
Erythromycin ethylsuccinate 800 mg orally four times a day for 7 days
Erythromycin ethylsuccinate 400 mg orally four times a day for 14 days

Source: Reproduced from Workowski KA, Bolan GA. Sexually transmitted diseases treatment guidelines, 2015. *MMWR Recomm Rep.* 2015 Jun 5;64(RR-03):1-137.

Gonorrhea

Table 7.35. 2015 CDC guidelines for treatment of gonorrhea

Pregnant and Non-pregnant Patient Recommended Regimens
Ceftriaxone 250 mg IM in a single dose
PLUS
Azithromycin 1 g orally in a single dose
Non-pregnant Patient Alternative Regimens
If ceftriaxone is not available:
Cefixime 400 mg orally in a single dose
PLUS
Azithromycin 1 g orally in a single dose

Source: Reproduced from Workowski KA, Bolan GA. Sexually transmitted diseases treatment guidelines, 2015. *MMWR Recomm Rep.* 2015 Jun 5;64(RR-03):1-137.

INFECTIOUS DISEASES

Bacterial Vaginosis

Table 7.36. 2015 CDC guidelines for treatment of bacterial vaginosis
Treatment is recommended for all symptomatic pregnant women.

Recommended Regimens
Metronidazole 500 mg orally twice a day for 7 days
Metronidazole gel 0.75%, one full applicator (5 g) intravaginally, once a day for 5 days
Clindamycin cream 2%, one full applicator (5 g) intravaginally at bedtime for 7 days

Alternative Regimens:
Tinidazole 2 g orally once daily for 2 days
Tinidazole 1 g orally once daily for 5 days
Clindamycin 300 mg orally twice daily for 7 days
Clindamycin ovules 100 mg intravaginally once at bedtime for 3 days*

*Clindamycin ovules use an oleaginous base that might weaken latex or rubber products (e.g., condoms and vaginal contraceptive diaphragms). Use of such products within 72 hours following treatment with clindamycin ovules is not recommended.

Source: Reproduced from Workowski KA, Bolan GA. Sexually transmitted diseases treatment guidelines, 2015. *MMWR Recomm Rep.* 2015 Jun 5;64(RR-03):1-137.

Trichomoniasis

Table 7.37. 2015 CDC guidelines for treatment of trichomoniasis

Non-pregnant Patient Recommended Regimens
Metronidazole 2 g orally in a single dose
Tinidazole 2 g orally in a single dose

Alternative Regimens:
Metronidazole 500 mg orally twice a day for 7 days

Pregnant Patient Recommended Regimens
Metronidazole 2 g orally in a single dose

Source: Reproduced from Workowski KA, Bolan GA. Sexually transmitted diseases treatment guidelines, 2015. *MMWR Recomm Rep.* 2015 Jun 5;64(RR-03):1-137.

ULCERATIVE LESIONS IN STI

Table 7.38. Ulcerative lesions in sexually transmitted diseases[a]

Characteristic	Herpes	Syphilis	Chancroid	LGV	Granuloma Inguinale
Organism	Herpes simplex virus	*Treponema pallidum*	*Haemophilus ducreyi*	*Chlamydia trachomatis*	*Calymmatobacterium granulomatis*
Incubation	3–7 days	10–60 days	2–6 days	1–4 wk	8–12 wk
Primary lesion	Vesicle	Papule	Papule/pustule	Papule/pustule/vesicle	Papule
Number	Multiple, coalescing	1–2	1–5	Single	Single or multiple
Pain	Yes	Rare	Often	No	Rare
Shape	Regular	Regular	Irregular	Regular	Regular
Margins	Flat	Raised	Red, undermined	Flat	Rolled, elevated
Depth	Superficial	Superficial	Excavated	Superficial	Elevated
Base	Red, smooth	Red, smooth	Yellow, gray	Variable	Red, rough
Induration	None	Firm	Rare, soft	None	Firm
Secretions	Serous	Serous	Purulent, hemorrhagic	Variable	Rare, hemorrhagic
Lymph nodes	Firm, tender	Firm, nontender	Tender, suppurative	Tender, suppurative	Pseudoadenopathy
Duration	5–10 days, recurrent	Weeks	Weeks	Days	Weeks
Diagnosis	Culture, PCR	Dark field, immunofluorescence, PCR	Culture, PCR	Culture, PCR	Giemsa staining

LGV, lymphogranuloma venereum; PCR, polymerase chain reaction.

[a]Scabies, molluscum contagiosum, *Candida* species, and other dermatologic conditions (e.g., hidradenitis suppurativa) also may cause genital lesions. Boldfaced items are of particular help in making a differential diagnosis.

Source: Modified from Beckmann CR, Ling FW, Herbert WNP, et al., eds. *Obstetrics and Gynecology*, 3rd Ed. Baltimore: Williams & Wilkins; 1998:349.

HERPES SIMPLEX VIRUS
Fast Facts
- 50 million adolescent and adult Americans are infected with genital herpes.
- Only 5–15% of infected individuals report recognition of infection.
- Type-specific HSV serologic assays might be useful in the following scenarios: (1) recurrent genital symptoms or atypical symptoms with negative HSV cultures; (2) a clinical diagnosis of genital herpes without laboratory confirmation; or (3) a partner with genital herpes. HSV serologic testing should be considered for persons presenting for an STD evaluation (especially for those persons with multiple sex partners), persons with HIV infection, and MSM at increased risk for HIV acquisition. Screening for HSV-1 and HSV-2 in the general population is not indicated.
- 80% of infected infants are born to mothers with no reported history of HSV infection.
  - 1/3 to ½ of neonatal HSV infections are from HSV-1
  - Infant mortality has been decreasing
  - 30% for disseminated disease
  - 4% for CNS disease
  - 20% of survivors have neurologic long-term sequelae
  - Risk of vertical transmission from mother to fetus (187).
    - 30–60% if primary genital HSV infection at time of delivery
    - 3% if recurrent genital lesion at time of delivery
    - 2/10,000 if history of HSV but no prodrome or lesions
    - "Very low" if nongenital HSV lesion in patient with history of HSV

HSV and Pregnancy
- Most mothers of infants who acquire neonatal herpes lack histories of clinically evident genital herpes.
- Prevention of neonatal herpes depends both on preventing acquisition of genital HSV infection during late pregnancy and during delivery.
  - The risk for herpes is high in infants of women who acquire genital HSV during late pregnancy; these women should be managed in consultation with an infectious disease specialist.
- Pregnant women without known genital herpes should abstain from intercourse during the third trimester with partners known or suspected of having genital herpes.
- Pregnant women without known orolabial herpes should be advised to abstain from receptive oral sex during the third trimester with partners known or suspected to have orolabial herpes.
- Some specialists believe that type-specific serologic tests are useful to identify pregnant women at risk for HSV infection and to guide counseling regarding the risk for acquiring genital herpes during pregnancy and that such testing should be offered to uninfected women whose sex partner has HSV infection.
- The effectiveness of antiviral therapy to decrease the risk for HSV transmission to pregnant women by infected partners has not been studied.
- All pregnant women should be asked whether they have a history of genital herpes.
- At the onset of labor, all women should be questioned carefully about symptoms of genital herpes, including prodromal symptoms, and all women should be examined carefully for herpetic lesions.
- Women without symptoms or signs of genital herpes or its prodrome can deliver vaginally.

- Women with recurrent genital herpetic lesions at the onset of labor should deliver by cesarean section to prevent neonatal HSV infection, but cesarean section does not completely eliminate the risk for HSV transmission to the infant.
- The safety of systemic acyclovir, valacyclovir, and famciclovir therapy in pregnant women has not been definitively established.
- Available data do not indicate an increased risk for major birth defects compared with the general population in women treated with acyclovir during the first trimester, but the data are too limited to provide useful information on pregnancy outcomes.
- Acyclovir can be administered orally to pregnant women with first episode genital herpes or severe recurrent herpes and should be administered IV to pregnant women with severe HSV infection. Acyclovir treatment late in pregnancy reduces the frequency of cesarean sections among women who have recurrent genital herpes by diminishing the frequency of recurrences at term.
- The effect of antiviral therapy late in pregnancy on the incidence of neonatal herpes is not known. No data support the use of antiviral therapy among HSV seropositive women without a history of genital herpes.

Source: Reproduced from Workowski KA, Bolan GA. Sexually transmitted diseases treatment guidelines, 2015. *MMWR Recomm Rep*. 2015 Jun 5;64(RR-03):1-137.

Table 7.39. 2015 CDC guidelines for treatment of HSV

First clinical episode of genital herpes	acyclovir	400 mg orally 3x/day for 7–10 days
	acyclovir	200 mg orally 5x/day for 7–10 days
	valacyclovir	1 g orally 2x/day for 7–10 days
	famciclovir	250 mg orally 3x/day for 7–10 days
Episodic therapy for recurrent genital herpes	acyclovir	400 mg orally 3x/day for 5 days
	acyclovir	800 mg orally 2x/day for 5 days
	acyclovir	800 mg orally 3x/day for 2 days
	valacyclovir	500 mg orally 2x/day for 3 days
	valacyclovir	1 g orally 1x/day for 5 days
	famciclovir	125 mg orally 2x/day for 5 days
	famciclovir	1,000 mg orally 2x/day for 1 day
	famciclovir	500 mg orally once, followed by 250 mg 2x/day for 2 days
Suppressive therapy[14] for recurrent genital herpes	acyclovir	400 mg orally 2x/day
	valacyclovir	500 mg orally 1x/day
	valacyclovir	1 g orally once a day
	famciclovir	250 mg orally 2x/day
Recommended regimens for episodic infection in persons with HIV infection	acyclovir	400 mg orally 3x/day for 5–10 days
	valacyclovir	1 g orally 2x/day for 5–10 days
	famciclovir	500 mg orally 2x/day for 5–10 days
Recommended regimens for daily suppressive therapy in persons with HIV infection	acyclovir	400–800 mg orally 2–3x/day
	valacyclovir	500 mg orally 2x/day
	famciclovir	500 mg orally 2x/day

Source: Reproduced from Workowski KA, Bolan GA. Sexually transmitted diseases treatment guidelines, 2015. *MMWR Recomm Rep*. 2015 Jun 5;64(RR-03):1-137.

SYPHILIS

Table 7.40. 2015 CDC guidelines for treatment of syphilis

	Recommended Regimens	Alternative Regimens:
Primary, secondary, or early latent <1 year	Benzathine penicillin G 2.4 million units IM in a single dose	Doxycycline 100 mg 2x/day for 14 days OR tetracycline 500 mg orally 4x/day for 14 days
Latent >1 year, latent of unknown duration	Benzathine penicillin G 2.4 million units IM in 3 doses each at 1-week intervals (7.2 million units total)	Doxycycline 100 mg 2x/day for 28 days OR tetracycline 500 mg orally 4x/day for 28 days
Neurosyphilis	Aqueous crystalline penicillin G 18–24 million units per day, administered as 3–4 million units IV every 4 hours or continuous infusion, for 10–14 days	Procaine penicillin G 2.4 MU IM 1x daily PLUS probenecid 500 mg orally 4x/day, both for 10–14 days.
Pregnancy	Pregnant women should be treated with the penicillin regimen appropriate for their stage of infection.	

Some evidence suggests that additional therapy is beneficial for pregnant women. For women who have primary, secondary, or early latent syphilis, a second dose of benzathine penicillin 2.4 million units IM can be administered 1 week after the initial dose.

When syphilis is diagnosed during the second half of pregnancy, management should include a sonographic fetal evaluation for congenital syphilis. However, this evaluation should not delay therapy. Sonographic signs of fetal or placental syphilis (i.e., hepatomegaly, ascites, hydrops, fetal anemia, or a thickened placenta) indicate a greater risk for fetal treatment failure; cases accompanied by these signs should be managed in consultation with obstetric specialists. Evidence is insufficient to recommend specific regimens for these situations.

Women treated for syphilis during the second half of pregnancy are at risk for premature labor and/or fetal distress if the treatment precipitates the Jarisch-Herxheimer reaction. These women should be advised to seek obstetric attention after treatment if they notice any fever, contractions, or decrease in fetal movements. Stillbirth is a rare complication of treatment, but concern for this complication should not delay necessary treatment. No data are available to suggest that corticosteroid treatment alters the risk for treatment-related complications in pregnancy.

Missed doses are not acceptable for pregnant women receiving therapy for late latent syphilis. Pregnant women who miss any dose of therapy must repeat the full course of therapy.

All women who have syphilis should be offered testing for HIV infection.

Source: Reproduced from Workowski KA, Bolan GA. Sexually transmitted diseases treatment guidelines, 2015. *MMWR Recomm Rep.* 2015 Jun 5;64(RR-03):1-137.

Table 7.41. Classification, clinical presentation, and adverse perinatal effects of syphilis

Stage of Disease	Clinical Presentation	Frequency of Perinatal Transmission
Primary	Painless chancre	40–50%
Secondary	Generalized maculopapular rash Mucous patches Condylomata lata	40–50%
Tertiary	Gumma formation Cardiac abnormalities Central nervous system abnormalities	≤10%
Early latent	Asymptomatic	40–50%
Late latent	Asymptomatic	≤10%

Source: Ling FW, Duff P, eds. *Obstetrics and Gynecology: Principles and Practice*. New York: McGraw-Hill; 2001:121.

Table 7.42. Oral desensitization protocol for pregnant women with allergies to penicillin[a]

Dose[b]	Penicillin V Suspension (U/mL)	Amount[c] mL	Amount[c] U	Cumulative Dose (U)
1	1,000	0.1	100	100
2	1,000	0.2	200	300
3	1,000	0.4	400	700
4	1,000	0.8	800	1,500
5	1,000	1.6	1,600	3,100
6	1,000	3.2	3,200	6,300
7	1,000	6.4	6,400	12,700
8	10,000	1.2	12,000	24,700
9	10,000	2.4	24,000	48,700
10	10,000	4.8	48,000	96,700
11	80,000	1.0	80,000	176,700
12	80,000	2.0	160,000	336,700
13	80,000	4.0	320,000	656,700
14	80,000	8.0	640,000	1,296,700

[a]Observation period: 30 mins before parenteral administration of penicillin.

[b]Interval between doses, 15 mins; elapsed time, 3 hr and 45 mins; cumulative dose, 13 million U.

[c]The specific amount of drug was diluted in approximately 30 mL of water and then given orally.

Source: Reproduced with permission from Wendel GD Jr., Stark BJ, Jamison RB, et al. Penicillin allergy and desensitization in serious infections during pregnancy. *N Engl J Med*. 1985;312:1230. Copyright © 1985 Massachusetts Medical Society. All rights reserved.

PELVIC INFLAMMATORY DISEASE AND SEXUALLY TRANSMITTED DISEASES
Fast Facts
- Sequela of pelvic inflammatory diseases (PID): adhesions, hydrosalpinx, 10 × increase in ectopic, 4 × increase in pelvic pain
- Starts most often with cervical gonococcal or chlamydia leading to ascending infection
- 90% with lower abdominal pain
- 75% with mucopurulent cervical discharge
- 75% have ESR >15 mm/hour
- 50% have WBC >10,000 mm^3
- Have low threshold to treat as inpatient

Diagnosis
All Three Should Be Present
- History of lower abdominal pain and the presence of lower abdominal tenderness with or without evidence of rebound
- Cervical motion tenderness
- Adnexal tenderness (may be unilateral)

Empiric Therapy
The requirement that all three minimum criteria be present before the initiation of empiric treatment could result in insufficient sensitivity for the diagnosis of PID. The presence of signs of lower genital tract inflammation (predominance of leukocytes in vaginal secretions, cervical exudates, or cervical friability), in addition to one of the three minimum criteria, increases the specificity of the diagnosis. Upon deciding whether to initiate empiric treatment, clinicians should also consider the risk profile of the patient for STDs.

Additional Criteria That Support a Diagnosis of PID
- Oral temperature >101° F (>38.3° C);
- Abnormal cervical or vaginal mucopurulent discharge;
- presence of abundant numbers of WBC on saline microscopy of vaginal fluid;
- Elevated erythrocyte sedimentation rate;
- Elevated C-reactive protein
- Laboratory documentation of cervical infection with N. gonorrhoeae or C. trachomatis.

Definitive Criteria for Diagnosing PID in Selected Cases
- Histopathologic evidence of endometritis on endometrial biopsy
- Transvaginal ultrasonography or other imaging techniques showing thickened fluid-filled tubes with or without free pelvic fluid or tubo-ovarian complex
- Laparoscopic abnormalities consistent with PID

Outpatient vs. Inpatient Treatment

In women with PID of mild or moderate clinical severity, outpatient therapy yields short- and long-term clinical outcomes similar to inpatient therapy. The decision of whether hospitalization is necessary should be based on the judgment of the provider and whether the patient meets any of the following suggested criteria:

- Surgical emergencies (e.g., appendicitis) cannot be excluded;
- The patient is pregnant;
- The patient does not respond clinically to oral antimicrobial therapy;
- The patient is unable to follow or tolerate an outpatient oral regimen;
- The patient has severe illness, nausea and vomiting, or high fever; or
- The patient has a tubo-ovarian abscess.

No evidence is available to suggest that adolescents benefit from hospitalization for treatment of PID. The decision to hospitalize adolescents with acute PID should be based on the same criteria used for older women. Younger women with mild-to-moderate acute PID have similar outcomes with either outpatient or inpatient therapy, and clinical response to outpatient treatment is similar among younger and older women.

For women with PID of mild or moderate severity, parenteral and oral therapies appear to have similar clinical efficacy. Many randomized trials have demonstrated the efficacy of both parenteral and oral regimens. Clinical experience should guide decisions regarding transition to oral therapy, which usually can be initiated within 24–48 hours of clinical improvement. In women with tubo-ovarian abscesses, at least 24 hours of direct inpatient observation is recommended.

Table 7.43. 2015 CDC guidelines for treatment of pelvic inflammatory disease (PID)

Parenteral Regimens
Cefotetan 2 g IV every 12 hours PLUS Doxycycline 100 mg orally or IV every 12 hours
Cefoxitin 2 g IV every 6 hours PLUS Doxycycline 100 mg orally or IV every 12 hours
Clindamycin 900 mg IV every 8 hours PLUS Gentamicin loading dose IV or IM (2 mg/kg), followed by a maintenance dose (1.5 mg/kg) every 8 hours. Single daily dosing (3–5 mg/kg) can be substituted.
Alternative Parenteral Regimen:
Ampicillin/Sulbactam 3 g IV every 6 hours PLUS Doxycycline 100 mg orally or IV every 12 hours
Recommended Intramuscular/Oral Regimens
Ceftriaxone 250 mg IM in a single dose
PLUS
Doxycycline 100 mg orally twice a day for 14 days
WITH* or WITHOUT
Metronidazole 500 mg orally twice a day for 14 days
Cefoxitin 2 g IM in a single dose and Probenecid, 1 g orally administered concurrently in a single dose
PLUS
Doxycycline 100 mg orally twice a day for 14 days
WITH or WITHOUT
Metronidazole 500 mg orally twice a day for 14 days
Other parenteral third-generation cephalosporin (e.g., ceftizoxime or cefotaxime)
PLUS
Doxycycline 100 mg orally twice a day for 14 days
WITH* or WITHOUT
Metronidazole 500 mg orally twice a day for 14 days

* The recommended third-generation cephalsporins are limited in the coverage of anaerobes. Therefore, until it is known that extended anaerobic coverage is not important for treatment of acute PID, the addition of metronidazole to treatment regimens with third-generation cephalosporins should be considered.

If allergy precludes the use of cephalosporin therapy, if the community prevalence and individual risk for gonorrhea are low, and if follow-up is likely, use of fluoroquinolones for 14 days (levofloxacin 500 mg orally once daily, ofloxacin 400 mg twice daily, or moxifloxacin 400 mg orally once daily) with metronidazole for 14 days (500 mg orally, twice daily) can be considered

Source: Reproduced from Workowski KA, Bolan GA. Sexually transmitted diseases treatment guidelines, 2015. *MMWR Recomm Rep.* 2015 Jun 5;64(RR-03):1-137.

EXTERNAL GENITAL WARTS

Table 7.44. 2015 CDC guidelines for external anogenital warts

Patient-applied:
Imiquimod 3.75% or 5% cream[†] OR **Podofilox** 0.5% solution or gel OR **Sinecatechins** 15% ointment[†]
Provider-administered:
Cryotherapy with liquid nitrogen or cryoprobe OR Surgical removal either by tangential scissor excision, tangential shave excision, curettage, laser, or electrosurgery OR **Trichloroacetic acid** (TCA) or **bichloroacetic acid** (BCA) 80%–90% solution

*Many persons with external anal warts also have intra-anal warts. Thus, persons with external anal warts might benefit from an inspection of the anal canal by digital examination, standard anoscopy, or high-resolution anoscopy.

[†]Might weaken condoms and vaginal diaphragms.

Source: Reproduced from Workowski KA, Bolan GA. Sexually transmitted diseases treatment guidelines, 2015. *MMWR Recomm Rep.* 2015 Jun 5;64(RR-03):1-137.

Table 7.45. Comparison of treatment modalities for external anogenital warts

Method	Cost	4+ Disease	Pain/Rx	Pain/PO	Healing	Scar
Cryotherapy	Low	Possible	Moderate	Mild[b]	4 days–4 wk	Little
Laser	High	Excellent	Great/none[a]	Mild[b]	2–4 wk	Little[c]
Imiquimod	Low	Good	None	Mild/moderate	2–3 wk	Rarely
Liquid nitrogen	Low	Poor	Some	Mild	4 days–3 wk	Little
TCA/BCA	Low	Poor	Sharp	Some	1–2 wk	Little
Podophyllin	Low	Poor	None	Some	1–2 wk	Little
Cautery	Low	Possible	Great/none	Mild	2–6 wk	Possible
Interferon	High	Possible	Some	None	None	None

4+ Disease, severe or widespread; Pain/Rx, pain requiring prescription medication; Pain/PO, postoperative pain; TCA/BCA, trichloroacetic acid/bichloroacetic acid.

[a]If general or extensive local anesthesia used.

[b]Mild for small areas, can be very painful for large areas.

[c]If done expertly.

Source: Reproduced with permission from APGO Educational Series on Women's Health Issues. *Sexually transmitted infections human papillomavirus: the Ob/Gyn's role.* 2002:3–11.

Table 7.46. Reported clearance and recurrence rates for EGW therapies

Therapy	Range of Clearance Rates (%)	Rates of Recurrence (%)
CO_2 laser	27–82	7–72
Cryotherapy	68	38
Imiquimod (female)	72–84	5–19
Interferon (intralesional)	32–60	65–67
Interferon (systemic)	17–21	Not reported
Podofilox	45–88	33–60
Podophyllin	32–79	27–65
TCA/BCA	70–81	Not reported

TCA/BCA, trichloroacetic acid/bichloroacetic acid; EGW, external genital warts.

Source: Reproduced with permission from APGO Educational Series on Women's Health Issues. *Sexually transmitted infections human papillomavirus: the Ob/Gyn's role.* 2002:3–11.

TETANUS PROPHYLAXIS

Table 7.47. Recommendations for tetanus prophylaxis in routine wound management

History of Adsorbed Tetanus Toxoid	Clean, Minor Wounds		All Other Wounds[a]	
	TD[b]	TIG	TD	TIG
Unknown or <3 doses	Yes	No	Yes	Yes
≥3 doses[c]	No[d]	No	No[e]	No

TD, tetanus and diphtheria; TIG, tetanus immune globulin.

[a]Such as, but not limited to, wounds contaminated with dirt, feces, soil, or saliva; puncture wounds; avulsions; and wounds resulting from missiles, crushing, burns, or frostbite.

[b]For children older than 7 years, the TD toxoids and acellular pertussis vaccines (DtaP) or the TD toxoids and whole-cell pertussis vaccines (DTP)—or pediatric TD toxoids, if pertussis vaccines contraindicated—is preferred to tetanus toxoid (TT) alone. For children aged 7 years or less, the TD toxoids for adults is preferred to TT alone.

[c]If only three doses of fluid toxoid have been received, a fourth dose of toxoid—preferably an adsorbed toxoid—should be administered.

[d]Yes, if >10 yr have elapsed since the last dose.

[e]Yes, if >5 yr have elapsed since the last dose. More frequent boosters are not needed and can accentuate side effects.

Source: Bardenheier B, Prevots DR, Khetsuriani N, Wharton M. Tetanus surveillance—United States, 1995–1997. *MMWR CDC Surveill Summ.* 1998;47(2):1-13.

ANTIBIOTIC PROPHYLAXIS

Table 7.48. Antimicrobial prophylactic regimens by procedure

Procedure	Antibiotic	Dose (Single Dose)
Hysterectomy	Cefazolin[†]	1 g or 2 g[‡] IV
Urogynecology procedures, including those involving mesh	Clindamycin[§] plus gentamicin or quinolone[‖] or aztreonam	600 mg IV 1.5 mg/kg IV 400 mg IV 1 g IV
	Metronidazole[§] plus gentamicin or quinolone[‖]	500 mg IV 1.5 mg/kg IV 400 mg IV
Laparoscopy Diagnostic Operative Tubal Sterilization	None	
Laparotomy	None	
Hysteroscopy Diagnostic Operative Endometrial ablation Essure	None	
Hysterosalpingogram or Chromotubation	Doxycycline[¶]	100 mg orally, twice daily for 5 days
IUD insertion	None	
Endometrial biopsy	None	
Induced abortion/dilation and evacuation	Doxycycline Metronidazole	100 mg orally 1 hour before procedure and 200 mg orally after procedure 500 mg orally, twice daily for 5 days
Urodynamics	None	

IV, intravenously; IUD, intrauterine device.

*A convenient time to administer antibiotic prophylaxis is just before induction of anesthesia.

[†]Acceptable alternatives include cefotetan, cefoxitin, cefuroxime, or ampicillin-sulbactam.

[‡]A 2-g dose is recommended in women with a body mass index greater than 35 or weight greater than 100 kg or 220 lb.

[§]Antimicrobial agents of choice in women with a history of immediate hypersensitivity to penicillin.

[‖]Ciprofloxacin or levofloxacin or moxifloxacin.

[¶]If patient has a history of pelvic inflammatory disease or procedure demonstrates dilated fallopian tubes. No prophylaxis is indicated for a study without dilated tubes.

Source: Reproduced with permission from ACOG Committee on Practice Bulletins—Gynecology. ACOG Practice Bulletin No. 104: Antibiotic prophylaxis for gynecologic procedures. *Obstet Gynecol.* 2009 May;113(5):1180-9. Copyright © 2009 The American College of Obstetricians and Gynecologists.

MRSA INFECTIONS

Table 7.49. Rates of resistance and dosing of oral agents for treatment of community acquired MRSA infections

Antimicrobial Agent	Resistance Rates	Typical Adult Oral Dosing	Comments
Clindamycin	3–24%	300 TID	D-test should be performed. Excellent activity against strep. Increasing resistance a concern.
Doxycycline Minocycline	[1]9–24%	100 mg BID 100 mg BID	Doxycycline and minocycline, probably active against tetracycline resistant strains.
Trimethoprim-sulfamethoxazole	0–10%	1–2 DS (160/800 mg) BID	Low resistance rates in community, reasonable option for empiric therapy.
Rifampin	<1%	600 mg QD	Should not be used alone; potential for significant drug interactions.
Fusidic acid	<5%	500 mg TID	Should not be used alone; limited experience in children.
Linezolid	<1%	600 mg PO BID	Expensive.

[1]Rates shown are for tetracycline and are likely to be <5% or less for doxycycline and minocycline.

Source: Reproduced with permission from DeLeo FR, Otto M, Kreiswirth BN, Chambers HF. Community-associated methicillin-resistant *Staphylococcus aureus*. Lancet. 2010 May 1;375(9725):1557-68. Copyright © 2010 Elsevier.

C. DIFFICILE INFECTIONS

Table 7.50. Diagnostic testing for *C. difficile*

Test	Sensitivity	Specificity	Availability	Expense[a]	Utilization
C. difficile culture	Low	Moderate	Limited	$5–10	No diagnostic use; only toxigenic organisms cause disease
Toxigenic culture	High	High	Limited	$10–30	Reference method; epidemiologic tool; limited diagnostic use
CCNA	High	High	Limited	$15–25	Reference method; limited diagnostic use
GDH	High	Low	Widely	$5–15	Diagnostically as a screening test; must be confirmed
Toxin EIA tests	Low	High	Widely	$5–15	Must detect toxins A + B; inferior sensitivity
NAATs	High	High	Widely	$20–50	Use only in acute disease; false positives of concern

CCNA, *C. difficile* cytotoxin neutralization assay; GDH, glutamate dehydrogenase; EIA, enzyme immunoassay; NAAT, nucleic acid amplification tests

[a]Cost of goods; does not reflect laboratory changes.

Source: Reproduced with permission from Macmillan Publishers Ltd:Surawicz CM, Brandt LJ, Binion DG, et al. Guidelines for diagnosis, treatment, and prevention of *Clostridium difficile* infections. *Am J Gastroenterol.* 2013;108:478.

Table 7.51. CDI severity scoring system and summary of recommended treatments

Severity	Criteria	Treatment	Comment
Mild-to-moderate disease	Diarrhea plus any additional signs or symptoms not meeting severe or complicated criteria	Metronidazole 500 mg orally three times a day for 10 days. If unable to take metronidazole, vancomycin 125 mg orally four times a day for 10 days	If no improvement in 5–7 days, consider change to vancomycin at standard dose (vancomycin 125 mg four times a day for 10 days)
Severe disease	Serum albumin <3 g/dL plus ONE of the following: WBC ≥15,000 cells/mm³, Abdominal tenderness	Vancomycin 125 mg orally four times a day for 10 days	
Severe and complicated disease	Any of the following attributable to CDI: Admission to intensive care unit for CDI; Hypotension with or without required use of vasopressors; Fever ≥38.5 °C; Ileus or significant abdominal distention; Mental status changes; WBC ≥35,000 cells/mm³ or <2,000 cells/mm³; Serum lactate levels >2.2 mmol/l; End organ failure (mechanical ventilation, renal failure, etc.)	Vancomycin 500 mg orally four times a day and metronidazole 500 mg IV every 8 hr, and vancomycin per rectum (vancomycin 500 mg in 500 mL saline as enema) four times a day	Surgical consultation suggested
Recurrent CDI	Recurrent CDI within 8 weeks of completion of therapy	Repeat metronidazole or vancomycin pulse regimen	Consider FMT after 3 recurrences

CDI, *Clostridium difficile* infection; FMT, fecal microbiota transplant; IV, intravenous; WBC, white blood cell.

Source: Reproduced with permission from Macmillan Publishers Ltd: Surawicz CM, Brandt LJ, Binion DG, et al. Guidelines for diagnosis, treatment, and prevention of *Clostridium difficile* infections. *Am J Gastroenterol.* 108:478, 2013.

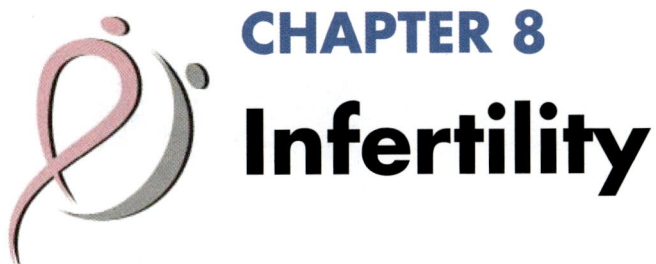

CHAPTER 8
Infertility

BASIC INFERTILITY
Fast Facts
- Impaired fecundity (the inability have a child) affects 6.7 million women in the U.S.—about 11% of the reproductive-age population (Chandra 2013).
- In a survey of married women, the CDC found that 1.5 million women in the US (6%) are infertile (Chandra 2013).
- Infertility affects men and women equally.
- 25% of infertile couples have more than one factor that contributes to their infertility.
- In approximately 40% of infertile couples, the male partner is either the sole cause or a contributing cause of infertility.
- Irregular or abnormal ovulation accounts for approximately 25% of all female infertility problems.
- Prolonged infertility suggests a poorer prognosis for spontaneous pregnancy.
  - Monthly pregnancy rate (PR) in couples with unexplained subfertility after 18 months duration → 1.5–3.0%.
    - Cumulative PRs for couples with unexplained subfertility 1 year and 3 years after the first visit are 13% and 40%, respectively.
- Approximately 50% of healthy women become clinically pregnant during the first two cycles, and between 80% and 90% during the first 6 months (Gnoth 2003; Wang 2003).
- Nearly all pregnancies can be attributed to intercourse during a 6-day window ending on the day of ovulation:

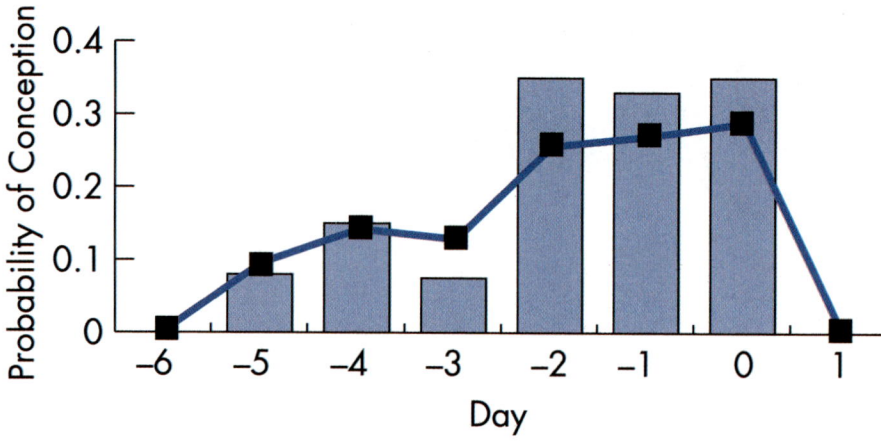

Figure 8.1. Probability of conception as a function of timing of intercourse
"0" denotes the day of ovulation.
Source: Reproduced with permission from Wilcox AJ, et al. Timing of sexual intercourse in relation to ovulation. Effects on the probability of conception, survival of the pregnancy, and sex of the baby. *N Engl J Med.* 1995; 333:1517–1521. Copyright © 1995 Massachusetts Medical Society.

Definitions
- **Infertility:** failure to conceive after 12 months (regular cycles) of unprotected intercourse
- **Subfertility:** failure to conceive after 6 months (regular cycles) of unprotected intercourse (Gnoth 2005)
- **Fecundability:** conception rate, usually *per month*
- **Fecundity:** birth rate per 1 month

Etiology
Table 8.1. Etiology of infertility

Cause of Infertility	%
Male Factor	30%
Female Factor	30%
Unexplained	25%
Combined	10%
Other	5%

Source: Data from Expert Group on Commissioning NHS Infertility Provision. Regulated fertility services: a commissioning aid. UK Department of Health, 2009.

Basic Infertility

Table 8.2. Prevalence of infertility

Age	Infertile (%)
≤30 years old	5
30–35 years old	9
35–40 years old	20
>40 years old	>30

Source: Data from Expert Group on Commissioning NHS Infertility Provision. Regulated fertility services: a commissioning aid. UK Department of Health, 2009.

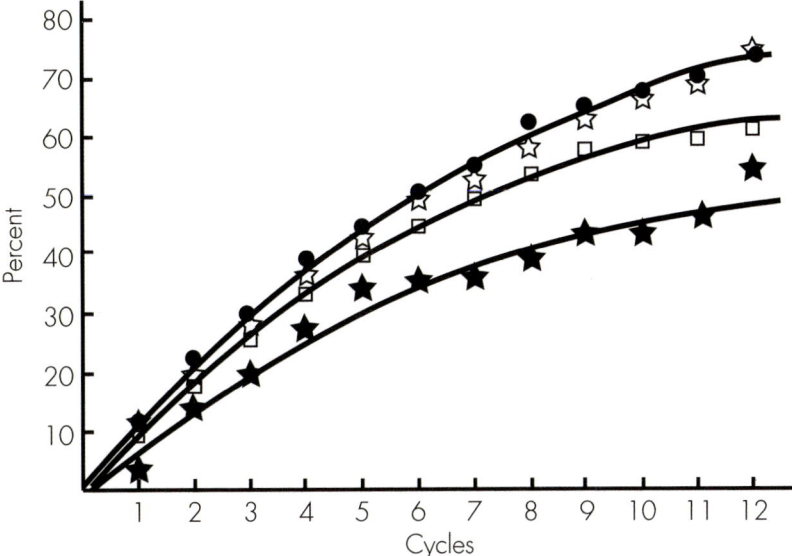

Figure 8.2. Effect of age on the cumulative pregnancy rate in a donor insemination program
The younger age groups (<31 years) were significantly different from the older groups.
- ● < 25 years
- ☆ 26–30
- □ 31–35
- ★ > 35

Source: Reproduced with permission from Schwartz D, Mayaux MJ. Female fecundity as a function of age: results of artificial insemination in 2193 nulliparous women with azoospermic husbands. Federation CECOS. N Engl J Med. 1982;306:404. Copyright © 1982 Massachusetts Medical Society.

Impact of Duration of Infertility
- Since fertile patients become pregnant and leave the cohort of patients still trying to conceive, the duration of a couple's infertility influences their continued odds of success.
  - Young patients with prolonged infertility in the face of normal testing have a poorer monthly rate of fertility than may be expected and aggressive therapy may be justified.

Table 8.3. Probability for natural conception by age and month of trying

	Month				
	1	2	3	6	12
<25 yo	50%	40%	30%	20%	4%
25–34 yo	40%	30%	20%	10%	2%
35–40 yo	30%	20%	10%	5%	1%

Source: Data from Gnoth C, Godehardt D, Godehardt E, et al. Time to pregnancy: results of the German prospective study and impact on the management of infertility. *Hum Reprod.* Sep;18(9):1959-66, 2003.

Diagnostic Evaluation
History
- Family history of endometriosis, early menopause
- Previous surgeries
- Menstrual irregularity
- Dysmenorrhea, dyspareunia
- Sexual dysfunction

Physical Exam/Transvaginal Ultrasound
- Uterine appearance, presence of fibroids/polyps/adenomyosis
- Ovarian morphology and antral follicle count
- Presence of ovarian cysts especially endometriomas

Laboratory Testing
- Prolactin (see page 554): routine testing in the absence of irregular cycles or galactorrhea is not supported by the medical literature
- TSH (see page 564–569)
- Assessment of ovarian reserve (see page 468)
  - D3 FSH and estradiol
  - AMH
  - Antral follicle count
  - Clomiphene citrate challenge test (CCCT)
- Semen analysis (see page 473)

Evaluation of Tubal Patency
- Hysterosalpingogram (HSG)
  - Perform CD 6–12

- ○ Consider prophylactic antibiotics in high-risk patients
  - ■ Azithromycin 1 g PO qhs night before HSG
  - ■ Doxycycline 100 mg PO bid night before and day of HSG
- ○ Treat with extended antibiotics (doxycycline 100 mg bid × 7–10 days) if HSG reveals hydrosalpinx given 4% chance of significant infection including tubo-ovarian abscess
- Laparoscopy
  - ○ Consider early in evaluation in patient with sonographic evidence of endometrioma or in patients who do not desire ART
  - ○ Removal of endometrioma prior to IVF may not improve outcome and may negatively impact ovarian reserve
  - ○ Useful in patients planning to undergo ART who have a hydrosalpinx
    - ■ removal will increase IVF success rates (see page 495)

OVARIAN RESERVE
Ovarian Reserve Tests
Day 3 Follicle-Stimulating Hormone
- FSH on day 3 of <10 IU/L is normal. Levels between 10 IU/L and 14 IU/L are a gray zone with decreasing fertility as levels rise.
- Most centers consider CD 3 FSH >10 IU/L as worrisome and ≥15–20 IU/L as abnormal and unlikely to benefit from stimulated cycle IVF.
- Variability does not affect the prognostic category (Buyalos 1998; Scott 1990; Abdalla 2006).
- Valid to test basal FSH on CD 2–5 (Hansen 1996).
- Basal FSH screening may not be of value in the general subfertility population with ovulatory menstrual cycles (Van Montfrans 2000).
- Threshold values of D3 FSH (Scott 2007):

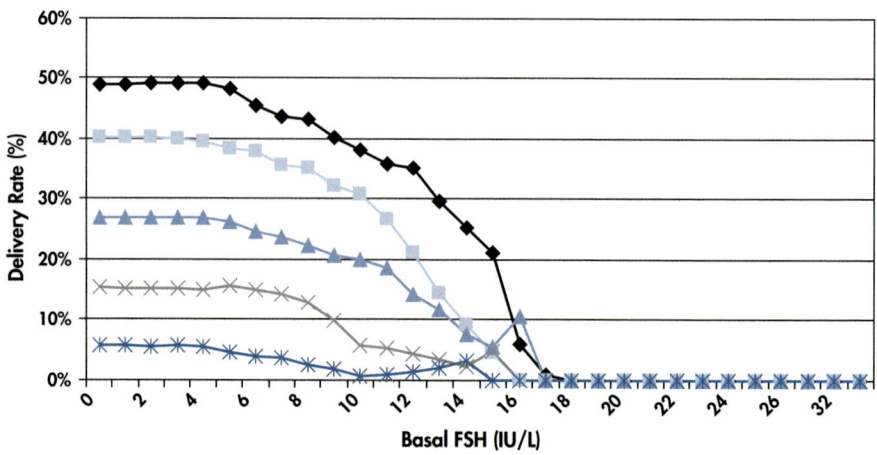

Figure 8.3. Threshold values for FSH in IVF
Source: Reproduced with permission from Scott RT Jr., Elkind-Hirsch KE, Styne-Gross A, et al. The predictive value for in vitro fertility delivery rates is greatly impacted by the method used to select the threshold between normal and elevated basal follicle stimulating hormone. *Fertil Steril.* Apr;89(4):868-78, 2008. Copyright © 2008 The American Society for Reproductive Medicine.

Day 3 Estradiol
- Levels typically nadir at CD 3 (Sharara 1998).
- Elevated E2 levels on CD 3 indicate advanced follicular phase; this is due to a premature rise in FSH in the luteal phase and reflects DOR (Sharara 1998).
- Inappropriately high E2 can suppress FSH back into the normal range by CD 3, and therefore may mask DOR.

- E2 >80 pg/mL have higher cancellation rates with IVF (Smotrich 1995).
- CD 3 E2 <20 pg/mL or ≥80 pg/mL have an ↑ risk for canceled IVF cycles, but these levels do not seem to predict pregnancy outcome nor correlate with ovarian response in those patients not canceled (Frattarelli 2000).

Clomiphene Citrate Challenge Test (CCCT)
- A dynamic test of ovarian reserve that has been supplanted by AMH and Antral Follicle Count.
- Indicated for women >35 yr old, smokers, those with one ovary or unexplained infertility:, and patients in whom decreased ovarian reserve is suspected.
- Involves standard day 3 laboratory tests, as described above, along with the administration of clomiphene citrate, 100 mg days 5–9, and a repeat FSH on day 10. Day 10 FSH thresholds should be the same as those on day 3.
    - Day 3 FSH <10 IU/L and Day 10 FSH <10 IU/L: Reassuring result, good prognosis.
    - Day 3 FSH >10 IU/L and Day 10 FSH >10 IU/L: Poor prognosis, high cancellation rate.
    - Day 3 FSH <10 IU/L and Day 10 FSH >10 IU/L: Poor stimulation possible in spite of normal Day 3 FSH level.
    - Day 3 FSH >10 IU/L and Day 10 FSH <10 IU/L: Better odds than expected for adequate stimulation given poor Day 3 FSH result.

Understanding How the CCCT Works
- Clomiphene blocks the effects of E2 at the hypothalamus and pituitary, mimicking a hypoestrogenic state; the hypothalamic-pituitary axis responds by releasing a flood of FSH.
- A woman with a normal, healthy cohort of follicles will produce enough E2 and inhibin B to dislodge the clomiphene and suppress FSH.
- A woman with a poor cohort and aging follicles cannot generate enough E2 or inhibin B to clear the clomiphene or suppress FSH, respectively; therefore, FSH stays high.
- A meta-analysis of CCCT studies concluded that there was too little difference between basal FSH(D3) and CCCT prediction to justify the additional cost and drug exposure (Jain et al. 2004).

Anti-Müllerian Hormone (AMH)
- AMH is produced by granulosa cells of all follicles beyond the primordial follicle stage but not yet entered selection for dominance (Weenan 2004).
- AMH seems to be influenced by combined contraception (oral contraceptives, transdermal patches, and vaginal rings) with significant decreases in serum AMH levels after 9 weeks of continuous use (~50% decline from baseline values; Kallio 2013).
- Measuring AMH on day 7 of the pill-free interval seems to reflect accurate levels (Van den Berg 2010).
- <1.26 mg/mL was predictive of reduced ovarian reserve (IVF) ≤4 oocytes retrieved (Gnoth 2008).
- Measuring AMH at the onset of FSH stimulation for IVF cycles was predictive of pregnancy rates per initiated cycle (P<0.0001; Blazar 2011):
    - <1 ng/mL –23.4%
    - >3 ng/mL –60.3%
- There is reason to believe AMH may be a more useful measure of diminished ovarian reserve than FSH (Toner 2013).

Table 8.4. Clinical usefulness of AMH values

AMH (ng/mL)	Clinical Situation	Implications for Management
Low (<0.5)	Impending onset of menopause	Counseling; consider possible options of HRT, DEXA
	Impending POF	Above, plus option for donated eggs
	Impending cancer treatment	Fertility preservation
	Test for ovarian reserve	Realistic expectations
		Option of aggressive OI, DHEA, CoQ10, vitamin D
Midrange (1.0–3.5)	Ovarian reserve testing	Guide dose selection for OI/IVF
		Consideration of fertility preservation if having treatment for cancer or for social reasons
		Provide insight into options for exclusive vs. split egg donors (i.e., the higher the AMH, the more likely to split donor)
Elevated (>3.5)	PCO or PCO-like ovaries	Consider possible option of metformin
	Increased risk for OHSS	Gentle stimulation protocols; consider GnRH agonist trigger; consideration of transferring fewer good quality embryos

Source: Reproduced with permission from Toner JP, Seifer DB. Why we may abandon basal follicle-stimulating hormone testing: a sea change in determining ovarian reserve using anti-Müllerian hormone. *Fertil Steril*. 2013 Jun;99(7):1825-30. Copyright © 2013 The American Society for Reproductive Medicine.

Table 8.5. Comparison of ovarian reserve markers FSH and AMH

Feature	FSH	AMH
Site of secretion	Anterior pituitary	Granulosa of pre- and small antral follicles
Temporal change indicating ovarian aging	Latest	Earliest
Timing requirement	Cycle day 2–4 only	Any cycle day
Need for concomitant assay	E2	None
Cycle to cycle variability	High	Low
Sensitivity for low response	Moderate	Moderate
Sensitivity for high response (risk of OHSS)	None	High
Specificity for low response	High	High
Specificity for high response	None	High
Age-specific values	Limited	Extensive information
Methodology	Automated (1 hr)	ELISA (6 hr)

Source: Reproduced with permission from Toner JP, Seifer DB. Why we may abandon basal follicle-stimulating hormone testing: a sea change in determining ovarian reserve using anti-Müllerian hormone. *Fertil Steril*. 2013 Jun;99(7):1825-30. Copyright © 2013 The American Society for Reproductive Medicine.

Antral Follicle Count (AFC)

- Antral follicles 2–10 mm in diameter should be measured on days 2–4 of the menstrual cycle using transvaginal sonography.
- AFC is a reproducible measure of remaining follicle pool and is directly correlated with likelihood of pregnancy after assisted reproductive technology treatments and inversely correlated with cancellation rates. No antral follicle count, however, can be used as an absolute predictor of pregnancy or cancellation during ART treatments.
- An antral follicle count of <4 is associated with a high (41–69%) cancellation rate.

- There is a negative linear correlation between antral follicle counts and gonadotropin dose required to achieve response (Change 1998; Frattarelli 2000; Frattarelli 2003).
- Antral follicle numbers ↓ with advancing chronologic age. The rate of this decline is biphasic, with mean yearly decline of 4.8% in women <37 years of age and increasing to a mean of 11.7% thereafter (Scheffer 1999).

Diminished Ovarian Reserve

Definition
- Diminished ovarian reserve (DOR) refers to the condition of having a low number of normal oocytes or having poor quality oocytes (Scott 1995).

Background
- ↑ age is associated with ↓ fecundity (ability to get pregnant), ↓ live birth rate, ↑ early follicular phase follicular-stimulating hormone (FSH) levels, ↓ antimüllerian hormone (AMH), ↑ miscarriage rates, and ↑ in vitro fertilization (IVF) cancellation rates due to poor stimulation (Pearlstone 1992; Pellestor 2003; Stein 1985).

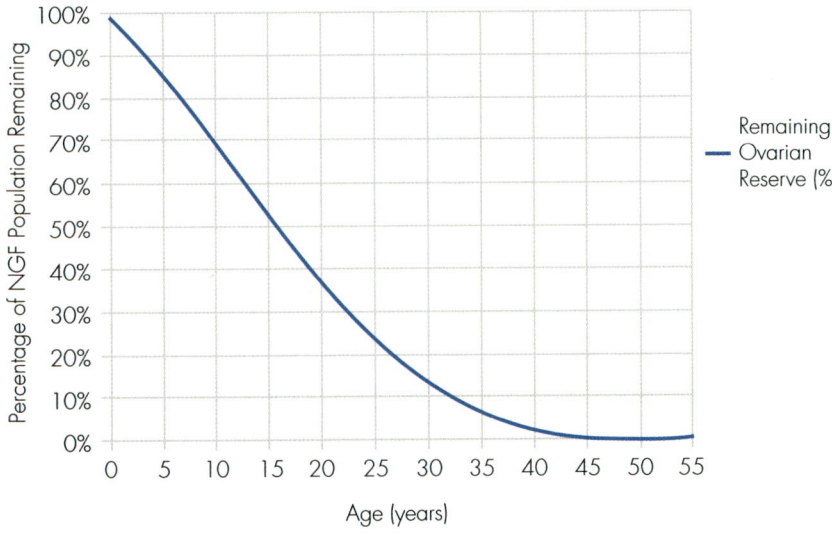

Figure 8.4. Percentage of ovarian reserve related to increasing age
NGF, nongrowing follicle.
Source: Reproduced from Wallace WH, Kelsey TW. Human ovarian reserve from conception to the menopause. *PLoS One*. 2010 Jan 27;5(1):e8772.

- For ~95% of women, by the age of 30 years only 12% of their maximum prebirth nongrowing follicles population is present, whereas for those at age 40 years only 3% of these follicles remain (Wallace 2010).

Implications
- Fragile X carrier screening (FMRI premutation) should be considered in women with diminished ovarian reserve (ACOG Committee Opinion No. 469, October 2010).
- Women with low ovarian reserve have ↓ fecundity with stimulated IVF cycles.
- The combination of an abnormal ovarian reserve test AND a poor ovarian response in the first IVF cycle predicts a very low response in subsequent cycles (Klinkert 2004).
- This **does not mean** that they do not ovulate, that they will not respond to gonadotropins or oral ovulation induction, or that there are **no** good eggs remaining within the ovary.
- It does mean, however, that there are no means by which to selectively stimulate the good eggs to ovulate and recruitment of additional follicles is unlikely.
- Before embarking on aggressive surgery or infertility treatment to enhance fertility, it is a good idea for some patients to undergo ovarian reserve testing.
- There is no significant decline in ovarian response in patients undergoing up to 3 repetitive IVF cycles (Luk 2010).
- Natural cycle IVF may be a reasonable alternative (Schimberni 2009).
- Adjuvant therapy that may improve success rates with IVF or those with diminished ovarian reserve include Coenzyme Q10, dehydroepiandrosterone, growth hormone, microdose GnRH agonist flare protocol, transdermal testosterone, and vitamin D (Bosdou 2012; Duffy 2010; Kahraman 2009; Rudick 2012; Turi 2010; Urman 2012).
- DOR testing has been found to correlate with embryonic aneuploidy (Katz-Jaffe 2013).

EVALUATION OF MALE FACTOR INFERTILITY
Semen Analysis
- Collect × 2 if first one is abnormal; one test is not enough. Patient must be abstinent for 2–3 days before collection of semen.
- Collected by masturbation or by intercourse using special semen collection condoms that do not contain substances detrimental to sperm.
- Collected at home or in the laboratory; should be kept at room temperature during transport and examined within 1 hour of collection.
- Parameters can vary widely over time, even among fertile men, and exhibit seasonal variation.

Table 8.6. Normal values for semen analysis

Parameter	Reference Value (5th %Ile)	50th %Ile	Possible Pathologies
Volume	1.5 mL	3.7	Low: ejaculatory dysfunction, hypogonadism, poor collection technique
Concentration	>15 million/mL	73	Azoospermia or oligospermia: varicocele, genetic, cryptorchidism, endocrinopathy, drugs, infections, toxins or radiation, obstruction, idiopathic
Total motile count	≥10 million	≥165	10–20 would warrant IUI therapy
Motility	>40%	61%	Asthenospermia: prolonged abstinence, antisperm antibodies, partial obstruction, infection, sperm structural defects, idiopathic
Normal morphology	>4% normal	15%	Teratospermia: varicocele, genetic, cryptorchidism, drugs, infections, toxins or radiation, idiopathic

Source: Adapted from Cooper TG, Noonan E, von Eckardstein S, et al. World Health Organization reference values for human semen characteristics. *Hum Reprod Update*. 2010; May-Jun;16(3):231-45.

Total Motile Count
- Total motile count (TMC) before processing (million = volume × concentration × percent motility):
  - 10–20 million: IUI helpful
  - 5–10 million: IVF
  - <5 million: intracytoplasmic sperm injection (ICSI)

Antisperm Antibodies
- SperMAR >20% necessitates obtaining immunobead testing wherein head-binding antibodies are worse than tail, and >50% head-binding antibodies are worrisome (Clarke 1985).
- Pregnancy rates are lower when >50% of sperm are antibody-bound (Ayvaliotis 1985).
- ICSI can circumvent adverse effects of antisperm antibodies (ASAs).
- Screen for ASA when there is isolated asthenospermia with normal sperm concentration, sperm agglutination, or an abnormal postcoital test.
- ASAs found on the surface of sperm by direct testing are more significant than ASAs found in the serum or seminal plasma by indirect testing.
- ASA testing is not needed if sperm are to be used for ICSI.

Round Cells
- Leukocytes and immature germ cells appear similar and are properly termed *round cells*.
- When >5 million/mL or >10/high power fields (high power fields = 40× magnification), must differentiate using cytologic staining and immunohistochemical techniques.
- Mild prostatitis, epididymitis? (Treatment: doxycycline 100 mg b.i.d. or ciprofloxacin 500 mg b.i.d. × 14–21 days + ibuprofen 600 mg t.i.d. × 7 days)

Hormones
- Evaluation of the pituitary-gonadal axis (1.7% incidence of abnormalities); evaluate if <10 million/mL sperm concentration, impaired sexual function, or other clinical findings suggestive of a specific endocrinopathy.
- Testosterone: ↓ in presence of prolactinoma or hypogonadotropism.
  - If low, obtain a repeat measurement of total and free testosterone.
- FSH: ↑ in germ cell aplasia.
- Prolactin: ↓ libido/impotence.
- Thyroid-stimulating hormone: hypothyroidism leads to hyperprolactinemia.

Table 8.7. Hormone profiles of men with normal and abnormal spermatogenesis

Clinical Condition	Follicle-Stimulating Hormone	Luteinizing Hormone	Testosterone	Prolactin
Normal spermatogenesis	Normal	Normal	Normal	Normal
Hypogonadotropic hypogonadism	Low	Low	Low	Normal
Abnormal spermatogenesis[a]	High/normal	Normal	Normal	Normal
Complete testicular failure/hypergonadotropic hypogonadism	High	High	Normal/low	Normal
Prolactin-secreting pituitary tumor	Normal/low	Normal/low	Low	High

[a]Many men with abnormal spermatogenesis have a normal serum follicle-stimulating hormone, but a marked elevation of serum follicle-stimulating hormone is clearly indicative of an abnormality in spermatogenesis.

GENETICS OF MALE SUBFERTILITY
Cystic Fibrosis Gene Mutations (Autosomal Recessive)
- Congenital bilateral absence of vas deferens (CBAVD) is strongly associated with mutations of the cystic fibrosis (CF) transmembrane regulator gene on chromosome 7.
  - CBAVD is associated with mutations within the CF gene in 70–80% of men.
  - CBAVD is present in 1% of infertile males.
- CBAVD is one of the more common diagnoses in patients with obstructive azoospermia.
- The female partner should be carefully screened for CF (genetic sequencing preferable) before performing a treatment that uses his sperm because of the risk that his partner may be a CF carrier.

Chromosomal Abnormalities Resulting in Impaired Testicular Function
- The prevalence of karyotypic abnormalities in infertile men is 7%.
- The frequency is inversely proportional to sperm count:
  - 10–15% in azoospermic men
  - 5% in oligospermic men
  - <1% in normospermic men
- Klinefelter's syndrome (47,XXY or 46,XY/47,XXY) accounts for 2/3 of the chromosomal abnormalities observed in subfertile men.
- Structural abnormalities of the autosomal chromosomes, such as inversions and translocations, are also observed at a higher frequency in infertile men than in the general population.
- A couple is at an increased risk for miscarriages and children with chromosomal and congenital defects when the male has gross karyotypic abnormalities.
- Karyotyping should be offered to men who have nonobstructive azoospermia (NOA) or severe oligospermia (<5 million/mL) before IVF with ICSI.
- Genetic counseling should be provided whenever a genetic abnormality is detected.

Y-Chromosome Microdeletions Associated with Isolated Spermatogenic Impairment
- Y-chromosome analysis should be offered to men who have NOA or severe oligospermia (<5 million/mL) before ICSI.
- Found in approximately 10% of men with azoospermia or severe oligospermia.
- Too small to be detected by standard karyotyping but can be found by using polymerase chain reaction.
- The intervening large segment of the Y chromosome, known as the male specific Y, contains many genes involved in spermatogenesis.
- The regions prone to microdeletion are the AZFa, AZFb, and AZFc.

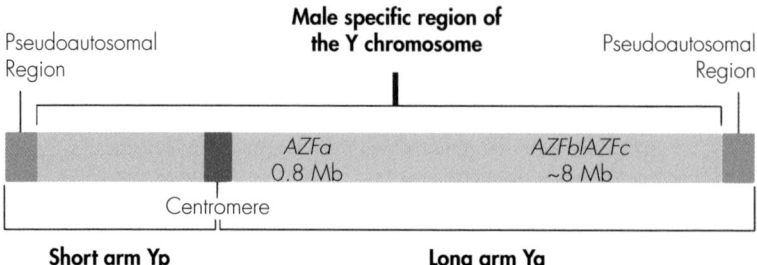

Figure 8.5. Location of Y chromosome deletions related to azoospermia (DAZ)
Source: Adapted from Oates RD. The genetics of male reproductive failure: what every clinician needs to know. *Sexuality, Reproduction and Menopause.* 2004;2(4):213.

- There is microdeletion in AZFc region in 1 in 4000 men; it is the most common molecular cause of NOA.
  - Approximately 70% of men with an AZFc microdeletion possess sperm.
  - 13% of men with NOA are AZFc microdeleted.
  - Approximately 6% of men with severe oligospermia (<5 million/mL) are AZFc microdeleted.

BASIC FERTILITY TREATMENT: OVULATION INDUCTION
Fast Facts
- Treatment of anovulation requires correct identification of underlying etiology.
  - Polycystic ovarian syndrome: ovulation induction with oral or injectable medications
  - Thyroid dysfunction: thyroid hormone therapy
  - Hyperprolactinemia: dopamine agonist therapy
  - Functional hypothalamic amenorrhea: lifestyle modification or low dose gonadotropin injections after low dose estrogen priming
- Prior to ovulation induction, it may be prudent to rule out other potential causes of infertility.
- In a couple in whom the woman is diagnosed with PCOS, the prevalence of additional infertility factors are as follows (McGovern 2007):
  - 10% oligospermia
  - 4% nonpatency of tubes
  - 1% hyperprolactinemia
  - 1% uncontrolled thyroid disease

Treatment Options for PCOS Patients: Initial Approach
Lifestyle Modification/Weight Loss
- Guzick (1994) compared weight loss to no weight loss in obese, hyperandrogenic, anovulatory women.
  - Women in the treatment group displayed SHBG, ↓ free T, and ↓ fasting insulin levels.
  - Four of six spontaneously ovulated.
- As little as a 7% ↓ in body weight significantly improves hyperandrogenism (Kiddy 1992).
- 5–10% ↓ in body weight is enough to restore ovulation in 55–100% within 6 months (Kiddy 1992).

Metformin (see page 545)
- A popular adjuvant therapy that may assist in weight loss and may improve responsiveness to ovulation induction agents

Clomiphene (SERM) or Letrozole (Aromatase Inhibitors)
- These are the treatments of choice for ovulation induction.
- If nonresponsive, a higher dose of CC or AI may be initiated without inducing menses ("stair-step" protocol; Hurst 2009).
- Metformin in addition to CC may not improve pregnancy rates (Legro 2007) in spite of increasing ovulation rates. Other studies have shown a benefit (Morin-Papunen 2012).
- Aromatase inhibitors may have better efficacy than clomiphene citrate (Legro NEJM 2014) when used with intercourse:
  - Both CC and AI require intact hypothalamic-pituitary-ovarian axis.
  - Letrozole's terminal elimination half-life is approximately 2 days.
  - Letrozole use for ovulation induction is off-label as it is not FDA approved for fertility treatment.
  - Compared to clomiphene citrate, there was no difference in rate of congenital malformations (Zulaudi 2006; Badawy 2008).
  - Letrozole seems more effective than clomiphene for PCOS.

Table 8.8. Live birth rates in PCOS patients using clomiphene vs. letrozole

	Aromatase Inhibitor	Clomiphene Citrate
Cumulative live birth rate over 5 cycles	27.5%*	19.1%
Live birth rate/cycle	6.2%	4%

Source: Data from Legro RS, Brzyski RG, Diamond MP et al; NICHD Reproductive Medicine Network. Letrozole versus clomiphene for infertility in the polycystic ovary syndrome. *N Engl J Med.* 2014 Jul 10;371(2):119-29.

Table 8.9. "Rule of 5s" and "rule of 7s" for ovulation induction

Rule of 5s	Check estradiol and progesterone to rule out recent or imminent ovulation
	(E2 <100 pg/mL and progesterone <3 ng/dL)
	Oral progestin 10 mg q day × 5 days (after negative β-hCG)
	Begin clomiphene (or letrozole) on day 5 of bleeding
	50 mg clomiphene (or 5 mg of letrozole) q day × 5 days
	Timed coitus 5 days later and for 5 days every other day
Rule of 7s (only valid for patients taking clomiphene)	Check estradiol 7 days after last pill (CD#16) to assess recruitment
	Check progesterone 7 days after estradiol to confirm ovulation
	Check β-hCG 7 days after progesterone and perform pelvic exam/sonogram to assess prior to next clomiphene cycle
Other Rules	Increase clomiphene by 50 mg until ovulation obtained, 50% will ovulate on 50 mg. No dose adjustment for letrozole
	Follow follicular size with ultrasound
	Consider IUI especially in couple with unexplained infertility:
	Give 5000–10,000 mIU hCG when follicle 20–22 mm
	Ovulation will occur about 41 hours after hCG
	15% of patients develop poor cervical mucus
	Treatment usually limited to 4 ovulatory cycles as most pregnancies occur during first 4 cycles

Treatment Options: Patients Resistant to Clomiphene or Letrozole at Standard Doses

Gonadotropins

- PCOS patients are highly susceptible to hyperstimulation; start with low doses.

Glucocorticoids

- Steroid treatment appears to be related to the suppression of excessive androgen levels (Steinberger 1979).
- Three randomized trials demonstrated reasonable pregnancy rates (40–75% vs. 4–35%) in CC-resistant women (Daly 1984; Elnashar 2006; Parsanezhad 2002).
- A response was seen for those with or without elevated DHEA-S levels.
- One protocol is to utilize **2 mg dexamethasone from cycle days 5 through 14** in conjunction with ovulation induction medicine (Parsanezhad 2002).

Laparoscopic Ovarian Cautery/Drilling:

- Restores spontaneous ovulation in ~50% of CC-resistant hyperandrogenic women (Gjønnæss 1984; Daniell and Miller 1989; Abdel Gadir 1990; Gjønnæss 1998; Lazovic 1998; Vegetti 1998).
- Consider the balance between reducing androgen levels and potential negative effects:
  - Postoperative adhesion formation
  - General endotracheal anesthesia
  - Iatrogenic diminished ovarian reserve
- Spontaneous abortion (SAB) rate may be lower for ovarian cautery compared with medical induction of ovulation (Abdel Gadir 1992).
- Predictors of success:
  - Good responders:
    - Women with hyperinsulinemia respond better to ovarian drilling than do those with normoinsulinemia with respect to lowered glucose and insulin values (Saleh 2001).
    - LH >10 IU/L (Amer 2004)
    - Lean PCOS women (<25 kg/m^2 BMI; Baghdadi 2012)
  - Poor responders (Amer 2004):
    - BMI ≥35 kg/m^2
    - Total T ≥4.5 nmol/L or 130 ng/dL
    - Duration of infertility >3 years
- In women with PCOS, the pregnancy rate at 12 and 18 months after drilling is 55% and 70%, respectively (Felemban 2000).
- Approximately 20 years after ovarian cauterization in anovulatory PCOS women, 74% were still ovulating (Gjønnaess 1998).
- Randomized, controlled trial for CC-resistant women with PCOS: ovarian cauterization or recombinant FSH

Table 8.10. Use of electrocautery and/or recombinant FSH for ovulation induction in the PCOS patient

Technique	Pregnancies (%)	Live Births (%)
r-hFSH	67	60
Ovarian cauterization	34	34
Ovarian cauterization → anovulatory women given CC	29	29
Ovarian cauterization → anovulatory women given r-hFSH after failed CC	65	52

CC, clomiphene citrate (Clomid); r-hFSH, recombinant human follicle-stimulating hormone.

Source: Data from Bayram N, Van Wely M, et al. Using an electrocautery strategy or recombinant follicle stimulating hormone to induce ovulation in polycystic ovary syndrome: randomised controlled trial. *BMJ*. 2004 328(7433):192.

Cochrane Library Review Concluding Statement concerning Ovarian Drilling

There is a lack of controlled data, and relatively few RCTs of this surgical technique have been carried out. With such a small number of patients studied in a controlled way and underpowered studies, conclusions about the effectiveness of laparoscopic treatment of the polycystic ovarian syndrome remain uncertain. Although observational data show that it is likely that ovarian drilling has a beneficial effect on ovulation and pregnancy rates for anovulatory PCOS patients wishing to conceive, more data on the short- and long-term safety of the procedure are required.

ADVANCED FERTILITY TREATMENT: SUPEROVULATION AND INTRAUTERINE INSEMINATION (IUI) FOR UNEXPLAINED INFERTILITY

Fast Facts
- As goal is the recruitment of multiple follicles, consider changing dosing clomiphene to 100 mg CD #3–7 or combining oral and injectable medications or utilizing gonadotropins as a single agent.
- Ultrasound monitoring of ovarian response required.
- Risk of hyperstimulation and multiple pregnancy may be problematic, especially in patients <35 years old.
- Best candidates are those with previous conception as a couple and no significant male factor nor peritoneal issues like adhesions or endometriosis.
- Non-ART options for unexplained infertility:
  - clomiphene/IUI
  - letrozole/IUI
  - gonadotropin/IUI

Table 8.11. Live birth, multiple live birth, clinical pregnancy, multiple clinical pregnancy, and conception rates per cycle

Variable	Gonadotropin Group (n = 301)	Clomiphene Group (n = 300) No./Total No. (%)	Letrozole Group (n = 299)
Live birth per treatment cycle			
Pre-treatment cycle 1	1/301(0.3)	0/300(0)	0/299(0)
Treatment cycle 1	47/292(16.1)	31/294(10.5)	25/288(8.7)
Treatment cycle 2	23/217(10.6)	15/235(6.4)	10/242(4.1)
Treatment cycle 3	19/160(11.9)	11/195(5.6)	10/204(4.9)
Treatment cycle 4	7/110(6.4)	13/163(8.0)	11/172(6.4)
Clinical pregnancy per treatment cycle			
Pre-treatment cycle 1	1/301(0.3)	0/300(0)	1/299(0.3)
Treatment cycle 1	50/292(17.1)	38/294(12.9)	28/288(9.7)
Treatment cycle 2	26/217(12.0)	18/235(7.7)	13/242(5.4)
Treatment cycle 3	23/160(14.4)	13/195(6.7)	13/204(6.4)
Treatment cycle 4	7/110(6.4)	16/163(9.8)	12/172(7.0)

Source: Data from Diamond MP, Legro RS, Coutifaris C, Alvero R, et al., Gonadotropin, or Clomiphene for Unexplained infertility:. N Engl J Med. 2015 Sep 24;373(13):1230-40.

Fast Track and Standard Treatment Trial (FASTT)
- Couples were randomized to receive either conventional treatment (n = 247) with three cycles of clomiphene citrate (CC)/IUI, three cycles of FSH/IUI, and up to six cycles of IVF or an accelerated treatment (n = 256) that omitted the three cycles of FSH/IUI.
- An increased rate of pregnancy was observed in the accelerated arm (hazard ratio [HR], 1.25; 95% confidence interval [CI], 1.00–1.56) compared with the conventional arm. Median time to pregnancy was 8 and 11 months in the accelerated and conventional arms, respectively.

- Per cycle pregnancy rates for CC/IUI, FSH/IUI, and IVF were 7.6%, 9.8%, and 30.7%. Average charges per delivery were $9,800 lower (95% CI, $25,100 lower to $3,900 higher) in the accelerated arm compared to conventional treatment. The observed incremental difference was a savings of $2,624 per couple for accelerated treatment and 0.06 more deliveries.

Source: Reindollar RH, et al. A randomized clinical trial to evaluate optimal treatment for unexplained infertility: the fast track and standard treatment (FASTT) trial. *Fertil Steril.* 2010;94(3):888-899.

ASSISTED REPRODUCTIVE TECHNOLOGIES
Fast Facts
- ART, by definition, are any fertility treatments in which both egg and sperm are handled. Accordingly, ART procedures involve the surgical removal of eggs, known as egg retrieval.
- IVF is the most common ART procedure; IVF has been used in the United States since 1981, and data are collected by the Centers for Disease Control and Prevention and published annually (http://www.cdc.gov/reproductivehealth/art.htm).
  - In 2013, 190,773 ART cycles were performed in over 460 fertility clinics.
    - 47,818 live births yielding 67,996 babies

Definitions
- **IVF:** ovulation induction, oocyte retrieval, and fertilization of the oocytes in the laboratory; embryos are then cultured for 3–5 days with subsequent transfer transcervically under abdominal ultrasound guidance into the uterine cavity.
- **Gamete intrafallopian transfer:** ovarian stimulation and egg retrieval along with laparoscopically guided transfer of a mixture of unfertilized eggs and sperm into the fallopian tubes.
- **Zygote intrafallopian transfer:** ovarian stimulation and egg retrieval followed by fertilization of the eggs in the laboratory and laparoscopic transfer of the day 1 fertilized eggs (zygotes) into the fallopian tubes.
- **Donor egg IVF:** used for patients with poor egg numbers or egg quality; involves stimulation of an egg donor with typical superovulation followed by standard egg retrieval; eggs are then fertilized by the sperm of the infertile woman's partner, and embryos are transferred to the infertile woman in a standard IVF-like process.
- **ICSI:** developed in the early 1990s to help couples with severe male factor infertility; one sperm is injected directly into each mature egg, typically resulting in a 50–70% fertilization rate.

Table 8.12. Gonadotropin preparations

Trade Name, Manufacturer	Source
FSH/LH-*containing preparations*	
Menopur, Ferring	Urine of menopausal women
Repronex, Ferring	Urine of menopausal women
FSH-*containing preparations*	
Bravelle, Ferring	Urine of menopausal women
Follistim AQ, Merck & Co.	Recombinant, Chinese hamster ovary cells
Gonal-F, EMD Serono	Recombinant, Chinese hamster ovary cells

FSH, follicle-stimulating hormone; LH, luteinizing hormone.

Assisted Reproductive Technologies

Table 8.13. Gonadotropin-releasing hormone agonist/antagonist preparations

Trade Name, Manufacturer	Formulations
Cetrotide, EMD Serono (antagonist)	250 μg/1 mL SC
Ganirelex, Merck & Co. (antagonist)	250 μg/0.5 mL SC
Leuprolide (agonist)	1 mg/0.2 mL = 20 U SC
Synarel, Pfizer (agonist)	2 mg/mL intranasal
Zoladex, AstraZeneca (agonist)	3.6 mg SC

Stimulation Protocols and Doses

- Estimating the patient's responsiveness to the fertility agents should guide choice of protocol:
  - Age, body mass index, day 3 FSH, AMH, antral follicle count, response to prior ovarian stimulation

Oral Contraceptive—Gonadotropin-Releasing Hormone Agonist Stimulation Protocol

Oral contraceptives (OCs) can help with scheduling of IVF cycles and may help synchronize the ovary and result in a better cohort size. OCs typically increase the amount of medications required during stimulation and may decrease the number of eggs in older women.

1. Start OCs between days 1 and 3 of menstrual cycle. Typically administer for 15–21 days.
2. Start GnRH-a 3–5 days before the completion of the OCs. This overlap of OCs and GnRH-a helps to prevent ovarian cyst formation.
3. Spontaneous menses expected 10–12 days after the first day of GnRH-a.
4. Start ovarian stimulation and continue GnRH-a. Stimulation can be with FSH, human menopausal gonadotropin (HMG), or a combination of FSH and HMG.
5. Serial ultrasounds and E2 levels monitor follicular development; E2 should ↑ by ~50% each day of stimulation.
6. Once several follicles reach 18–22 mm, administer hCG, typically 5,000–10,000 U SC or IM.
7. Check serum hCG day after hCG injection to verify.
8. Oocyte retrieval is 36 hours after hCG.

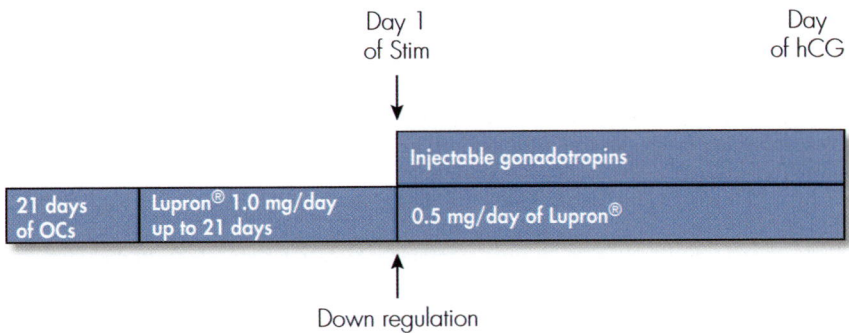

Figure 8.6. OCP/LTL protocol for IVF

OC, oral contraceptive; Stim, gonadotropin-stimulating hormone agonist stimulation; hCG, human chorionic gonadotropin.

INFERTILITY — Assisted Reproductive Technologies

Luteal Gonadotropin-Releasing Hormone Agonist Stimulation Protocol
1. Start GnRH-a on day 21 of menstrual cycle. The luteal start is typically confirmed by a serum progesterone level >5 ng/mL. The luteal start of GnRH-a helps to prevent ovarian cyst formation.
2. Spontaneous menses expected 10–12 days after the first day of GnRH-a.
3. Start ovarian stimulation and continue Lupron at lower dose. Stimulation can be with FSH, HMG, or a combination of FSH and HMG.
4. Serial ultrasounds and E2 levels monitor follicular development; E2 should ↑ by ~50% each day of stimulation.
5. Once several follicles reach 18–22 mm, administer hCG, typically 10,000 U SC or IM.
6. Check serum hCG day after hCG injection to verify.
7. Oocyte retrieval 36 hours after hCG.

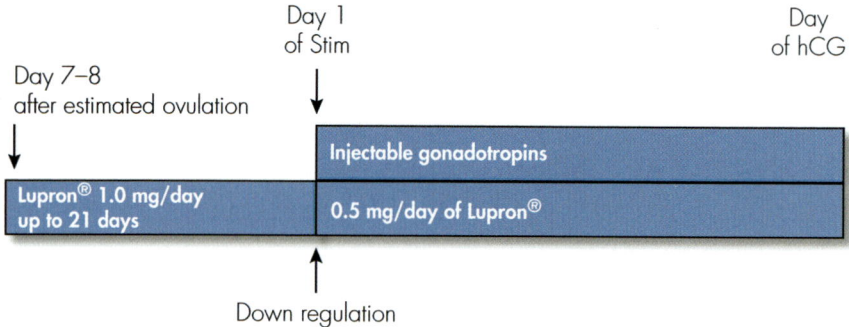

Figure 8.7. LTL protocol for IVF
Stim, gonadotropin-releasing hormone agonist stimulation; hCG, human chorionic gonadotropin.

Microdose Gonadotropin-Releasing Hormone Agonist Flare Stimulation Protocol
1. Start of OCs between days 1 and 3 of menstrual cycle and administer for 21 days. (Note: Many programs do not use OCs at all for this protocol.)
2. Start Lupron, 40 μg SC q12 hours, 3 days after the end of the OC course (i.e., day 24).
3. Start ovarian stimulation with FSH, HMG, or a combination of FSH and HMG 3 days after the start of Lupron (i.e., day 27) and continue Lupron. (Note: Many programs start the gonadotropins on the same day as the microdose Lupron.)
4. Serial ultrasounds and E2 levels monitor follicular development; E2 should ↑ by ~50% each day of stimulation.
5. Once several follicles reach 18–22 mm, administer hCG, typically 5,000–10,000 units SC or IM.
6. Check serum hCG day after hCG injection to verify.
7. Oocyte retrieval is 36 hours after hCG.

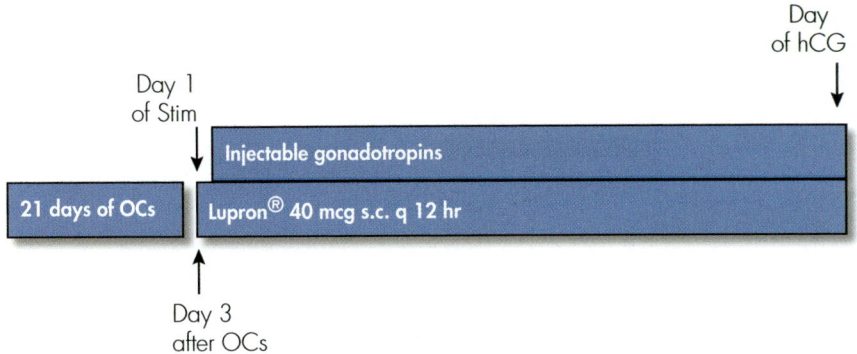

Figure 8.8. OCP/microdose GnRH-agonist protocol for IVF
Stim, gonadotropin-releasing hormone agonist flare stimulation; hCG, human chorionic gonadotropin; OCs, oral contraceptives.

Oral Contraceptive—Gonadotropin-Releasing Hormone Antagonist Stimulation Protocol

1. Start of OCs between days 1 and 3 of menstrual cycle. Typically, administer for 15–21 days.
2. Start ovarian stimulation 3–5 days after discontinuing OCs. Stimulation can be with FSH, HMG, or a combination of FSH and HMG.
3. Serial ultrasounds and E2 levels to monitor follicular development; E2 should rise ~50% per day.
4. On stimulation day 6, start GnRH antagonist. Administration of the GnRH antagonist can lower endogenous E2 levels. Typically, no further decrease in gonadotropin dose is recommended. Rather, most clinicians add back FSH/LH drugs at time of antagonist start. Could use GnRH agonist trigger to decrease incidence of OHSS.
5. Once several follicles 18–22 mm, administer hCG, typically 5,000–10,000 U SC or IM or 4 mg SC leuprolide (some programs repeat dose in 12 hours).
6. To ensure an adequate response to the trigger, check hCG for the hCG trigger or serum LH and P4 if GnRH-agonist utilized (adequate if LH ≥15 mIU/mL and P4 ≥3 ng/mL).
7. Oocyte retrieval is 36 hours after hCG. or GnRH-a.
8. Some evidence suggests that cryopreservation of all embryos following GnRH-a trigger is appropriate given difficulty in providing adequate luteal support. Ovarian hyperstimulation is almost never seen following GnRH-a trigger. Some clinics use dual trigger with minimal HCG dose given in addition to GnRH-a trigger.

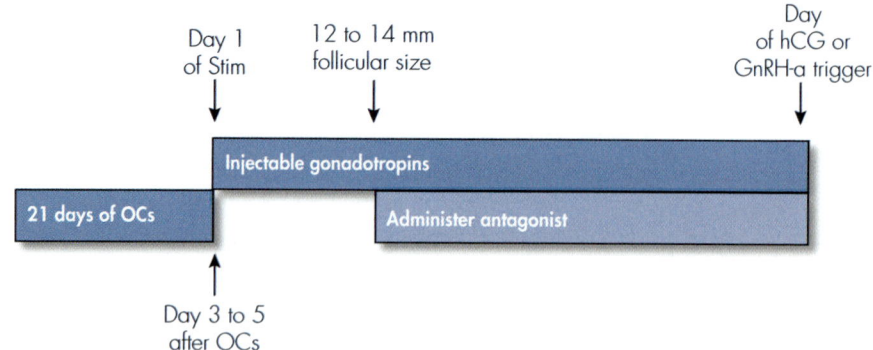

Figure 8.9. OCP/GnRH-antagonist protocol for IVF
Stim, gonadotropin-releasing hormone antagonist stimulation; hCG, human chorionic gonadotropin; OCs, oral contraceptives.

Natural Cycle IVF
1. Baseline ultrasound between cycle days 2 and 4 of menstrual cycle.
2. Monitoring ultrasound on cycle day 7 and serial ultrasounds and E2 levels thereafter.
3. When E2 >125 pg/mL and follicle >15.5 mm, administer hCG 10,000 U IM.
4. Oocyte retrieval is 36 hours later; aspirate follicle and flush until oocyte is obtained.

- Benefits to natural cycle IVF:
  - Lower costs per cycle but lower pregnancy rates as well
  - Elimination of OHSS
  - Single embryo transfer in >99% of cases
  - Obviates ethical concerns of patients regarding frozen embryos

Oocyte Retrieval
- This is typically performed under IV sedation using a 5-MHz vaginal transducer with associated needle guide 36 hours after hCG.
- A 17-gauge, 35-cm aspiration needle is inserted transvaginally into multiple preovulatory follicles with sequential aspiration (low-grade suction <100 mm Hg) of oocytes. The aspirate is then given to the embryologist for evaluation.
- Complications can include intraabdominal bleeding and infection, typically occurring in <1% of IVF cases.

Assisted Reproductive Technologies   **INFERTILITY**

Embryology Primer

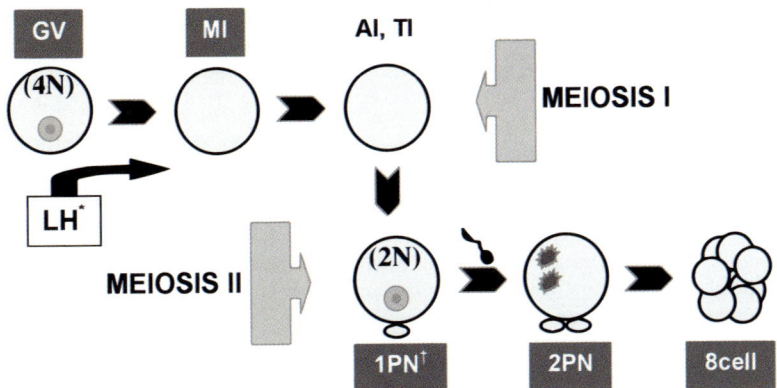

Figure 8.10. Sequence of oocyte maturation, fertilization, and embryo development
AI, anaphase I; GV, germinal vesicle; MI, metaphase I; N, nuclei; PN, pronuclei; TI, telophase I.
*Arrested at prophase I until luteinizing hormone (LH) surge.
†Arrested at metaphase II until fertilization.

- Retrieved eggs are identified in the follicular aspirate. Once they are identified, they are removed from the aspirate and placed in culture dishes.
- A standard IVF insemination is performed by culturing the identified eggs for approximately 16 hours with ~50,000 sperm/mL. The next morning, the eggs are identified and evaluated for fertilization. The first sign of fertilization is two pronuclei within the cytoplasm.
- ICSI is performed in cases of severe male factor infertility, failed fertilization in a previous cycle, or severe antisperm antibody levels. After identification of the eggs in the follicular aspirate, the eggs are then placed into culture dishes. The cumulus cell complex surrounding the eggs is then removed in a process called stripping. Once the eggs are stripped, they are evaluated for maturity. Only metaphase 2 (MII) eggs can be fertilized. All MII eggs are then inseminated by taking one motile, morphologically normal-appearing sperm and injecting it into each mature egg.
- Fertilization. rate with standard insemination is approximately 70%. With ICSI fertilization, rates range from 50–70%.
- Embryos are then cultured, typically for 3–5 days, in incubators maintained at body temperature and media specific for human embryo culture. Embryos are typically evaluated on day 3 for their cell number and overall morphology.
- According to the most recent data from the CDC ART Summary, blastocyst transfer (day 5 or beyond) is now more commonly performed than day 2 or day 3 ET.
- Extended embryo culture to the blastocyst stage may help to identify embryos with the highest prognosis for pregnancy. In addition, vitrification of blastocyst stage embryos yields excellent frozen embryo transfer pregnancy rates and trophectoderm biopsy can be performed prior to vitrification to allow preimplantation genetic testing of the embryo.
- Blastocyst embryo transfer seems to increase the risk of monozygotic twins compared to day 2–3 embryo transfers (Behr et al. 2000).

Postretrieval Hormonal Management

- Due to the use of GnRH-a and antagonists, there is concern about diminished progesterone secretion by the corpus luteum. Accordingly, the vast majority of ART cycles use supplemental progesterone via IM progesterone or vaginally administered progesterone. This is typically continued until 9–12 weeks of pregnancy.
- Some centers also replace E2, which is also concomitantly secreted by the corpus luteum.

Embryo Transfer

- Most commonly on day 5, the embryo(s) are transferred transcervically into the uterine cavity.
- The number of embryos transferred is ultimately based on the patient's age, prior IVF history, egg quality, embryo quality, and the IVF center's success rates.
- Embryo transfer is typically performed under ultrasound guidance. A full bladder helps provide acoustic window and decreases the anterior bend of the cervix in patients with an anteverted uterus. This can ease embryo transfer.
- Patients are typically asked to rest for 12–24 hours after embryo transfer, although there is little scientific evidence to support this practice.

Table 8.14. Criteria for number of embryos to transfer in IVF[a]

Prognosis	Age <35	Age 35–37	Age 38–40	Age >40
Favorable[b]	1–2	2	3	5
All others	2	3	4	5
Blastocysts[a]				
Favorable[b]	1	2	2	3
All others	2	2	3	3

[a]See text for more complete explanations. Justification for transferring more than the recommended number of embryos should be clearly documented in the patient's medical record.

[b]Favorable = first cycle of in vitro fertilization, good embryo quality, excess embryos available for cryopreservation, or previous successful *in vitro* fertilization cycle.

Source: Reproduced from Practice Committee of American Society for Reproductive Medicine; Practice Committee of Society for Assisted Reproductive Technology. Criteria for number of embryos to transfer: a committee opinion. *Fertil Steril.* 2013 Jan;99(1):44-46. Copyright © 2013 The American Society for Reproductive Medicine.

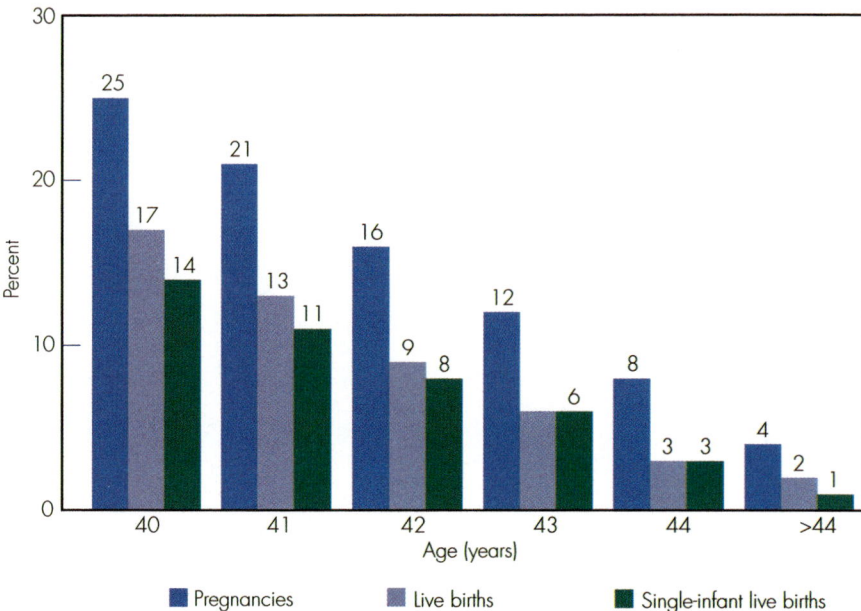

* For consistency, all percentages are based on cycles started.

Figure 8.11. Percentages of ART cycles using fresh nondonor eggs or embryos that resulted in pregnancies, live births, and singleton live births, by age of woman, 2013
Source: Centers for Disease Control and Prevention, American Society for Reproductive Medicine, Society for Assisted Reproductive Technology. *2013 Assisted Reproductive Technology National Summary Report.* Atlanta: US Department of Health and Human Services; 2015.

Preimplantation Genetic Screening in IVF

- Allows for genetic testing to be performed on a cell or cells from a developing embryo created through IVF.
  - Biopsy/testing can take place at various stages of development:
    - polar bodies, blastomeres, and blastocysts can be biopsied and analyzed; current trends appear to favor trophectoderm biopsy of 5–10 cells per embryo (Forman 2013).
- Healthy embryos, free of the tested disorder, are selectively transferred.
- Can be performed for all single gene disorders as long as the DNA mutations are known. Can also test embryos for HLA matching, chromosome rearrangements, aneuploidy screening. Testing for multiple indications is often possible.
- Limitations:
  - Not 100% accurate and prenatal testing is still recommended.
  - Biopsy is an invasive procedure that can damage embryos although data is thus far reassuring.

- Gamete/embryo donation represents an alternative pathway to parenthood.
  - Using gametes from a donor reduces the risk of passing on a genetic disorder. This is an option for dominant, X-linked, and recessive genetic disorders.

Risk of Birth Defects Following IVF

- Subfertile women should be aware that there is an increased risk of birth defects whether or not they undergo fertility treatment.

Table 8.15. Risk of birth defects following IVF or IVF/ICSI

Singleton Births	AOR (CI)	# Defects*	% Defects*	Per 100
Spont and fertile	1.00	16,841/293,314	5.7%	6
Spont and infertility	**1.37** (1.02–1.83)	52/600	**8.7%**	**9**
IVF + ICSI	**1.28** (1.14–1.43)	361/4,333	**8.3%**	**8**
IVF fresh ET	1.05 (0.82–1.35)	71/1,005	7.1%	7
FET from IVF	1.08 (0.76–1.53)	34/479	7.1%	7
ICSI fresh ET	**1.73** (1.35–2.21)	76/713	**10.7%**	**11**
FET from ICSI	1.10 (0.65–1.85)	15/226	6.6%	7

AOR, adjusted odds ratio.
*Unadjusted.
Source: Data from Davies MJ, Moore VM, Willson KJ, Van Essen P, Priest K, Scott H, Haan EA, Chan A. Reproductive technologies and the risk of birth defects. N Engl J Med. 2012 10;366(19):1803-13.

Risk of Cancer in Women Undergoing Fertility Treatment

- Studies from the 1990s reported an increased risk of breast, endometrial, and ovarian cancer with more recent studies refuting this (Sergentanis 2013; Siristatidis 2013).
- By and large, infertility itself seems to be an important risk factor for ovarian cancer rather than infertility treatment increasing the risk.
- A retrospective cohort study in 87,403 Israeli women undergoing VF found no significant increase in breast, endometrial, or ovarian cancer in a ≤7 year time span (Brinton 2013). Note: Borderline ovarian tumors were not included.
- A historical cohort study (with ~15 years of follow-up) in 19,146 women undergoing IVF compared to 6,006 subfertile women not treated with IVF (van Leeuwen 2011) found the following:
  - The incidence of borderline ovarian tumors was higher in the IVF cohort when compared with the general population and when compared with the subfertility group.
  - The rate of invasive ovarian cancer was not increased when compared with the subfertile group.
- The largest systematic review evaluating the risk of borderline ovarian tumors following the use of fertility drugs demonstrated no significant increased risk for borderline ovarian tumors with CC alone, CC and gonadotropins, or gonadotropins alone (Rizzuto 2013).

OVARIAN HYPERSTIMULATION SYNDROME (OHSS)
Incidence
- Iatrogenic complication of superovulation with gonadotropins (rarely oral fertility medications) with a varied spectrum of clinical and laboratory manifestations
- Incidence in superovulation cycles:
  - Mild ovarian hyperstimulation syndrome (OHSS) →33%
  - Moderate OHSS → 3%
  - Severe OHSS → 0.1%

Risk Factors
- <33 years old
- Aggressive response to ovarian stimulation (≥18 follicles and/or E2 ≥5,000 ng/dL)
- Anovulatory women with polycystic ovary syndrome (PCOS)
- High antral follicle count
- High basal antimüllerian hormone (>3.36 ng/mL; Lee 2008)
- History of OHSS
- hCG trigger (use of Luprolide [GnRH-a trigger nearly completely eliminates risk of OHSS])

Pathophysiology
- Ovarian enlargement with multiple cysts
- Stromal edema
- ↑ capillary permeability (marked arteriolar vasodilation) with acute fluid shift out of intravascular space
- ↑ permeability secondary to a factor secreted by corpora lutea? Factors: Prostaglandins (PGs)? Endothelin-I? Vascular endothelial growth factor? Angiotensin-II?
- Shift of fluid from intravascular space into the abdominal cavity → massive third spacing
- At time of oocyte retrieval, follicular aspirations of even smaller follicles offer partial protection against OHSS by removing granulosa cells
- Early vs. late form (Papanikolaou 2004):
  - Early-onset:
    - OHSS is related to exogenous hCG and is associated with a higher risk for preclinical miscarriage
    - presents 3–7 days after hCG administration
  - Late-onset:
    - OHSS is more likely associated with pregnancy and tends to be more severe with a relatively low risk for miscarriage presents 12–17 days after hCG administration

Management
- Conservative management leading to spontaneous resolution with time:
  - 7 days in nonpregnant women
  - 10–20 days in pregnant women
- Have patient drink ≥1 L fluid/day (Gatorade)
- ↓ physical activity
- Pelvic rest; in fact, bimanual examination may lead to ovarian rupture and hemorrhage

INFERTILITY — Ovarian Hyperstimulation Syndrome (OHSS)

- Laboratory tests:
  - Electrolytes, creatinine (Cr)
  - Complete blood count (CBC) with platelets (PLTs)
  - Prothrombin time (PT)/partial thromboplastin time (PTT)
- Hospitalize if:
  - Dehydration secondary to intolerance of food/liquid and/or persistent nausea/vomiting
  - Severe abdominal pain
  - Physical examination demonstrates:
    - Tachycardia
    - Hypotensive blood pressure (BP)
    - ↓ breath sounds
    - Tense, distended abdomen
    - Peritoneal signs
  - Blood tests demonstrate:
    - Hematocrit (Hct) >48% (more than 30% increment over baseline value)
    - Na^+ <135 mEq/L
    - K^+ >5.0 mEq/L
    - Cr >1.5 mg/dL

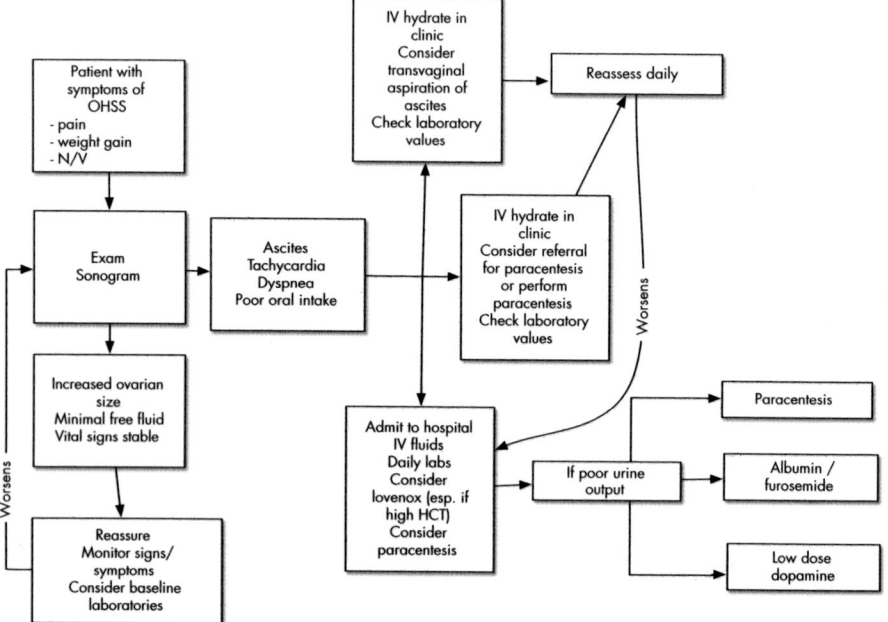

Figure 8.12. Algorithm for the management of ovarian hyperstimulation syndrome (OHSS)

Ovarian Hyperstimulation Syndrome (OHSS)

Hospital Management
Admission Orders for Severe Ovarian Hyperstimulation Syndrome
- Daily weight
- Strict intake and output (I&O)
- CBC, PT/PTT, electrolytes, liver function tests (LFTs), and β-human chorionic gonadotropin (β-hCG) on admission and p.r.n.
- Chest X-ray (CXR) and arterial blood gas (ABG) if short of breath
- Bed rest with bathroom privileges
- Enoxaparin* (Lovenox) if hemoconcentrated:
  - Prophylaxis: 40 mg SC once daily
  - Treatment: 1 mg/kg SC q12 hours
  - Adjust dose if renal impairment: GFR <30 mL/min
- Regular diet
- Fluid replacement management (remember strict I&O)
  - Initial: 1 L of normal saline (NS) × 1 hr (Lactated Ringer solution [LR] not recommended, as patients with severe OHSS are hyponatremic)
  - Maintenance: D5NS at 125–150 mL/hr without added potassium (see below)
  - On diuresis: Restrict oral fluids to 1 L/day and stop IV fluid
- Continue progesterone for luteal support
- Acetaminophen with narcotics as needed; avoid nonsteroidal antiinflammatory drugs (NSAIDs)
- Paracentesis/transvaginal aspiration for discomfort, shortness of breath (SOB), and/or persistent oliguria
- If hypovolemic, oliguric (<30 cc/hr), see treatment algorithm on the previous page
- Other management tips to consider:
  - No pelvic/abdominal examinations secondary to fragility of ovaries (can precipitate ovarian rupture and hemorrhage)
  - CXR if SOB present
  - White blood cell count (WBC) >22,000 is an ominous sign of imminent thromboembolism (Kodama 1995)
  - K-exchange resins (i.e., Kayexalate) p.r.n.; no diuretics; electrocardiogram (ECG) p.r.n. for elevated K⁺
  - A falling Hct associated with diuresis is an indication of resolution, not hemorrhage
  - Patient may be given indomethacin, or perhaps captopril or antihistamines
  - Surgery if suspicion of intraperitoneal bleeding (↓ Hct without diuresis) or torsion of ovarian cyst

Prevention
- Choice of stimulation protocol may help avoid this situation.
- Dopamine agonist cabergoline can reduce the incidence of moderate OHSS (likely by ↓ VEGF-mediated vascular permeability; Alvarez 2007; Youssef 2010).
  - Start 0.5 mg cabergoline or per vagina the evening of hCG for a total of 8 days.
- Cancel cycle, withhold hCG.
- Give hCG, aspirate, then cryopreserve all embryos (Imudia 2013; Maheshwari 2013).

- Aspiration of follicles has a protective effect (decreasing volume of granulosa cells and subsequent vascular endothelial growth factor [VEGF] production for Late-onset: OHSS but not necessarily for early-onset OHSS).
- Induce ovulation/oocyte maturation with:
  - Minimal effective dose of hCG: 5,000 IU and avoid hCG in luteal phase
  - Gonadotropin-releasing hormone agonist (GnRH-a)
    - Acceptable in cycles without GnRH agonist or in those using GnRH antagonist.
    - 4 mg SC leuprolide (= 80 units = 0.8 mL), some programs repeat dose in 12 hours; retrieval is done 36 hours later.
    - Check serum LH and P4 following day (should be LH ≥15 mIU/mL and P4 ≥3 ng/mL to suggest an adequate response).
    - Using GnRH agonist to trigger may be associated with lower pregnancy rates with fresh embryo transfer but has a significantly lower rate of OHSS (Kolibianakis 2005; Melo 2009), so consider cryopreservation of all embryos; frozen embryo transfer may result in higher pregnancy rates (Roque 2013).

SURGICAL TREATMENT OF INFERTILITY

Uterine Polyps and Fibroids
- Removal of intracavitary polyps or fibroids clearly beneficial in the infertile patient.
- Diagnostic/operative hysteroscopy preferred over "blind" D&C.
- Intramural fibroids without a submucous component may also decrease fertility but criteria to determine specific recommendations as to which fibroids require removal remains to be determined.

Tubal Reversal
- For patients over 37 years old, IVF may be more appropriate than tubal reversal.
- Tubal length (≥4 cm) after reanastomosis is most important; duration of Sterilization not important; laparoscopic tubal anastomosis has a 50% PR at 6 months (Bissonnette 1999).
- Consider female age and presence of male factor when counseling.
- Pregnancy success rates after microsurgical tubal reversal: clip > ring > coagulation = Pomeroy (Gordts 2009).

Tubal Factor—Hydrosalpinges
- Operative laparoscopy prior to ART in order to remove a hydrosalpinx is recommended.
  - Meta-analysis: hydrosalpinx ↓ PR by 50% and ↑ spontaneous abortion × 2 (Camus 1999)
  - Ligation of the hydrosalpinx or salpingectomy restores normal PR (Johnson 2002; Strandell 2001).
  - Number needed to treat calculation: Seven to eight women would need to have a salpingectomy before in vitro fertilization (IVF) to gain one additional live birth (Johnson 2002); a cost-effectiveness analysis of salpingectomy prior to IVF proved this to be a reasonable intervention (Strandell 2005).
  - No compromise of ovarian stimulation is seen following salpingectomy (Strandell 2001).

Table 8.16. Mechanism of adverse effect of hydrosapinx upon ART success

↓ nutrients in hydrosalpinx fluid
Toxic effect of fluid on embryos (Sachdev 1997) and/or sperm (Ng 2000)
↓ endometrial: $\alpha_v\beta_3$, LIF, HOXA10 (Meyer 1997)
Embryo wash-out effect from fluid
Endometrial peristalsis due to hydrosalpinx fluid
↓ endometrial and subendometrial blood flow (Ng 2006)
Endometrial inflammatory cells (Copperman 2006)

Source: From Strandell A, Lindhard A. Why does hydrosalpinx reduce fertility? The importance of hydrosalpinx fluid. Hum Reprod. 2002;17(5):1141.

Removal of Endometrioma Prior to IVF
- Laparoscopic cystectomy for endometrioma (>3 cm) before an IVF cycle does not improve fertility outcomes; likewise, conservative surgical treatment of endometriomas does not impair IVF success rates (Garcia-Velasco 2004).
- Ovarian reserve as judged by antral follicle count may be less impaired by sutured ovaries after cystectomy than in those electrocoagulated for hemostasis (Coric 2011).

- Endometriomas are associated with a reduced responsiveness (mean diameter follicles >15 mm) to gonadotropins (Somilgiana 2006); however, the pregnancy rates seem unaffected (Banaglia 2013).
- IVF outcome is impaired in women having excision of bilateral ovarian endometriomas (4% vs. 17% delivery rate for controls; Somigliana 2008).
- Removal of unilateral endometriomas prior to IVF compared with no treatment has no significant effect on IVF pregnancy rates (Tsoumpou 2009).
- The mere presence of an endometrioma is associated with lower AMH values; excision of endometriomas may have a further negative impact on AMH with a mean decline in AMH by ~1–1.5 ng/mL (Raffi 2012; Uncu 2013).

RECURRENT PREGNANCY LOSS
Fast Facts
- Fetal viability is only achieved in 30% of all human conceptions, 50% of which are lost before the first missed menses (Edmonds 1982).
- **15–20%** of clinically diagnosed pregnancies are lost in the first or early second trimester (TM) (Warburton 1964; Alberman 1988).
- Risk of loss:
  - 12% after one successful pregnancy
  - 24% after two consecutive losses
  - 30% after three consecutive losses
  - 40% after four consecutive losses
- Risk of a fourth loss after three prior losses depends on past reproductive history:
  - If no prior live birth → 40–45%
  - If ≥1 prior live birth → 30%
- The rate of pregnancy loss increases with advanced maternal age (most common cause is isolated nondisjunction)
- 80% of spontaneous abortions (SABs) occur within first 12 weeks of pregnancy, and 60–75% of these are due to chromosome abnormalities.
- Recurrent pregnancy loss (RPL) is a risk factor for ectopic pregnancy (2.5%), complete molar gestation (5 in 2,500), and neural tube defects (Adam 1995).
- Advanced paternal age may be associated with spontaneous abortion: For fathers age 40 years or older, there is an approximately threefold increase in SAB compared with women conceiving with men <25 years old (Kleinhaus 2006).

Table 8.17. Incidence of sporadic miscarriage (SM) or recurrent miscarriage (RM) in different age groups

Age Groups (Years)	Sporadic Miscarriage (%)[a]	RM Occurring by Chance[b] % (CI)	RM Occurring in Total (%)
20–24	11	0.13 (0.13–.013)	—
25–29	12	0.17 (0.17–0.17)	~0.4
30–34	15	0.34 (0.34–0.34)	~1
35–39	25	1.56 (1.56–1.56)	~3
40–44	51	13.3 (13.29–13.31)	—

CI, confidence intervals for binomial proportions.

[a]Data from Nybo Andersen AM, Wohlfahrt J, et al. Maternal age and fetal loss: population based register linkage study. *BMJ.* 2000 Jun 24;320(7251):1708–12.

[b]Calculated based on the assumption that if sporadic miscarriage rate = μ, recurrent miscarriage rate occurring by chance = μ^3.

Definition

American College of Obstetricians and Gynecologists (2001)
Two or three or more consecutive losses. (ACOG Practice Bulletin No. 24: Management of recurrent pregnancy loss. 2001 Feb. This practice bulletin has been withdrawn and not yet replaced).

American Society for Reproductive Medicine (2012)
Two or more failed pregnancies. (Practice Committee of the American Society for Reproductive Medicine. Evaluation and treatment of recurrent pregnancy loss: a committee opinion. *Fertil Steril*. 2012;98[5]:1103–1111).

Royal College of Obstetrics and Gynecology (2012)
Loss of three or more consecutive pregnancies. (National Collaborating Centre for Women's and Children's Health [UK]. *Ectopic Pregnancy and Miscarriage: Diagnosis and Initial Management in Early Pregnancy of Ectopic Pregnancy and Miscarriage*. London: Royal College of Obstetrics and Gynecology; 2012 December [NICE Clinical Guidelines, No. 154]).

Table 8.18. Prognostic value of transvaginal ultrasound observation of embryonic heart activity

Maternal Age (Years)	Risk of Loss (%)
≤35	<5
36–39	10
≥40	29
History of recurrent pregnancy loss	15–25

Source: Adapted from Van Leeuwen I, Branch DW, et al. First-trimester ultrasonography findings in women with a history of recurrent pregnancy loss. *Am J Obstet Gynecol*. 1993;168(1 Pt 1):111; Laufer MR, Ecker JL, et al. Pregnancy outcome following ultrasound-detected fetal cardiac activity in women with a history of multiple spontaneous abortions. *J Soc Gynecol Investig*. 1994;1(2):138; and Deaton JL, Honore GM, et al. Early transvaginal ultrasound following an accurately dated pregnancy: the importance of finding a yolk sac or fetal heart motion. *Hum Reprod*. 1997;12(12):2820.

Etiology Overview

Table 8.19. Etiologies of evidence-based tests when evaluating recurrent pregnancy loss

Control Frequency (%)	Abnormal Test Result	2 Prior Losses (n = 447)	3 Prior Losses (n = 343)	≥4 Prior Losses (n = 230)	P Value (2 vs. 3 vs. >3)
0.4	Parental genetics	2.8%	5.4%	5.2%	NS
7.5	Uterine anatomy	18.7%	18.2%	16.7%	NS
0.5	Lupus anticoagulant	5.0%	2.9%	1.9%	NS
6.7	Anticardiolipin antibodies	15.6%	13.1%	17.1%	NS
3.9	Thyroid-stimulating hormone	8.1%	6.5%	6.2%	NS
6.8	Factor V Leiden mutation	4.2%	8.1%	10.3%	NS

Frequency of abnormal test results in 1,020 women with recurrent pregnancy loss. Control frequency based on the percent of reproductive-aged, nonpregnant women without a history of miscarriage who had an abnormal test result.

Data modified from Jaslow CR, Carney JL, Kutteh WH. Diagnostic factors identified in 1020 women with two versus three or more recurrent pregnancy losses. *Fertil Steril*. 2010;93(4):1234-43.

Source: Reproduced with permission from Kutteh WH. Novel strategies for the management of recurrent pregnancy loss. *Semin Reprod Med*. 2015 May;33(3):161-68. Copyright © Georg Thieme Verlag KG.

Genetic Factors
Parental Chromosome Abnormality
- Approximately 4% in couples with RPL (vs. 0.2% in normal population).
- The maternal to paternal ratio is 3:1.
- One aneuploid SAB increases the risk of a subsequent loss to aneuploidy (Golbus 1981).
- 4% probability that either parent is a carrier of a balanced translocation if there are ≥2 SABs or one SAB + a malformed fetus.
- Majority of abnormalities are balanced translocations (no DNA is lost and phenotype of the parent is normal), resulting in an unbalanced translocation in the fetus. However, with no intervention there is still a 70% chance of a live birth.
- Breakdown of prevalence of balanced translocations found in RPL couples:
  - 40% Robertsonian (any)
  - 60% Reciprocal (any)

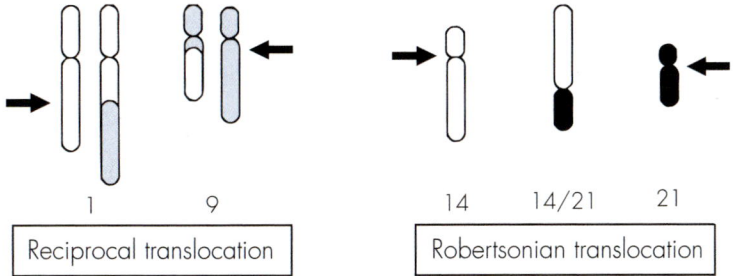

Figure 8.13. Reciprocal and Robertsonian translocations

- **Reciprocal translocation:** even exchange of chromatin between two nonhomologous.
- **Robertsonian translocation:** involves group D (13–15) and G (21 and 22) chromosomes (i.e., 14/21 translocation = long arms join up, but some short-arm material may be lost; breakage occurs close to the centromere; there are 45 chromosomes present [one normal 14 and 21, along with the balanced 14/21]).

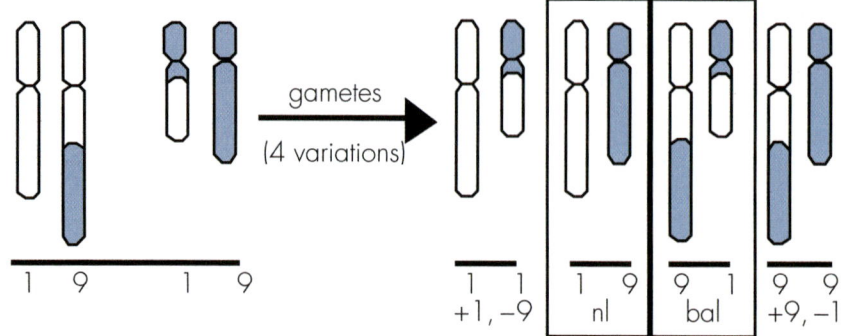

Figure 8.14. Gamete permutations in reciprocal translocation
Bal, balanced; nl, normal.

- Reciprocal translocation: ½ of gamete pairs are normal (including balanced).

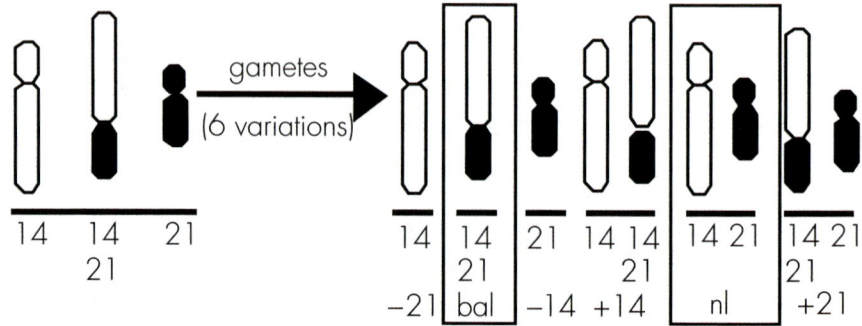

Figure 8.15. Gamete permutations in Robertsonian translocation
Bal, balanced; nl, normal.

- Robertsonian translocation: ⅓ of gamete pairs are normal (including balanced).

Table 8.20. Risk of an abnormal live birth in a patient with a translocation

	Risk for Live Birth Trisomy
Reciprocal translocations	**0–30%**, varies depending on chromosomes involved, breakpoints and amount of material translocated
Robertsonian translocations as a group	**<1%**
t(13,14) = 75% of all Robertsonian translocations	**<0.4%**
t(14;21) = 10% of all Robertsonian translocations	**10%** (21') if mother is carrier **1%** (21') if father is carrier

21', trisomy 21.

- Robertsonian translocation of homologous chromosomes (incidence of 1 in 2,500 with RPL) necessitates donor gametes for the affected partner.
    - *De novo* translocations (Warburton 1991):
        - Reciprocal translocation: 1 in 2,000
        - Robertsonian translocation: 1 in 9,000
- Turner mosaics are more susceptible to spontaneous miscarriages (Tarani 1998)
    - Out of 160 pregnancies:
        - 29%: spontaneous loss
        - 20%: malformed babies (Turner syndrome [TS], trisomy 21, and so forth)
        - 7%: perinatal death

Fetal Chromosomal Abnormality
- Chromosomal abnormalities make up approximately 60–75% of SABs (Fritz 2001).
- Karyotyping of the conceptus may reveal need for parental karyotype testing.
    - The survival rate of 45,X embryos is ~1 in 300.
    - Chromosomally normal embryos tend to abort later in gestation (~12–13 weeks) than aneuploid embryos.
- It is generally held that fetal chromosomal abnormalities play a prominent role in affecting single pregnancy losses but not recurrent losses; in fact, as the number of losses increases, the chance of a fetal chromosomal aberration decreases (Ogasawara 2000; Christiansen 2002).
- As a group, the trisomies are the most common anomaly, and of these, trisomy 16 is the most common trisomy found in abortuses, although the single most common aneuploidy for first TM losses is 45,XO.

Table 8.21. Estimating the probability of a miscarried embryo/fetus with an abnormal karyotype according to the number of previous miscarriages and maternal age

Miscarriages, n	Maternal Age, %			
	18–29	30–35	36–39	>40
≥7	**21**	**23**	**43**	**50**
6	**27**	**29**	**49**	56
5	**37**	**39**	59	64
4	53	55	75	82
3	57	59	79	86

Bold figures: high risk of miscarriage of a karyotypically normal embryo.

Source: Data from Christiansen OB, Steffensen R, Nielsen HS, et al. Multifactorial etiology of recurrent miscarriage and its scientific and clinical implications. *Gynecol Obstet Invest.* 66(4):257-67, 2008. Ogasawara M, Aoki K, Okada S, Suzumori K. Embryonic karyotype of abortuses in relation to the number of previous miscarriages. *Fertil Steril.* 2000;73:300-304; Stephenson MD, Awartani KA, Robinson WP. Cytogenetic analysis of miscarriages from couples with recurrent miscarriage: a case-control study. *Hum Reprod.* 2002;17:446-51.

Anatomic Factors
Congenital Uterine Anomalies
- A bicornuate uterus may not be associated with RPL (Proctor 2003).
- Incomplete caudal to cephalad septum reabsorption, type V (septate) anomaly, is associated with a 60% rate of RPL (Buttram 1983).
- The vascular density in uterine septa removed at the time of metroplasty is similar to that of the normal uterine wall (Dabirashrafi 1995).
- Pregnancy loss is more common among women with diethylstilbestrol (DES) exposure (Kaufman 2000).
- Benefit of metroplasty on pregnancy outcome is currently being assessed by an RCT study in the Netherlands.
- Repair of a uterine septum for a nulligravid women is not recommended (Branch 2010).

Table 8.22. Comparison of congenital and acquired uterine anomalies identified in women (primary vs. secondary RPL)

	Primary RPL (n = 479)	Secondary RPL (n = 425)	P Value
All uterine anomalies	22.8 (109)	15.8 (67)	0.009
Congenital anomalies	8.8 (42)	4.5 (19)	0.011
Bicornuate uterus	1.0 (5)	0.5 (2)	NS
Didelphic uterus	0.2 (1)	0.2 (1)	NS
Septate uterus	6.3 (30)	3.1 (13)	0.028
Unicornuate uterus	0.8 (4)	0.5 (2)	NS
Acquired anomalies	14.6 (71)	11.7 (50)	NS
Adhesions	4.0 (19)	4.2 (18)	NS
Fibroids	7.3 (35)	5.4 (23)	NS
Polyps	4.0 (19)	2.4 (10)	NS

RPL, recurrent pregnancy loss.

Values represent percent occurrence with number of cases in parentheses. Primary recurrent pregnancy loss means that there had never been a live birth. Secondary recurrent pregnancy loss means that a series of losses followed a live birth.

Data modified from Jaslow CR, Carney JL, Kutteh WH. Diagnostic factors identified in 1020 women with two versus three or more recurrent pregnancy losses. *Fertil Steril.* 2010;93(4):1234-43.

Source: Reproduced with permission from Kutteh WH. Novel strategies for the management of recurrent pregnancy loss. *Semin Reprod Med.* 2015 May;33(3):161-68. Copyright © Georg Thieme Verlag KG.

Acquired Uterine Anomalies

- Intrauterine synechiae (also known as Asherman syndrome) from vigorous uterine curettage have been found to occur in ~5% of women with RPL.
- Submucosal leiomyomas may cause an unfavorable implantation site by interfering with vascularization or by reducing the intrauterine cavity size; likewise, subserosal and intramural fibroids may cause reproduction failure if they distort the uterine cavity.
- Pregnancy losses are reduced after the removal of large intramural fibroids (>5 cm; Bajekal 2000).
- Uterine polyps may induce an inflammatory milieu that may be unfavorable for implantation.

Diagnosis

- Hysterosalpingogram/hysteroscopy/hysterosonography/laparoscopy/magetic resonance imaging (MRI); 3D transvaginal sonography.
- Imaging for septate uterus (Pellerito 1992):
  - Transvaginal sonography (TVS) has a sensitivity of 100% and specificity of 80%; addition of 3D transvaginal scanning may increase accuracy.
  - MRI has a sensitivity and specificity of 100%.

Treatment

- **Primary method of treatment in all cases is corrective surgery.** In the case of congenital anomalies, unification procedures such as the Strassman procedure are rarely undertaken. Septum resection may be warranted. In the case of Asherman syndrome, hysteroscopy to lyse adhesions is advisable. Hysteroscopic myomectomy, when feasible, is recommended for submucosal fibroids.
- IVF with gestational carrier should be considered as effective treatment.

Endocrine Factors
Luteal Phase Deficiency
- A large multicenter study failed to demonstrate any benefit from progesterone supplementation for unexplained RPL (Coomarasamy 2015).
- The insufficient level of progesterone, presumably from a deficient corpus luteum in the second half of the menstrual cycle, is hypothesized to prevent implantation of conceptus or impair maintenance of pregnancy; luteal phase deficiency (LPD) is more clearly associated with RPL than subfertility; histologic differences between fertile and infertile women are not significant (Coutifaris 2004); consider LPD if duration of luteal phase is <13 days (from positive luteinizing hormone [LH] kit to start of menses).
  - Normal women have endometrial histology suggestive of LPD in up to 50% of single menstrual cycles and 25% of sequential cycles (Davis 1989).
  - If progesterone deficiency is the cause of a miscarriage, the pregnancy is usually lost before the 6th week of gestation.
  - Suggested treatment options include aromatase inhibitor, clomiphene citrate, recombinant human follicle-stimulating hormone (rhFSH), human chorionic gonadotropin (hCG), and progesterone supplementation (beginning 3 days after positive ovulation prediction kit [OPK] until 10 weeks EGA).
  - **Hyperprolactinemia** has been shown to induce luteal phase insufficiency (possibly by progesterone from luteal cells).

Polycystic Ovary Syndrome
- Sonographic evidence of polycystic-appearing ovaries (PCAOs) in women with RPL does not predict worse pregnancy outcome than in women with RPL without PCOS (Rai 2000).

Insulin
- Prevalence of **insulin resistance** in women with RPL (Craig 2002):
  - 27.0% vs. 9.5%; odds ratio (OR), 3.55; 95% confidence interval (CI), 1.40–9.01
- Insulin resistance confers a greater than eightfold risk of miscarriage during IVF than those without insulin resistance (Tian 2007); intervention with appropriate **insulin sensitizing therapy** has been suggested to reduce miscarriage risk among women with PCOS (Glueck 2002). A free androgen index (FAI) <5 was associated with a significantly higher miscarriage rate and women with PCOS are more prone to have elevated FAI (Cocksedge 2008).

Thyroid Dysfunction
- **Hyper-** and **hypothyroidism** have been associated with pregnancy loss; no direct causal relationship specifically known toward RPL.
- Euthyroid women with TSH >2.5 mIU/L have increased pregnancy loss rates when compared to those with TSH <2.5 mIU/L.

Obesity
- Obesity (body mass index >30 kg/m^2) is associated with risk of first TM and recurrent miscarriage (Lashen 2004).
  - Early miscarriage OR 1.2; 95% CI, 1.01–1.46
  - RPL OR 3.5; 95% CI, 1.03–12.01

Microbiologic Factors
- Several infectious agents have been implicated as etiologic factors in sporadic pregnancy loss, but no infectious agent has been clearly proven to cause RPL.
- Studies of women with RPL show an increased colonization with *Ureaplasma urealyticumas* well as evidence of chronic endometritis (9.3% incidence for RPL) in the endometrium (Kundsin 1981; Kitaya 2011).
- Other commonly linked infections include *Toxoplasma gondii*, rubella, herpes simplex virus (HSV), measles, cytomegalovirus (CMV), coxsackie virus, *Listeria monocytogenes*, and *Mycoplasma hominis*, although none has been convincingly associated with RPL.
- Bottom line: it is more cost effective and time efficient to empirically treat each partner with azithromycin (1 g × 1 dose) or doxycycline (100 mg b.i.d. × 10 days) than to pursue multiple and repeated cultures.
- It is reasonable to omit infectious testing or treatment.

Inherited Thrombophilia (also see pages 219–224)
- Who should be tested? (Lockwood 2011)
    - Screening is appropriate for non-RPL indications that would lead to altered management decisions (see below). There is insufficient evidence of a causal relationship between inherited thrombophilia and RPL. Also, there is insufficient evidence of anticoagulant therapy efficacy.
        - Personal history of venous thromboembolism (VTE) associated with a nonrecurrent risk factor
        - First degree relative having a VTE before age 50
        - First degree relative with a history of a high risk thrombophilia (antithrombin III (AT) deficiency; double heterozygous for prothrombin G20210A mutation and factor V Leiden; factor V Leiden homozygous or prothrombin G20210A mutation)
- **Factor V Leiden (FVL)** and **prothrombin G20210A (ProG)** mutations are found in approximately 9% (1% of these are homozygous for the FVL mutation) and 3%, respectively, of white women in the United States; these mutations are associated with ~25% of isolated thrombotic events and ~50% of familial thrombosis.
- Although all who carry the FVL mutation show phenotypic resistance to activated protein C (PC), approximately 15% of all cases of activated PC resistance are not related to FVL mutation.
- The majority of large prospective studies have not found an association between fetal loss and inherited thrombophilia (Lockwood 2011).
- Bottom line: there is no evidence-based benefit of universal hereditary thrombophilia screening for early RPL.
- Other less common thrombophilias include autosomal-dominant deficiencies of the anticoagulants **PC, protein S (PS**; bad if <60%, then test antigenic levels of PS), and antithrombin deficiency.
- It is believed that women with inherited thrombophilia may be susceptible to local microthrombosis affecting syncytiotrophoblast invasion of maternal vessels at the site of implantation; however, since maternal blood does not perfuse the intervillous space until later in the first trimester, implantation failure cannot be explained solely on a thrombophilia disorder (Stern 2006).

Immunologic Factors—Antiphospholipid Antibody Syndrome
- **Antiphospholipid-Ab syndrome** (APS or Hughes syndrome) is present in approximately 5% of women with RPL; fetal loss more commonly occurs >10 weeks of gestation (Simpson 1998). It is characterized by the following:
  - Antiphospholipid antibodies (Abs) (anticardiolipin- or anti-b2 glycoprotein-immunoglobulins (IgG or IgM) [Katsuragawa 1997]) or **lupus anticoagulant** with one or more clinical features:
    - RPL, thrombosis, autoimmune thrombocytopenia
  - APS is actually composed of two syndromes:
    - Not associated with another illness (*primary APS*)
    - Additional burden of systemic lupus erythematosus or other rheumatic disease (*secondary APS*)
  - One-third of patients with lupus have antiphospholipid antibodies (Abs).
  - Possible mechanism: uteroplacental thrombosis and vasoconstriction secondary to immunoglobulin binding to platelets and vascular endothelial membrane phospholipids.
    - Note: True blood flow through placental vasculature does not occur until 9 to 10 weeks' EGA (Jaffe 1997).

Table 8.23. Revised classification criteria for the antiphospholipid syndrome

Antiphospholipid antibody syndrome is present if at least one of the clinical criteria and one of the laboratory criteria that follow are met.[a]

Clinical Criteria

1. Vascular thrombosis[b]

One or more clinical episodes[c] of arterial, venous, or small vessel thrombosis,[d] in any tissue or organ. Thrombosis must be confirmed by objective validated criteria (i.e., unequivocal findings of appropriate imaging studies or histopathology). For histopathologic confirmation, thrombosis should be present without significant evidence of inflammation in the vessel wall.

2. Pregnancy morbidity
   (a) One or more unexplained deaths of a morphologically normal fetus at or beyond the 10th wk of gestation, with normal fetal morphology documented by ultrasound or by direct examination of the fetus, or
   (b) One or more premature births of a morphologically normal neonate before the 34th wk of gestation because of (i) eclampsia or severe preeclampsia defined according to standard definitions or (ii) recognized features of placental insufficiency,[e] or
   (c) Three or more unexplained consecutive spontaneous abortions before the 10th wk of gestation, with maternal anatomic or hormonal abnormalities and paternal and maternal chromosomal causes excluded.

In studies of populations of patients who have more than one type of pregnancy morbidity, investigators are strongly encouraged to stratify groups of subjects according to a, b, or c above.

Laboratory Criteria[f]

1. Lupus anticoagulant present in plasma, on two or more occasions at least 12 wk apart, detected according to the guidelines of the International Society on Thrombosis and Haemostasis (Scientific Subcommittee on LAs/phospholipid-dependent antibodies).
2. Anticardiolipin antibody of IgG and/or IgM isotype in serum or plasma, present in medium or high titer (i.e. >40 IgG antiphospholipid or IgM antiphospholipid, or > the 99th percentile), on two or more occasions, at least 12 wk apart, measured by a standardized enzyme-linked immunosorbent assay.
3. Anti-β_2 glycoprotein-I antibody of IgG and/or IgM isotype in serum or plasma (in titer > the 99th percentile), present on two or more occasions, at least 12 wk apart, measured by a standardized enzyme-linked immunosorbent assay, according to recommended procedures.

[a]Classification of antiphospholipid antibody syndrome should be avoided if less than 12 wk or more than 5 yr separate the positive antiphospholipid test and the clinical manifestation.

[b]Coexisting inherited or acquired factors for thrombosis are not reasons for excluding patients from APS trials. However, two subgroups of APS patients should be recognized according to (a) the presence and (b) the absence of additional risk factors for thrombosis. Indicative (but not exhaustive) such cases include age (>55 in men and >65 in women) and the presence of any of the established risk factors for cardiovascular disease (hypertension, diabetes mellitus, elevated LDL or low HDL cholesterol, cigarette smoking, family history of premature cardiovascular disease, body mass index ≥30 kg m^{-2}, microalbuminuria, estimated glomerular filtration rate <60 mL min^{-1}), inherited thrombophilias, oral contraceptives, nephrotic syndrome, malignancy, immobilization, and surgery. Thus, patients who fulfill criteria should be stratified according to contributing causes of thrombosis.

[c]A thrombotic episode in the past could be considered as a clinical criterion, provided that thrombosis is proved by appropriate diagnostic means and that no alternative diagnosis or cause of thrombosis is found.

[d]Superficial venous thrombosis is not included in the clinical criteria.

[e]Generally accepted features of placental insufficiency include (i) abnormal or nonreassuring fetal surveillance test(s) (e.g., a nonreactive nonstress test, suggestive of fetal hypoxemia), (ii) abnormal Doppler flow velocimetry waveform analysis suggestive of fetal hypoxemia (e.g., absent end-diastolic flow in the umbilical artery), (iii) oligohydramnios (e.g., an amniotic fluid index of 5 cm or less), or (iv) a postnatal birth weight less than the 10th percentile for the gestational age.

[f]Investigators are strongly advised to classify APS patients in studies into one of the following categories: (I) more than one laboratory criteria present (any combination), (IIa) LA present alone, (IIb) aCL antibody present alone, (IIc) anti-β_2 glycoprotein-I antibody present alone.

Source: Reproduced with permission from Miyakis S, Lockshin MD, Atsumi T, et al. International consensus statement on an update of the classification criteria for definite antiphospholipid syndrome (APS). *J Throm Haemost.* 2006;4:295-306. Copyright © 2006 International Society on Thrombosis and Haemostasis.

INFERTILITY — Recurrent Pregnancy Loss

Treatment of APS

- Low-molecular-weight heparin (LMWH) may be an effective alternative to unfractionated heparin (Rai 1997; Greer 2002); initiate along with low-dose aspirin (81 mg/day) at positive pregnancy test, should stop at 36 weeks and potentially convert to unfractionated heparin to reduce risk of epidural hematoma.
  - Efficacy: Low-dose aspirin (81 mg/day) and unfractionated heparin (with a positive BhCG) compared to aspirin alone led to decreased pregnancy loss by 54% (RR 0.46, 0.29–0.71; Empson 2002).
- Some experts (Branch 2011) believe that unfractionated heparin therapy is superior to LMWH. Head-to-head comparisons are recommended.

Table 8.24. Treatment of pregnant women with APS

	Antepartum	Postpartum
APS with prior arterial or venous thrombosis	LMWH	Warfarin
APS with prior arterial or venous thrombosis and APS-defining pregnancy morbidity	LMWH and low-dose ASA	Warfarin
APS based on laboratory criteria for aPL and APS-defining pregnancy morbidity of ≥1 fetal losses ≥10 weeks of gestation or ≥3 unexplained consecutive spontaneous pregnancy losses <10 weeks of gestation, but no history of arterial or venous thrombosis	LMWH and low-dose ASA	LMWH and low-dose ASA
APS based on laboratory criteria for aPL and APS-defining pregnancy morbidity of ≥1 preterm deliveries of a morphologically normal infant before 34 weeks of gestation due to severe preeclampsia, eclampsia, or other findings consistent with placental insufficiency. No history of arterial or venous thrombosis.	Low-dose ASA LMWH with low-dose ASA in cases of ASA failure or when placental examination shows extensive decidual inflammation and vasculopathy and/or thrombosis	None LMWH with low-dose ASA
Laboratory criteria for aPL but no clinical criteria for APS	Low-dose ASA	None

APS, antiphospholipid syndrome; aPL, antiphospholipid antibodies; ASA, aspirin; LMWH, low-molecular-weight heparin.

Graphic 91501 Version 2.0

Source: Reproduced with permission from Park L, Lockwood CJ, Lockshin MD. Pregnancy in women with antiphospholipid syndrome. In: Post, TW, ed. *UpToDate*. Waltham, MA: UpToDate (accessed on February 19, 2016). Copyright © 2016 UpToDate, Inc. For more information, visit www.uptodate.com.

- Monitoring:
  - Consider antifactor Xa levels: goal = 0.6–1 U/mL 4 hours after injection (LMWH only).
  - Check platelets monthly.
- Risk of thrombosis presumably highest first 6 weeks postpartum. Continue anticoagulation through 6–12 weeks postpartum; some recommend long-term anticoagulation.
  - Initiating heparin before conception is potentially dangerous because of the risk of hemorrhage at the time of ovulation.
  - Need close maternal and fetal surveillance secondary to high risk for complications (i.e., preeclampsia, fetal distress, intrauterine growth restriction [IUGR], preterm labor [PTL], and so forth).
  - If surgery planned while on LMWH, stop 18–24 hours before procedure and restart 12 hours postprocedure. If emergent, may try to reverse with **protamine sulfate** (1 mg/100 anti-Xa

units of LMWH; though not as effective as with UFH); **slow infusion, no need to reverse if >18 hours from last dose.** For enoxaparin, use 1 mg protamine sulfate per 1 mg enoxaparin, for dalteparin, use 1 mg protamine sulfate per 100 units dalteparin.
- If surgery planned while on UFH, stop 12 hours preprocedure, restart 8–12 hours after the procedure. UFH can be rapidly reversed with protamine sulfate (1 mg protamine sulfate/100 units heparin; not greater than 20 mg/minute and no more than 50 mg over any 10-minute period).

Summary of Treatment Options for RPL
- Antiphospholipid antibody syndrome and history of RPL: ASA + LMWH or UFH.
- Patients with RPL are anxious and desperate to have a "take-home baby." Support and counseling are important.
- Remember, 60–70% of women with unexplained RPL have a successful subsequent pregnancy (Jeng 1995).
- Oocyte donation has been efficacious in treating RPL (Remohi 1996).
- In vitro fertilization (IVF) with preimplantation genetic screening (PGS) may eventually prove to benefit RPL patients, although studies to date do not indicate that PGS improves the live birth rate (Fanssen 2011).
  - If, however, the goal is to minimize recurrence of a loss, then PGS may be an option while pointing out that the LBR is not necessarily improved.
  - There may be single gene defects present that are not detected by karyotyping; consider offering IVF/ICSI and preimplantation genetic diagnosis. The parents should be referred to genetic counseling/prenatal diagnosis.

Table 8.25. Rate of pregnancy loss in subsequent pregnancy in patients with a history of recurrent pregnancy loss

RPL (Number of Prior Losses)	Loss Rate with Subsequent Pregnancy				
	20 yo	25 yo	30 yo	35 yo	40 yo
2	8%	11%	16%	23%	31%
3	10%	14%	20%	27%	36%
4	12%	18%	24%	32%	42%
5	15%	21%	29%	29%	48%

RPL, recurrent pregnancy loss; yo, years old.

Source: Adapted from Brigham SA, Conlon C, Farquharson RG. A longitudinal study of pregnancy outcome following idiopathic recurrent miscarriage. *Hum Reprod.* 1999 Nov;14(11):2868-71.

Table 8.26. Prognosis for livebirth in patients with recurrent pregnancy loss

Status	Intervention	Viable Births (%)
Genetic factors	Timed intercourse and supportive care	20–90
Anatomic factors	Surgery and supportive care	60–90
Endocrine Factors		
Luteal phase deficiency	Progesterone ± ovulation induction and supportive care	80–90
Hypothyroidism	Thyroid replacement and supportive care	80–90
Hyperprolactinemia	Dopamine agonist	80–90
Infections	Antibiotics and supportive care	70–90
Antiphospholipid syndrome	Aspirin, heparin, and supportive care	70–90
Unknown factors	Timed intercourse and supportive care	60–90

Source: Derived from >1,000 cases at Boston's Brigham and Women's Hospital. Adapted from Hill JA. *Recurrent Pregnancy Loss: Male and Female Factor, Etiology and Treatment.* Frontiers in Reproductive Endocrinology. Washington, DC: Serono Symposia USA; 2001.

GAMETE PRESERVATION
Male Gamete Preservation
Indications
- Chemotherapy—affects germinal epithelium
- Radiotherapy—affects germinal epithelium, Leydig cell function, and sperm DNA integrity
- Retroperitoneal surgery
- Postmortem

Options
Sperm Cryopreservation
- Most reliable option for adolescent and adult males
- If time before treatment allows, 3 samples are produced at least 48 hours apart (Holoch 2011)
- For azoospermic men, testicular extraction of sperm for future IVF/ICSI

Embryo Cryopreservation
- Viable option for reproductive-aged male and partner
- Requires IVF

Female Gamete Preservation
- Medical indications
- Gonadotoxic therapies for cancer and other medical diseases
  - Radiotherapy
  - Autoimmune/collagen vascular disease
  - Oophorectomy for benign/malignant conditions (i.e., endometriosis, ovarian cancer)
- Genetic conditions
  - Women with *BRCA* mutations may undergo prophylactic oophorectomy
  - Mosaic Turner syndrome (efficacy of oocyte banking unknown)
  - Fragile X permutation (efficacy of oocyte banking unknown)
- Failure to obtain sperm for IVF on day of oocyte retrieval
- Those unable to cryopreserve embryos (moral or religious concerns)
- Elective cryopreservation to defer childbearing

Gonadotoxicity
- Chemotherapy damages the ovaries' steroid-producing cells (granulosa and theca cells) and oocytes → primary ovarian insufficiency (POI) → premature menopause → infertility
- Chemotherapy drugs and their potential for gonadal damage (alkylating agents have the highest risk):
  - **High potential:** cyclophosphamide (RR between 4–9.3; Sonmezer 2004), chlorambucil, melphalan, busulfan, nitrogen mustard and procarbazine
  - **Moderate potential:** cisplatin and adriamycin
  - **Mild or no potential:** bleomycin, actinomycin D, vincristine, methotrexate and 5-fluorouracil
- Radiotherapy depletes the primordial follicle pool in a dose-dependent manner (Gosden 1997)
  - Six Gy results in permanent ovarian failure (Howell 1998)

INFERTILITY — Gamete Preservation

Options for Female Gamete Preservation

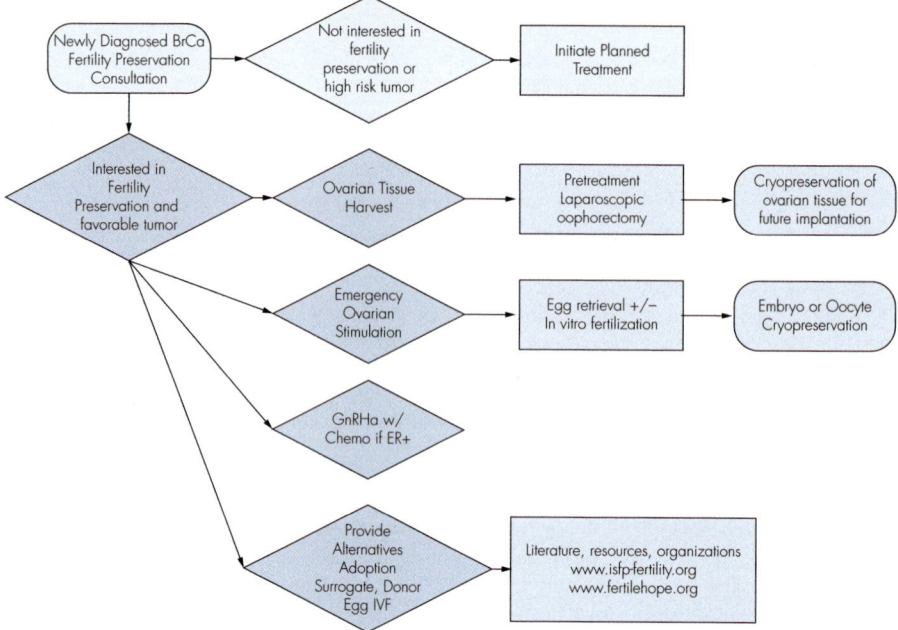

Figure 8.16. Options for female gamete preservation
Source: Reproduced with permission from Kim SS, Klemp J, Fabian C. Breast cancer and fertility preservation. *Fertil Steril.* 2011 Apr;95(5):1535-43. Copyright © 2011 The American Society for Reproductive Medicine.

Embryo Cryopreservation
- Well-established technique
- Requires IVF protocol; therefore, controlled ovarian stimulation and egg retrieval may delay disease treatment
- Good option for women with a partner and time for an IVF cycle
- Not acceptable to single women who decline the use of donor sperm
- Not an option for pediatric/prepubertal females
- Ethical/legal concern: disposition of cryopreserved embryos in the case of the patient's death

Letrozole Protocol
- For patients with estrogen-sensitive breast cancer, letrozole is a more desirable option (Kim 2011; Rodriguez-Wallberg 2010).
  - Letrozole 5 mg starting on cycle day 2 until day of trigger
  - FSH 150–300 IU/day starting on cycle day 4
  - 0.25 mg GnRH antagonist started when lead follicle reaches 14 mm or E2 ≥250 pg/mL
  - 5,000–10,000 IU HCG or 250 mg recombinant HCG or 4 mg GnRH-agonist trigger
  - Restart letrozole on day of retrieval for 5 more days

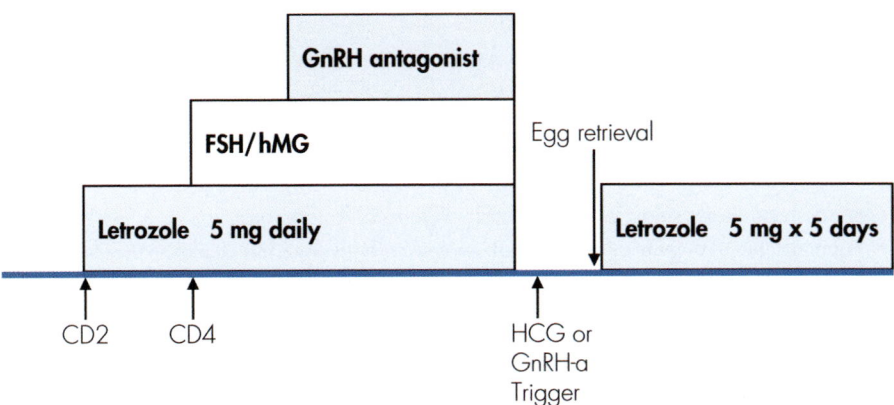

Figure 8.17. Letrozole/gnRH-antagonist protocol for ART patients with estrogen-sensitive cancer
CD, cycle day.
Source: Modified from original protocol described in Rodriguez-Wallberg KA, Oktay K. Fertility preservation in women with breast cancer. *Clin Obstet Gynecol.* 2010 Dec;53(4):753-62.

Oocyte Cryopreservation
- Egg freezing is no longer considered experimental (ASRM 2013).
- Requires IVF protocol; therefore, controlled ovarian stimulation and egg retrieval may delay cancer treatment.
- Does not require a male partner but not considered a routine procedure due to current pregnancy rates being significantly lower than those with embryo cryopreservation.
- First report of successful pregnancy from thawed oocytes (Chen 1986) → more than 900 babies born to date.
- Vitrification (ultrarapid freezing) eliminates ice crystal formation and growth leading to improved outcomes over slow freezing.
- Post-thaw survival rates in vitrified oocytes have improved and fertilization rates are similar to those of fresh oocytes (Cobo 2010; Rienzi 2010).
- Online age-specific individualized oocyte freezing live birth success rates: http://www.i-fertility.net/probability-calc.

Ovarian Tissue Cryopreservation and Transplantation
- Experimental, under auspices of IRB; an area of extensive research with great potential (Donnez 2013).
- Future applications include patients with cancer and those who decline donor oocytes.
- Tissue ischemia and risk for reintroduction of cancerous cells are two crucial issues (Kim 2006; Dolmans 2013).

Oophoropexy (Ovarian Transposition)
- Technique involves dividing the utero-ovarian ligament and laterally transposing the ovary (Tulandi 1998).
- Pelvic irradiation at doses >300 cGy can result in loss of ovarian function.
- Total lymph node irradiation in patients with Hodgkin's lymphoma exposes the ovaries to 2,000–4,000 cGy, invariably causing POF (Williams 1999).

Gonadotropin-Releasing Hormone (GnRH) Agonists/Antagonists
- Administered to downregulate hypothalamic-pituitary-ovarian (HPO) axis to decrease susceptibility to gonadotoxicity, although no GnRH receptor has been identified as yet on human primordial follicles or oocytes.
- Efficacy is controversial.
- Possible mechanism(s) include mediation of antiproliferative effects by GnRH receptors on ovarian cells (Volker 2002), a decrease in gonadotropin concentrations, decreased ovarian perfusion due to hypoestrogenic milieu, antiapoptotic effect mediated by sphingosine-1-phosphate, and germline stem cell preservation.
- Benefit of GnRH-a demonstrated in one study (Blumenfeld 1996) of young women with lymphoma who received chemotherapy: in GnRH-agonist-treated group, 94% had spontaneous menses within 3–8 months of completing chemotherapy treatment; in the control group, 61% had POI.
- Randomized trial of 281 patients with breast cancer who received chemotherapy (anthracycline, cyclophosphamide, methotrexate, fluorouracil; Del Mastro 2011):
  - 3.75 mg GnRH-agonist administered at least 1 week before the start of chemotherapy and then every 4 weeks for the duration of chemotherapy.
  - 8.9% premature menopause in GnRH-agonist treated group compared with 25.9% in the control group (P<0.01) with **NNT=6**.
- One protocol adapted from ClinicalTrials.gov #NCT01257802:
  - 3.75 mg GnRH-agonist monthly throughout course of chemotherapy with transdermal E2 add-back (0.05–1 mg) beginning 1 month into the Lupron.

Table 8.27. Fertility preservation options

	Timeframe for Referral/Initiation	Potential for Success
Male patients		
Sperm cryopreservation	Anytime before cancer treatment	Established
Testicular tissues/spermatogonial cryopreservation	Anytime before cancer treatment	No clinical experience
Hormonal therapy	Anytime before cancer treatment	Unsuccessful
Female patients		
Embryo cryopreservation	Before chemotherapy begins	Established
Surgical transposition	Before pelvic radiation begins if no chemotherapy administered	Established
Oocyte cryopreservation	Needs minimum of 2 weeks for stimulation	Over 200 live births; success rate lower than with fresh oocytes
Transplantation of cryopreserved ovarian tissue	Can be performed at any time before, and sometimes after, chemotherapy	Successful return of ovarian function and fertility shown in case studies
Ovarian stimulation with aromatase inhibitors	Requires minimum of 2 weeks	Controlled studies show equal success rates in standard IVF; no increase in recurrence in short-term follow-up
GnRH agonist administration	During chemotherapy treatment	Mixed results; no benefit in women undergoing high-dose chemotherapy with HSCT

GnRH, gonadotropin-releasing hormone; HSCT, hematopoietic stem cell transplant; IVF, in vitro fertilization

Source: Modified from Oktay K, Meirow D. Planning for fertility preservation before cancer treatment. *Sexuality, Reproduction and Menopause.* 2007;5(1):17–22

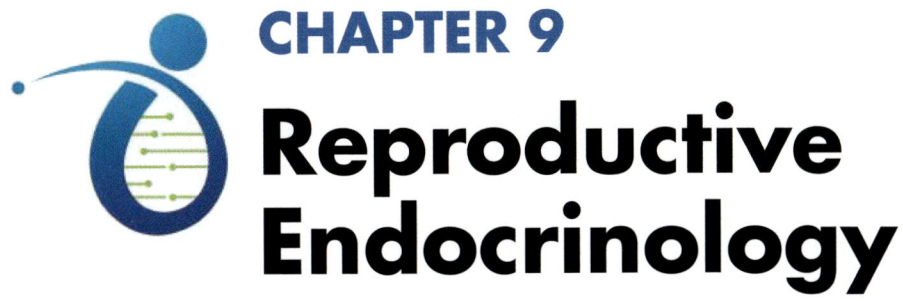

CHAPTER 9
Reproductive Endocrinology

MENSTRUAL CYCLE
Fast Facts
- Mean age of menarche = 12.8 years old; mean age of menopause = 51 years old
- Cycle day 1 = first day of vaginal bleeding; mean duration of flow = 4 ± 2 days
- Cycle length:
  - Least variable between ages 20 and 40 years (gradual decrease in length)
  - 90% have menstrual cycles between 24 and 35 days; 15% have 28-day cycles.
- Irregular cycles: just after menarche (2 years); just before menopause (3 years)
- Menstrual cycle phases:
  - Follicular phase: variable length (7–21 days); key determinant of cycle length
  - Ovulation
  - Luteal phase: more constant (~12 days)

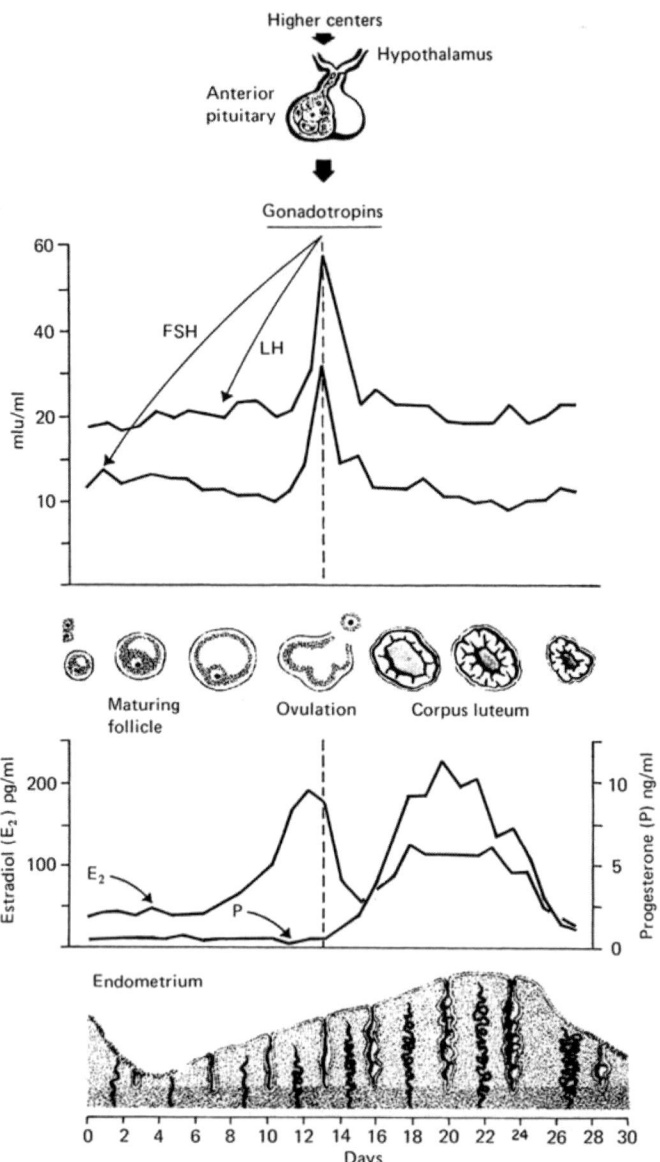

Figure 9.1. The normal reproductive cycle
Source: Reproduced with permission from Couchman GM, Hammond CB. Physiology of reproduction. In: Scott JR, DiSaia PD, Hammond CB, Spellacy WN, ed. *Danforth's Obstetrics and Gynecology*, 7th Ed. Philadelphia: Lippincott; 1994.

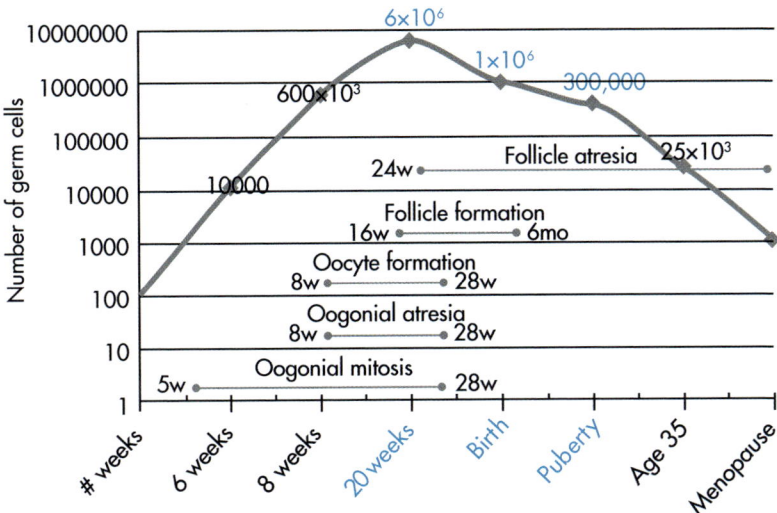

Figure 9.2. The life history of germ cells
Source: Reproduced with permission from Oktem O, Urman B. Understanding follicle growth in vivo. *Hum Reprod.* 2010;25(12)2944-54. Copyright © 2010 Oxford University Press.

Table 9.1. Suggested normal limits for menstrual parameters in the midreproductive years

Clinical Dimensions of Menstruation and Menstrual Cycle	Descriptive Terms	Normal Limits (5th–95th Percentiles)
Frequency of menses (days)	Frequent	<24
	Normal	24–38
	Infrequent	>38
Regularity of menses (cycle to cycle variation over 12 months; in days)	Absent	—
	Regular	Variation ±2 to 20 days
	Irregular	Variation greater than 20 days
Duration of flow (days)	Normal	4.5–8.0
	Prolonged	>8.0
	Shortened	<4.5
Volume of monthly blood loss (mL)	Heavy	>80
	Normal	5–80
	Light	<5

Source: Reproduced with permission from Munro MG, Critchley HO, Fraser IS. The FIGO systems for nomenclature and classification of causes of abnormal uterine bleeding in the reproductive years: who needs them? *Am J Obstet Gynecol.* 2012 Oct;207(4):259-65. Copyright © 2012 Elsevier.

PUBERTY

Definition
- Puberty is the process of biologic and physical development through which sexual reproduction first becomes possible.
- Progression:
  - thelarche → adrenarche → peak growth spurt → menarche → ovulation

Factors That Influence the Onset of Puberty
- Genetics: average interval between menarche in monozygotic twins is 2.2 months compared with 8.2 months in dizygotic twins (McDonough 1998)
- Race: African American girls enter puberty 1.0–1.5 years before white girls (Herman-Giddens 1997)
- Nutritional state: earlier with moderate obesity; delayed with malnutrition
- General health
- Geographic location: urban, closer to the equator, lower altitudes earlier than rural, farther from the equator, higher altitudes
- Exposure to light: blind earlier than sighted
- Psychological state

Physical Changes during Puberty
- Thelarche to menarche requires approximately 2–3 years.
  - Accelerated growth
  - Breast budding (thelarche)
  - Pubic and axillary hair growth (pubarche and adrenarche)
  - Peak growth velocity
  - Menarche
  - Ovulation—half the cycles are ovulatory approximately 1–3 years after menarche (McDonough 1998)
- Adrenarche can precede thelarche
  - Prevalent in girls of African descent (McDonough 1998)

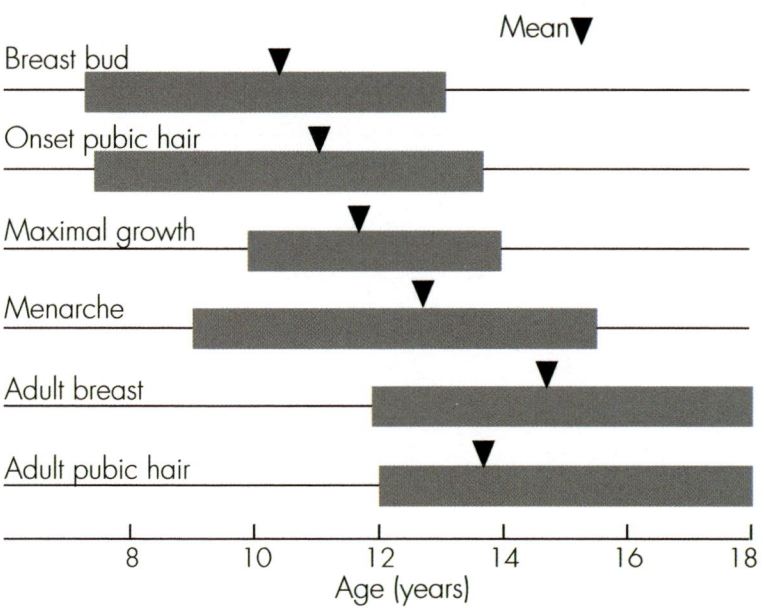

Figure 9.3. Average age of appearance of pubertal events
Source: Reproduced with permission from Gordon JD, Speroff L. Abnormal puberty and growth problems. In: *Handbook for Clinical Gynecologic Endocrinology and Infertility*, 6th Ed. Philadelphia: Lippincott–Raven; 2002.

Table 9.2. Tanner staging of breast and pubic hair

Classification	Description
Breast growth	
B1	Prepubertal: elevation of papilla only.
B2	Breast budding.
B3	Breast with glandular tissue, without separation of breast contours.
B4	Second mound formed by areola.
B5	Single contour of breast and areola.
Pubic hair growth	
PH1	Prepubertal: no pubic hair.
PH2	Labial hair present.
PH3	Labial hair spreads over mons pubis.
PH3	Slight lateral spread.
PH4	Further lateral spread to form inverse triangle and reach medial thighs.

B, breast; PH pubic hair.

Source: Reproduced with permission from Gordon JD, Speroff L. Abnormal puberty and growth problems. In: *Handbook for Clinical Gynecologic Endocrinology and Infertility*, 6th Ed. Philadelphia: Lippincott–Raven; 2002.

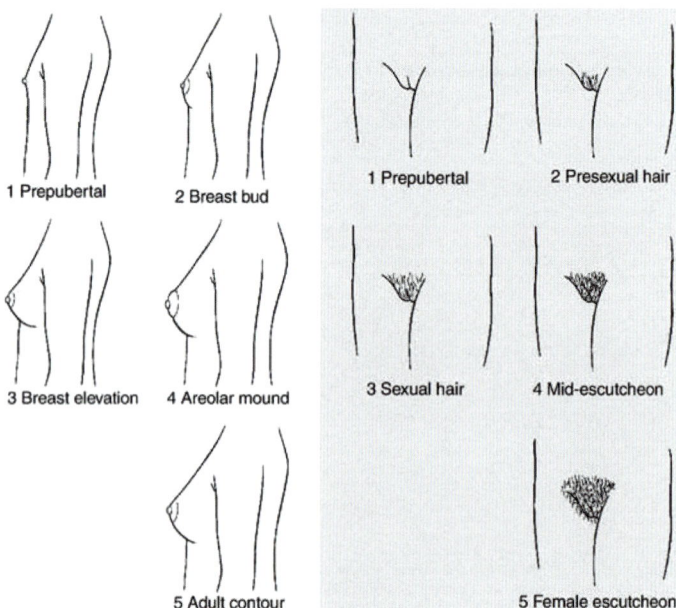

Figure 9.4. Tanner staging of breast and pubic hair
Source: Reproduced with permission from Gordon JD, Speroff L. Abnormal puberty and growth problems. In: *Handbook for Clinical Gynecologic Endocrinology and Infertility*, 6th Ed. Philadelphia: Lippincott–Raven; 2002.

DELAYED OR INTERRUPTED PUBERTY
- Difficult to define due to wide variation in normal development (most girls should enter puberty by 13 years; mean age of menarche is 16 years)

Eugonadal
- Well-estrogenized (26%)
  - Müllerian agenesis or Mayer-Rokitansky-Kuster-Hauser syndrome (14%)
    - Second most common cause of primary amenorrhea after gonadal dysgenesis
      - Amenorrhea aside, pubertal development is normal (ovaries present)
      - 11–50% have skeletal abnormalities (scoliosis, phocomelia, lobster claw)
      - Up to 30% have unilateral renal agenesis or a single pelvic kidney
    - Diagnosis: normal pubic hair (to differentiate from androgen insensitivity syndrome), ultrasound reveals absence of uterus and presence of ovaries
    - Treatment: counseling, creation of a neovagina (through dilators or surgery), possible assisted reproductive technology with use of a surrogate
    - Karyotype 46,XX
  - Vaginal septum (3%)
  - Imperforate hymen (0.5%)
  - Androgen insensitivity syndrome (1%)
    - Etiology: receptor absence, receptor defect, postreceptor defect
    - Complete: testes, female external genitalia, blind vaginal pouch, no Müllerian derivatives
    - Incomplete: above features as well as clitoral enlargement, labioscrotal fusion
    - Diagnosis: absent or significantly reduced pubic hair, male testosterone levels (to differentiate from Müllerian agenesis), karyotype
    - Treatment: gonadectomy after breast development, estrogen replacement therapy
    - Karyotype 46,XY
  - Inappropriate positive feedback (7%): constitutional delay

Hypogonadal
- Hypoestrogenic (74%)
  - Hypergonadotropic hypogonadism (follicle-stimulating hormone [FSH] >30 mIU/mL) (43%)
    - Turner syndrome (45,X or mosaic)
      - Lymphedema at birth, short stature, webbed neck, nevi and heart/kidney/skeletal/great vessel problems, streak ovaries secondary to oocyte depletion
      - Check karyotype, complete physical exam, thyroid function tests, glucose, liver function tests, and intravenous pyelogram or renal ultrasound
      - Treatment: growth hormone (GH) for height, then estrogen (gradually increase to 2× postmenopausal dose); later, progestins; counseling
    - Pure gonadal dysgenesis
      - 46,XX
        - ▶ Idiopathic
        - ▶ FSH and luteinizing hormone (LH) receptor mutations
        - ▶ Steroidogenic acute regulatory protein, CYP17 (congenital adrenal hyperplasia [CAH]), and CYP19 mutations
      - 46,XY

- ▶ Swyer syndrome: point mutations in sex-related Y (SRY) or deletion of SRY
  - ▷ No secondary sexual development, normal (or above average) height, normal but infantile female genitalia
- ▶ Wilms' tumor suppressor gene mutations
  - ▷ Hypogonadism, nephropathy, and Wilms' tumor
- ▶ Camptomelic dysplasia (SOX9 gene), SF-1, DAX1, Leydig cell hypoplasia
- ☐ Treatment: estrogen, gonadectomy if XY (20–30% risk of developing a gonadal tumor)
  - ▶ Must differentiate Swyer syndrome (–SRY) from LH-R mutation, as the latter involves a more technically challenging surgery because of the lack of landmarks
- ○ Hypogonadotropic hypogonadism (LH and FSH <5 mIU/mL; 31%)
  - ▪ Physiologic or constitutional delay is most common, but it is important to exclude other causes
    - ☐ Sustained malnutrition: gastrointestinal malabsorption, anorexia nervosa, excessive exercise
    - ☐ Endocrine disorders: hypothyroidism, Cushing syndrome, CAH, hyperprolactinemia
  - ▪ Hypothalamic-pituitary etiologies:
    - ☐ Kallmann syndrome (anosmia, hypogonadism)
      - ▶ Absence of gonadotropin-releasing hormone (GnRH) neurons in hypothalamus
    - ☐ Pituitary insufficiency
    - ☐ Pituitary tumors
      - ▶ Craniopharyngioma
        - ▷ Signs: headache, visual changes, growth failure, delayed puberty
        - ▷ Treatment: surgical, radiation treatment

Table 9.3. Relative frequency of delayed pubertal abnormalities

Classification			
Hypergonadotropic hypogonadism	43%		
Ovarian failure, abnormal karyotype		26%	
Ovarian failure, normal karyotype		17%	
46,XX			15%
46,XY			2%
Hypogonadotropic hypogonadism	31%		
Reversible		18%	
Physiologic delay			10%
Weight loss/anorexia			3%
Primary hypothyroidism			1%
Congenital adrenal hyperplasia			1%
Cushing syndrome			0.5%
Prolactinomas			1.5%
Irreversible		13%	
GnRH deficiency			7%
Hypopituitarism			2%
Congenital CNS defects			0.5%
Other pituitary adenomas			0.5%
Craniopharyngioma			1%
Malignant pituitary tumor			0.5%
Eugonadism	26%		
Müllerian agenesis		14%	
Vaginal septum		3%	
Imperforate hymen		0.5%	
Androgen insensitivity syndrome		1%	
Inappropriate positive feedback		7%	

GnRH, gonadotropin-releasing hormone.

Source: Reproduced with permission from Gordon JD, Speroff L. Abnormal puberty and growth problems. In: *Handbook for Clinical Gynecologic Endocrinology and Infertility*, 6th Ed. Philadelphia: Lippincott–Raven; 2002.

PUBERTAL VARIANTS AND PRECOCIOUS PUBERTY
Fast Facts
- Traditional definition of precocious puberty: thelarche before 8 years, pubarche before 9 years.
- New definition of precocious puberty (Kaplowitz 1999):
  - Pubarche or thelarche before 7 years (white girls) or 6 years (African American girls)
  - After ages 7 (white) or 6 (African American) in conjunction with
    - Rapid progression of puberty
    - Central nervous system (CNS) findings: headache, neurologic symptoms, seizures
    - Pubertal progression that affects the emotional health of the family or girl
- Most patients with Tanner stage 2 breast or pubic hair can be evaluated with only a history, physical exam, and review of the growth chart, without the need for hormonal studies and an estimate of bone age, provided that growth is normal (Kaplowitz 2004).

Table 9.4. Distribution of diagnoses in 80 girls referred for precocious puberty

Diagnosis	%
Premature adrenarche	46
Premature thelarche	11
True precocious puberty	11
Early breast development	11
Pubic hair of infancy	6
Premature menses	6
No puberty	6

Source: Adapted from Kaplowitz P. Clinical characteristics of 104 children referred for evaluation of precocious puberty. *J Clin Endocrinol Metab.* 2004;89(8):3644.

Table 9.5. Types of benign pubertal variants

Etiology	Clinical Features	Bone Age	Additional Evaluation
Premature adrenarche (boys or girls)	Isolated pubarche. Gonads are prepubertal in size and there is no breast development in girls. Typical age of onset 4 to 8 years. Seen more commonly in African American and Hispanic girls and in children with obesity and insulin resistance.	↑ to ↑↑*	Further investigations needed only if there is significant progressive virilization to help exclude peripheral precocity. Mild elevation in DHEAS for chronological age (but appropriate for bone age). Prepubertal concentrations of 17-hydroxyprogesterone and testosterone.
Premature thelarche (girls)	Isolated breast development with normal growth velocity. Most commonly seen in girls less than 3 years of age.	Normal (prepubertal)	No further evaluation needed in most cases, unless evidence of pubertal progression. Basal LH concentrations typically <0.2 to 0.3 mIU/L.¶
Non-progressive or intermittently progressive precocious puberty (boys or girls)	Development of gonadarche (breast or testicular enlargement) with pubarche (pubic and/or axillary hair), with either no progression or intermittent slow progression in clinical pubertal signs.	Normal to ↑	Basal LH concentrations typically <0.2 to 0.3 mIU/L, although can be in early pubertal range in some children. Lower stimulated LH/FSH ratio compared with children with progressive central precocious puberty.◊ Patients with nonprogressive precocious puberty do not need treatment with GnRH agonist, because final height untreated is concordant with midparental height.

↑, elevated for chronological age; DHEAS, dehydroepiandrosterone sulfate; LH, luteinizing hormone; FSH, follicle-stimulating hormone; GnRH; gonadotropin-releasing hormone.

If further evaluation is needed and performed, patients with benign pubertal variants typically have prepubertal basal LH concentrations (<0.2 to 0.3 mIU/L) and/or stimulated LH concentration post GnRHa of <3.3 to 5.0 mIU/L.

*Up to 30% of children with premature adrenarche can have a bone age more than 2 years advanced than their chronological age (DeSalvo 2013).

¶Interpretation of basal LH and stimulated LH concentrations can be difficult in girls younger than 2 years of age because normal gonadotropin concentrations can be elevated as part of the mini-puberty of infancy (Bizzarri 2014).

◊A peak LH/FSH ratio <0.66 suggests nonprogressive precocious puberty, whereas a ratio >0.66 is typically seen with central precocious puberty (Oerter 1990).

Source: Reproduced with permission from Harrington J, Palmert MR. Definition, etiology, and evaluation of precocious puberty. In: Post, TW, ed. *UpToDate*. Waltham, MA: UpToDate (accessed on March 6, 2016). Copyright © 2016 UpToDate, Inc. For more information, visit www.uptodate.com.

Table 9.6. Clinical characteristics of forms of early pubertal development

	Nonprogressive Precocious Puberty	Central Precocious Puberty (CPP)	Peripheral Precocity
Physical examination: Advancement through pubertal stages (Tanner stage)	No progression in Tanner staging during 3 to 6 months of observation	Progression to next pubertal stage in 3 to 6 months	Progression
Growth velocity	Normal for bone age	Accelerated (>6 cm per year)*	Accelerated*
Bone age	Normal to mildly advanced	Advanced for height age	Advanced for height age
Serum estradiol concentration (girls)¶	Prepubertal	Prepubertal to increased	Increased in ovarian causes of peripheral precocity, or with exogenous estrogen exposure
Serum testosterone concentration (boys, or girls with virilization)¶	Prepubertal	Prepubertal to pubertal	Pubertal and increasing
Basal (unstimulated) serum LH concentration¶	Prepubertal◻	Pubertal◻	Suppressed or prepubertal◻
GnRH (or GnRHa) stimulation test¶	LH peak in the prepubertal range✧ Lower stimulated LH to FSH ratio§	LH peak elevated (in the pubertal range)✧ Higher stimulated LH to FSH ratio§	No change from baseline, or LH peak in the prepubertal range

CPP, central precocious puberty (also known as gonadotropin-dependent precocious puberty); LH, luteinizing hormone; GnRH, gonadotropin-releasing hormone; GnRHa, gonadotropin-releasing hormone agonist; FSH, follicle-stimulating hormone.

*UNLESS the patient has concomitant growth hormone deficiency (as in the case of a neurogenic form of CPP), or has already passed his or her peak height velocity at the time of evaluation, in which case growth velocity may be normal or decreased for chronological age.

¶Using most commercially available immunoassays, serum concentrations of gonadal steroids have poor sensitivity to differentiate between prepubertal and early pubertal concentrations.

◻Using ultrasensitive assays with detection limit of LH <0.1 mIU/L, prepubertal basal LH concentrations are <0.2 to 0.3 mIU/L.

✧In most laboratories, the upper limit of normal for LH after GnRH stimulation is 3.3 to 5.0 mIU/mL. Stimulated LH concentrations above this normal range suggests CPP.

§A peak stimulated LH/FSH ratio <0.66 usually suggests nonprogressive precocious puberty, whereas a ratio >0.66 is typically seen with CPP.

Source: Reproduced with permission from Harrington J, Palmert MR. Definition, etiology, and evaluation of precocious puberty. In: Post, TW, ed. *UpToDate*. Waltham, MA: UpToDate (accessed on March 6, 2016). Copyright © 2016 UpToDate, Inc. For more information, visit www.uptodate.com.

Table 9.7. Etiologies of GnRH-independent and GnRH-dependent precocious puberty

Classification	Female	Male
GnRH independent (true precocity)		
Idiopathic	74%	41%
CNS problem	7%	26%
GnRH independent (precocious pseudopuberty)		
Ovarian (cyst or tumor)	11%	—
Testicular	—	10%
McCune-Albright syndrome:	5%	1%
Adrenal feminizing	1%	0%
Adrenal masculinizing	1%	22%
Ectopic gonadotropin production	0.5%	0.5%

GnRH, gonadotropin-releasing hormone.

Source: Reproduced with permission from Gordon JD, Speroff L. Abnormal puberty and growth problems. In: *Handbook for Clinical Gynecologic Endocrinology and Infertility, 6th Ed*. Philadelphia: Lippincott–Raven; 2002.

Central or True Precocious Puberty
- Premature stimulation by GnRH (GnRH-dependent)
- Idiopathic is the most common.
- CNS tumors, infection, congenital abnormality, trauma, juvenile primary hypothyroidism, Russell-Silver syndrome

Table 9.8. Central (gonadotropin-dependent) precocious puberty

Etiology	Clinical Features	Bone Age	Additional Evaluation
Idiopathic (80 to 90% of girls with CPP, and 25 to 60% of boys with CPP)	Early progressive pubertal development, but proceeds in normal sequence.	↑↑	Increased ovarian and uterine volumes on ultrasound may help differentiate girls with CPP from those with premature thelarche.
Secondary to CNS lesions (e.g., hypothalamic hamartomas, other CNS tumors and lesions, cranial radiation)	Early progressive pubertal development, but proceeds in normal sequence. Central precocious puberty secondary to a CNS lesion occurs more commonly in boys and younger children.	↑↑	Contrast enhanced MRI to rule out CNS abnormality.
Post early exposure to sex steroids (after treatment for peripheral precocity)	History of treatment of peripheral precocity. Progressive pubertal development with breast development in girls and testicular enlargement in boys.	↑↑	Basal and stimulated LH concentrations are pubertal.

↑↑, significantly advanced for chronological age (e.g., ≥ 2 standard deviations); CPP, central precocious puberty; CNS, central nervous system; LH, luteinizing hormone; MRI, magnetic resonance imaging; GnRH, gonadotropin-releasing hormone; GnRHa, gonadotropin-releasing hormone agonist.

Central precocious puberty is characterized by basal LH concentrations >0.2 to 0.3 mIU/L, and/or stimulated LH concentration post GnRH or GnRHa of >3.3 to 5.0 mIU/L.

Source: Reproduced with permission from Harrington J, Palmert MR. Definition, etiology, and evaluation of precocious puberty. In: Post, TW, ed. *UpToDate*. Waltham, MA: UpToDate (accessed on March 6, 2016). Copyright © 2016 UpToDate, Inc. For more information, visit www.uptodate.com.

Peripheral Precocious Puberty

- GnRH independent.
- Peripheral precocious puberty may result in GnRH-dependent precocious puberty if left untreated.
- McCune-Albright syndrome:
  - Gene mutation of the G protein α-subunit (leads to hormone receptor activation in absence of the hormone); toxic multinodular goiter, pituitary gigantism, Cushing syndrome, polyostotic fibrous dysplasia, café-au-lait spots
  - Treat with testolactone (aromatase inhibitor)
- Neoplasms (adrenal or gonadal); 11% of girls with precocious puberty have an ovarian tumor.
- Exogenous hormones (drugs, food)

Table 9.9. Peripheral precocity (gonadotropin-independent precocious puberty)

Etiology	Clinical Features	Bone Age	Additional Evaluation
Girls only			
Ovarian cysts	Breast development and/or vaginal bleeding. Occasionally presents with ovarian torsion and abdominal pain.	↑ to ↑↑	Pelvic ultrasound may visualize the cyst, although in some cases the cyst may have involuted by the time of the study. Vaginal bleeding is indicative of estrogen withdrawal. Recurrent ovarian cysts suggest McCune Albright syndrome:.
Ovarian tumor	Development of either isosexual or contrasexual sexual precocity, depending of tumor type.	↑↑	Pelvic ultrasound
Boys only			
Leydig cell tumor	Asymmetrical enlargement of the testes.	↑↑	Pubertal testosterone concentrations. Testicular ultrasound aids in diagnosis.
hCG-secreting germ cell tumors	Symmetric testicular enlargement to an early pubertal size, but testes remain smaller than expected for degree of pubertal development. Peripheral precocity is seen only in boys, because hCG only activates LH receptors (estrogen biosynthesis in the ovaries requires both FSH and LH receptor activation).	↑↑	These tumors may occur in gonads, brain, liver, retroperitoneum, or mediastinum. When a tumor is identified in the anterior mediastinum, a karyotype must be performed because of an association of this finding with Klinefelter syndrome.
Familial male-limited precocious puberty	Symmetric testicular enlargement to an early pubertal size, but testes remain smaller than expected for degree of pubertal development; spermatogenesis may occur. Familial: Male-limited autosomal dominant trait. Peripheral precocity is seen only in boys, because there is only activation of the LH receptors (ovarian estrogen biosynthesis requires both FSH and LH receptor activation).	↑↑	Genetic testing for mutations of the LH receptor gene (LHCGR).
Girls and boys			
Exogenous sex steroids (estradiol and testosterone creams)	Estrogen preparations cause feminization, while topical androgens cause virilization in both sexes.	↑↑	Clinical history explores use of exogenous sex steroids and folk remedies by caretakers.

(continued)

Etiology	Clinical Features	Bone Age	Additional Evaluation
Girls and boys			
McCune-Albright syndrome: (girls>boys)	In girls, may present with recurrent episodes of breast development, regression and vaginal bleeding. In boys, sexual precocity less common. Skin: Multiple irregular-edged café-au-lait spots. Bone: Polyostotic fibrous dysplasia.	↑ to ↑↑	Ultrasound: Ovaries enlarged, with follicular cysts. In boys, testicular ultrasound can demonstrate hyper- and hypoechoic lesions (most likely representing areas of leydig cell hyperplasia), microlithiasis and focal calcifications. May have other hyperactive endocrine disorders (i.e., thyrotoxicosis, glucocorticoid excess and/or gigantism).
Primary hypothyroidism	Girls: vaginal bleeding, breast development, and galactorrhea. Boys: testicular enlargement. Other clinical features of hypothyroidism such as short stature.	↓	Elevated TSH
Congenital adrenal hyperplasia (untreated)	Boys have prepubertal testes with enlarged phallus and pubic hair development. Girls with "nonclassic" CAH may present with early pubic and/or axillary hair and other signs of androgen excess.	↑↑	Sex hormone levels vary depending on the adrenal enzyme block. An early morning 17-OHP >200 ng/dL (6 nmol/L) has a high sensitivity and specificity for congenital adrenal hyperplasia secondary to 21 hydroxylase deficiency. ACTH stimulation test is recommended to confirm the diagnosis of CAH if the 17-OHP level is intermediate (e.g., between 200 and 1500 ng/dL). After therapy with glucocorticoids, CPP may develop.
Virilizing adrenal tumor	Boys: pubic and/or axillary hair and penile growth with prepubertal testes. Girls: pubic and/or axillary hair, other significant signs of androgen excess (acne and clitoromegaly). May present with signs of glucocorticoid excess. May be associated with hereditary cancer syndromes.	↑↑	High DHEA or DHEAS, androstenedione and testosterone. CT and/or ultrasound of adrenal glands to locate tumor.

↑, advanced for chronological age; ↓, delayed for chronological age; hCG, human chorionic gonadotropin; LH, luteinizing hormone; FSH, follicle-stimulating hormone; LHCGR, luteinizing hormone/choriogonadotropin receptor; CPP, central precocious puberty; TSH, thyroid-stimulating hormone; CAH, congenital adrenal hyperplasia; 17-OHP, 17-hydroxyprogesterone; ACTH, adrenocorticotropic hormone; DHEA, dehydroepiandrosterone; DHEAS, dehydroepiandrosterone sulfate; CT, computed tomography.

Peripheral precocity is characterized by low or suppressed gonadotropin concentrations with elevated sex hormone levels. Pubertal status should be monitored for 3 to 6 months after treatment, because treatment of peripheral precocity can trigger central precocious puberty (CPP).

Source: Reproduced with permission from Harrington J, Palmert MR. Definition, etiology, and evaluation of precocious puberty. In: Post, TW, ed. *UpToDate*. Waltham, MA: UpToDate (accessed on March 6, 2016]. Copyright © 2016 UpToDate, Inc. For more information, visit www.uptodate.com.

AMENORRHEA
Primary Amenorrhea
Definition
- This is the absence of menses by 16 years old in the presence of normal growth and secondary sexual development (breasts).
- If by age 13 menses has not occurred and the onset of puberty, such as breast development, is absent, a workup for primary amenorrhea is appropriate.

Table 9.10. Distribution of causes of primary amenorrhea

Category	Frequency (%)
No breast development: high FSH	43
45,X and variants	27
46,XX	14
46,XY	2
Breast development (eugonadal)	30
Müllerian agenesis	15
PCOS	7
Vaginal septum	3
Cushing syndrome and thyroid disease	2
Imperforate hymen	1
Androgen insensitivity	1
CAH	1
No breast development: low FSH	27
Constitutional delay	14
Prolactinomas	5
Kallmann syndrome	5
Stress, weight loss, anorexia	2
Other central nervous system disorder	1

FSH, follicle-stimulating hormone.

Source: Adapted from Reindollar RH, Byrd JR, McDonough PG. Delayed sexual development: a study of 252 patients. *Am J Obstet Gynecol.* 1981;140(4):371. Copyright © 1981 Elsevier.

Table 9.11. Mnemonic for primary amenorrhea differential diagnosis: XMAS

Diagnosis	Incidence
XO, Turner Syndrome	1:2,500
Müllerian Agenesis	1:4,000–1:10,000
Androgen Insensitivity (complete)	1:40,000
Swyer Syndrome	1:80,000

Table 9.12. Mayer-Rokitansky-Kuster-Hauser syndrome (müllerian agenesis) vs. androgen insensitivity syndrome

	Mayer-rokitansky-kuster-hauser Syndrome	Complete Androgen Insensitivity Syndrome
Vagina	Absent	Absent
Pubic hair	Present	Absent
Breasts	Present	Present
Gonads	Ovaries	Testes
Uterus	Absent	Absent
Karyotype	46,XX	46,XY
Other anomalies (renal, cardiac)	Increased	Not increased

Secondary Amenorrhea

Definition
- Absence of menses for 3 cycles or months
- Oligomenorrhea <9 cycles/year
- Most commonly → PCOS, hypothalamic amenorrhea, hyperprolactinemia, and ovarian failure

Table 9.13. Distribution of causes of secondary amenorrhea

Category Frequency	(%)
Low or normal FSH	**67.5**
Chronic anovulation (PCOS)	28
Nonspecific hypothalamic	18
Weight loss/anorexia/stress	15.5
Pituitary tumor/empty sella	2
Hypothyroidism	1.5
Sheehan syndrome	1.5
Cushing syndrome	1
High prolactin	**13**
High FSH: Gonadal failure	**10.5**
46,XX	10
Abnormal karyotype	0.5
Anatomic	**7**
Asherman syndrome	7
Hyperandrogenic states	**2**
Ovarian tumor	1
Nonclassic CAH	0.5
Undiagnosed	0.5

Source: Reproduced with permission from Reindollar RH, Novak M, Thos SP, et al. Adult-onset amenorrhea: a study of 262 patients. *Am J Obstet Gynecol.* 1986;155(3):531. Copyright © 1986 Elsevier.

Table 9.14. Causes of intrauterine adhesions

%	Antecedent Event
46	Hysteroscopic resection of multiple fibroids
40	Retained products of conception
39	Recurrent miscarriage
31	Late (fibrotic villi and no blood vessels) spontaneous miscarriage D&C
31	Hysteroscopic resection of single fibroid
23	Postpartum D&C (second–fourth week)
13	Elective abortion D&C
7	Infertility
7	Hysteroscopic metroplasty
6	Early (villi contain blood vessels) spontaneous abortion D&C
4	Postpartum D&C (anytime)
3	Post-cesarean delivery
2	Secondary amenorrhea

Source: Reproduced with permission from March CM. Asherman's syndrome. *Semin Reprod Med.* 2011 Mar;29(2):83-94. Copyright © Georg Thieme Verlag KG.

REPRODUCTIVE ENDOCRINOLOGY — Secondary Amenorrhea

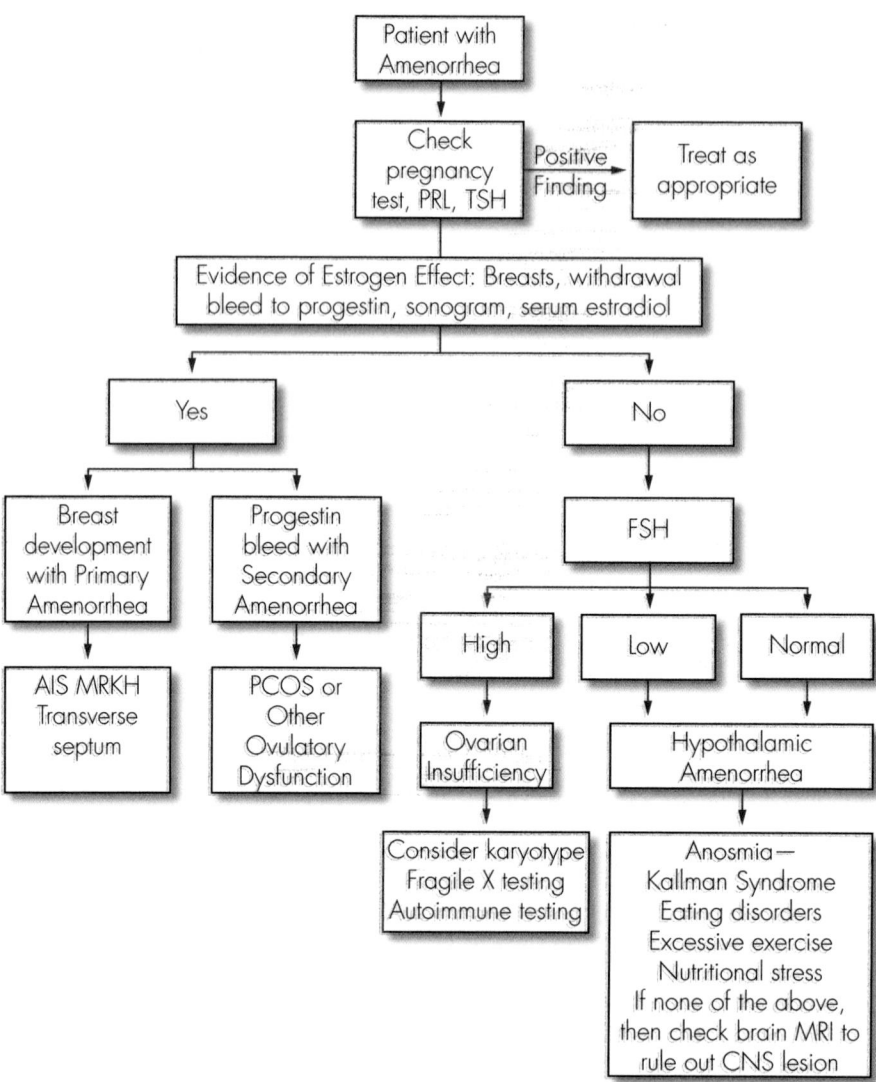

Figure 9.5. Algorithm for the evaluation of amenorrhea

POLYCYSTIC OVARY SYNDROME (PCOS)
Fast Facts
- 10–15% of reproductive-aged women have PCOS.
- Mothers of women with PCOS have elevated low-density lipoprotein/androgen levels as well as markers of insulin resistance (IR) consistent with a heritable trait (Sam 2006).
- PCOS patients frequently develop regular menstrual cycles when aging (Elting 2000), possibly resulting from ↓ size of the follicle cohort or from ↓ inhibin.
- Theory of etiology: enhanced serine phosphorylation unification theory → CYP17 activity in the ovary (hyperandrogenism) and ↓ insulin receptor activity peripherally (insulin resistance [IR]; Dunaif 1995) lead to the endocrine dysfunction of PCOS.

Diagnostic Criteria

Table 9.15. Recommended diagnostic schemes for polycystic ovary syndrome by varying expert groups

Signs and Symptoms*	National Institutes of Health Criteria[†] 1990 (Both Are Required for Diagnosis)	Rotterdam Consensus Criteria[‡] 2003 (Two Out of Three Are Required for Diagnosis)	Androgen Excess Society[§] 2006 (Hyperandrogenism Plus One Out of Remaining Two Are Required for Diagnosis)
Hyperandrogenism[‖]	R	NR	R
Oligoamenorrhea or amenorrhea	R	NR	NR
Polycystic ovaries by ultrasound diagnosis		NR	NR

R, required for diagnosis; NR, possible diagnostic criteria but not required to be present.

*All criteria recommend excluding other possible etiologies of these signs and symptoms and more than one of the factors present to make a diagnosis.

[†]Dunaif A, Givens JR, Haseltine FP, Merriam GR, eds. *Polycystic Ovary Syndrome.* Boston, MA: Blackwell Scientific Publications; 1992.

[‡]Rotterdam ESHRE/ASRM-Sponsored PCOS Consensus Workshop Group. Revised 2003 consensus on diagnostic criteria and long-term health risks related to polycystic ovary syndrome. *Fertil Steril.* 2004;81:19–25.

[§]Azziz R, Carmina E, Dewailly D, Diamanti-Kandarakis E, Escobar-Morreale HF, Futterweit W, et al. Positions statement: criteria for defining polycystic ovary syndrome as a predominantly hyperandrogenic syndrome: an Androgen Excess Society guideline. Androgen Excess Society. *J Clin Endocrinol Metab.* 2006;91:4237–45.

[‖]Hyperandrogenism may be either the presence of hirsutism or biochemical hyperandrogenemia.

Source: Reproduced with permission from ACOG Practice Bulletin No. 108: Polycystic ovary syndrome. *Obstet Gynecol.* 2009 Oct;114(4):936-49. Copyright © 2009 The American College of Obstetricians and Gynecologists.

Ultrasound Criteria for PCOS

The Androgen Excess-Polycystic Ovary Syndrome Society Task Force reviewed the literature and released recommendations for the diagnosis of polycystic ovarian morphology in 2014. These new criteria are as follows:

1. At least one ovary with ≥25 follicles 2–9 mm in diameter.
2. At least one ovary with volume >10 mL.

Ovarian volume should only be used to diagnose polycystic ovarian morphology if the ovaries are not optimally visualized, such as in the following situations:

1. The ovaries are only visualized transabdominally.
2. The ovaries are partially obscured by bowel gas.
3. An endovaginal transducer with frequency less than 8 MHz is used.

Source: Dewailly D, et al. Definition and significance of polycystic ovarian morphology: a task force report from the Androgen Excess and Polycystic Ovary Syndrome Society. *Hum Reprod Update*. 2014;20(3):334–52.

Table 9.16. Other diagnoses to exclude in all women before making a diagnosis of PCOS

Disorder	Test	Abnormal Values	Reference for Further Evaluation and Treatment of Abnormal Findings (First Author, Year)
Thyroid disease	Serum TSH	TSH > the upper limit of normal suggests hypothyroidism; TSH < the lower Limit, usually <0.1 mIU/L, suggests hyperthyroidism	Ladenson, 2000
Prolactin excess	Serum prolactin	> Upper limit of normal for the assay	Melmed, 2011
Nonclassical congenital adrenal hyperplasia	Early morning (before 8 AM) serum 17-OHP	200–400 ng/dL depending on the assay (applicable to the early follicular phase of a normal menstrual cycle as levels rise with ovulation), but a cosyntropin stimulation test (250/ µg) is needed if levels fall near the lower limit and should stimulate 17-OHP >1000 ng/dL	Speiser, 2010

Source: Reproduced with permission from Legro RS, Arslanian SA, Ehrmann DA, Hoeger KM, Murad MH, Pasquali R, Welt CK; Endocrine Society. Diagnosis and treatment of polycystic ovary syndrome: an Endocrine Society clinical practice guideline. *J Clin Endocrinol Metab*. 2013 Dec;98(12):4565-92. Copyright © 2013 The Endocrine Society.

Table 9.17. Diagnoses to consider excluding in select women, depending on presentation

Other Diagnoses[a]	Suggestive Features in the Presentation	Tests to Assist In the Diagnosis	Reference for Further Evaluation and Treatment of Abnormal Findings (First Author, Year)
Pregnancy	Amenorrhea (as opposed to oligomenorrhea), other signs and symptoms of pregnancy including breast fullness, uterine cramping, etc.	Serum or urine hCG (positive)	Morse, 2011
HA including functional HA	Amenorrhea, clinical history of low body weight/BMI, excessive exercise, and a physical exam in which signs of androgen excess are lacking; multifollicular ovaries are sometimes present	Serum LH and FSH (both low to low normal), serum estradiol (low)	Wang, 2008
Primary ovarian insufficiency	Amenorrhea combined with symptoms of estrogen deficiency including hot flashes and urogenital symptoms	Serum FSH (elevated), serum estradiol (low)	Nelson, 2009
Androgen-secreting tumor	Virilization including change in voice, male pattern androgenic alopecia, and clitoromegaly; rapid onset of symptoms	Serum T and DHEAS levels (markedly elevated), ultrasound imaging of ovaries, MRI of adrenal glands (mass or tumor present)	Carmina, 2006
Cushing syndrome	Many of the signs and symptoms of PCOS can overlap with Cushing (i.e., striae), obesity, dorsocervical fat (i.e., buffalo hump, glucose intolerance); however, Cushing is more likely to be present when a large number of signs and symptoms, especially those with high discriminatory index (e.g., myopathy, plethora, violaceous striae, easy bruising) are present, and this presentation should lead to screening	24-hr urinary collection for urinary free cortisol (elevated), late night salivary cortisol (elevated), overnight dexamethasone suppression test (failure to suppress morning serum cortisol level)	Nieman, 2008
Acromegaly	Oligomenorrhea and skin changes (thickening, tags, hirsutism, hyperhidrosis) may overlap with PCOS. However, headaches, peripheral vision loss, enlarged jaw (macrognathia), frontal bossing, macroglossia, increased shoe and glove size, etc., are indications for screening	Serum free IGF-1 level (elevated), MRI of pituitary (mass or tumor present)	Melmed, 2009

DHEAS, dehydroepiandrosterone sulfate; HA, hypothalamic amenorrhea; hCG, human chorionic gonadotropin; MRI, magnetic resonance imaging.

[a]Additionally there are very rare causes of hyperandrogenic chronic anovulation that are not included in this table because they are so rare, but they must be considered in patients with an appropriate history. These include other forms of congenital adrenal hyperplasia (e.g., 11β-hydroxylase deficiency, 3 β-hydroxysteroid dehydrogenase), related congenital disorders of adrenal steroid metabolism or action (e.g., apparent/cortisone reductase deficiency, apparent DHEA sulfotransferase deficiency, glucocorticoid resistance), virilizing congenital adrenal hyperplasia (e.g., adrenal rests, poor control, fetal programming), syndromes of extreme IR, drugs, portohepatic shunting, and disorders of sex development.

Source: Reproduced with permission from Legro RS, Arslanian SA, Ehrmann DA, Hoeger KM, Murad MH, Pasquali R, Welt CK; Endocrine Society. Diagnosis and treatment of polycystic ovary syndrome: an Endocrine Society clinical practice guideline. *J Clin Endocrinol Metab.* 2013 Dec;98(12):4565-92. Copyright © 2013 The Endocrine Society.

Table 9.18. Suggested evaluation for patients with polycystic ovary syndrome

Physical

Blood pressure

BMI (weight in kg divided by height in m^2)

    25–30 = overweight, greater than 30 = obese

    Waist circumference to determine body fat distribution

    Value greater than 35 inches = abnormal

Presence of stigmata of hyperandrogenism and insulin resistance

    Acne, hirsutism, androgenic alopecia, acanthosis nigricans

Laboratory

Documentation of biochemical hyperandrogenemia

    Total testosterone and sex hormone–binding globulin or bioavailable and free testosterone

Exclusion of other causes of menstrual irregularity

    Thyroid-stimulating hormone levels (thyroid dysfunction)

    Prolactin (hyperprolactinemia)

Exclusion of other causes of hyperandrogenism

    17-hydroxyprogesterone (nonclassical congenital adrenal hyperplasia due to 21 hydroxylase deficiency); random normal level less than 4 ng/mL or morning fasting level less than 2 ng/mL

    Consider screening for Cushing syndrome and other rare disorders such as acromegaly

Evaluation for metabolic abnormalities

    Two-hour oral glucose tolerance test (fasting glucose less than 110 mg/dL = normal, 110–125 mg/dL = impaired, greater than 126 mg/dL = type 2 diabetes) followed by 75 g oral glucose ingestion and then 2-hour glucose level (less than 140 mg/dL = normal glucose tolerance, 140–199 mg/dL = impaired glucose tolerance, greater than 200 mg/dL = type 2 diabetes)

    Fasting lipid and lipoprotein level (total cholesterol, high density lipoproteins less than 50 mg/dL abnormal, triglycerides greater than 150 mg/dL abnormal, [low density lipoproteins usually calculated by Friedewald equation])

Ultrasound Examination

Determination of polycystic ovaries: in one or both ovaries, either 12 or more follicles measuring 2–9 mm in diameter, or increased ovarian volume (greater than 10 cm^3). If there is a follicle greater than 10 mm in diameter, the scan should be repeated at a time of ovarian quiescence in order to calculate volume and area. The presence of one polycystic ovary is sufficient to provide the diagnosis.

Identification of endometrial abnormalities

Optional Tests to Consider

Gonadotropin determinations to determine cause of amenorrhea

Fasting insulin levels in younger women, those with severe stigmata of insulin resistance and hyperandrogenism, or those undergoing ovulation induction

24-hour urinary free-cortisol excretion test or a low dose dexamethasone suppression test in women with late onset of polycystic ovary syndrome symptoms or stigmata of Cushing syndrome

Source: Reproduced with permission from ACOG Practice Bulletin No. 108: Polycystic ovary syndrome. *Obstet Gynecol.* 2009 Oct;114(4):936-49. Copyright © 2009 The American College of Obstetricians and Gynecologists.

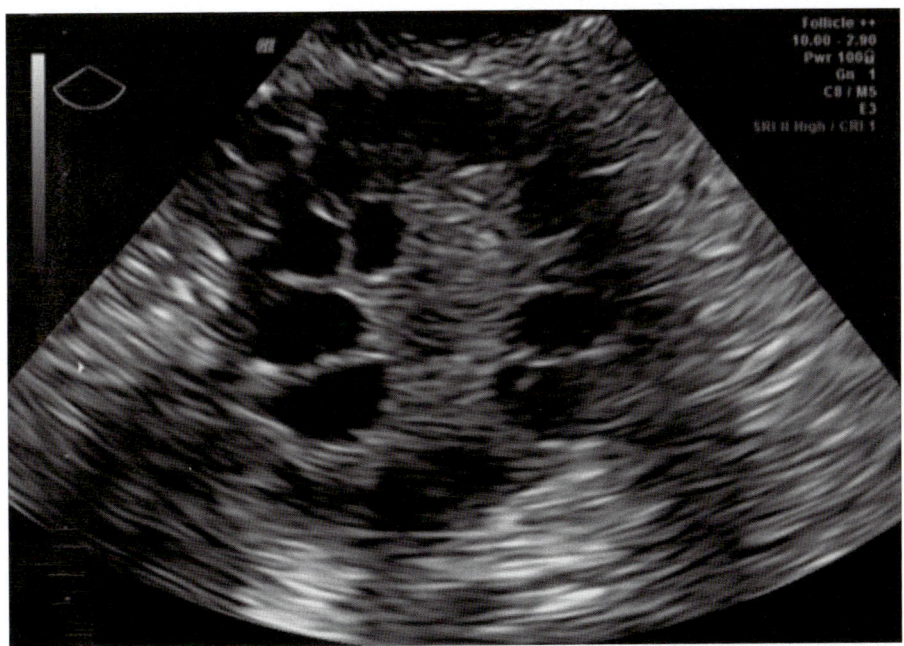

Figure 9.6. Ultrasonographic appearance of the PCOS ovary

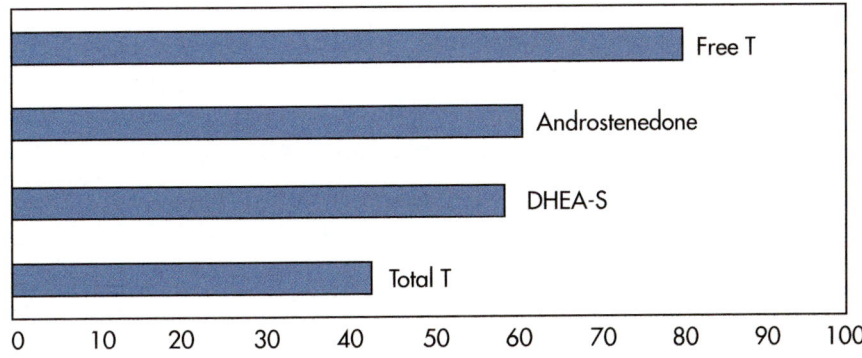

Figure 9.7. Frequency of elevated androgens in women with PCOS
Frequency of elevation of each of the androgens in 138 women with polycystic ovary syndrome listed as a percentage.
DHEA-S, dehydroepiandrosterone sulfate; T, testosterone.
Source: Reproduced with permission from Wild RA, Umstot ES, Andersen RN, et al. Androgen parameters and their correlation with body weight in one hundred thirty-eight women thought to have hyperandrogenism. *Am J Obstet Gynecol.* 1983;146(6):602. Copyright © 1983 Elsevier.

Glucose Tolerance Testing
- Insulin resistance is present in both lean and obese PCOS.
- Screening ought to be done every 2 years for those with normal values and every year if insulin resistant.
- Hemoglobin A1C:
  - 5.7–6.4% = insulin resistance
  - ≥6.5% = diabetes (confirm with repeat test)
- Incidence of IR or NIDDM in women with PCOS (Legro 1999):
  - IR: 31.1%
  - Type II DM: 7.5%

Table 9.19. Accepted values for glucose tolerance testing

	Fasting Plasma Glucose (mg/dL)	2-hr Plasma Glucose (mg/dL)
Normal	≤99	≤139
Impaired	100–125	140–199
Type II diabetes mellitus	≥126	≥200

Source: Adapted from American Diabetes Association. Diagnosis and classification of diabetes mellitus. *Diabetes Care.* 2010;33(Suppl1):S62-S69.

Virilizing Ovarian or Adrenal Tumor
- *Rapid* onset and *progressive* course of virilizing symptoms
- *Severe* hirsutism: male pattern balding, clitoromegaly, weight gain
- Total T >200 ng/dL (6.9 nmol/L) or DHEA-S >700 µg/dL (19 µmol/L)
  - Positive predictive value of a repeat total T >250 ng/dL → 9%; negative predictive value of 100% (Waggoner 1999)
- Computed tomography (CT) of pelvis and adrenals with contrast if tumor suspected (may require selective venous catheterization of ovarian/adrenal veins)
- Most common virilizing ovarian tumor: *arrhenoblastoma*
- Adrenal tumor: suspected if DHEA-S >700 µg/dL (19 µmol/L) and markedly elevated total testosterone

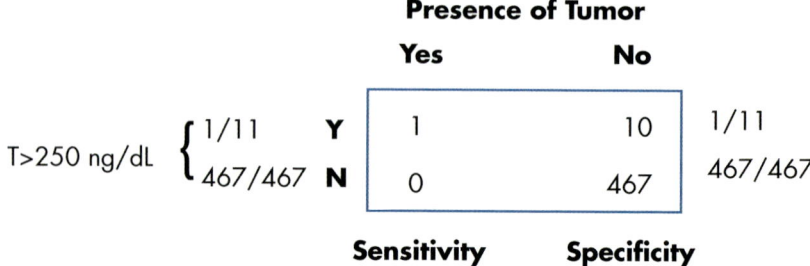

Figure 9.8. Predictive value of elevated testosterone for presence of a virilizing ovarian or adrenal tumor

Source: Data from Waggoner W, Boots LR, Azziz R. Total testosterone and DHEAS levels as predictors of androgen-secreting neoplasms: a populational study. *Gynecol Endocrinol.* 1999 Dec;13(6):394-400.

Table 9.20. Prevalence of different androgen excess disorders in 950 women referred because of clinical hyperandrogenism organ dysfunction

	Number of Patients	% of Total Number of Patients
Classic PCOS	538	56.6
Ovulatory PCOS	147	15.5
Idiopathic hyperandrogenism	150	15.8
Idiopathic hirsutism	72	7.6
NCAH	41	4.3
Androgen-secreting tumors	2	0.2

Source: Reproduced with permission from Carmina E, Rosato F, Janni A, et al. Extensive clinical experience: relative prevalence of different androgen excess disorders in 950 women referred because of clinical hyperandrogenism. *J Clin Endo Metab.* 2006;91(1):2–6 Copyright © 2006 The Endocrine Society.

Treatment of PCOS
Goals
- Prevent endometrial hyperplasia/cancer
- Restore normal menstruation; resolution of anovulation/infertility
- Improve hirsutism and acne
- Reduce long-term consequences to patient's health

Table 9.21. Potential long-term consequences of polycystic ovary syndrome

Definite or Very Likely Consequences of Polycystic Ovary Syndrome	Possible Consequences of Polycystic Ovary Syndrome
Insulin resistance; type II diabetes mellitus (greater than weight-matched controls)	Hypertension
	Dyslipidemia
Coronary heart disease	Ovarian cancer (conflicting data)
Endometrial hyperplasia/atypia	Spontaneous abortion (may not be greater than for subfertility population)
Gestational diabetes	
Sleep apnea (even when controlled for body mass index)	
Depression	

Weight Reduction
- As little as 5–7% of body weight reduction can reduce hyperandrogenism, improve insulin sensitivity, and restore spontaneous ovulation and fertility in 75% of women with PCOS (Kiddy 1992).
    - Low-calorie diet (1,000–1,500 kcal/day)
    - Waist-hip ratio >0.85 at greater risk for morbidity
    - Metformin may promote weight loss

Oral Contraceptives
- First line of drug treatment (use at least 30 mcg of ethinyl estradiol and avoid norgetrel and levonorgestrel).
- Method of action: SHBG, suppression of LH, inhibition of 5α-reductase and androgen receptor binding.
- Greatest efficacy against acne (hirsutism usually requires the addition of antiandrogens).
- Avoid levonorgestrel-containing oral contraceptives (OCs), due to the androgenic properties of the progestin (e.g., Alesse, Levlen, Nordette, Triphasil).
- OCs ↓ LH but not to normal levels (Polson 1988).
- Gonadotropin-releasing hormone (GnRH) agonist plus add-back no better than OCs alone (Carr 1995).

Progestins
- Give progestins q month or q 2–3 months to prevent endometrial hyperplasia.

Antiandrogens
- Antiandrogens are effective in the treatment of hirsutism after 6–9 months; however, cessation of antiandrogen therapy is followed by recurrence (Yucelten 1999).
  - **Spironolactone** (Aldactone, 100–200 mg/day) plus OCs (Lobo 1985; Young 1987). Contraception is mandatory with the use of spironolactone, as incomplete virilization of a male fetus may occur. Wait ≥2 months after discontinuance of spironolactone before beginning attempts at conception.
    - Aldosterone antagonist, K⁺-sparing diuretic:
      - Inhibits steroidogenic enzymes and binds the DHT receptor at the hair follicle
      - Can cause irregular uterine bleeding
      - 25-mg tablets are generic and inexpensive
  - **Finasteride** (Proscar, 5 mg/day), type II 5α-reductase inhibitor; shows signs of being an excellent and safe antiandrogen
    - ↓ Circulating DHT levels; not effective topically (Price 2000); not approved by the Food and Drug Administration (FDA) for this purpose
    - Low dose (2.5 mg) every 3 days is as effective as continuous administration in ↓ hirsutism (Tartagni 2004)
    - *Contraception is mandatory* (Ciotta 1995; Wong 1995; Fruzzetti 1999) because its use during the late first trimester may risk of hypospadias and other genital abnormalities in male fetuses
  - **Cyproterone acetate (Androcur)**, not approved in the United States (used extensively in Europe [Diane 35] and Israel for hirsutism)
    - Androgen receptor antagonist, decreases 5α-reductase activity, impairs androgen synthesis
    - Reports of liver tumors in beagles have kept this effective drug from the U.S. market
  - **Eflornithine** (Vaniqa, 13.9% topical cream b.i.d.)
    - Irreversibly inhibits ornithine decarboxylase (ODC) to inhibit follicle polyamine synthesis necessary for hair growth
    - Effect seen over 4–8 weeks; *reversible* if medicine is stopped
    - <1% systemic absorption; skin irritation may occur

Hair-Removal Systems
- Systemic treatment of hyperandrogenism and hirsutism should be combined with hair removal (shaving, waxing, depilatories [short-acting], or electrolysis or laser [long-acting]) for maximum effect on existing hair.

Electrolysis
- Electric current (through needle in hair follicle) destroys hair follicle.
- Blend most effective: galvanic electrolysis and thermolysis.
- Expensive, painful, and time-consuming but can be permanent.
- Scarring if not done correctly.

Laser-Assisted Hair Removal
- Thermal injury targeted to follicular melanin ("selective photothermolysis") destroys hair follicle (Hobbs 2000).
- Works best for those with light skin and dark hair, although newer lasers are better at light hair.
- May cause pigment changes: hypo- or hyperpigmentation.
- Requires multiple (4–6) treatments; effect may be improved by waxing before procedure.
- Avoid in patients who form keloids or hypertrophic scars or who are on retinoids.
- For dark skin, choose longer wavelength: Nd:YAG and Diode; avoid long-pulsed Ruby (Lanigan 2003).
- Types of lasers:
  - **Nd:YAG:** 1,064 nm, Q-switched or long-pulsed, temporary hair loss, uses carbon solution massaged into hair follicles.
  - **Ruby:** 694 nm, long-pulsed, long-term reduction in hirsutism, pigment changes can occur.
  - **Alexandrite:** 755 nm, long-pulsed, may have fewer pigment changes, long-term reduction.
  - **Diode:** 800 nm, long-term hair loss, fewer pigment changes, works less well on fine hair.

Insulin Sensitizing Drugs—Metformin (Glucophage)
- Biguanide oral hypoglycemic agent
- Inhibits hepatic glucose production; increases peripheral tissue insulin sensitivity; ↓ LH, free T, and PAI-I
  - Avoid metformin if: creatinine >1.4 mg/dL (124 μmol/L); liver function tests (LFTs) are elevated → risk of lactic acidosis; severe congestive heart failure; history of alcohol abuse
  - Metformin may cause dizziness and/or gastrointestinal (GI) discomfort (10–25% of patients) and should not be taken with IV contrast dye (e.g., hysterosalpingogram [HSG])
  - Metformin XR regimen (no consensus regarding optimal dose but most use 1000–1500 mg daily [Nestler 2001])
  - Stop after first trimester, although preliminary studies suggest no teratogenicity

REPRODUCTIVE ENDOCRINOLOGY

CONGENITAL ADRENAL HYPERPLASIA

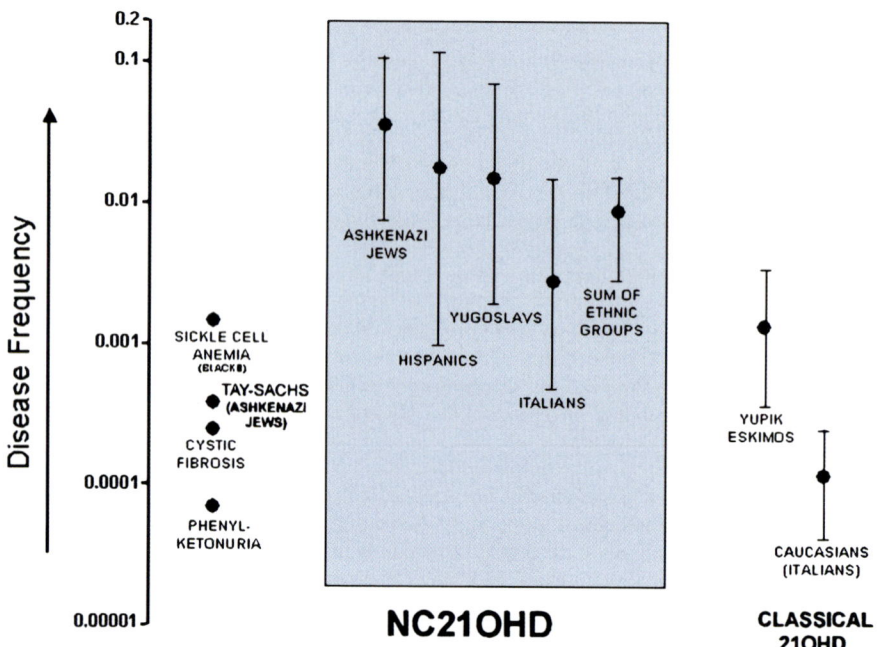

Figure 9.9. Prevalence of autosomal recessive genetic disorders by ethnic group
Source: Reproduced with permission from New MI. Nonclassical 21-hydroxylase deficiency. *J Clin Endo Metab.* 2006;91:4205–4214. Copyright © 2006. The Endocrine Society.

Congenital Adrenal Hyperplasia

Table 9.22. Prevalence of nonclassic congenital adrenal hyperplasia (NCCAH) by ethnic group

Ethnic Group	n	Disease Frequency	Carrier Frequency
Ashkenazi Jews	56	1:27	1:3
Hispanics	9	1:40	1:4
Slavics[1]	8	1:50	1:5
Italians	12	1:300	1:10
Heterogeneous population of New York City	249	1:100	1:6

[1] From Croatia.

Source: Reproduced with permission from New MI. Nonclassical 21-hydroxylase deficiency. *J Clin Endo Metab.* 2006;91:4205–4214. Copyright © 2006. The Endocrine Society.

Table 9.23. Interpretation of Cortrosyn stimulation test in evaluation of CAH

17-hydroxyprogesterone (17-OHP) (ng/dL)	Diagnosis
<200	Polycystic ovary syndrome
200–400	Cortrosyn stimulation test[a]
>400	Nonclassic congenital adrenal hyperplasia

[a] Cortrosyn stimulation test: Measure 17-OHP at t = 60 after 0.25 mg IV adrenocorticotropic hormone administration (see list below).

T = 60 17-Hydroxyprogesterone (ng/dL):

>1,500 ng/dL = NCCAH.

>1,000 ng/dL = Likely NCCAH.

<1,000 ng/dL = Polycystic ovary syndrome.

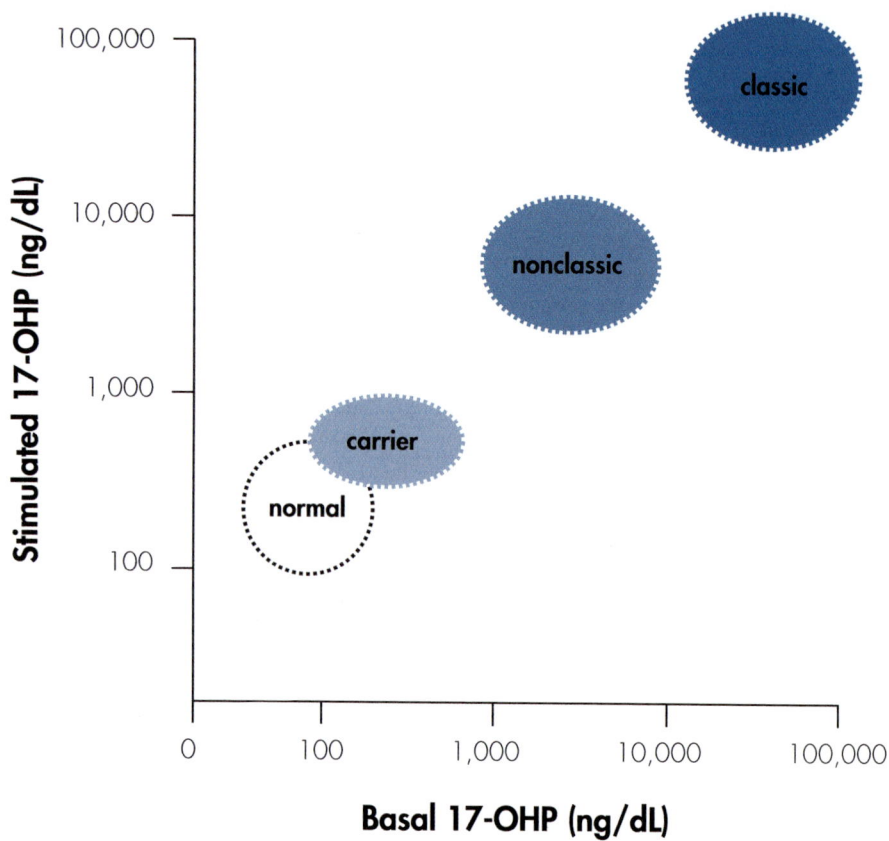

Figure 9.10. Nomogram for ACTH stimulation test
Nomogram for comparing 17-hydroxyprogesterone (17-OHP) ratio before and after administration of 0.25-mg IV cosyntropin (carriers = heterozygotes).
Source: Reproduced with permission from White PC, Speiser PW. Congenital adrenal hyperplasia due to 21-hydroxylase deficiency. *Endocr Rev.* 2000;21(3):2454. Copyright © 2000. The Endocrine Society.

Treatment of Patient at Risk for an Infant with CAH
Mother Is a Carrier and Had a Previous Child with CAH
- If she becomes pregnant with the same partner, the fetus has a 1-in-4 chance of having CAH.
- Consider IVF with PGD to test embryos for CAH.
- Dexamethasone (not inactivated by placental enzymes and thus provides more effective suppression of fetal adrenals) if PGD is not performed and the gender and CAH status of the current fetus are unknown (Lo 1999). The goal here is to suppress endogenous androgen production by the fetal adrenal and thus prevent virilization.

- o Dexamethasone 20 mg/kg in divided oral doses t.i.d. (it is unclear why such a high dose is needed).
- o Since maternal estriol (E3) is derived from the placental metabolism of fetal adrenal androgens, serum E3 levels can be used to monitor glucocorticoid therapy: Aim for E3 between 0.2–10 nmol/L.
- Nevertheless, ~15% of female fetuses who receive glucocorticoid treatment will still have some virilization.
- Since genitalia begin virilization just 6 weeks after conception, to be effective, corticosteroid treatment (see below for dosage recommendations) must be started before 9 weeks, although this is controversial. Informed consent is suggested (see Rationale for Withholding Glucocorticoid Replacement). Steroids are continued until genetic diagnosis from chorionic villous biopsy or cell-free circulating DNA at 10–12 weeks. If the results show a CAH-affected female fetus, dexamethasone is continued in order to diminish fetal virilization from high maternal androgen exposure.

Mother Has CAH or NCCAH
- Screen the father for CAH/NCCAH.
- Start glucocorticoid replacement before 9 weeks of gestation using prednisolone or hydrocortisone to lower maternal androgens and avoid virilization of female fetus; prednisolone or hydrocortisone is inactivated by placental enzymes and hence do not suppress fetal adrenal androgens, but they do reduce maternal androgen production. If a male karyotype is determined, corticosteroids can be discontinued.
  - o Prednisolone 7 mg/day, range from 4–10 mg/day
  - o Hydrocortisone 30 mg/day, range from 15–40 mg/day
- Aggressive suppression of maternal androgens in pregnancy is **probably not warranted** since the placenta can effectively aromatize maternal androgens. However, if the aromatase enzyme is saturated by extremely high androgen levels, then theoretically, virilization of a female fetus could occur. This is extremely rare with maternal CAH (Oglivie 2006).

Rationale for Withholding Glucocorticoid Replacement
- Adverse effects to the mother: weight gain, edema, striae, signs of Cushing syndrome.
- Adverse effects to the fetus:
  - o Glucocorticoids are increasingly recognized as having potent genomic imprinting effects in utero with the following potential adverse effects to the fetus: postnatal failure to thrive, psychomotor developmental delay, neuropsychological dysfunctions, increased risk of orofacial clefts.
- Clinical practice guidelines statement for CAH due to 21-hyroxylase deficiency published in 2010 by the Endocrine Society: "We recommend that prenatal therapy continue to be regarded as experimental" (Speiser 2010).
- Conundrum treating all at risk for only 1 in 8 affected female fetus (Miller 2013):
  - o Since only 1 in 4 will be affected, and only half of the affected fetuses will be females (those most benefiting from treatment), then treatment would be directed toward only 1 in 8 fetuses. Put another way, one would be exposing 7 of 8 fetuses (4 of 4 males and 3 of 4 females) to high-dose dexamethasone to treat the one affected female.
  - o Maternal blood testing for fetal Y-chromosomal DNA can determine fetal sex and thus improve the probability of treating an affected female fetus from 1 in 8 to 1 in 4.

STEROID HORMONE BIOSYNTHESIS

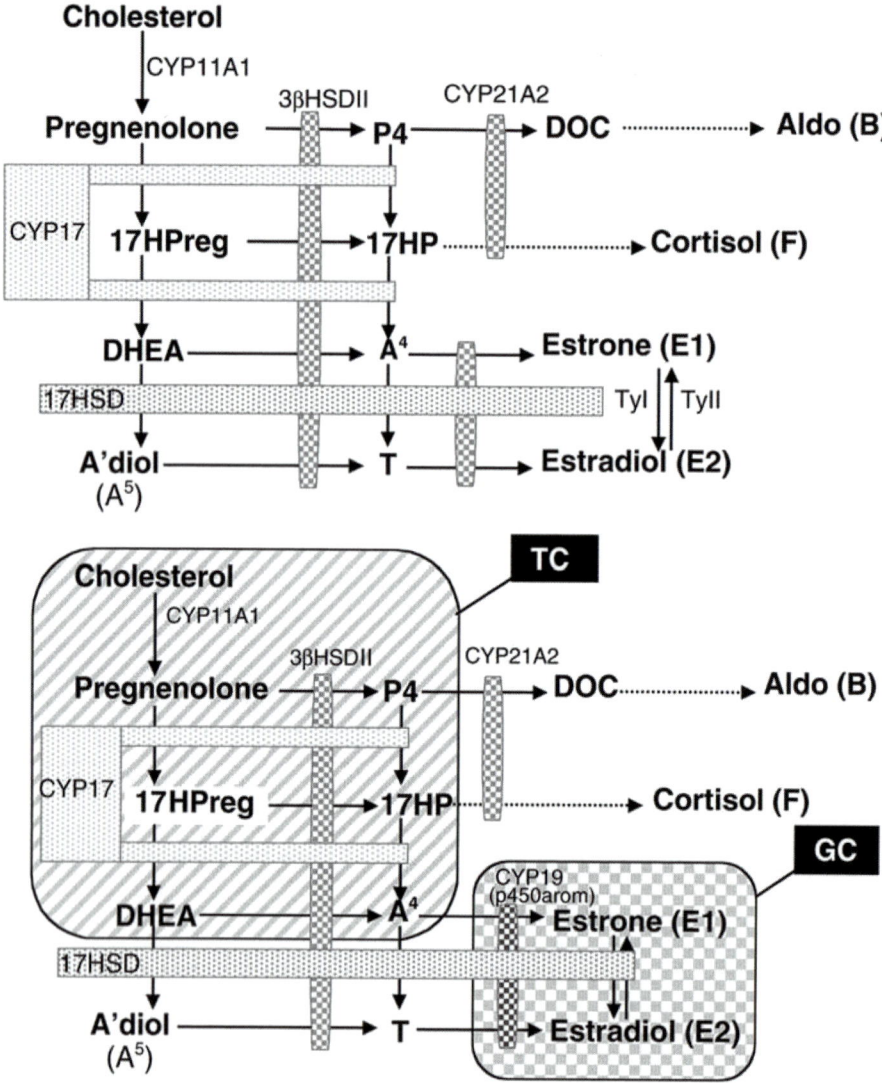

Figure 9.11. Steroid hormone synthesis
A⁴, androstenedione; A'diol, androstenediol; Aldo (B), aldosterone; DHEA, dehydro-epiandrosterone; DOC; 17HP, 17OH-progesterone; GC, granulosa cell; HSD, hydroxysteroid dehydrogenase; 17-HPreg, 17OH-pregnenolone; P4, progesterone; T, testosterone; TC, theca cell; TyI, type I; TyII, type II.

Steroid Hormone Biosynthesis

REPRODUCTIVE ENDOCRINOLOGY

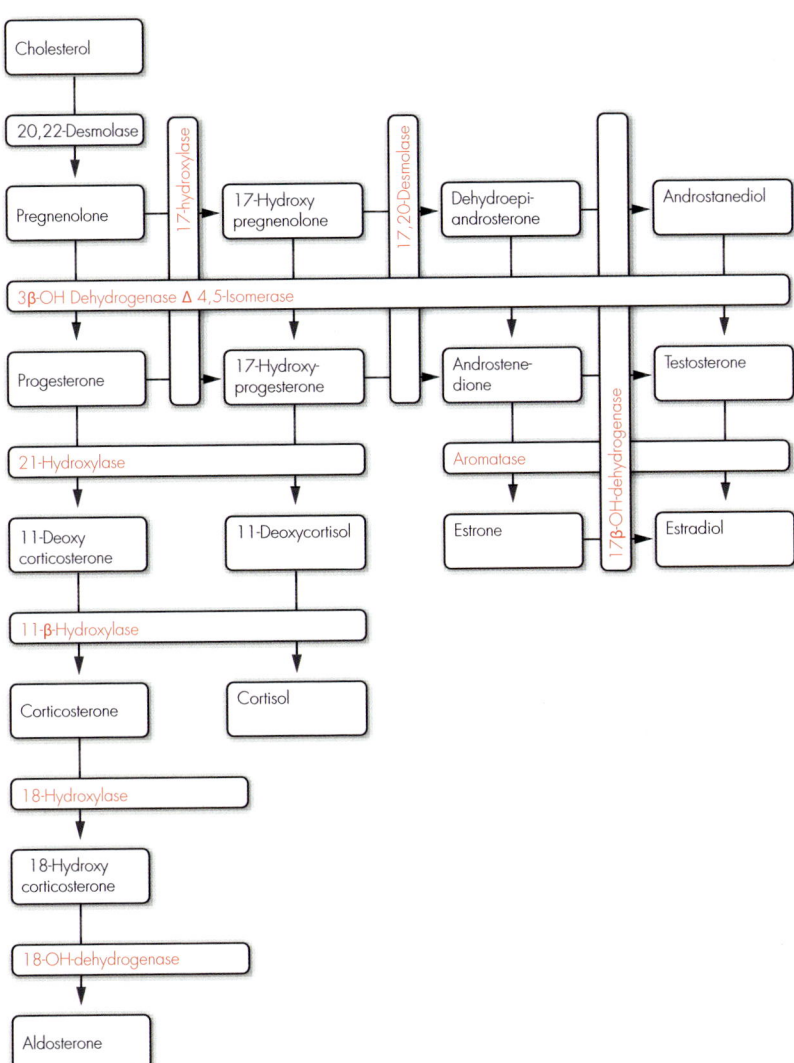

Figure 9.12. Steroid hormone synthesis
Source: Reproduced with permission from Fritz MA, Speroff L. Abnormal growth and puberty. In: *Clinical Gynecologic Endocrinology and Infertility*, 8th Ed. Philadelphia: Lippincott Williams & Wilkins; 2011.

HIRSUTISM
Fast Facts
- Definition: male type body hair distribution (sexual hair areas)
  - Face—mustache, beard, sideburns
  - Body—chest, circumareolar, linea alba, abdominal trigone, inner thighs
- One-third of women age 14–45 have excessive upper lip hair.
- 6–9% have unwanted chin/sideburn hair.
- Hair follicles laid down at 8 weeks gestation.

Cyclic Hair Growth
- Anagen: growing phase
- Catagen: rapid involution phase
- Telogen: resting phase

Differential Diagnosis
- Polycystic ovarian syndrome
- Androgen-secreting adrenal tumors
- Androgen-secreting ovarian tumors
- Congenital adrenal hyperplasia
- Exogenous androgens
- Iatrogenic Cushing syndrome
- Idiopathic hirsutism
- Medications (phenytoin, streptomycin, steroids, penicillamine, diazoxide, minoxidil)

Initial Laboratory Studies
- Testosterone (>200 ng/dL possible ovarian or adrenal tumor)
- DHEAS (>700 mg/dL adrenal hyperplasia or tumor)
  - According to Dr. Leon Speroff (personal communication), adrenal androgen producing tumors always have elevated testosterone associated with elevated DHEAS. Increased DHEAS as an isolated finding is nonspecific and frequently seen in PCOS patients.
- 17-OH progesterone (<300 ng/dL or perform ACTH stimulation test if >300 ng/dL)
  - See page 547

Androgens
- The majority of androgens are synthesized by the adrenal glands and ovaries:
  - Pro-hormones: A, androstenedione; DHEA, dehydroepiandrosterone; DHEA-S, dehydroepiandrosterone sulfate
  - Potent androgens: T, testosterone and the nonaromatizable dihydrotestosterone (DHT)

Hirsutism

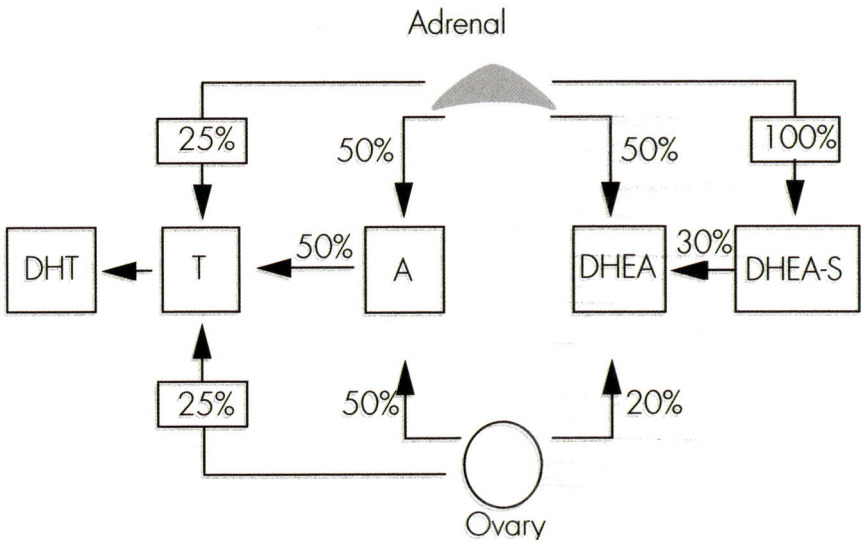

Figure 9.13. Sources of androgen production
Source: Reproduced with permission from Gordon JD, Speroff L. Abnormal puberty and growth problems. In: *Handbook for Clinical Gynecologic Endocrinology and Infertility*, 6th Ed. Philadelphia: Lippincott–Raven; 2002.

HYPERPROLACTINEMIA

Definition
- Consistently elevated fasting serum prolactin in the absence of pregnancy or postpartum lactation; nonpuerperal lactation

Prolactin Biochemistry
- Little PRL = polypeptide hormone of 198 amino acids, but there are several different circulating forms.
- Circulating big PRL can be converted to little PRL by disulfide bond reduction.
- In the vast majority of cases, big-big PRL (bbPRL) consists of a complex of PRL and an anti-PRL IgG autoantibody and is referred to as macroprolactin. Less commonly, bbPRL is composed of either covalent or noncovalent polymers of monomeric PRL. This may account for 10% of hyperprolactinemia, but this is not symptomatic (Gibney 2005).
- Macroprolactin (or bbPRL) should be suspected when the clinical history or MRI findings are inconsistent with the elevated PRL (D'Ercole 2010).
- Synthesized and stored in the pituitary gland in lactotrophs (also synthesized in decidua and endometrium, although not under dopaminergic control).
- Mean levels of 8 ng/dL in adult women; $t_{1/2}$ = 20 minutes.
- Cleared by the liver and kidney (hence PRL with renal failure).
- Functions:
    - Mammogenic → stimulates growth of the mammary tissue
    - Lactogenic → stimulates mammary tissue to produce and secrete milk

Table 9.24. Different forms of the prolactin hormone

Name	Molecular Weight	Biologically Active	Immunologically Active
Little PRL	22 kd	Yes	Yes
Glycosylated little PRL	25 kd	Yes, but decreased	No
Big PRL	50 kd	No	Yes
Big-big PRL	>100 kd	No	Yes

PRL, prolactin.

Physiology
- Synthesis and release controlled by central nervous system (CNS) neurotransmitters (usually inhibitory).
- Dopamine (DA; PRL-inhibiting factor) and cannabinoids inhibit secretion through D2 DA receptors (DA-Rs) on lactotrophs (Pagotto 2001).
- PRL-releasing peptide (PrRP), thyrotropin-releasing factor, and estrogen stimulate release (Rubinek 2001).
- FSH may be suppressed by ↑ PRL through GnRH suppression; in addition to a direct action on GnRH neurons, PRL may modify these neurons through afferent pathways via GABAergic and kisspeptin neurons in the arcuate nucleus (Anderson 2008; Kokay 2011).
- Episodic secretion varying throughout the day and cycle (PRL at time of luteinizing hormone [LH] surge; Djahanbakhch 1984).

Hyperprolactinemia

REPRODUCTIVE ENDOCRINOLOGY

- ↑ PRL induces a dose-dependent ↑ DA secretion, which in turn inhibits GnRH pulsatile release through the D1 receptor on GnRH neurons and by the activation of the a-endorphin neuronal system that further inhibits GnRH release (Seki 1986).
- Autopsy: pituitary adenomas in 27% of women (Burrow 1981; **PRL-secreting** incidence in autopsies: 11%).
- No clinically relevant changes over the menstrual cycle, although there is a significant albeit subtle midcycle peak in PRL (Fujimoto 1990).
- Changes in pregnancy:
  - Steadily increases during pregnancy, reaching 200 ng/mL in the third trimester (TM)
  - Returns to normal in nonlactating women 2–3 weeks postpartum
  - Returns to normal in lactating women 6 months postpartum

Table 9.25. Prevalence of increased prolactin with the following signs and symptoms

Sign/Symptom	Chance of Prolactin (%)
Anovulation	15
Amenorrhea	15
Galactorrhea	30
Amenorrhea + galactorrhea	75
Infertility	34

Source: Reproduced with permission from Molitch ME, Reichlin S. Hyperprolactinemic disorders. *Dis Mon.* 1982;28(9):1. Copyright © 1982 Elsevier.

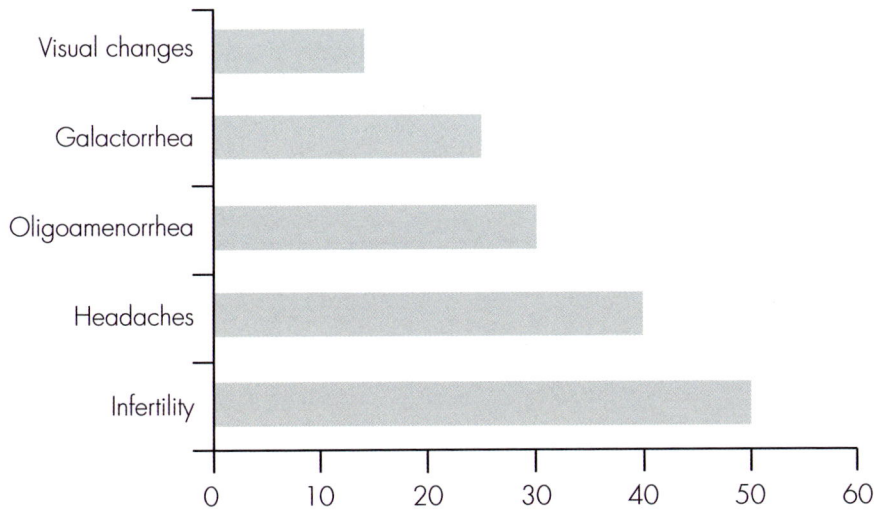

Figure 9.14. Most commonly reported symptoms in patients with hyperprolactinemia
Source: Adapted from Bayrak A, Saadat P, Mor E, et al. Pituitary imaging is indicated for the evaluation of hyperprolactinemia. *Fertil Steril.* 2005;84(1):181-85. Copyright © 2005 The American Society for Reproductive Medicine.

Table 9.26. Potential causes of hyperprolactinemia

Cause	Example	Mechanism
Physiological	Pregnancy	Increasing estrogen levels
	Breast stimulation	Inhibition of dopamine via the autonomic nervous system
	Breastfeeding	
	Stress	Reduced dopamine stimulation
	Exercise	
	Sleep	
Pituitary disorders	Pituitary tumors: micro- or macroprolactinoma, adenoma, hypothalamic stalk interruption, hypophysitis (inflammation)	Disruption of dopamine delivery from the hypothalamus and/or secretion of growth hormone and prolactin
	Acromegaly	Prolactin secretion from a growth hormone adenoma
	Cushing syndrome	Prolactin secretion from a corticotroph adenoma
	Empty sella syndrome	Damage to/regression of the pituitary
	Rathke cysts	Compressed pituitary
	Infiltrative diseases (tuberculosis, sarcoidosis)	Infiltration of pituitary
Hypothalamic disorders	Primary hypothyroidism	Increased hypothalamic thyrotrophin-releasing hormone and decreased metabolism
	Adrenal insufficiency	
Medications	Anti-psychotics (phenothiazines, haloperidol, butyrophenones, risperidone, monoamine oxidase inhibitors, fluoxetine, sulpiride)	Inhibition of dopamine release
	Anti-emetics (metoclopramide, domperidone)	
	Antihypertensives (methyldopa, calcium channel blockers, reserpine)	
	Tricyclic antidepressants	Stimulation of hypothalamic opioid receptors
	Opiates	Positive action on lactotrophs
	Estrogens	Unknown
	Verapamil	
	Protease inhibitors	
Neurogenic	Chest wall injury	Peripheral triggers of autonomic control that interrupt central neurogenic pathways that attenuate dopamine release into the hypophyseal portal circulation; may act via the same nerves affected by nipple stimulation
	Spinal cord lesions	
Increased prolactin production	Polycystic ovary syndrome	Usually transient
Reduced prolactin elimination	Renal failure	Less rapid clearance of prolactin from the systemic circulation plus central stimulation of prolactin
	Hepatic insufficiency	
Abnormal molecules	Macroprolactinemia	Polymeric form of prolactin formed following binding of prolactin to immunoglobulin G antibodies that cannot bind to the prolactin receptor
Idiopathic	Unknown	Unknown

Source: Reproduced with permission from Crosignani PG. Current treatment issues in female hyperprolactinemia. *Eur J Obstet, Gynecol and Reprod Biol.* 2006;125:152-64. Copyright © 2006 Elsevier.

Prolactin-Secreting Pituitary Adenomas
- Even with normal values or only mildly elevated PRL, patient may have a large tumor (Bayrak 2005).
- Prolactinomas rise most commonly from the lateral wings of the anterior pituitary where the lactotrophs predominate.
- Islands of pituitary lactotrophs may be released from the normal tonic inhibitory effect of DA through spontaneous or estradiol (E2)-dependent generation of arteriolar shunts (Elias 1984).
- Found in 10% of general population (most asymptomatic).
- **Found in 50% of women with hyperprolactinemia.**
- Incidence increases with (a) increasing PRL levels and (b) severity of symptoms.
- Microadenoma <1 cm.
  - Prevalence of up to 27% in autopsy series (Burrow 1981)
  - Enlargement uncommon (≤5%; Schlechte 1989)
  - Most regress spontaneously
- Macroadenoma >1 cm and usually PRL >200 ng/mL
  - The risk of diminished secretion of other pituitary hormones due to the presence of a prolactinoma is based on their proximity to the prolactinoma mass and their overall cell number: mnemonic for the adenohypophyseal hormones with the greatest to least propensity to be affected → **GnTAG** (% relates to the number of cells):
    - Gonadotropins (Gns; 5%, close to lactotrophs), thyroid-stimulating hormone (TSH; 5%), adrenocorticotropic hormone (ACTH; 20%), growth hormone (GH; 50%), antidiuretic hormone (ADH; rare, posterior pituitary)

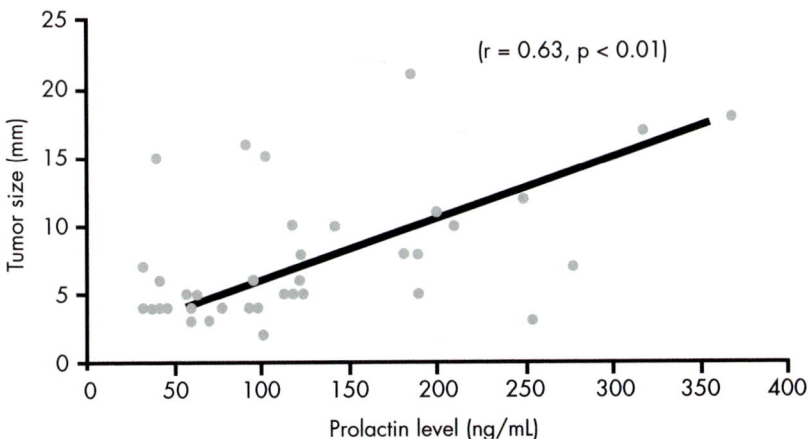

Figure 9.15. Correlation between the pituitary size and serum PRL level (ng/mL)
Source: Reproduced with permission from Bayrak A, Saadat P, Mor E, et al. Pituitary imaging is indicated for the evaluation of hyperprolactinemia. *Fertil Steril.* 2005;84(1):181-85. Copyright © 2005 The American Society for Reproductive Medicine.

Other Pituitary Etiologies of Hyperprolactinemia

Cushing Disease
- Diagnosis: elevated 24-hr urinary free cortisol excretion and failure of cortisol to suppress with dexamethasone suppression tests:
  - **Low-dose dexamethasone suppression test**: differentiates patients with Cushing syndrome of any cause from patients without Cushing syndrome:
    - Overnight 1 mg test—1 mg dexamethasone at 11 p.m. to 12 a.m., measurement of serum cortisol at 8 a.m. the next day. Cushing syndrome if >1.8 mg/dL (50 nmol/L).
    - At least one other test should be performed to confirm the diagnosis.
  - **High-dose dexamethasone suppression test**: differentiates patients with Cushing disease (pituitary hypersecretion of ACTH) from those with ectopic ACTH syndrome:
    - Two-day 2 mg test—0.5 mg dexamethasone every 6 hours × 8 doses, measurement of serum cortisol either 2 or 6 hours after the last dose. Cushing disease if >1.8 mg/dL (50 nmol/L).
- Adenoma secretes ACTH.
- Patients present with hypertension, hirsutism, weakness and proximal muscle wasting, coarse facial features, arthritis, and supraclavicular/posterior dorsal fat.
- 10% secrete PRL.

Other Pituitary Tumors
- Clinically nonfunctioning microadenoma (~80% are gonadotroph adenomas), lymphocytic hypophysitis, craniopharyngioma, Rathke's cleft cyst, TSH-pituitary adenoma. (rarest)
- Growth of nonfunctioning pituitary adenomas: ~13% of microadenomas and ~50% of macroadenomas over 5 years (for review, please see Dekkers 2008)

Empty Sella Syndrome
- Congenital or acquired defect in the sella diaphragm.
- Intrasellar extension of the subarachnoid space results in compression of the pituitary gland and an enlarged sella turcica.
- 5–10% have hyperprolactinemia (usually <100 ng/mL).
- Diagnose with MRI.
- Benign course, although headaches (mostly localized anteriorly) are a frequent symptom (Catarci 1994).

Hyperprolactinemia

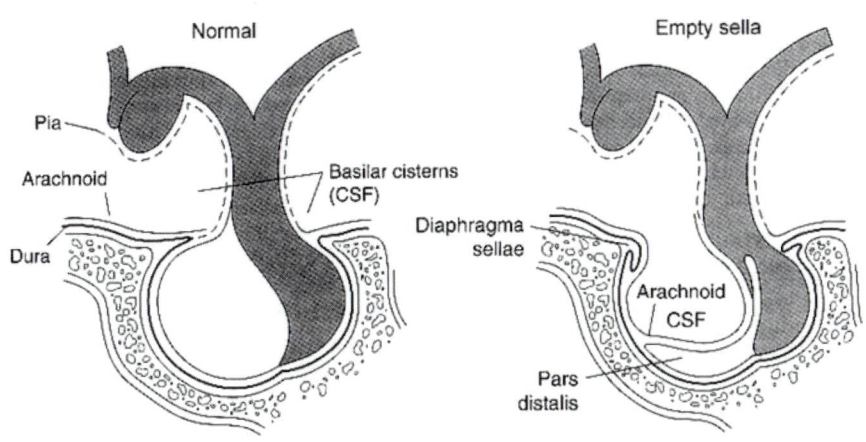

Figure 9.16. Anatomic changes resulting in empty sella syndrome
CSF, cerebrospinal fluid.
Source: Reproduced with permission from Jordan RM, Kendall JW, Kerber CW. The primary empty sella syndrome: analysis of the clinical characteristics, radiographic features, pituitary function and cerebrospinal fluid adenohypophysial hormone concentrations. *Am J Med.* 1977;62(4):569. Copyright © 1977 Elsevier.

Treatment of Hyperprolactinemia

- Microadenoma or functional hyperprolactinemia: risk of progression for PRL secreting tumors to macroadenomas is <7% (Gillam 2005).
  - Most patients with microadenomas verified by MRI may be monitored by serial PRL as it is very rare for a prolactinoma to grow significantly without an increase in PRL (Hofle 1998).
- Macroadenomas should be treated no matter the severity of symptoms.
- Without treatment of microadenomas, there is a 24% chance of PRL normalization within 5 years, and 95% do not grow (Schlechte 1989).
- Microadenoma follow-up: measure PRL yearly and do not repeat an MRI unless there is a marked rise in PRL or there are clinical signs of tumor expansion.
- Macroademona follow-up: repeat MRI 2–3 years after PRL normalized to confirm tumor suppression (Schlechte 2007).

Goals of Treatment

IF Low E2 (<40 pg/mL)
Estrogen treatment or oral contraceptives (OCs; no size of microadenoma or [serum PRL])
Yearly PRL levels

IF Normal E2
Normal cycles
Yearly PRL levels

IF Oligomenorrhea or amenorrhea and E2 >40 pg/mL
Progestin withdrawal or OCs
Yearly PRL levels

Pregnancy and Prolactinomas

- 70% increase in pituitary size during normal pregnancy due to lactotroph hypertrophy.
  - Microadenoma: 1.6%
  - Macroadenoma: 15.5%; check visual-field testing, a.m. cortisol, and TSH every trimester.
- Complete remission of hyperprolactinemia occurs in 17–37% of women after pregnancy.
- Risk of symptomatic tumor enlargement during pregnancy (Molitch 1985):
  - Only 4 of the 246 women with microadenomas (1.6%) had symptoms of tumor enlargement (headaches or visual disturbances or both), and 11 (4.5%) had asymptomatic tumor enlargement (as evidenced by radiologic techniques). In no case was surgical intervention necessary.
  - Of the 45 women with macroadenomas, 7 (15.5%) had symptomatic tumor enlargement, and 4 (8.9%) had asymptomatic enlargement (radiologic evidence only). During pregnancy, surgery was required in four patients, and bromocriptine in two. Of the 46 women with macroadenomas had been treated with irradiation or surgery before pregnancy, only 2 of the 46 (4.3%) had symptomatic tumor enlargement, and none had asymptomatic enlargement during gestation.

Table 9.27. Dopamine agonists commonly used in the treatment of hyperprolactinemia

	Bromocriptine	Cabergoline (Dostinex)	Quinagolide (Norprolac)[a]
Dopamine receptor target sites	D_1 and D_2	D_1 (low affinity) and D_2 (high affinity)	D_2
Duration of action	8–12 hours	7–14 days	24 hours
Half-life (hours)	3.3	65	22
Available doses	1.0 and 2.5 mg scored tablets; 5 and 10 mg capsules	0.5 mg scored tablets	25, 50, 75, and 150 μg tablets
Typical dose	2.5 mg/day in divided doses	0.5 mg/week or 0.25 mg twice weekly	75 μg/day
Dosing regimens, starter packs, dosage	Start at 1.25–2.5 mg/day at bedtime. Gradually increase to a median of 5.0–7.5 mg/day and a maximum of 15–20 mg/day	Start at 0.25–0.5 mg twice weekly. Adjust by 0.25 mg twice weekly up to 1 mg twice weekly every 2–4 months according to serum prolactin levels	Start at 25 μg/day. Increase over 1 week up to 75 μg/day. Starter pack (3× 25 μg tablets + 3× 50 μg tablets) allows quick and convenient titration
Advantages	Long history of use; does not appear to be teratogenic; inexpensive	Good efficacy; low frequency of adverse events; may be useful in bromocriptine-resistant patients; weekly or twice-weekly dose	Good efficacy and tolerability; once-daily dosing; simple titration; pituitary selective; use to the time of confirmed pregnancy
Disadvantages	Tolerance; recurrence; resistance; multiple daily dosing	Not yet indicated for use during pregnancy	Not currently available in the United States or Japan
Common side effects	Nausea, headache, dizziness, abdominal pain, syncope, orthostatic hypotension, fatigue	Milder and less frequent compared with bromocriptine	Milder and less frequent compared with bromocriptine

[a] Quinagolide is not approved for treatment of hyperprolactinemia in the United States or Japan.

Source: Reproduced with permission from Crosignani PG. Current treatment issues in female hyperprolactinemia. *Eur J Obstet, Gynecol and Reprod Biol.* 2006;125:152-64. Copyright © 2006 Elsevier.

Hyperprolactinemia — REPRODUCTIVE ENDOCRINOLOGY

Dopamine Agonist Medical Therapy
- Bromocriptine
    - DA agonists do not restore bone mass to a clinically meaningful degree (Colao 2000)
    - Discontinue after 2 years in patients treated for galactorrhea to assess for remission (11% after 1 year, 22% after 2 years; Ciccarelli 1996)
    - Measure PRL 4–6 weeks after initiating treatment
    - No risk for pituitary insufficiency (including diabetes insipidus [DI]) as opposed to surgical or radiation treatment
    - Response occurs in 6 weeks in ⅔ and can take up to 6 months in ⅓
    - No need to repeat MRI if microadenoma and ↓ PRL; if ↑ PRL, repeat MRI after 3 months of treatment, if PRL normalized then repeat MRI in 2–3 years
    - Follow PRL every 6–12 months once stabilized—no need to repeat MRI scans; visual field testing is more sensitive than MRI for detecting tumor shrinkage
    - Advise patients to take medicine in the middle of a bulk meal
    - Alternate route: 2.5 mg **per vagina** q.d. (fewer side effects; Jasonni 1991)
    - Depot form (q month injection) not yet available
- Cabergoline is a more specific D_2 agonist; approximately ½ of those who do not respond to bromocriptine respond to cabergoline (Verhelst 1999)
    - Follow-up after cabergoline withdrawal (Colao 2003):
        - 2–5 years after normalization of hyperprolactinemia:
            - ↑ PRL in 24% of nontumoral hyperprolactinemia
            - ↑ PRL in 31% with microadenomas
            - ↑ PRL in 36% with macroadenomas
            - 22% showed gonadal dysfunction
            - 0% renewed tumor growth
            - Rate for recurrence of hyperprolactinemia was 19% for each mm increment in the maximal tumor diameter
            - Before discontinuation of cabergoline, decrease by 0.25 mg of the weekly dose in 3-month intervals, check PRL after each dose reduction and obtain an MRI 6 months after initiation of tapering (Schlechte 2007)

Nonmedical Treatment Options
Transsphenoidal Microsurgical Resection
- Mortality: <0.5%
- Pituitary insufficiency rate: 19%
- Temporary DI: 10–40%; permanent DI: <2%
- 3.9% require glucocorticoid replacement therapy (Feigenbaum 1996)
- 3% chronic sinusitis; 2% septal defect (i.e., epistaxis; Feigenbaum 1996)
- Initial cure rate (Amar 2002):
    - Microadenoma: 65–91%
    - Macroadenoma: 20–40%
- Effect on reproductive function (those actively attempting postoperatively):
    - 6 months: 82% pregnancy rate
    - 12 months: 88% pregnancy rate
- Better prognosis: PRL <100 ng/mL
- Poor prognosis: PRL >200 ng/mL, >26 years old, amenorrhea >6 months

- Cure rates based on pre- and postoperative PRL levels (Feigenbaum 1996):
  - Preoperative levels <100 ng/mL: 69% cure rate
  - Preoperative levels <200 ng/mL: 60% cure rate
  - Immediate postoperative levels <5 ng/mL: 84% cure rate
  - Immediate postoperative levels <20 ng/mL: 74% cure rate
- Recommended after failure of medical treatment (i.e., cabergoline) or if patient is intolerant of side effects.
- Transsphenoidal approach provides a decompression of the bony confines of the sella turcica, so that recurrence of the tumor tends to follow the path of least resistance into the sphenoid sinus rather than the intracranial compartment.

Radiation Therapy
- Cobalt, proton beam, heavy particle therapy, or brachytherapy
- Inconsistent results; takes years to ↓ tumor growth
- Delay in symptom resolution
- Only used in adjunctive management with surgery for large tumors

Other Possible Therapies
- Gamma knife: inconclusive data but may be preferred over conventional radiation treatment for patients not responding to DA with residual tumor after surgery

Acromegaly
- GH-secreting pituitary adenoma.
- Associated symptoms: acral changes, macrognathia (enlarged jaw), macroglossia, spread teeth, sweaty palms, carpal tunnel syndrome.
- Affected patients experience symptoms of the disease ~7 years before diagnosis.
- GH can bind to PRL receptors (but PRL does not bind to GH receptors).
- ~20% of GH-secreting pituitary adenomas secrete PRL (Vance 2004).
- Check serum insulin-like growth factor-I (IGF-I) (need age-adjusted and sex-adjusted IGF-I levels) as GH-secreting pituitary adenomas may not be visible on magnetic resonance imaging (MRI); IGF-I is produced primarily by the liver in response to GH. GH levels may appear normal since this hormone is released in pulses.
- Diagnosis: Elevated basal fasting GH and IGF-I; 1-hr glucose (75 mg) challenge reveals GH concentration >1 ng/mL in patients with acromegaly.
- Currently, surgery is the first choice for acromegaly; if the adenoma is not fully resectable, then utilize a long-acting somatostatin analog (i.e., octreotide).
- Hormonal assessment to rule out:
  - Pituitary hormone excess from clinically silent adenoma.
  - Pituitary hormone deficiency attributable to a pituitary tumor/infiltrative disease with mass effects.

Table 9.28. Hormonal assessment of the clinically nonfunctional pituitary mass

Axis	Hypersecretion Assessment	Reserve Assessment
Somatotropic	100 mg oral glucose suppression test	GH level does not decrease to <2 ng/mL if there is a GH-producing adenoma
PRL	a.m. PRL (normal range, 1.4–24.2 ng/mL)	TRH stimulation test → PRL should 2× 15–30 minutes after TRH
Gonadotropic	LH, FSH, E2, free α-subunit	E2 should be >30 pg/mL; TRH stimulation test with 500 μg TRH → abnormal result if there is more than a 2-fold increase in free alpha-subunit at 30 to 60 minutes
Corticotropic	Low-dose dexamethasone test (normal if cortisol <1.8 μg/dL)	Metyrapone test (normal if 11-deoxycortisol >10 μg/L)
Thyrotropic	Free T_4, free T_3, TSH	Free T_4, free T_3, TSH; TRH stimulation test

E2 estradiol; FSH, follicle-stimulating hormone; GH, growth hormone; LH, luteinizing hormone; PRL, prolactin; T_3, triiodothyronine; T_4, thyroxine; TRH, thyroid-releasing hormone; TSH, thyroid-stimulating hormone.

THYROID DISORDERS

Fast Facts
- Evaluation and treatment of thyroid disorders is important given the prevalence of thyroid disorders in women.
- Although both hyperthyroidism and hypothyroidism are found in reproductive-aged women, the former is less common.
- Recently there has been a confusing array of recommendations regarding the definition, evaluation, and management of patients with hypothyroidism.
- See the obstetrics section for additional management issues during pregnancy.

Algorithm for the Evaluation of Thyroid Dysfunction

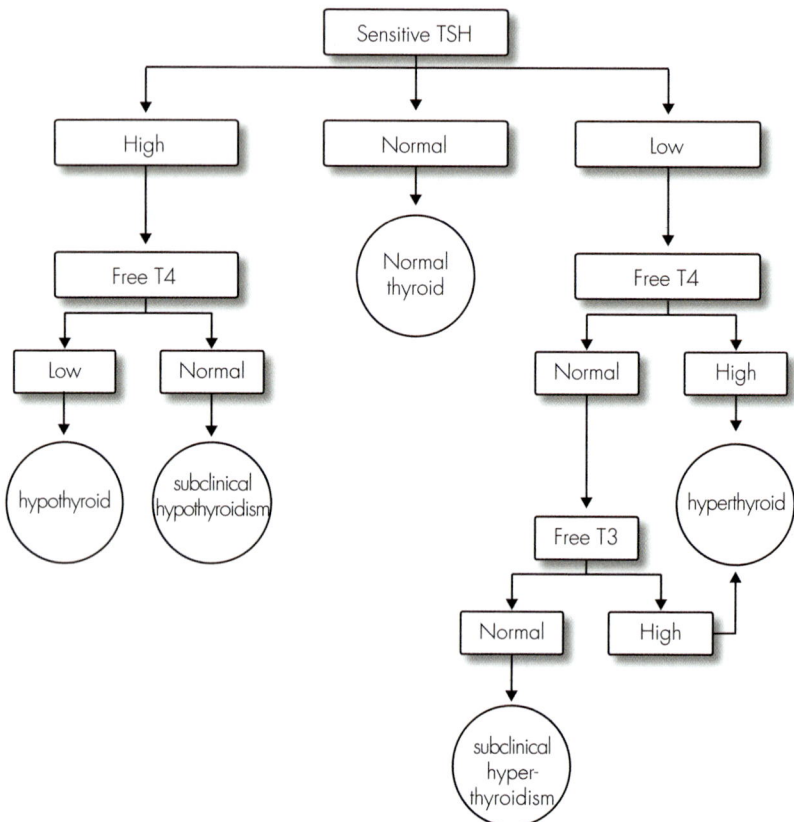

Figure 9.17. Algorithm for the evaluation of thyroid dysfunction
Source: Reproduced with Permission from Speroff L, Glass RH, Kase NG. Reproduction and the thyroid. In: *Clinical Gynecologic Endocrinology and Infertility, 6th Ed.* Philadelphia: Lippincott Williams & Wilkins; 1999. Reproduced with the permission of the publisher.

Thyroid Function Tests

Table 9.29. Changes in thyroid function test results in normal pregnancy and in thyroid disease

Maternal Status	TSH	Free T_4
Pregnancy	Varies by trimester*	No change
Overt hyperthyroidism	Decrease	Increase
Subclinical hyperthyroidism	Decrease	No change
Overt hypothyroidism	Increase	Decrease
Subclinical hypothyroidism	Increase	No change

T_4, thyroxine; TSH, thyroid-stimulating hormone.

*The level of TSH decreases in early pregnancy because of weak TSH receptor stimulation due to substantial quantities of human chorionic gonadotropin during the first 12 weeks of gestation. After the first trimester, TSH levels return to baseline values.

Source: Reproduced with permission from ACOG Practice Bulletin No. 148: Thyroid disease in pregnancy. *Obstet Gynecol.* 2015 Apr;125(4):996-1005. Copyright © 2015 The American College of Obstetricians and Gynecologists.

Table 9.30. Comparison of the recommendations of different organizations in evaluation and treatment of hypothyroidism

ACOG	ASRM	ATA	Endocrine Society
Screening of non-pregnant patients who are planning to conceive			
Universal screening for thyroid disease in/before pregnancy is not recommended	Currently available data support that it is reasonable to test TSH in infertile women attempting pregnancy	Universal screening is not recommended for patients who are pregnant or are planning pregnancy, including assisted reproduction	Universal screening of healthy women for thyroid dysfunction before pregnancy is not recommended
		There is insufficient evidence to recommend for or against TSH testing preconception in women at high risk for hypothyroidism	Test high-risk women for elevated TSH concentrations by the 9th week or at the time of their first visit before or during pregnancy
If universal screening is not performed who is in the high-risk group that should be screened.			
Indicated testing of thyroid function should be performed in women with a personal history of thyroid disease or symptoms of thyroid disease	Infertility is an indication for testing TSH	Women over age 30 yr	Same as ATA
		Women with a family history or autoimmune thyroid disease or hypothyroidism	
		Women with a goiter	
		Women with thyroid antibodies, primarily thyroid peroxidase antibodies	
		Women with symptoms or clinical signs suggestive of thyroid hypofunction	
		Women with type 1 DM or other autoimmune disorders	
		Women with infertility	
		Women with a prior history of miscarriage or preterm delivery	
		Women with prior therapeutic head or neck irradiation or prior thyroid surgery	
		Women currently receiving levothyroxine replacement	
		Women living in a region with presumed iodine deficiency	

(continued)

Thyroid Disorders — REPRODUCTIVE ENDOCRINOLOGY

ACOG	ASRM	ATA	Endocrine Society
In patients seeking to conceive (and for whom there is no prior history of thyroid disease) what level of TSH requires action?			
Overt hypothyroidism (high TSH and low FT4) should be treated with adequate thyroid hormone replacement to minimize the risk of adverse outcomes Identification and treatment of maternal subclinical hypothyroidism has not been shown to result in improved neurocognitive function in offspring	There is good evidence that levothyroxine treatment in women with SCH defined as TSH >4.0 mIU/L is associated with improvement in pregnancy and miscarriage rates There is insufficient evidence that levothyroxine therapy in women with TSH levels between 2.5 and 4 mIU/L is associated with improvement in pregnancy and miscarriage rates Treating when the TSH is between 2.5 mIU/L and the upper range of normal prior to pregnancy remains controversial. However, given that there appears to be benefit in some subgroups and minimal risk, it is reasonable to treat even though the evidence is weak. Alternatively, it is reasonable to monitor levels and treat above nonpregnant and pregnancy ranges	Treatment with L-thyroxine should be considered in women of childbearing age with serum TSH levels between 2.5 mIU/L and the upper limit of normal for a given laboratory's reference range if they are planning a pregnancy including assisted reproduction in the immediate future	If TSH is above 2.5 mIU/liter, the test should be confirmed by repeat assay. Although no randomized controlled trials are available to guide a response, the committee believes it is appropriate to give low-dose T4 treatment to bring TSH below 2.5 mIU/liter. This treatment can be discontinued if the woman does not become pregnant
Is testing for anti-thyroid antibodies recommended?			
There currently is no evidence to support routine testing of these antibodies	While thyroid antibody testing is not routinely recommended, one might consider testing antithyroperoxidase (TPO) antibodies for repeated TSH values >2.5 mIU/L or when other risk factors for thyroid disease are present	TPOAb measurement should be considered when evaluating patients with recurrent miscarriage, with or without infertility	Universal screening for the presence of anti-TPO antibodies either before or during pregnancy is not recommended However, women with elevated anti-TPO antibodies are at increased risk for miscarriage, preterm delivery, progression of hypothyroidism, and PPT Therefore, if identified, such women should be screened for serum TSH abnormalities before pregnancy, as well as during the first and second trimesters of pregnancy

(continued)

REPRODUCTIVE ENDOCRINOLOGY — Thyroid Disorders

ACOG	ASRM	ATA	Endocrine Society
What treatment is recommended for women with anti-thyroid antibodies?			
	There is good evidence that thyroid autoimmunity is associated with miscarriage and fair evidence that it is associated with infertility. Levothyroxine treatment may improve pregnancy outcomes in women with positive thyroid antibodies, especially if the TSH level is over 2.5 mIU/L	Treatment with L-thyroxine should be considered in women of childbearing age with normal serum TSH levels when they are pregnant or planning a pregnancy, including assisted reproduction in the immediate future, if they have or have had positive levels of serum TPOAb, particularly when there is a history of miscarriage or past history of hypothyroidism	Women of childbearing age who are pregnant or planning a pregnancy, including assisted reproduction in the immediate future, should be treated with L-thyroxine if they have or have had positive levels of serum TPOAb and their TSH is greater than 2.5 mIU/L. If serum TSH is greater than 2.5 mIU/liter at the time of testing (or >3.0 mIU/liter in the second trimester), levothyroxine therapy should be instituted
Treatment of hypothyroidism (overt and SCH) in pregnancy.			
Overt hypothyroidism should be treated in pregnancy	Overt hypothyroidism should be treated in pregnancy	Overt hypothyroidism should be treated in pregnancy	Overt hypothyroidism should be treated in pregnancy
Currently, there is no evidence that identification and treatment of subclinical hypothyroidism during pregnancy improves these outcomes	There is good evidence that levothyroxine treatment in women with SCH defined as TSH >4.0 mIU/L is associated with improvement in pregnancy and miscarriage rates	Due to the lack of randomized controlled trials there is insufficient evidence to recommend for or against universal LT4 treatment in TAB negative pregnant women with SCH (TSH>2.5 mIU/L)	T4 replacement is recommended in women with SCH (TSH>2.5 mIU/L) who are TPO-Ab negative subjects
There currently is no evidence to support routine testing of these antibodies	Levothyroxine treatment may improve pregnancy outcomes in women with positive thyroid antibodies, especially if the TSH level is over 2.5 mIU/L	Women who are positive for TPOAb and have SCH (TSH>2.5 mIU/L) should be treated with LT4	The same
The goal of LT4 treatment is to normalize maternal serum TSH values within the trimester-specific pregnancy reference range (first trimester, 0.1–2.5 mIU/L; second trimester, 0.2–3 mIU/L; third trimester, 0.3–3 mIU/L)	The same	The same	The same

(continued)

Thyroid Disorders — REPRODUCTIVE ENDOCRINOLOGY

ACOG	ASRM	ATA	Endocrine Society
Treatment of hypothyroidism (overt and SCH) in pregnancy.			
Currently, there is no evidence that identification and treatment of subclinical hypothyroidism during pregnancy improves these outcomes	No recommendation	Women with SCH (TSH>2.5 mIU/L) in pregnancy who are not initially treated should be monitored for progression to OH with a serum TSH and FT4 approximately every 4 weeks until 16–20 weeks gestation and at least once between 26 and 32 weeks' gestation	No recommendation
Significant hypothyroidism may develop early in women without thyroid reserve, such as those with a previous thyroidectomy or prior radioiodine ablation. Anticipatory 25% increases in T4 replacement at pregnancy confirmation will reduce this likelihood. All other women with hypothyroidism should undergo TSH testing at initiation of prenatal care	No recommendation	Treated hypothyroid patients (receiving LT4) who are newly pregnant should independently increase their dose of LT4 by ~25%–30% upon a missed menstrual cycle or positive home pregnancy test and notify their caregiver promptly. One means of accomplishing this adjustment is to increase LT4 from once daily dosing to a total of nine doses per week (29% increase)	The same

Sources: American College of Obstetricians and Gynecologists ACOG Practice Bulletin No. 148: Thyroid Disease in Pregnancy. *Obstet Gynecol.* 2015;125:996-1005; Practice Committee of the American Society for Reproductive Medicine. Subclinical hypothyroidism in the infertile female population: a guideline. *Fertil Steril.* 2015 Sep;104(3):545-53; Garber JR, Cobin RH, Gharib H, et al. American Association of Clinical Endocrinologists and American Thyroid Association Taskforce on Hypothyroidism in Adults. Clinical practice guidelines for hypothyroidism in adults: cosponsored by the American Association of Clinical Endocrinologists and the American Thyroid Association. *Thyroid.* 2012 Dec;22(12):1200-35; De Groot L, Abalovich M, Alexander EK, et al. Management of thyroid dysfunction during pregnancy and postpartum: an Endocrine Society clinical practice guideline. *J Clin Endocrinol Metab.* 2012 Aug;97(8):2543-65.

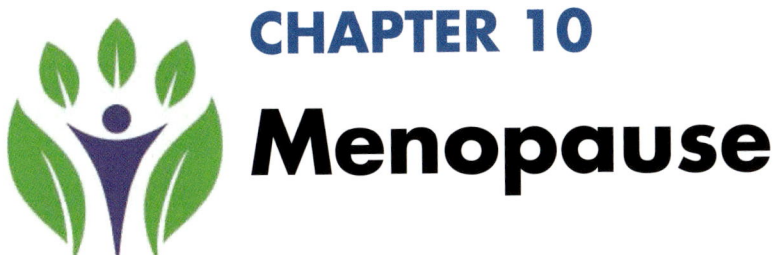

CHAPTER 10
Menopause

FAST FACTS

- Menopause is strictly defined as 1 year without menses.
- Approximately 70 million women in the United States are 50 years of age.
- 85% of menopausal women experience hot flashes, sweating, insomnia, and vaginal dryness/discomfort.
- Menopausal symptoms typically cease within 5 years.

Table 10.1. Stages of the menopausal transition

Variable	Reproductive Years			Menopausal Transition (Perimenopause)		Postmenopausal Years	
	Early	Peak	Late	Early	Late	Early	Late
Menstrual cycle	Regular or variable	Regular		Variable cycle length; 1 or 2 missed cycles per yr	3 or more missed cycles per yr	None	
Range of steroid hormones (pg/mL)							
Estradiol		50–200		50–200 or slightly higher		40	0–15
Testosterone		400		400		400	400
Range of pituitary hormones (mu/mL)							
Follicle-stimulating hormone		10 on days 2–4		10 or higher on days 2–4		>100	
Luteinizing hormone		10 on days 2–4		10 or higher on days 2–4		>100	
Prevalence of hot flushes (%)			10	40	65	50	10–15

Source: Reproduced with permission from Grady D. Clinical practice: management of menopausal symptoms. *N Engl J Med.* 2006 Nov 30;355(22):2338-47. Copyright © 2006 Massachusetts Medical Society.

Table 10.2. Definitions of the spectrum of menopause

Menopause
: Clinical status after the final menstrual period, diagnosed retrospectively after cessation of menses for 12 mo in a previously cycling woman and reflecting complete or nearly complete permanent cessation of ovarian function and fertility.

Spontaneous menopause
: Cessation of menses that occurs at an average age of 51 yr in the absence of surgery or medication.

Menopausal transition (or perimenopause)
: An interval preceding the menopause characterized by variations in menstrual cycle length and bleeding pattern, mood shifts, vasomotor, and vaginal symptoms and with rising FSH levels and falling antimüllerian hormone and inhibin B levels, which starts during the late reproductive stage and progresses during the menopause transition.

Climacteric
: The phase in the aging of women marking the transition from the reproductive phase to the nonreproductive state. This phase incorporates the perimenopause by extending for a longer variable period before and after the perimenopause.

Climacteric syndrome
: When the climacteric is associated with symptomatology.

Menopause after hysterectomy without oophorectomy
: Spontaneous cessation of ovarian function without the clinical signal of cessation of menses.

Induced menopause
: Cessation of ovarian function induced by chemotherapy, radiotherapy, or bilateral oophorectomy.

Early menopause
: Cessation of ovarian function occurring between ages 40 and 45 in the absence of other etiologies for secondary amenorrhea (pregnancy, hyperprolactinemia, and thyroid disorders).

POI
: Loss of ovarian function before the age of 40 yr with waxing and waning course and potential resumption of menses, conception, and pregnancy. The prevalence of POI is approximately 1% and is differentiated into idiopathic, autoimmune (associated with polyglandular autoimmune syndromes), metabolic disorders, and genetic abnormalities (including Fragile X premutation).

Source: Reproduced with permission from Stuenkel CA, Davis SR, Gompel A, et al. Treatment of symptoms of the menopause: an endocrine society clinical practice guideline. *J Clin Endocrinol Metab.* 2015 Nov;100(11):3975-4011. Copyright © 2015 The Endocrine Society.

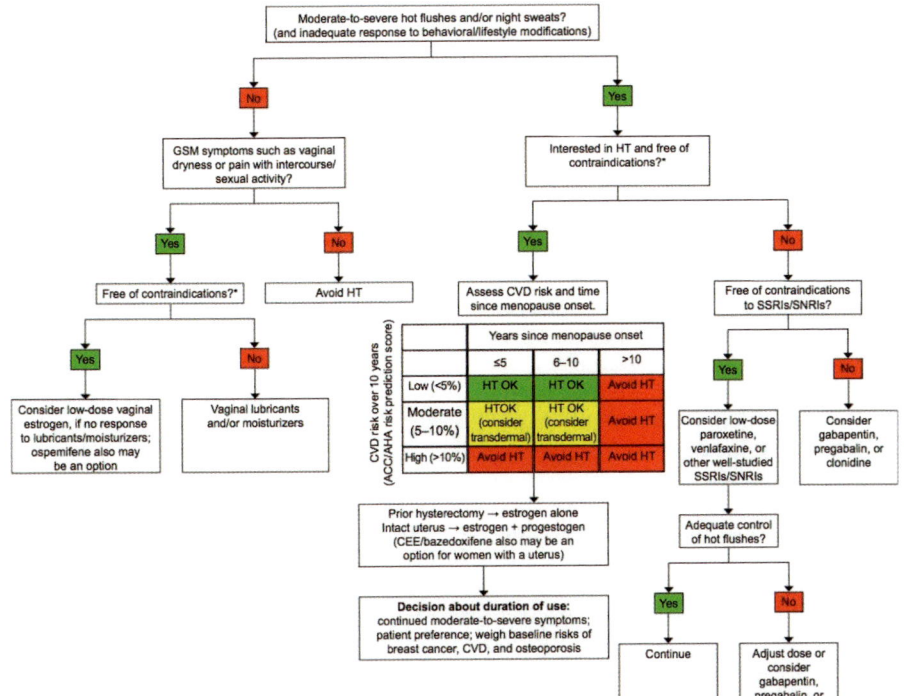

Figure 10.1. Algorithm for menopausal symptom management
GSM, genitourinary syndrome of menopause; HT, hormone therapy; CVD, cardiovascular disease; SSRIs, selective serotonin reuptake inhibitors; SNRIs, serotonin-norepinephrine reuptake inhibitors; ACC, American College of Cardiology; AHA, American Heart Association.
Algorithm developed in collaboration with the North American Menopause Society and available in a free mobile app called MenoPro (dual mode for clinicians and patients).
Source: Modified from Manson JE, Ames JM, Shapiro M, Gass ML, Shifren JL, Stuenkel CA, et al. Algorithm and mobile app for menopausal symptom management and hormonal/non-hormonal therapy decision making: a clinical decision-support tool from the North American Menopause Society. *Menopause.* 2015;22:247-53. Reproduced with permission from: Kaunitz AM, Manson JE. Management of Menopausal Symptoms. *Obstet Gynecol.* 2015 Oct;126(4):859-76. Copyright © 2015 The American College of Obstetricians and Gynecologists.

HOT FLUSHES
Incidence
- Overall incidence:
  - Premenopausal: 25%
  - Late perimenopausal: 69%
  - Late postmenopause: 39%

Background
- Usually a sensation of heat, sweating, flushing, dizziness, palpitations, irritability, anxiety, and/or panic.
- Classic hot flash (HF): head-to-toe sensation of heat, culminating in perspiration.
- Large cross-cultural variability in prevalence:
  - 0% Mayan women in Mexico
  - 18% Chinese factory workers in Hong Kong
  - 70% North American women (black women > white women)
  - 80% Dutch women
- Despite these vast differences, some trends are seen:
  - HFs usually last 0.5–5.0 years (but may last up to 15 years); one study reported that among women who had experienced moderate to severe HFs, 58% persisted at 5 years, 12% at 8 years, and 10% at 15 years subsequent to reaching menopause.
  - Generally more severe in women who undergo surgical menopause; one study reported that 100% of patients undergoing surgical menopause had vasomotor symptoms, and 90% of them had continuing symptoms for 8.5 years. It is postulated that slower, continuous reductions of gonadal steroid levels result in downward regulation of hormone receptors in the hypothalamus in women undergoing natural (vs. surgical) menopause.
  - The lack of correlation between HFs and sleep disturbance seems counterintuitive and challenges the dogma that HFs cause insomnia (Freedman 2004).
  - HFs have been associated with a diminished sense of well-being (likely as a result of fatigue, irritability, poor concentration, anxiety-type symptoms).
  - Premenopausal/early perimenopausal women with symptoms may be more likely to report a ↓ sense of well-being than late perimenopausal and late postmenopausal women.
  - Some studies estimate that approximately 50% of breast cancer survivors list HF as their most prominent complaint.

Table 10.3. Onset and duration of hot flushes in the menopausal transition

Onset of HFs	Median Duration of HFs (Years)
Near entry of menopausal transition	>11.5
Early transition stage	7.4
Late transition stage	3.8

Most common ages at onset of moderate-to-severe HFs = 45–49 years.

Source: Data from Freeman EW, Sammel MD, Lin H, et al. Duration of menopausal hot flushes and associated risk factors. *Obstet Gynecol.* 2011 May;117(5):1095-1104

Etiology

- Believed to be related to estrogen withdrawal (not seen in 45,XO patients).
- Estrogen modulates the firing rate of thermosensitive neurons in the preoptic area of the hypothalamus in response to thermal stimulation in the rat.
- Responsiveness of arterioles to catecholamines is greater in women with HFs than in those without HFs. Estrogen enhances α2-adrenergic activity, and estrogen withdrawal may therefore lead to vasomotor flushes as a result of ↓ α2-adrenergic activity. Thermogenic changes occurring during a HF may be baroreflex-related since there is **acute** hypotension and a brisk increase in heart rate in both HFs and baroreflex responses to acute hypotensive episodes.
- Women who experience HFs have a significantly smaller thermoneutral zone than women without HF (0.0°C vs. 0.4°C, respectively); small elevations in core body temperature have been shown to precede most HFs.
- Other causes: thyroid disease, epilepsy, infection, insulinoma, pheochromocytoma, carcinoid syndromes, leukemia, pancreatic tumors, autoimmune disorders, and mast-cell disorders.

Table 10.4. Approved oral estrogen products for menopausal symptoms
(Providers should check the full prescribing information for appropriate dosages for the indication and any updates or information that is not provided here, such as warnings and contraindications.)

Active Ingredient(s)	Product Name(s)	Dosages (mg/d)
17β-estradiol*	Estrace[†]	0.5, 1.0, 2.0
	Generic(s) available	
Conjugated estrogens	Premarin	0.3, 0.45[‡], 0.625, 0.9[‡], 1.25
Synthetic conjugated estrogens, B	Enjuvia[‡]	0.3, 0.45, 0.625, 0.9, 1.25
Conjugated estrogens, CSD[‡] (synthetic)	C.E.S.	0.3, 0.625, 0.9, 1.25
	pms-Conjugated estrogens, CSD	
Esterified estrogens	Menest[‡] Estragyn[†]	0.3, 0.625, 1.25, 2.5 (administer cyclically)
		0.3, 0.625
Estropipate	Generic(s) available[‡]	0.625 (0.75 estropipate), 1.25 (1.5), 2.5 (3.0)

*Bioidentical: defined as compounds that have the same chemical and molecular structure as hormones that are produced in the body.
[†]Available in Canada but not the United States.
[‡]Available in the United States but not Canada.
Product names not marked are available in both the United States and Canada.

Source: Reproduced with permission from the North American Menopause Society (NAMS) website. http://www.menopause.org/docs/default-source/2014/nams-ht-tables.pdf. Accessed on March 5, 2016. Copyright © 2016 The North American Menopause Society (NAMS).

Table 10.5. Treatment options for menopausal vasomotor symptoms

Treatment	Dosage/Regimen	Evidence of Benefit*	FDA Approved
Hormonal			
Estrogen-alone or combined with progestin			
Standard Dose	Conjugated estrogen 0.625 mg/d	Yes	Yes
	Micronized estradiol-17β 1 mg/d	Yes	Yes
	Transdermal estradiol-17β 0.0375–0.05 mg/d	Yes	Yes
Low Dose	Conjugated estrogen 0.3–0.45 mg/d	Yes	Yes
	Micronized estradiol-17β 0.5 mg/d	Yes	Yes
	Transdermal estradiol-17β 0.025 mg/d	Yes	Yes
Ultra-Low Dose	Micronized estradiol-17β 0.25 mg/d	Mixed	No
	Transdermal estradiol-17β 0.014 mg/d	Mixed	No
Estrogen combined with estrogen agonist/antagonist	Conjugated estrogen 0.45 mg/d and bazedoxifene	Yes 20 mg/d	Yes
Progestin	Depot medroxyprogesterone acetate	Yes	No
Testosterone		No	No
Tibolone	2.5 mg/d	Yes	No
Compounded bioidentical hormones		No	No
Nonhormonal			
SSRIs and SSNRIs		No	No
Paroxetine	7.5 mg/d	Yes	Yes
Clonidine	0.1 mg/d	Yes	No
Gabapentin	600–900 mg/d	Yes	No
Phytoestrogens		No	No
Herbal Remedies		No	No
Vitamins		No	No
Exercise		No	No
Acupuncture		No	No
Reflexology		No	No
Stellate-ganglion block		Yes	No

FDA, Food and Drug Administration; SSRIs, selective serotonin reuptake inhibitors; SSNRIs, selective serotonin norepinephrine reuptake inhibitors.

*Compared with placebo.

Source: Reproduced with permission from ACOG Practice Bulletin No. 141: Management of menopausal symptoms. *Obstet Gynecol.* 2014 Jan;123(1):202-216. Copyright © 2014 The American College of Obstetricians and Gynecologists.

Table 10.6. Treatment options for menopausal vaginal symptoms

Treatment			Dosage	Evidence of Benefit*	FDA Approved
Hormonal					
Estrogen					
	Systemic				
		Standard Dose	Conjugated estrogen 0.625 mg/d	Yes	
			Micronized estradiol-17β 1 mg/d	Yes	
			Transdermal estradiol-17β 0.0375–0.05 mg/d	Yes	
		Low Dose	Conjugated estrogen 0.3–0.45 mg/d Micronized estradiol-17β 0.5 mg/d	Yes Yes	Yes Yes
			Transdermal estradiol-17β 0.025 mg/d	Yes	Yes
		Ultra-Low Dose	Micronized estradiol-17β 0.25 mg/d	Mixed	No
			Transdermal estradiol-17β 0.014 mg/d	Mixed	No
	Vaginal/Local		Estradiol-17β ring 7.5 micrograms/d	Yes	Yes
			Estradiol vaginal tablet 25 micrograms/d	Yes	Yes
			Estradiol ring 0.05 mg/d	Yes	
			Estradiol-17β cream 2 g/d	Yes	
			Conjugated estrogen cream 0.5–2 g/d	Yes	
Nonhormonal					
Estrogen agonists–antagonists					
	Raloxifene and tamoxifen			No	No
	Ospemifene		60 mg/d	Yes	Yes
Vaginal lubricants				Yes	No
Vaginal moisturizers				Yes	No
Herbal remedies and soy products				No	No

FDA, Food and Drug Administration.

*Compared with placebo.

Source: Reproduced with permission from ACOG Practice Bulletin No. 141: Management of menopausal symptoms. Obstet Gynecol. 2014 Jan;123(1):202-216. Copyright © 2014 The American College of Obstetricians and Gynecologists.

Table 10.7. Approved transdermal estrogen products for menopausal symptoms
(Providers should check the full prescribing information for appropriate dosages for the indication and any updates or information that is not provided here, such as warnings and contraindications.)

Active Ingredient(s)	Product Name	Dosage (mg E_2/Day)
Patch, film		
17β-estradiol*	Alora[†]	0.025, 0.05, 0.075, 0.1 twice/wk
	Climara	0.025, 0.0375,[†] 0.05, 0.06,[†] 0.075, 0.1 once/wk
	Estraderm[†]	0.05, 0.1 twice/wk
	Estradot[‡]	0.025, 0.0375, 0.05, 0.075, 0.1 twice/wk
	Minivelle[†]	0.025, 0.0375, 0.05, 0.075, 0.1 twice/wk
	Oesclim[‡]	0.025, 0.0375, 0.05, 0.075, 0.1 twice/wk
	Vivelle-Dot[†]	0.025, 0.0375, 0.05, 0.075, 0.1 twice/wk
	Generic(s) available	
Transdermal gel		
17β-estradiol*	Divigel	0.25, 0.5, 1.0
	EstroGel	0.75 (*US:* single approved dose, *Canada:* adjust to control symptoms)
	Elestrin[†]	0.52 (adjust based on clinical response)
Transdermal spray		
17β-estradiol*	Evamist[†]	1.53 (1 spray/d initially, adjust dosage by clinical response)

*Bioidentical: defined as compounds that have the same chemical and molecular structure as hormones that are produced in the body.

[†] Available in the United States but not Canada.

[‡] Available in Canada but not the United States.

Product names not marked are available in both the United States and Canada.

Source: Reproduced with permission from the North American Menopause Society (NAMS) website. http://www.menopause.org/docs/default-source/2014/nams-ht-tables.pdf. Accessed on March 5, 2016. Copyright © 2016 The North American Menopause Society (NAMS).

Table 10.8. Approved vaginal estrogen products for menopausal symptoms
(Providers should check the full prescribing information for appropriate dosages for the indication and any updates or information that is not provided here, such as warnings and contraindications.)

Active Ingredient(s)	Product Name *Indication*	Dosage
Creams		
17β-estradiol*	Estrace Vaginal Cream[†] *Vulvar and vaginal atrophy*	Initial: 2–4 g/d for 1–2 wk Maintenance: 1 g 1–3 times/wk (0.1 mg estradiol/g)
Conjugated estrogens	Premarin Vaginal Cream *Atrophic vaginitis Kraurosis vulvae* *Dyspareunia (US: Moderate to severe)*	US: For atrophic vaginitis and kraurosis vulvae: 0.5–2 g/d (0.625 mg conjugated estrogens/g) for 21 d then off 7 d For moderate to severe dyspareunia: 0.5 g twice weekly continuous or for 21 d then off 7 d Canada: Low dose: 0.5 g intravaginal or topical twice/wk Maximum recommended dose: 0.5 g/d intravaginally or topically for 21 d then off 7d. Start with 0.5 g/d. Dosage adjustments (0.5 to 2 g) may be made based on individual response
Estrone*	Estragyn Vaginal Cream[‡] *Vulvovaginal atrophy*	2–4 g/d (1 mg active ingredient/g) adjusted to lowest amount that controls symptoms. Usually cyclic (for 21 d then off 7 d)
Rings		
17β-estradiol*	Estring US: Moderate to severe symptoms of vulvar and vaginal atrophy due to menopause Canada: Postmenopausal urogenital complaints due to estrogen deficiency	2 mg (releases 7.5 μg/d) for 90 days Canada: Maximum recommended duration of continuous therapy is 2 years
Estradiol acetate*	Femring[†] Moderate to severe vasomotor symptoms due to menopause Moderate to severe vulvar and vaginal atrophy due to menopause	0.05 mg/d, 0.10 mg/d for 90 days (both strengths release systemic levels and require consideration of a progestogen if the uterus is intact)

(continued)

MENOPAUSE — Hot Flushes

Active Ingredient(s)	Product Name *Indication*	Dosage
Tablet		
Estradiol hemihydrate*	Vagifem[†] *Atrophic vaginitis due to menopause* Vagifem 10[‡] *Symptoms of vaginal atrophy due to estrogen deficiency*	10 μg, 25 μg Initial: 1 tablet/d for 2 wk Maintenance: 1 tablet twice/wk 10 μg Initial: 1 tablet/d for 2 wk Maintenance: 1 tablet twice/wk

*Bioidentical: defined as compounds that have the same chemical and molecular structure as hormones that are produced in the body.
[†]Available in the United States but not Canada.
[‡]Available in Canada but not the United States.
Products without asterisks are available in the United States and Canada.

Source: Reproduced with permission from the North American Menopause Society (NAMS) website. http://www.menopause.org/docs/default-source/2014/nams-ht-tables.pdf. Accessed on March 5, 2016. Copyright © 2016 The North American Menopause Society (NAMS).

POSTMENOPAUSAL OSTEOPOROSIS

Definition
- Low bone mass and microarchitectural deterioration with consequent ↑ bone fragility and susceptibility to fracture.
- Approximately 10–15% of women who take estrogen lose bone.
- Diagnosis requires bone densitometry.

Prevalence and Incidence
- 13–18% in women >50 years of age (Looker 1997).
- >1.3 million osteoporotic fractures/year in the United States.
- Postmenopausal women lose approximately 3% cortical and 8% trabecular bone/year.

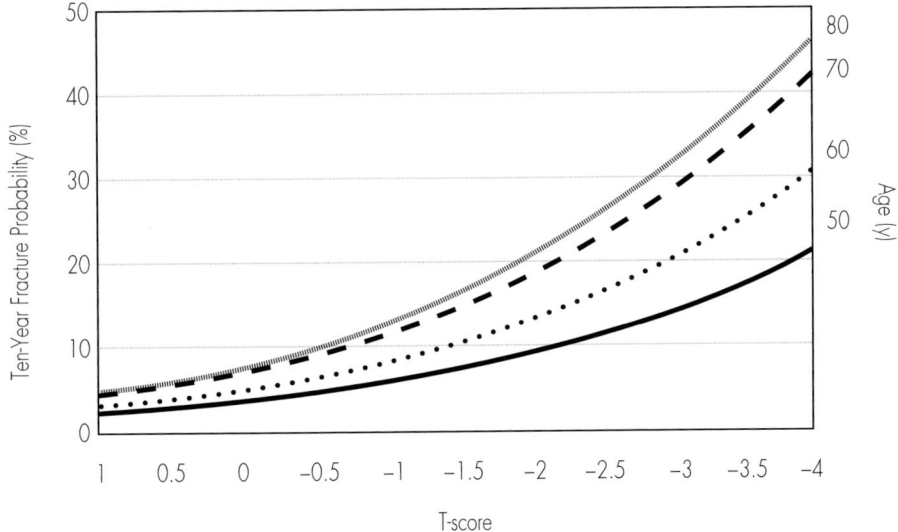

Figure 10.2. Ten-year probability of sustaining any osteoporotic fracture in women by age and T-score

Data from Kanis JA, Johnell O, Oden A, Dawson A, De Laet C, Jonsson B. Ten year probabilities of osteoporotic fractures according to BMD and diagnostic thresholds. *Osteoporos Int.* 2001;12(12):989–95.

Source: Reproduced with permission from. ACOG Practice Bulletin No. 129: Osteoporosis. *Obstet Gynecol.* 2012 Sep;120(3):718-34. Copyright © 2012 The American College of Obstetricians and Gynecologists.

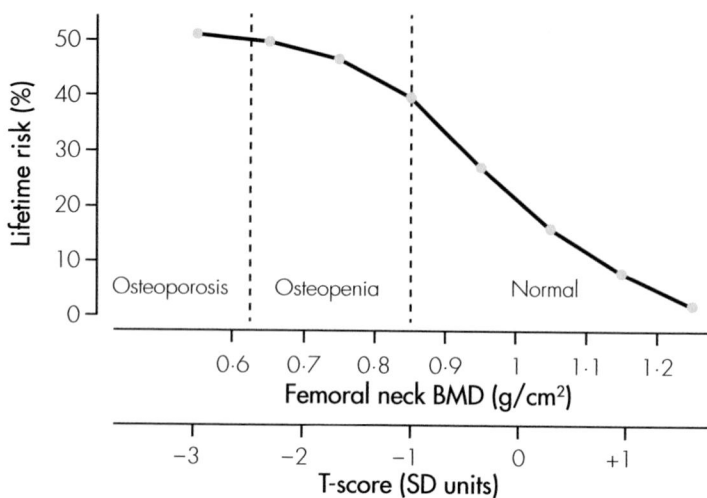

Figure 10.3. Lifetime risk of hip fractures in women aged 50 years according to bone mineral density or T-score at the hip
SD, standard deviation.
Source: Reproduced with permission from Kanis JA. Diagnosis of osteoporosis and assessment of fracture risk. *Lancet.* 2002;359(9321):1929. Copyright © 2002 Elsevier.

Fracture Risk Assessment Tool (FRAX)
- Developed in collaboration with the WHO to predict the risk of osteoporotic fracture for a person in the next 10 years (http://www.sheffield.ac.uk/FRAX/)
- Validated in 11 different cohorts studies
  - Risk factors used in FRAX:
    - Age, sex, body mass index, previous fragility fracture, parental hip fracture, current smoking status, corticosteroid use (greater than or equal to 5 mg prednisolone per day for 3 months), alcohol intake greater than or equal to 3 units per day (approximately three drinks), rheumatoid arthritis, and other secondary causes of osteoporosis
  - Results are specific for gender and race for various countries
  - FRAX has been most widely used as an aid in decision making regarding treatment initiation when the patient's BMD score is in the low bone mass (osteopenia) range
  - DXA reports are recommended to include a FRAX fracture risk score only when the patient's BMD is in the osteopenia zone
  - Consider treatment when there is a 3% risk of hip fracture or a 20% risk of a major osteoporotic fracture (defined as a fracture of the forearm, hip, shoulder, or clinical spine) or both in the next 10 years
  - FRAX is valid with or without the incorporation of the femoral neck BMD score

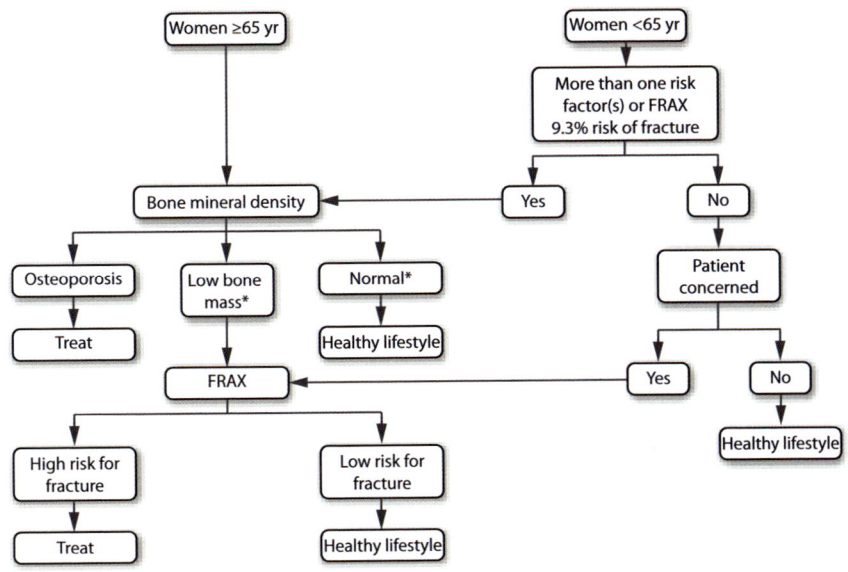

Figure 10.4. Algorithm for the management of osteoporosis
*Fragility fracture is an indication for treatment despite lack of osteoporosis on DXA.
Source: Reproduced with permission from ACOG Practice Bulletin No. 129: Osteoporosis. *Obstet Gynecol.* 2012 Sep;120(3):718-34. Copyright © 2012 The American College of Obstetricians and Gynecologists.

Table 10.9. Diagnostic tests in the work-up of secondary osteoporosis

Diagnostic Test	Purpose
History and physical exam	To identify risk factors for fractures, the underlying disease, and potential drugs
Dual-energy X-ray absorptiometry (lumbar spine and hip)	To quantify bone mineral density
Spinal X-rays	To detect prevalent vertebral fractures
	To exclude osteolytic lesions or tumors
Diagnostic test	*To detect or exclude*
Complete blood count	Anemia as in myeloma/celiac disease
	Leukocytosis in leukemia
Renal and liver function test	Renal or liver failure, alcohol abuse
Serum calcium and phosphate levels	Primary hyperparathyroidism, myeloma
Serum C-reactive protein	Chronic infection/inflammation
Serum bone-specific or total AP activity	Paget's disease; osteomalacia
Serum 25-hydroxyvitamin D	Vitamin D deficiency, osteomalacia
Serum levels of basal TSH	Hyperthyroidism
Serum free testosterone levels (in men)	Male hypogonadism
Fasting glucose levels	Diabetes mellitus
Intact parathyroid hormone	Primary hyperparathyroidism
Serum protein electrophoresis, immunofixation	MGUS, myeloma
24-hr urinary calcium excretion (with creatinine and sodium control)	Hypercalciuria
Anti-tissue transglutaminase antibodies	Celiac disease
Anti-HIV antibodies	HIV disease, AIDS
Morning fasting serum cortisol after dexamethasone suppression	Cushing syndrome
Serum tryptase levels, urinary histamine excretion	Systemic mastocytosis
COL1A genetic testing	Osteogenesis imperfecta
Iliac crest bone biopsy	Systemic mastocytosis, MGUS/myeloma, osteomalacia, lymphoma/leukemia

AP, alkaline phosphatase.

Source: Reproduced with permission from Hofbauer LC, Hamann C, Ebeling PR. Approach to the patient with secondary osteoporosis. *Eur J Endocrinol.* 2010 Jun;162(6):1009-20. Copyright © 2010 Bioscientifica.

Monitoring Response to Therapy
Repeat DXA
- First scan normal or mild osteopenia (T −1.5 or higher) → **rDXA in 15 years**
- First scan moderate osteopenia (T −1.5 to −1.99) → **rDXA in 5 years**
- First scan advanced osteopenia (−2.00 to −2.49) → **rDXA in 1 year**

   Source: Adapted from Gourlay ML, Fine JP, Preisser JS, et al. Study of Osteoporotic Fractures Research Group: Bone-density testing interval and transition to osteoporosis in older women. *N Engl J Med.* 2012 Jan 19;366(3):225-33.

DXA + Biochemical Markers of Bone Turnover
- Recommended approach:
  - Measure at baseline and repeat measurement of markers in 6 months.
  - If marker ↓ significantly (i.e., >50% of urine N-telopeptide [NTx] and >30% for serum C-telopeptide [CTx]) → therapy is having desired effect → repeat DXA after 2 years.
- Effective antiresorptive treatments induce a ↓ in bone turnover that reaches plateau within 1–3 months for oral bisphosphonates and usually up to 6 months for various types of estrogen, raloxifene, and nasal calcitonin, depending on the potency and route of administration of the drug and on the marker (Delmas 2000). Changes in bone turnover markers produced by raloxifene and calcitonin are generally smaller than those produced by the bisphosphonates and hormone therapy (HT; Delmas 2000).

Treatment of Osteoporosis

Table 10.10. Government-approved drugs for postmenopausal osteoporosis
(Providers should check the full prescribing information for appropriate dosages for the indication and any updates or information that is not provided here, such as warnings and contraindications.)

Active Ingredient Indications	Product Name(s)	Dosages
Bisphosphonates (oral unless otherwise specified)		
Alendronate Treatment Prevention	Fosamax Generic(s) available Binosto*	Treatment: 70 mg/wk, 10 mg/d Prevention: 35 mg/wk or 5 mg/d Treatment: 70 mg/wk (effervescent)
Alendronate + vitamin D3 Treatment	Fosamax Plus D* Fosavance† Generic(s) available†	70 mg + 2,800 IU/wk; 70 mg + 5,600 IU/wk
Risedronate (immediate release) Treatment Prevention	Actonel Generic(s) available	Treatment: 5 mg/d; 35 mg/wk; 75 mg on 2 consecutive d/mo; 150 mg/mo Prevention: 5 mg/d; 35 mg/wk; 75 mg on 2 consecutive d/mo; 150 mg/mo may be considered
Risedronate (delayed release) Treatment	Atelvia* Actonel DR†	35 mg/wk
Risedronate + calcium carbonate Treatment Prevention	Actonel Plus Calcium†	35 mg/wk (day 1) + 1,250 mg Ca (days 2–7)
Ibandronate Treatment Prevention	Boniva* Generic(s) available*	150 mg/mo
Ibandronate injection* Treatment	Boniva Injection* Generic(s) available*	3 mg every 3 mo IV
Etidronate and calcium carbonate† Treatment Prevention	Didrocal† Generic(s) available†	400 mg/d oral tablet for 14 d followed by 1,250 mg calcium/d for 76 d
Zoledronic acid Treatment Prevention	Reclast* Aclasta† Generic(s) available	Treatment: 5 mg/yr IV Prevention: 5 mg/2 yr IV Treatment: 5 mg/yr IV Prevention: single infusion of 5 mg
Estrogen agonist/antagonist		
Raloxifene Treatment Prevention	Evista Generic(s) available	60 mg/d

(continued)

Postmenopausal Osteoporosis

Active Ingredient Indications	Product Name(s)	Dosages
Calcitonin		
Calcitonin-salmon nasal spray (rDNA origin) Treatment (>5 yr postmenopause)	Fortical*	200 IU/d
Calcitonin-salmon nasal spray (synthetic) Treatment (>5 yr postmenopause)	Miacalcin* Generic(s) available*	200 USP Salmon Calcitonin units/d
Calcitonin-salmon injection* Treatment (>5 yr postmenopause)	Miacalcin*	100 IU/d SC or IM
Parathyroid hormone		
Teriparatide injection Treatment	Forteo	20 µg/d SC (maximum lifetime exposure 24 mo)
RANK ligand inhibitor		
Denosumab Treatment	Prolia	60 mg every 6 mo SC
Estrogen-only (oral)		
17β-estradiol Prevention	Estrace† Generic(s) available*	start with 0.5 mg/d† lowest effective dose not determined*
Conjugated estrogens Prevention	Premarin	start with 0.3 mg/d
Conjugated estrogens, CSD (synthetic)† Prevention Treatment (C.E.S. only)	pms-Conjugated estrogens, CSD† C.E.S.†	0.625 mg/d
Estropipate* Prevention	Generic(s) available	0.625 (0.75 estropipate) 25 d/31-d cycle
Estrogen-only (transdermal)		
17β-estradiol patch Prevention	Alora*	0.025 mg/d (twice/wk)
	Climara	US: start with 0.025 mg/d, Canada: 0.05 mg/d minimum approved (once/wk)
	Estraderm* Estradot†	start with 0.05 mg/d (twice/wk) not specified: ideally, maintain plasma levels at 183 pg/mL
	Menostar*	0.014 mg/d (once/wk)
	Minivelle*	start with 0.025 mg/d (twice/wk)
	Vivelle-Dot* Generic(s) available	start with 0.025 mg/d (twice/wk)

(continued)

MENOPAUSE Postmenopausal Osteoporosis

Active Ingredient Indications	Product Name(s)	Dosages
Estrogen-progestogen combinations		
Oral continuous-cyclic		
Conjugated estrogens + medroxyprogesterone acetate *Prevention*	Premphase*	0.625 mg E + 5.0 mg P/d (2 tablets: E and E+P; E alone days 1–14, E + P days 15–28)
Oral continuous-combined		
Conjugated estrogens (E) + medroxyprogesterone acetate (P) *Prevention*	Prempro*	0.3 or 0.45 mg E + 1.5 mg P/d; 0.625 mg E + 2.5 mg or 5.0 mg P/d
Ethinyl estradiol (E) + norethindrone acetate (P) *Prevention*	femhrt*, femHRT Lo† Generic(s) available femhrt*, femHRT† Generic(s) available	2.5 µg E + 0.5 mg P/d 5 µg E + 1 mg P/d
Oral intermittent combined		
17β-estradiol (E) + norethindrone acetate (P) *Prevention*	Activella* Generic(s) available* Activelle LD† Activelle†	0.5 mg E + 0.1 mg P/d; 1 mg E + 0.5 mg P/d 0.5 mg E + 0.1 mg P 1 mg E + 0.5 mg P
17β-estradiol (E)+ norgestimate (P) (intermittent-combined) *Prevention*	Prefest*	1 mg E and 1 mg E + 0.09 mg P (E alone for 3 d, followed by E + P for 3 d, repeated continuously)
Transdermal continuous combined		
17β-estradiol (E)+ levonorgestrel (P) *Prevention (indication only in United States)*	Climara Pro	0.045 mg E + 0.015 mg P (once/wk)
Estrogen agonist/antagonist combination		
Conjugated estrogens (E)+ bazedoxifene (P) *Prevention*	Duavee*	0.045 mg E + 20 mg bazedoxifene/d

IV, intravenous; sc, subcutaneous.
*Available in the United States but not Canada.
†Available in Canada but not the United States.
Products not marked are available in both the United States and Canada.

Source: Reproduced with permission from the North American Menopause Society (NAMS) website. http://www.menopause.org/docs/default-source/professional/nams-osteo-table-q1-2016.pdf Accessed on March 5, 2016. Copyright © 2016 The North American Menopause Society (NAMS).

HORMONE REPLACEMENT THERAPY
Global Consensus Statement on Menopausal Hormone Therapy

- Endorsed by The American Society for Reproductive Medicine, The Asia Pacific Menopause Federation, The Endocrine Society, The European Menopause and Andropause Society, The International Menopause Society, The International Osteoporosis Foundation, and The North American Menopause Society.
- Menopausal hormone therapy (MHT) is the most effective treatment for vasomotor symptoms associated with menopause at any age, but benefits are more likely to outweigh risks for symptomatic women before the age of 60 years or within 10 years after menopause.
- MHT is effective and appropriate for the prevention of osteoporosis-related fractures in at-risk women before age 60 years or within 10 years after menopause.
- Randomized clinical trials and observational data as well as meta-analyses provide evidence that standard-dose estrogen-alone MHT may decrease coronary heart disease and all-cause mortality in women younger than 60 years of age and within 10 years of menopause. Data on estrogen plus progestogen MHT in this population show a similar trend for mortality, but in most randomized clinical trials, no significant increase or decrease in coronary heart disease has been found.
- Local low-dose estrogen therapy is preferred for women whose symptoms are limited to vaginal dryness or associated discomfort with intercourse.
- Estrogen as a single systemic agent is appropriate in women after hysterectomy, but additional progestogen is required in the presence of a uterus.
- The option of MHT is an individual decision in terms of quality of life and health priorities as well as personal risk factors such as age, time since menopause and the risk of venous thromboembolism, stroke, ischemic heart disease, and breast cancer.
- The risk of venous thromboembolism and ischemic stroke increases with oral MHT, but the absolute risk is rare below age 60 years. Observational studies point to a lower risk with transdermal therapy.
- The risk of breast cancer in women over 50 years associated with MHT is a complex issue. The increased risk of breast cancer is primarily associated with the addition of a progestogen to estrogen therapy and related to the duration of use. The risk of breast cancer attributable to MHT is small, and the risk decreases after treatment is stopped.
- The dose and duration of MHT should be consistent with treatment goals and safety issues and should be individualized.
- In women with premature ovarian insufficiency, systemic MHT is recommended at least until the average age of the natural menopause.
- The use of custom-compounded bioidentical hormone therapy is not recommended.
- Current safety data do not support the use of MHT in breast cancer survivors.

Source: From de Villiers TJ, Gass ML, Haines CJ, et al. Global consensus statement on menopausal hormone therapy. *Climacteric*. 2013 Apr;16(2):203-204.

CHAPTER 11
Gyn-Oncology

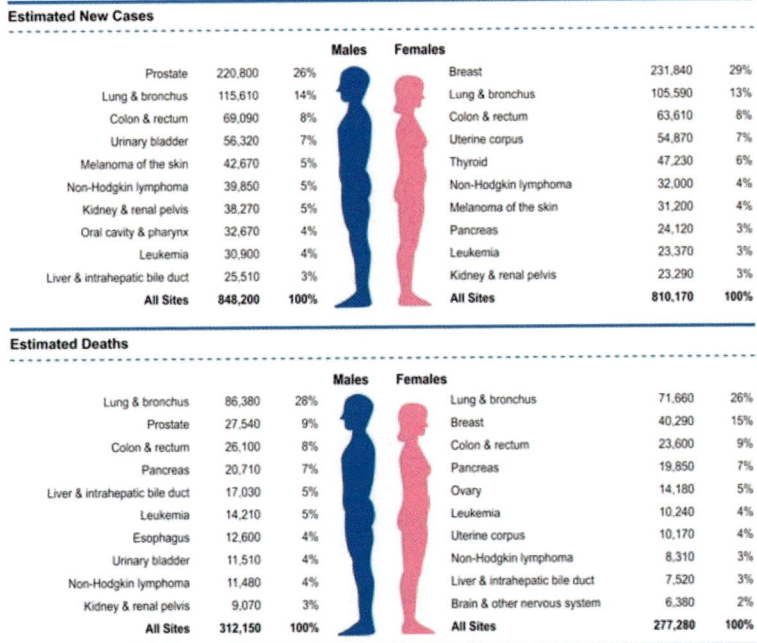

Figure 11.1. Cancer statistics 2015
Ten leading cancer types for the estimated new cancer cases and deaths, by sex, United States, 2015.
*Excludes basal and squamous cell skin cancers and in situ carcinoma except urinary bladder. In 2015, there will be 21,290 estimated new cases of ovarian cancer.
Source: Reproduced with permission from Siegel RL, Miller KD, Jemal A. Cancer statistics, 2015. *CA Cancer J Clin*. 2015;65(1):5-29. Copyright © 2015 American Cancer Society.

ENDOMETRIAL HYPERPLASIA

Fast Facts
- Precursor to endometrial carcinoma
- Associated with unopposed estrogen stimulation of uterine endometrium
- Usually presents with abnormal uterine bleeding
- Risk of progression related to presence/absence of atypia in both simple and complex hyperplasia
    - Use penny, nickel, dime, quarter rule:
        - Penny: 1% progression for simple
        - Nickel: 3–5% progression for complex hyperplasia
        - Dime: 8% progression for simple with atypia
        - Quarter: 29% progression for complex with atypia

Risk Factors
- Obesity
- Polycystic ovary syndrome with irregular or absent menses
- Early menarche/late menopause
- Unopposed estrogen therapy
- Tamoxifen

Table 11.1. Pathologic classification of endometrial hyperplasia

Classification	Description
Simple	Benign proliferation of endometrial glands that are irregular and perhaps dilated but do not display back-to-back crowding or cellular atypia. Mitoses may or may not be present.
Complex	Proliferation of endometrial glands with irregular outlines, architectural complexity, and back-to-back crowding but no atypia. Mitoses typically present.
Atypical	Varying degrees of nuclear atypia and loss of polarity. Found in both simple and complex hyperplastic lesions.

Table 11.2. Regression, persistence, and progression rates of endometrial hyperplasia

Type	N	% Regression	% Persistence	% Progression
Simple	93	80	19	1
Simple with atypia	13	69	23	8
Complex	29	80	17	3
Complex with atypia	35	57	14	29
All lesions with atypia	48	58	19	23

Data from Kurman RJ, et al. *Cancer*. 1985;56:403-412.

Source: Reprinted with permission from Childs AJ, Check WE, Hoskins WJ. Conservative management of endometrial hyperplasia: new strategies and experimental options. *OBG Management*. 2003;Sept:15-26.

Treatment for Atypical Hyperplasia
- Patient does not desire child bearing
  - Hysterectomy (there is a 17–52% risk of concurrent cancer)
- Patient desires child bearing or does not desire hysterectomy
  - Simple or complex hyperplasia without atypia
    - Progestins reverse hyperplasia by decreasing estrogen and progesterone receptors and cause stromal decidualization and thinning of endometrium.
      - Medroxyprogesterone acetate (MPA) 10 mg daily × 3–6 months
      - Megace 20–40 mg/day continuously × 3–6 months
      - MPA 10 mg daily × 14 days q month × 3–6 months
      - Levonorgestrel-releasing intrauterine device 20 mcg/day
    - Sample endometrium after completion of 3 months. If hyperplasia continues to show without atypia, consider hysterectomy or continue biopsies q6–12 months.
  - Complex atypical hyperplasia with atypia
    - Megestrol 40 mg bid × 3 months (Megestrol is more potent than MPA)
    - Sample endometrium 3–4 weeks after completion of 3 months of therapy
    - Abandon medical management if persistence after 6–12 months
    - Abandon treatment if progression to cancer after 3 months in most patients
      - If regression occurs, continue on low-dose progesterone therapy but will need endometrial biopsy every 6–12 months, indefinitely

ENDOMETRIAL CARCINOMA

Fast Facts
- Most common malignancy of the female genital tract, with 54,870 cases in 2015
  - Frequency of gynecologic cancers: endometrial > ovarian > cervical
  - Number of deaths: ovarian > endometrial > cervical
- >10,170 deaths in 2015 in United States
- Median age 60 years
- 90% of women have symptomatic bleeding leading to early diagnosis
- 72% stage I
- 12% stage II
- 13% stage III
- 3% stage IV

Bleeding Patterns That Should Prompt Endometrial Evaluation
- Any abnormal bleeding
  - Younger than 45 years—Persistent abnormal uterine bleeding in the setting of unopposed estrogen (obesity, chronic anovulation) or high risk of endometrial cancer (Lynch syndrome).
  - Older than 45 years—Any abnormal uterine bleeding, frequent episodes (less than 21 days), heavy (greater than 80 mL), prolonged (longer than 7 days), intermenstrual bleeding in women who are ovulatory, or prolonged amenorrhea (6 months or more) in women with anovulation.
  - Postmenopausal women—Any bleeding, spotting, or staining.
    - An estimated 3–20% of women with postmenopausal bleeding are found to have endometrial cancer and 5–15% with endometrial hyperplasia.
- Cervical cytology with the following findings:
  - Adenocarcinoma—Malignant cells can arise from the cervix or the endometrium; further evaluation with cervical and endometrial biopsy is required.
  - Atypical glandular cells—Atypical glandular cells detected by cervical cytology should be evaluated with an endometrial and endocervical biopsy.
  - Endometrial cells—Further evaluation appropriate in women with symptomatic bleeding. Endometrial cells on cytology in asymptomatic women do not need further evaluation.

Table 11.3. Risk factors for endometrial carcinoma

Factors Influencing Risk	Estimated Relative Risk
Older age	2–3
Residency in North America or Northern Europe	3–18
Higher level of education or income	1.5–2
White race	2
Nulliparity	3
History of infertility	2–3
Menstrual irregularities	1.5
Late age at natural menopause	2–3
Early age at menarche	1.5–2
Long-term use of high dosages of menopausal estrogens	10–20
Long-term use of high dosages of combination oral contraceptives	0.3–0.5
High cumulative doses of tamoxifen	3–7
Obesity	2–5
Stein-Leventhal disease or estrogen-producing tumor	>5
History of diabetes, hypertension, gallbladder disease, or thyroid disease	1.3–3
Cigarette smoking	0.5
Polycystic ovarian syndrome	3
Lynch syndrome (hereditary nonpolyposis colorectal cancer)	22 to 50%
Cowden syndrome (autosomal dom *PTEN* mutation—risk for endometrial, breast, thyroid, colorectal, and renal cancers)	13 to 19% lifetime risk

Relative risks depend on the study and referent group employed.
Women 50–70 years old have a 1.4% risk of endometrial cancer
Women in US have a 2.6% lifetime risk of developing uterine cancer

Adapted from data in Smith RA, von Eschenbach AC, Wender R, et al. American Cancer Society guidelines for the early detection of cancer: update of early detection guidelines for prostate, colorectal, and endometrial cancers. *CA Cancer J Clin.* 2001 Jan-Feb;51(1):38-75.

Source: Reprinted with permission from Gershenson DM, McGuire WP, Gore M, et al., eds. *Gynecologic Cancer: Controversies in Management.* Copyright © 2004 Elsevier.

Histologic Types

- Type I: estrogen dependent
    - Comprise 80% of endometrial cancers
    - Grade 1 or 2 tumors
    - Endometrioid histology
    - *PIK3CA, PTEN, ARID1A* mutations in endometrioid endometrial cancers
    - Good prognosis
- Type II: non–estrogen dependent
    - Grade 3 tumors
    - Non-endometrioid histology: serous, clear cell, mucinous, squamous histology
    - Tumor suppressor p53 mutations in serous endometrial carcinomas
    - Worse prognosis

Screening
- Routine screening of asymptomatic women not recommended.

Diagnosis
- Endometrial sample obtained by endometrial biopsy in office or dilation and curettage under anesthesia.
- Pelvic sonography, in postmenopausal women, can be used as an initial study, and endometrial biopsy can be deferred for an endometrial thickness <4mm. However, if a woman continues to have bleeding with a thickness <4 mm, an endometrial biopsy should be performed.
- In premenopausal women, ultrasound measurement of endometrial thickness cannot be used as an alternative to endometrial sampling.

Preoperative Evaluation
- Complete history and physical exam including rectovaginal exam.
- Chest X-ray for all endometrial cancers; computed tomography (CT) scan if metastatic disease is suspected.
- Complete blood count and liver and renal function tests as indicated.

Treatment
- Surgical staging includes total hysterectomy, bilateral salpingo-oophorectomy, +/- lymphadenectomy (for selected patient at risk for nodal metastases).
- Postoperative therapy may include observation, vaginal brachytherapy, external pelvic beam radiation, and/or chemotherapy.
- Lymphadenectomy for low-grade tumors is controversial.
- The rate of nodal spread varies with tumor stage and grade. Risk is 3–5% for those with well-differentiated, superficially invasive tumors and as high as 20% for poorly differentiated, deeply invasive tumors. Other risk factors for nodal metastases include serous, clear cell, or high-grade histology; myometrial invasion >50%; or large tumor (>2cm in diameter).

Endometrial Carcinoma

Table 11.4. Endometrial cancer: staging and treatment

Stage		Treatment
Stage I	Tumor Confined to Corpus Uteri	
IA	Tumor invades less than one-half of myometrium	Total hysterectomy, BSO, +/-pelvic lymph node dissection, cytology observe (if grade 2 or 3, consider vaginal brachytherapy)
IB	Tumor invades more than one-half of myometrium	Total hysterectomy, BSO, pelvic/para-aortic lymph node dissection, cytology + adjuvant treatment[*]
Stage II	Tumor invades cervix but does not extend beyond uterus	
II	Invades stromal connective tissue of the cervix	Total hysterectomy, BSO, pelvic/para-aortic lymph node dissection, cytology + adjuvant treatment[*]
Stage III	Local and/or regional spread	
IIIA	Tumor involves serosa and/or adnexa (direct extension or metastasis)	Total hysterectomy, BSO, pelvic/para-aortic lymph node dissection, cytology + adjuvant treatment[*]
IIIB	Vaginal involvement (direct extension or metastasis) or parametrial involvement	Total hysterectomy, BSO, pelvic/para-aortic lymph node dissection, cytology + adjuvant treatment[*]
IIIC1	Regional lymph node metastasis to pelvic lymph nodes	Total hysterectomy, BSO, pelvic/para-aortic lymph node dissection, cytology + adjuvant treatment[*]
IIIC2	Regional lymph node metastasis to para-aortic lymph nodes with or without pelvic lymph nodes	Total hysterectomy, BSO, pelvic/para-aortic lymph node dissection, cytology + adjuvant treatment[*]
Stage IV	Tumor invades outside of uterus, ovaries, and vagina	
Stage IVA	Tumor involves bladder mucosa and/or bowel mucosa	Total hysterectomy, BSO, pelvic/para-aortic lymph node dissection, cytology + adjuvant treatment[*]
Stage IVB	Distant metastasis including to inguinal lymph nodes, intraperitoneal disease, lung, liver, or bone.	Total hysterectomy, BSO, pelvic/para-aortic lymph node dissection, cytology + adjuvant treatment. If unresectable, RT +/- brachy, +/- chemo, +/- surgery.

BSO, bilateral salpingo-oophorectomy; RT, radiation therapy

[*] Adjuvant treatment such as vaginal brachytherapy vs. pelvic radiation therapy vs. +/- chemotherapy will be influenced by adverse risk factors (advanced age, positive lymphovascular invasion, depth of invasion, grade of tumor per GOG 99)

Cytology is no longer part of the 2009 FIGO staging, and treatment based on positive cytology is still under research.

FIGO = Féderation Internationale de Gynécologie et d'Obstétrique.

Source: Reproduced with permission from Pecorelli S. Revised FIGO staging for carcinoma of the vulva, cervix, and endometrium. *Int J Gynaecol Obstet.* 2009;105(2):103-104. Copyright © 2009 International Federation of Gynecology and Obstetrics.

Table 11.5. Frequency of nodal metastases in endometrial cancer

Risk Factor	No. of Patients	Pelvic Nodes (%)	Aortic Nodes (%)
Grade			
1 Well	180	5 (3%)	3 (2%)
2 Moderate	288	25 (9%)	14 (5%)
3 Poor	153	28 (18%)	17 (11%)
Myometrial invasion			
Endometrial	187	1 (1%)	1 (1%)
Superficial	279	15 (5%)	8 (3%)
Middle	116	7 (6%)	1 (1%)
Deep	139	35 (25%)	24 (17%)

Data from Creasman WT, Morrow CP, Bundy BN, et al. Surgical pathologic spread patterns of endometrial cancer. A Gynecologic Oncology Group study. *Cancer.* 1987; 60: 2035–2041.

Source: Reprinted with permission from Barakat RR. Current management of early-stage endometrial cancer. *OBG Management.* 2003;15(1):32

Endometrial Cancer Follow-up
- Five-year survival (Lewin 2010)
  - Stage I = 78–90%
  - Stage II = 74%
  - Stage III = 36–57%
  - Stage IV = 21–22%

Surveillance Post–Endometrial Cancer Treatment
- Physical and pelvic exam at each visit +/- Pap at vaginal cuff
  - Every 3–4 months for 2 years
  - Every 6 months for 3–5 years
  - Annually for >5 years

CERVICAL DYSPLASIA—CERVICAL INTRAEPITHELIAL NEOPLASIA
Fast Facts
- Ectocervix is covered in squamous epithelium and cervical intraepithelial neoplasia (CIN) refers to squamous abnormalities.
- Endodervix, including the cervical canal, is covered with glandular epithelium, and glandular cervical neoplasia includes adenocarcinoma in situ and adenocarcinoma.
- Transformation zone is a dynamic entity of metaplasia and the area where the glandular epithelium has been replaced by squamous epithelium.
- Squamocolumnar junction is where the squamous epithelium of the ectocervix meets the columnar epithelium of the endocervix. Squamocolumnar junction is part of the transformation zone.
- More exposure to carcinogens, such as breakdown products of cigarette smoke, increases CIN with increased chance of dysplasia.
- CIN 1 is a low-grade squamous intraepithelial lesion (koilocytotic atypia is often present).
- CIN2 and CIN3 are high-grade squamous intraepithelial lesions.
- High-grade lesions are typically diagnosed in 25–35 yo.
  - Untreated CIN III develops into cancer after 8–13 years.

Table 11.6. Risk factors associated with precancerous changes and cancer of the cervix

Human papillomavirus infection
Multiple sexual partners
Sexual activity begun at an early age
Parity
Human immunodeficiency virus (HIV)
Immune status
Smoking
History of other sexually transmitted diseases (e.g., herpes simplex, chlamydia, and bacterial vaginosis)
Oral contraceptive use
Low socioeconomic status
Poor diet (e.g., vitamin deficiency)
Alcoholism

Source: Reproduced with permission from APGO Educational Series on Women's Health Issues. Advances in the screening, diagnosis, and treatment of cervical disease. 2002.

GYN-ONCOLOGY — Cervical Dysplasia—Cervical Intraepithelial Neoplasia

Table 11.7. Common genital HPV genotypes

Lesions/Malignancies	HPV Genotypes Common	Less common
Anogenital lesions		
Condyloma acuminata	6	2, 11, 16, 30, 42, 43, 44, 54, 55, 61
CIN, VIN, VAIN, PAIN, PIN	16, 18, 31	6, 11, 30, 34, 35, 39, 45, 51, 52, 56, 59, 61, 62, 64, 66, 67, 69
Malignancies		
Cervical cancer	16, 18, 31, 45	6, 10, 11, 26, 33, 35, 39, 51, 52, 55, 56, 58, 59, 66, 68
Other anogenital cancers	6, 16, 18	11, 31, 33

CIN, cervical intraepithelial neoplasm; HPV, human papillomavirus; PIN, penile intraepithelial neoplasia; PAIN, perianal intraepithelial neoplasia; VAIN, vaginal intraepithelial neoplasia; VIN, vulvar intraepithelial neoplasia.

Source: Reproduced with permission from APGO Educational Series on Women's Health Issues. Advances in the screening, diagnosis, and treatment of cervical disease. 2002.

Pathophysiology

- Metaplasia progresses from columnar to squamous
- Lower 2/3 (cervical canal) = squamous epithelium, similar to vagina
- Upper 1/3 = columnar epithelium, similar to lining of lower uterine segment
- Junction is not static—moves up in cervical canal with age
- Critical periods for metaplasia:
  - Fetal life
  - Early adolescence
  - First pregnancy
- Low-risk types such as HPV 6 and 11 do not integrate into the host genome and only cause CIN1 and benign condylomatous genital warts
- High-risk HPV types, such as 16 and 18, are strongly associated with high-grade lesions; HPV 16 and 18 account for 25% of low-grade lesions, 50–60% of high-grade lesions, and 70% of cervical cancers

Four Major Steps in Cervical Cancer Development

1. Oncogenic HPV infection of the metaplastic epithelium at the cervical transformation zone.
2. Persistence of the HPV infection.
3. Progression of a clone of epithelial cells from persistent viral infection to precancer.
4. Development of carcinoma and invasion through the basement membrane.
    - Viral integration into host genome disrupts the E1 and E2 open reading frames and results in loss of transcriptional regulation of E6 and E7, leading to overexpression of oncoproteins E6 and E7.
    - HPV E6 protein binds to tumor suppressor p53 and induces cellular degradation of p53.
    - HPV E7 protein binds to tumor suppressor Rb and induces dissociation of transcription factor E2F and promotion of cell cycle progression.

Cervical Dysplasia—Cervical Intraepithelial Neoplasia — GYN-ONCOLOGY

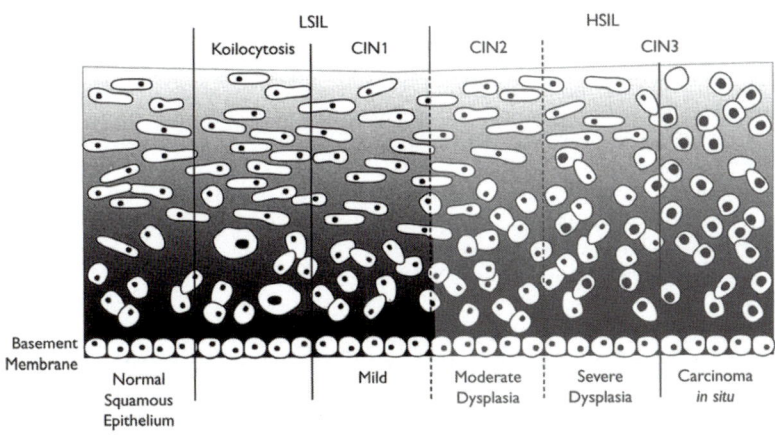

Figure 11.2. Progression from normal to dysplasia in the cervical epithelium
CIN, cervical intraepithelial neoplasia; CIN1, mild dysplasia; CIN2, moderate dysplasia; CIN3, severe dysplasia to carcinoma in situ (CIS); HSIL, high-grade squamous intraepithelial lesion; LSIL, low-grade squamous intraepithelial lesion.
Source: Reproduced with permission from APGO Educational Series on Women's Health Issues. Advances in the screening, diagnosis, and treatment of cervical disease. 2002.

Screening for Cervical Dysplasia
- Methods to detect preinvasive neoplasia—Pap test vs. HPV testing.
- Pap test collection device: Spatula + separate endocervical brush provides more endocervical cells vs. spatula alone. Broom is another option to insert central bristles into the endocervix and outer bristles into the ectocervix.
- Two methods for preparing Pap tests: conventional Pap smear or liquid-based, thin-layer prep. (Some liquid-based prep can test for HPV with same specimen for cytology.)
- Pap test evaluation of transformation zone
  - Satisfactory vs. absent endocervical cell/transformation zone (EC/TZ): clinical significance is controversial since patients are not at increased risk of cervical neoplasia with absent EC/TZ.
  - If negative cervical cytology but insufficient EC/TZ, should be managed according to HPV results:
    - HPV-positive: genotyping for HPV subtypes 16/18 or HPV and cytology cotesting in 1 year
    - HPV-negative: may resume routine screening
    - HPV unknown: either HPV testing (preferred) or cytology repeated in 3 years

Diagnosis

- Colposcopy is a diagnostic procedure. Primary goal is to identify precancerous and cancerous lesions.
- Colposcopic visualization needed for the following:
    - Persistent atypical cells of undetermined significance (ASC-US) or ASC-US with high-risk HPV subtypes
    - Atypical squamous cells: cannot exclude high-grade SIL (ASC-H)
    - Atypical glandular cells (AGC)
    - LSIL HPV unknown or HPV+ for >30 years of age
    - LSIL in those 25–29 years of age (CIN3+ risk of 5%)
    - HSIL
    - Malignant cells
- Repeat Pap if >6 wk prior to colposcopy (6 weeks are needed for cervical epithelium to regenerate after being sampled). Use 10 × magnification and 5% acetic acid. Acetic acid dehydrates, and squamous cells with large or dense nuclei that reflect light will appear white.
- Biopsy abnormal areas such as areas with atypical vessels or mosaicism.
- Colposcopy satisfactory if:
    - Transformation zone and entire lesion seen
    - Endocervical curettage (ECC) without dysplasia

Table 11.8. Risk of CIN2, CIN3, and cancer based on cytology and HPV status in women 30–64 years of age

Cytology (30–64 Yoa Unless Specified)	HPV Status	Risk of CIN2+	Risk of CIN3+/AIS	Risk of Cervical Cancer (SCC and AdenoCA)
Negative		0.68%	0.26%	0.025%
ASC-US	Unknown	6.9%	2.6%	0.18%
ASC-US	Positive	18%	6.8%	0.18%
ASC-US	Negative	1.1%	0.43%	
LSIL	Unknown	16%	5.2%	0.16%
LSIL	Positive	19%	6.1%	
LSIL	Negative	5.1%	2.0%	
LSIL (21–24 yoa)	Positive	3%		0
LSIL (25–29 yoa)	Positive	5%		0
ASC-H		35%	18%	2.6%
HSIL		69%	47%	7.3%
Atypical glandular cells		13%	8.5%	2.7%
Squamous cell cancer		84%	84%	68%

Source: Data from Katki HA, Schiffman M, Castle PE, et al. Five-year risks of CIN 3+ and cervical cancer among women with HPV testing of ASC-US Pap results. *J Low Genit Tract Dis.* 2013 Apr;17(5 Suppl 1):S36-42.

Table 11.9. Cervical cytology screening guideline recommendations

Timing	ACS (2012)	ACOG (2012)	USPTF (2012)	ASCCP/SGO (2015)
Initiate Screening	Age 21	Age 21	Age 21	Age 21
Screening 21–29 years	Pap test every 3 years	Pap test every 3 years	Pap test every 3 years	Can consider primary HPV testing every 3 years for ≥25 years of age
Screening age >30 years	Co-testing (pap test and HPV testing) every 5 years	Co-testing (pap test and HPV testing) every 5 years	Pap test every 3 years or cotesting every 5 years	Can consider primary HPV testing every 3 years
Cease screening	Age 65 with 3 consecutive negative cytology or 2 consecutive negative cotests in the past 10 years, with the most recent in the past 5 years	Age 65 with 3 or more negative cytology tests consecutively or 2 negative cotests in the past 10 years, with the most recent in the past 5 years	Age 65 with 3 consecutive negative cytology results or 2 consecutive negative cotests within the previous 10 years with the most recent test within the previous 5 years	N/A
Post–total hysterectomy (with cervix removed)	Not indicated for those with no history of CIN2, CIN3, or cervical cancer in the past 20 years. Evidence of adequate negative screening not required. Screening should not be resumed even with new partner	Not indicated for those with no history of CIN2, CIN3, or cervical cancer. Women in whom a negative history cannot be documented should continue to be screened	Not indicated for those with no history of CIN2, CIN3, or cervical cancer	N/A
HPV vaccination	Follow age-specific recommendation	Follow age-specific recommendation	Follow age-specific recommendation	N/A

HPV, human papillomavirus

Source: Saslow D, Solomon D, Lawson HW, et al. American Cancer Society, American Society for Colposcopy and Cervical Pathology, and American Society for Clinical Pathology screening guidelines for the prevention and early detection of cervical cancer. *J Low Genit Tract Dis.* 2012;16:175; Moyer VA. Screening for cervical cancer: U.S. Preventive Services Task Force recommendation statement. *Ann Intern Med.* 2012;156:880; ACOG Practice Bulletin No. 131: Screening for cervical cancer. *Obstet Gynecol.* 2012;120:1222; Huh WK, Ault KA, Chelmow D, et al. Use of primary high-risk human papillomavirus testing for cervical cancer screening: interim clinical guidance. *Gynecol Oncol.* 2015;136:178.

Table 11.10. Risk of progression and rate of regression

Papanicolaou Diagnosis	Regress to Normal (95% CI)	Progress To/Persist as HSIL In 24 Mo (95% CI)	Progress to Invasive Cancer In 24 Mo (95% CI)
ASC-US	68.19% (57.51, 78.86)	7.13% (0.8, 13.5)	0.25% (0, 2.25)
LSIL	47.39% (35.92, 58.86)	20.81% (6.08, 35.55)	0.15% (0, 0.71)
HSIL	35.03% (16.57, 53.49)	23.37% (12.82, 32.92)	1.44% (0, 3.95)

ASC-US, atypical squamous cells of undetermined significance; CI, confidence interval; HSIL, high-grade squamous intraepithelial lesion; LSIL, low-grade squamous intraepithelial lesion.

	Within 2 Yr	Within 5 Yr	Within 10 Yr
Progression			
Mild to moderate or worse	11.1%	20.4%	28.8%
Mild to severe or worse	2.1%	5.5%	9.9%
Moderate to severe or worse	16.3%	25.1%	32.0%
Regression			
Mild to first normal Pap	44.3%	74.0%	87.7%
Moderate to first normal Pap	33.0%	63.1%	82.9%
Mild to second normal Pap	8.7%	39.1%	62.2%
Moderate to second normal Pap	6.9%	29.0%	53.7%

Pap, Papanicolaou.

Source: Reprinted with permission from APGO Educational Series on Women's Health Issues. Advances in the screening, diagnosis, and treatment of cervical disease. 2002.

ASCCP: American Society for Colposcopy and Cervical Pathology
Definitions of Terms Utilized in the Consensus Guidelines

- *Colposcopy* is the examination of the cervix, vagina, and, in some instances, the vulva with the colposcope after the application of a 3–5% acetic acid solution, coupled with obtaining colposcopically-directed biopsies of all lesions suspected of representing neoplasia.
- *Endocervical sampling* includes obtaining a specimen for either histological evaluation using an endocervical curette or a cytobrush or for cytological evaluation using a cytobrush.
- *Endocervical assessment* is the process of evaluating the endocervical canal for the presence of neoplasia using either a colposcope or endocervical sampling.
- *Diagnostic excisional procedure* is the process of obtaining a specimen from the transformation zone and endocervical canal for histological evaluation and includes laser conization, cold-knife conization, loop electrosurgical excision procedure (i.e., LEEP), and loop electrosurgical conization.
- *Satisfactory colposcopy* indicates that the entire squamocolumnar junction and the margin of any visible lesion can be visualized with the colposcope.
- *Endometrial sampling* includes obtaining a specimen for histological evaluation using an endometrial biopsy or a dilatation and curettage or hysteroscopy.

Cervical Dysplasia—Cervical Intraepithelial Neoplasia GYN-ONCOLOGY

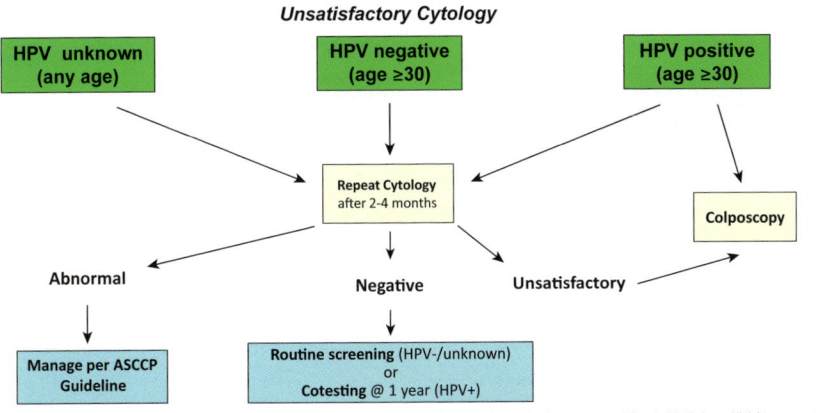

Figure 11.3. Unsatisfactory cytology
Source: Reproduced with permission from Massad LS, Einstein MH, Huh WK, et al. Guidelines for the management of abnormal cervical cancer screening test and cancer precursors. *J Low Genit Tract Dis.* 2013; 17(5):S1-S27. Copyright © 2013 ASCCP. All rights reserved.
Reprinted from *The Journal of Lower Genital Tract Disease* Volume 17, Number 5, with the permission of ASCCP © American Society for Colposcopy and Cervical Pathology 2013. No reproductions of the Work, in whole or in part, may be made without the prior written consent of ASCCP.

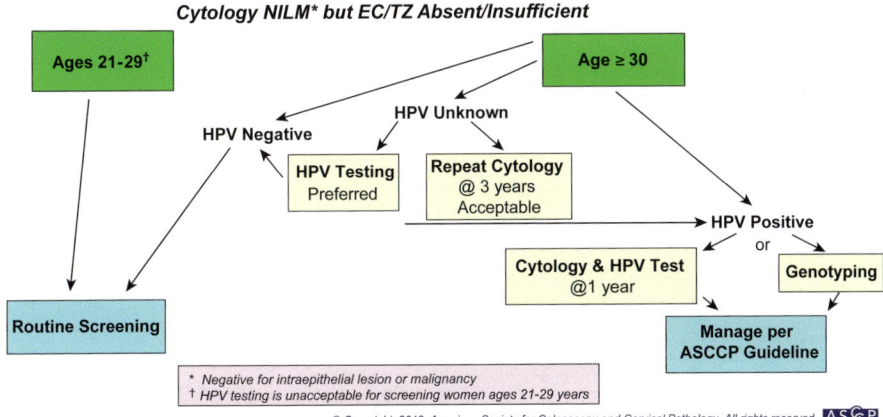

Figure 11.4. Cytology NILM* but EC/TZ Absent/Insufficient
Source: Reproduced with permission from Massad LS, Einstein MH, Huh WK, et al. Guidelines for the management of abnormal cervical cancer screening test and cancer precursors. *J Low Genit Tract Dis.* 2013; 17(5):S1-S27. Copyright © 2013 ASCCP. All rights reserved.
Reprinted from *The Journal of Lower Genital Tract Disease* Volume 17, Number 5, with the permission of ASCCP © American Society for Colposcopy and Cervical Pathology 2013. No reproductions of the Work, in whole or in part, may be made without the prior written consent of ASCCP.

GYN-ONCOLOGY — Cervical Dysplasia—Cervical Intraepithelial Neoplasia

Management of Women ≥ Age 30, who are Cytology Negative, but HPV Positive

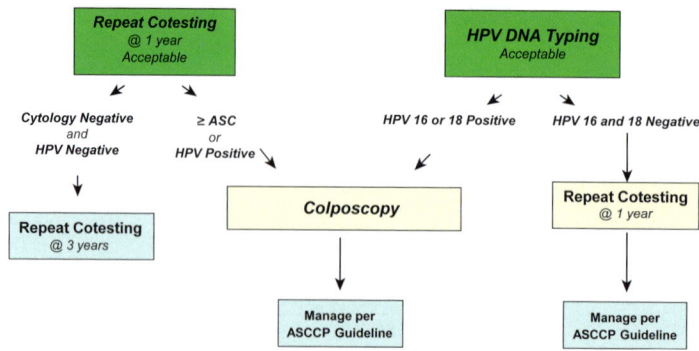

Figure 11.5. Management of women ≥ age 30 who are cytology negative but HPV positive
Source: Reproduced with permission from Massad LS, Einstein MH, Huh WK, et al. Guidelines for the management of abnormal cervical cancer screening test and cancer precursors. *J Low Genit Tract Dis* 2013; 17(5):S1-S27. Copyright © 2013 ASCCP. All rights reserved.
Reprinted from *The Journal of Lower Genital Tract Disease* Volume 17, Number 5, with the permission of ASCCP © American Society for Colposcopy and Cervical Pathology 2013. No reproductions of the Work, in whole or in part, may be made without the prior written consent of ASCCP.

Management of Women with Atypical Squamous Cells of Undetermined Significance (ASC-US) on Cytology*

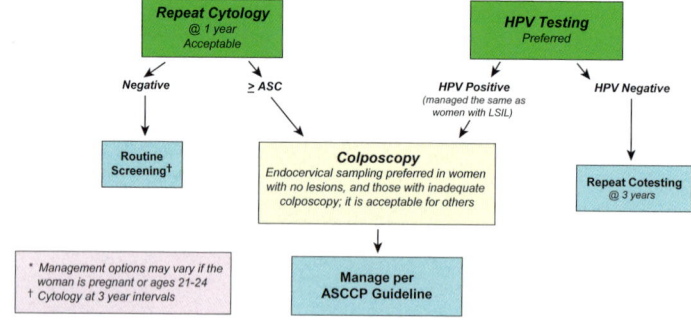

Figure 11.6. Management of women with atypical squamous cells of undetermined significance (ASC-US) on cytology
Source: Reproduced with permission from Massad LS, Einstein MH, Huh WK, et al. Guidelines for the management of abnormal cervical cancer screening test and cancer precursors. *J Low Genit Tract Dis* 2013; 17(5):S1-S27. Copyright © 2013 ASCCP. All rights reserved.
Reprinted from *The Journal of Lower Genital Tract Disease* Volume 17, Number 5, with the permission of ASCCP © American Society for Colposcopy and Cervical Pathology 2013. No reproductions of the Work, in whole or in part, may be made without the prior written consent of ASCCP.

Cervical Dysplasia—Cervical Intraepithelial Neoplasia   GYN-ONCOLOGY

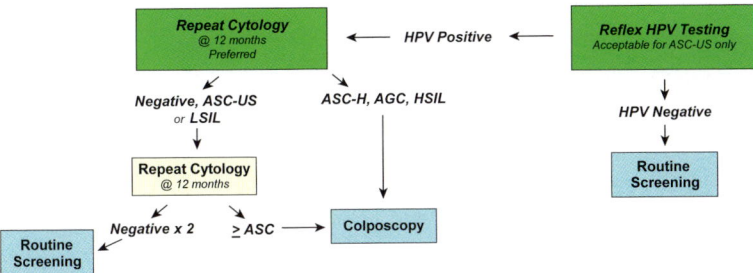

Figure 11.7. Management of women ages 21–24 years with either atypical squamous cells of undetermined significance (ASC-US) or low-grade squamous intraepithelial lesions (LSIL)
Source: Reproduced with permission from Massad LS, Einstein MH, Huh WK, et al. Guidelines for the management of abnormal cervical cancer screening test and cancer precursors. *J Low Genit Tract Dis* 2013; 17(5):S1-S27. Copyright © 2013 ASCCP. All rights reserved.
Reprinted from *The Journal of Lower Genital Tract Disease* Volume 17, Number 5, with the permission of ASCCP © American Society for Colposcopy and Cervical Pathology 2013. No reproductions of the Work, in whole or in part, may be made without the prior written consent of ASCCP.

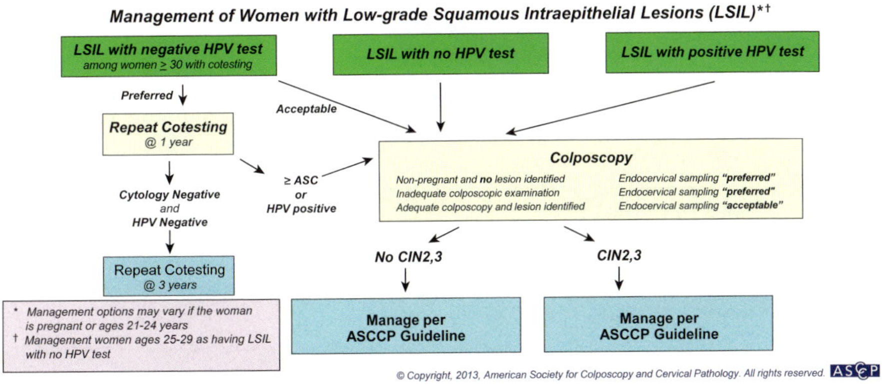

Figure 11.8. Management of women with low-grade squamous intraepithelial lesions (LSIL)
Source: Reproduced with permission from Massad LS, Einstein MH, Huh WK, et al. Guidelines for the management of abnormal cervical cancer screening test and cancer precursors. *J Low Genit Tract Dis* 2013; 17(5):S1-S27. Copyright © 2013 ASCCP. All rights reserved.
Reprinted from *The Journal of Lower Genital Tract Disease* Volume 17, Number 5, with the permission of ASCCP © American Society for Colposcopy and Cervical Pathology 2013. No reproductions of the Work, in whole or in part, may be made without the prior written consent of ASCCP.

GYN-ONCOLOGY
Cervical Dysplasia—Cervical Intraepithelial Neoplasia

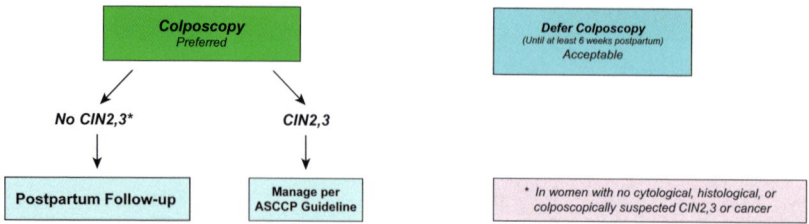

Figure 11.9. Management of pregnant women with low-grade squamous intraepithelial lesions (LSIL)

Source: Reproduced with permission from Massad LS, Einstein MH, Huh WK, et al. Guidelines for the management of abnormal cervical cancer screening test and cancer precursors. *J Low Genit Tract Dis* 2013; 17(5):S1-S27. Copyright © 2013 ASCCP. All rights reserved.

Reprinted from *The Journal of Lower Genital Tract Disease* Volume 17, Number 5, with the permission of ASCCP © American Society for Colposcopy and Cervical Pathology 2013. No reproductions of the Work, in whole or in part, may be made without the prior written consent of ASCCP.

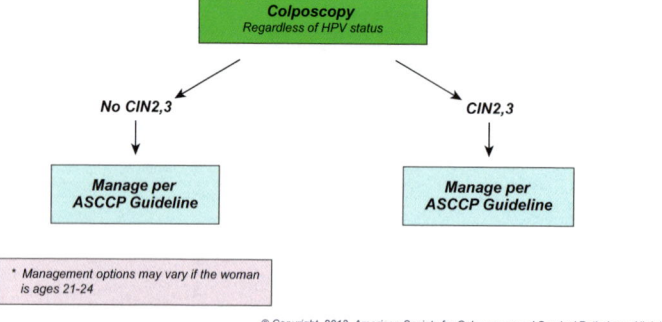

Figure 11.10. Management of women with atypical squamous cells: cannot exclude high-grade SIL (ASC-H)

Source: Reproduced with permission from Massad LS, Einstein MH, Huh WK, et al. Guidelines for the management of abnormal cervical cancer screening test and cancer precursors. *J Low Genit Tract Dis* 2013; 17(5):S1-S27. Copyright © 2013 ASCCP. All rights reserved.

Reprinted from *The Journal of Lower Genital Tract Disease* Volume 17, Number 5, with the permission of ASCCP © American Society for Colposcopy and Cervical Pathology 2013. No reproductions of the Work, in whole or in part, may be made without the prior written consent of ASCCP.

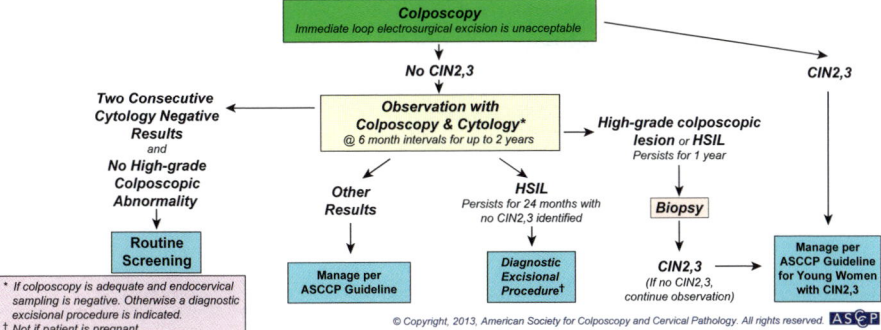

Figure 11.11. Management of women ages 21–24 yr with atypical squamous cells: cannot exclude high-grade SIL (ASC-H) and high-grade squamous intraepithelial lesion (HSIL)
Source: Reproduced with permission from Massad LS, Einstein MH, Huh WK, et al. Guidelines for the management of abnormal cervical cancer screening test and cancer precursors. *J Low Genit Tract Dis* 2013; 17(5):S1-S27. Copyright © 2013 ASCCP. All rights reserved.
Reprinted from *The Journal of Lower Genital Tract Disease* Volume 17, Number 5, with the permission of ASCCP © American Society for Colposcopy and Cervical Pathology 2013. No reproductions of the Work, in whole or in part, may be made without the prior written consent of ASCCP.

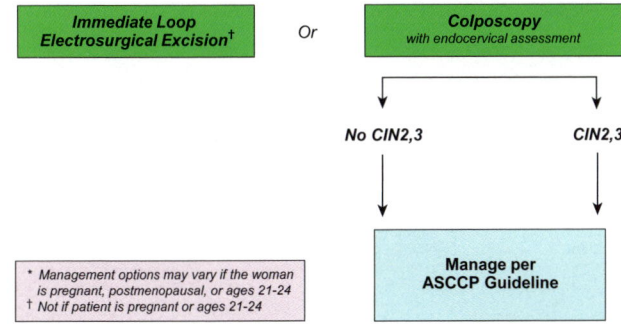

Figure 11.12. Management of women with high-grade squamous intraepithelial lesion (HSIL)
Source: Reproduced with permission from Massad LS, Einstein MH, Huh WK, et al. Guidelines for the management of abnormal cervical cancer screening test and cancer precursors. *J Low Genit Tract Dis* 2013; 17(5):S1-S27. Copyright © 2013 ASCCP. All rights reserved.
Reprinted from *The Journal of Lower Genital Tract Disease* Volume 17, Number 5, with the permission of ASCCP © American Society for Colposcopy and Cervical Pathology 2013. No reproductions of the Work, in whole or in part, may be made without the prior written consent of ASCCP.

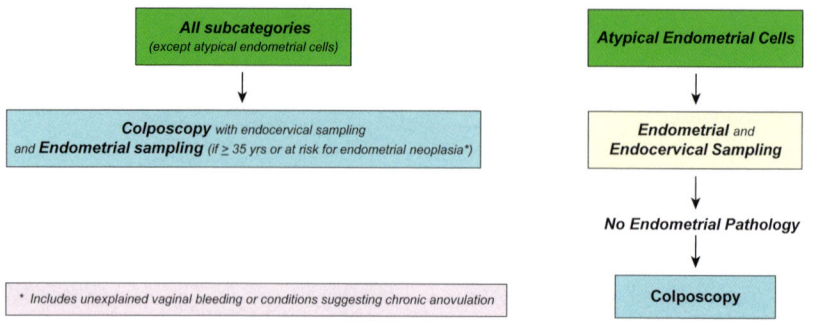

Figure 11.13. Initial workup of women with atypical glandular cells (AGC)
Source: Reproduced with permission from Massad LS, Einstein MH, Huh WK, et al. Guidelines for the management of abnormal cervical cancer screening test and cancer precursors. *J Low Genit Tract Dis* 2013; 17(5):S1-S27. Copyright © 2013 ASCCP. All rights reserved.

Reprinted from *The Journal of Lower Genital Tract Disease* Volume 17, Number 5, with the permission of ASCCP © American Society for Colposcopy and Cervical Pathology 2013. No reproductions of the Work, in whole or in part, may be made without the prior written consent of ASCCP.

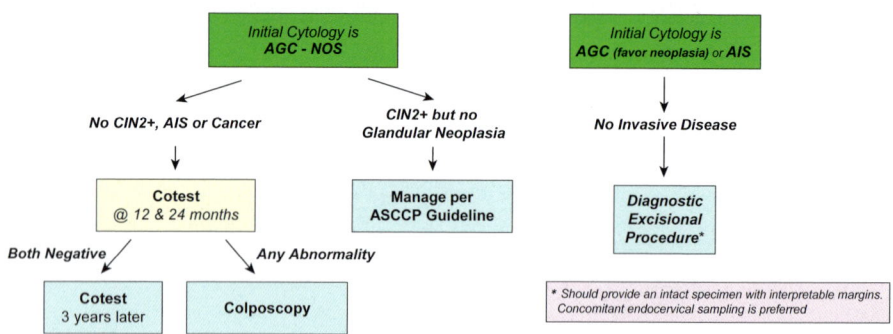

Figure 11.14. Subsequent management of women with atypical glandular cells (AGC)
Source: Reproduced with permission from Massad LS, Einstein MH, Huh WK, et al. Guidelines for the management of abnormal cervical cancer screening test and cancer precursors. *J Low Genit Tract Dis* 2013; 17(5):S1-S27. Copyright © 2013 ASCCP. All rights reserved.

Reprinted from *The Journal of Lower Genital Tract Disease* Volume 17, Number 5, with the permission of ASCCP © American Society for Colposcopy and Cervical Pathology 2013. No reproductions of the Work, in whole or in part, may be made without the prior written consent of ASCCP.

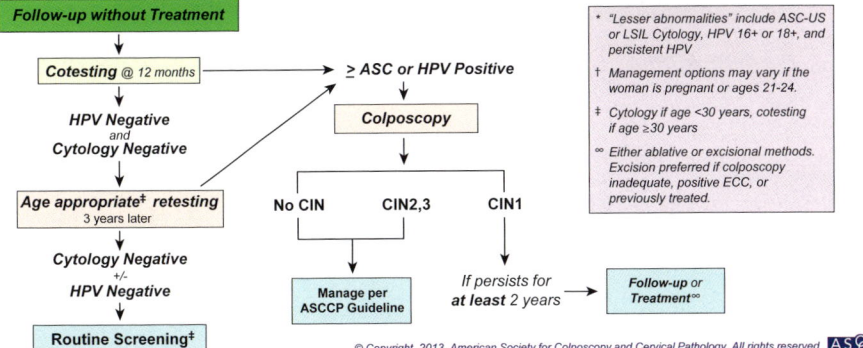

Figure 11.15. Management of women with no lesion or biopsy-confirmed cervical intraepithelial neoplasia—grade 1 (CIN1) preceded by "lesser abnormalities"

Source: Reproduced with permission from Massad LS, Einstein MH, Huh WK, et al. Guidelines for the management of abnormal cervical cancer screening test and cancer precursors. *J Low Genit Tract Dis* 2013; 17(5):S1-S27. Copyright © 2013 ASCCP. All rights reserved.

Reprinted from *The Journal of Lower Genital Tract Disease* Volume 17, Number 5, with the permission of ASCCP © American Society for Colposcopy and Cervical Pathology 2013. No reproductions of the Work, in whole or in part, may be made without the prior written consent of ASCCP.

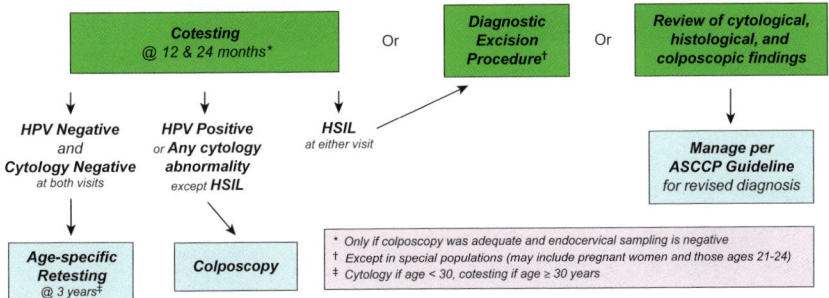

Figure 11.16. Management of women with no lesion or biopsy-confirmed cervical intraepithelial neoplasia—grade 1 (CIN1) preceded by ASC-H or HSIL cytology

Source: Reproduced with permission from Massad LS, Einstein MH, Huh WK, et al. Guidelines for the management of abnormal cervical cancer screening test and cancer precursors. *J Low Genit Tract Dis* 2013; 17(5):S1-S27. Copyright © 2013 ASCCP. All rights reserved.

Reprinted from *The Journal of Lower Genital Tract Disease* Volume 17, Number 5, with the permission of ASCCP © American Society for Colposcopy and Cervical Pathology 2013. No reproductions of the Work, in whole or in part, may be made without the prior written consent of ASCCP.

GYN-ONCOLOGY — Cervical Dysplasia—Cervical Intraepithelial Neoplasia

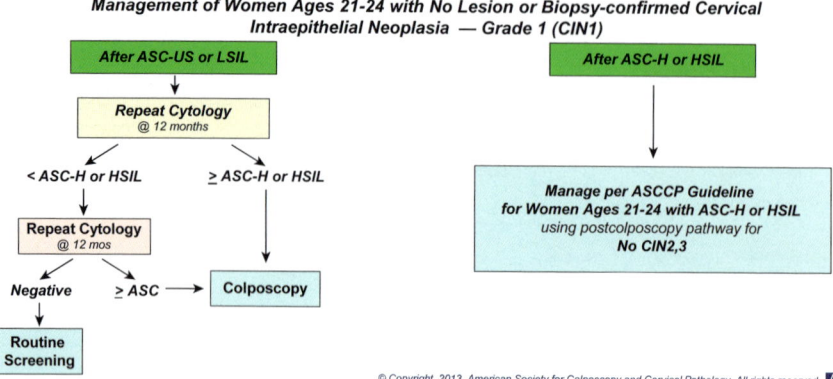

Figure 11.17. Management of women with no lesion or biopsy-confirmed cervical intraepithelial neoplasia—grade 1 (CIN1)
Source: Reproduced with permission from Massad LS, Einstein MH, Huh WK, et al. Guidelines for the management of abnormal cervical cancer screening test and cancer precursors. *J Low Genit Tract Dis* 2013; 17(5):S1-S27. Copyright © 2013 ASCCP. All rights reserved.
Reprinted from *The Journal of Lower Genital Tract Disease* Volume 17, Number 5, with the permission of ASCCP © American Society for Colposcopy and Cervical Pathology 2013. No reproductions of the Work, in whole or in part, may be made without the prior written consent of ASCCP.

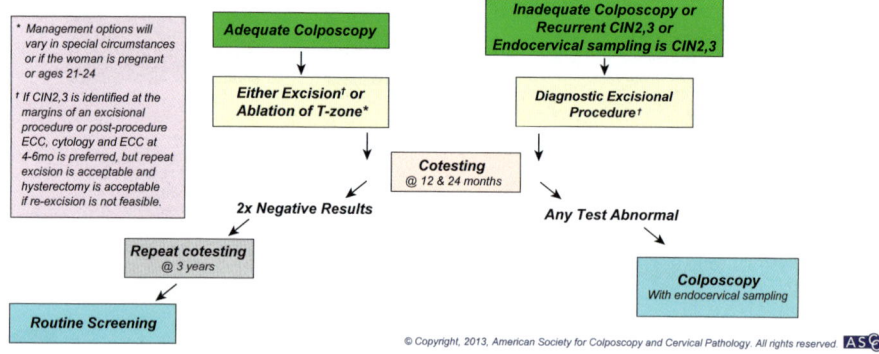

Figure 11.18. Management of women with biopsy-confirmed cervical intraepithelial neoplasia—grades 2 and 3 (CIN2, 3)
Source: Reproduced with permission from Massad LS, Einstein MH, Huh WK, et al. Guidelines for the management of abnormal cervical cancer screening test and cancer precursors. *J Low Genit Tract Dis* 2013; 17(5):S1-S27. Copyright © 2013 ASCCP. All rights reserved.
Reprinted from *The Journal of Lower Genital Tract Disease* Volume 17, Number 5, with the permission of ASCCP © American Society for Colposcopy and Cervical Pathology 2013. No reproductions of the Work, in whole or in part, may be made without the prior written consent of ASCCP.

Cervical Dysplasia—Cervical Intraepithelial Neoplasia **GYN-ONCOLOGY**

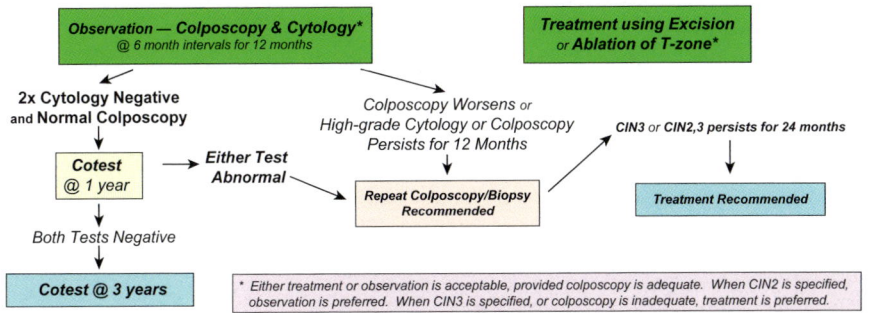

Figure 11.19. Management of young women with biopsy-confirmed cervical intraepithelial neoplasia—grades 2 and 3 (CIN2, 3) in special circumstances

Source: Reproduced with permission from Massad LS, Einstein MH, Huh WK, et al. Guidelines for the management of abnormal cervical cancer screening test and cancer precursors. *J Low Genit Tract Dis* 2013; 17(5):S1-S27. Copyright © 2013 ASCCP. All rights reserved.

Reprinted from *The Journal of Lower Genital Tract Disease* Volume 17, Number 5, with the permission of ASCCP © American Society for Colposcopy and Cervical Pathology 2013. No reproductions of the Work, in whole or in part, may be made without the prior written consent of ASCCP.

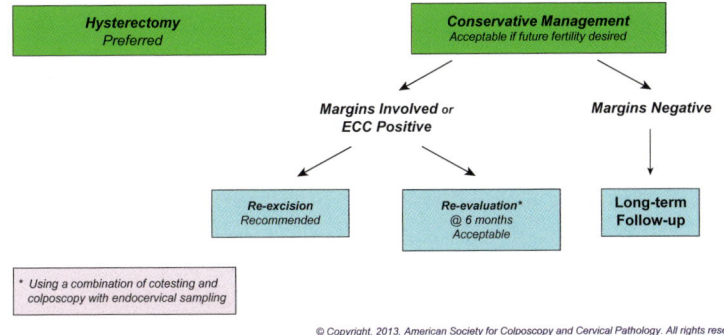

Figure 11.20. Management of women diagnosed with adenocarcinoma in situ (AIS) during a diagnostic excisional procedure

Source: Reproduced with permission from Massad LS, Einstein MH, Huh WK, et al. Guidelines for the management of abnormal cervical cancer screening test and cancer precursors. *J Low Genit Tract Dis* 2013; 17(5):S1-S27. Copyright © 2013 ASCCP. All rights reserved.

Management of Cervical Dysplasia in Pregnancy
- Women 20 years of age and younger with ASC-US or LSIL will have a 90% rate of spontaneous resolution. Colposcopy during pregnancy can be omitted, but cytology should be repeated postpartum.
- For women over 20 years of age, ASC-US and LSIL can be managed as in the nonpregnant patient with the exception that it is acceptable to defer colposcopy to at least 6 weeks postpartum.
- For ASC-H, HSIL, or AGC, colposcopy is recommended for all ages.
- At colposcopy, biopsy areas suspicious for CIN 2/3.
- Okay to use Monsel's solution or suture for any bleeding encountered during the biopsy.
- If colposcopy is unsatisfactory early in pregnancy, repeat the procedure in 6–12 weeks since the transformation zone may have migrated to the ectocervix, allowing a satisfactory exam by 20 weeks of gestation.
- Do not perform endocervical curettage in pregnant women.
- Diagnostic conization is only indicated in pregnancy if confirmation of invasive disease will later the timing or mode of delivery; otherwise postpone conization until the postpartum period.
- If conization needs to be performed, optimal time appears to be in the 2nd trimester between 14 and 20 weeks of gestation. Avoid cervical conization within 4 weeks of estimated date of delivery to prevent conization area to bleed or extend.
- Consider performing a "coin"-shaped specimen instead of a "cone"-shaped to limit disruption of endocervical canal.

CERVICAL CANCER

Fast Facts
- Incidence in United States has declined by 1/3 over the past 20 years.
  - 12,000 new cases in 2014
  - 4000 cancer related deaths in 2014
- Worldwide, cervical cancer is second only to breast cancer.
  - 86% of cases are in developing countries.

Risk Factors
- Early onset of sexual activity
- Multiple sexual partners, high parity
- History of other sexually transmitted diseases
- Smoking—associated with squamous cell carcinoma of cervix and not adenocarcinoma of cervix
- OCPs—may be associated with metabolite of estradiol, 16 alpha-hydroxyestrone, which can act as a cofactor with oncogenic HPV to promote cell proliferation
- Human papillomavirus (HPV) infection
  - Most important risk factor—over 70 distinct HPV subtypes
  - 75–80% sexually active adults have evidence of HPV infection by age 50
  - HPV DNA is present in 99.7% of cervical cancers
  - Subtypes determine clinical disease
  - HPV 6, 11: majority of genital warts (condyloma acuminate)
  - HPV 16, 18: found in 70% of cervical cancer cases
  - Squamous cell carcinoma —HPV 16 (59% of cases), 18 (13%), 58 (5%), 33 (5%), 45 (4%)
  - Adenocarcinoma—HPV 16 (36%), 18 (37%), 45 (5%), 31 (2%), 33 (2%)
  - Most HPV infections are transient, virus alone is not sufficient to cause cervical neoplasia. Takes an average of 15 years from time of initial infection to high-grade CIN to invasive cancer.
  - See page 439 for information regarding HPV vaccine

Symptoms
- Vaginal discharge, abnormal bleeding (pre- or postmenopausal), postcoital bleeding, pelvic pain/mass

Histolopathology
- Squamous cell cancer (69%)
  - Large cell, small cell, and verrucous
- Adenocarcinoma (25%)
  - Endocervical, endometrioid, clear cell, adenoid cystic, adenoma malignum
- Other histologies (6%)

Diagnosis
- Screening Pap—Identifies preinvasive and invasive neoplasia, scraping superficial cells from squamocolumnar junction and endocervix.

- Colposcopy—This is a direct biopsy. Use 3–5% acetic acid on cervix. Green filter accentuates vascular pattern. Adequate colpo entire transformation zone is visualized. Acetowhite changes—acetic acid reacts with nuclei so more cellular areas reflect white.
- Cone biopsy/loop electrosurgical excision procedure—Procedure allows adequate evaluation if colposcopy is inadequate.

Workup for Cervical Cancer
- Complete history and physical, including rectovaginal exam. Palpate right-upper quadrant, inguinal, and supraclavicular to assess for metastatic disease.
- To establish extent of disease: Cystoscopy, proctoscopy, intravenous pyelogram, radiographic examination of lungs and bones (approved as tests for FIGO staging).
- PET/CT scan for retroperitoneal and upper abdominal disease (results will not affect FIGO staging). PET/CT has a sensitivity of 93–96% and specificity of 93–95%.
- Complete blood count and renal and liver function tests.
- Remember that staging for cervical cancer is clinical not surgical.

Cervical Cancer

Table 11.11. Cervical cancer staging and treatment

STAGE	Cervical Carcinoma Confined to Uterus	Treatment
Stage I		
IA	Diagnosed only by microscopy	
IA1	Stromal invasion ≤3 mm in depth and ≤7 mm in horizontal spread	Cone biopsy or extrafascial hysterectomy + pelvic lymph nodes (LN) if cone margins are positive*
IA2	Stromal invasion >3 mm and ≤5 mm in depth and ≤7 mm in horizontal spread	Modified radical hysterectomy +/- adjuvant RT#
IB	Clinically visible lesion confined to the cervix or microscopic lesion greater than IA1/IA2	
IB1	Clinically visible lesion ≤4 cm	Radical hysterectomy + pelvic LN +/- adjuvant pelvic RT#
IB2	Clinically visible lesion >4 cm	Radical hysterectomy + pelvic LN +/- para-aortic LN +/- adjuvant RT# vs. definitive pelvic chemoradiation + brachytherapy vs. pelvic chemoradiation + adjuvant hysterectomy
Stage II	Cervical carcinoma invades beyond the uterus but not to the pelvic wall or to the lower 1/3 of the vagina	
IIA	Tumor without parametrial invasion or involvement of the lower 1/3 of the vagina	
IIA1	Clinically visible lesion ≤4 cm with involvement of less than the upper 2/3 of the vagina	Radical hysterectomy + pelvic LN +/- para-aortic LN +/- adjuvant RT# vs. primary pelvic chemoradiation + brachytherapy
IIA2	Visible lesion >4 cm with involvement of less than upper 2/3 of the vagina	Primary chemoradiation + brachytherapy vs. radical hysterectomy + pelvic LN +/- para-aortic LN vs. pelvic chemoradiation + brachytherapy + adjuvant hysterectomy
IIB	Tumor with parametrial invasion	Primary pelvic chemoradiation + brachytherapy
Stage III	Tumor extends to pelvic wall and/or involves lower 1/3 of vagina and/or causes hydronephrosis or nonfunctioning kidney	
IIIA	Tumor involves lower 1/3 of vagina with no extension to pelvic wall	Primary pelvic chemoradiation + brachytherapy
IIIB	Tumor extends to pelvic wall and/or causes hydronephrosis or nonfunctioning kidney	Primary pelvic chemoradiation + brachytherapy
Stage IVA	Tumor invades mucosa of bladder or rectum and/or extends beyond true pelvis (bullous edema is not sufficient to classify as stage IV)	Primary pelvic chemoradiation + brachytherapy
Stage IVB	Distant metastasis (including peritoneal spread, involvement of supraclavicular, mediastinal, or paraaortic lymph nodes, lung, liver, or bone)	Platinum-based regimen + paclitaxel + bevacizumab^

Source: Pecorelli S. Revised FIGO staging for carcinoma of the vulva, cervix, and endometrium. *Int J Gynaecol Obstet.* 2009;105(2):103-104. Copyright © 2009 International Federation of Gynecology and Obstetrics.

*Treatment option for women with no evidence of intermediate-risk (tumor size >2 cm, presence of LVSI, and/or deep cervical stromal invasion) or high-risk features (pathologically involved lymph nodes, parametrial invasion, positive surgical margins).

^Based on GOG 240 (Tewari 2014).

Lymphovascular Space Invasion (LVSI)	Stromal Invasion	Tumor Size
Present	Deep 1/3 cervical stromal invasion	Any size
Present	Middle 1/3 stromal invasion	≥2 cm
Present	Superficial 1/3 stromal invasion	≥5 cm
None	Deep or middle 1/3 stromal invasion	≥4 cm

- Adjuvant radiation therapy should be administered based on **Sedlis criteria** to define those at intermediate risk:

Radical Trachelectomy
- Indication: Desire for future childbearing + any of the following: stage IA1 +/-LVSI, stage IA2 disease, stage IB1, ≤2 cm lesion size with limited endocervical extension, no metastasis to lymph nodes. LVSI is a risk factor for lymph node recurrence but not a contraindication for trachelectomy.
  - Procedure: Cervix and parametria resected with placement of cerclage. Can be performed transvaginally or transabdominally or combined with laparoscopic pelvic, para-aortic lymphadenectomy.
    - Complications: Vascular and urinary tract trauma. Estimated 10–17% planned procedures are abandoned due to extensive disease found at time of surgery.
  - Survival: 97% recurrence-free survival, 98% overall survival; 20% risk of preterm delivery and 50% rate of vaginal delivery.

Radical Hysterectomy
- Indication: IB1, IB2, IIA1, IIA2.
- Procedure: Excision of uterus, upper 1/3 vagina, uterosacral ligaments divided near sacral origin, parametria pelvic node dissection, dissection of uterine artery to origin on hypogastric, and ovaries can be preserved.
- Complications: Most common is bladder dysfunction.
  - Fistula in 0–3%.
- Survival: 90% at 5 years, 75% for stage I.

Radiation Therapy (XRT)
- External beam and intracavitary radium.
  - Small bowel tolerates 4000–5000 rads.
  - External beam can deliver only 4000–5000 rads but can give 6000 in intracavitary sources.
  - Point A: 2 cm superior and 2 cm lateral to external os. This area is parametrial tissues.
  - Point B: 3 cm lateral to point A. This area is pelvic nodes.
- Survival: 90% at 5 years for stage I.

Follow-up
- Recurrent cervical cancer.
- Symptoms: Weight loss, leg edema, vaginal discharge, symptoms of ureteral obstruction (pain, uremia).
- Estimated 95% post-therapy ureteral obstructions are recurrent disease. Treatment with placement of ureteral stent.

Cervical Cancer

- About 75% occur in first 2 years following treatment. Most recurrences are local.
- Central recurrences may be treated with pelvic exenteration.
  - Operative mortality is 5%.
  - Survival: 30% at 5 years.
- Survival (following appropriate treatment) at 5 years
  - Stage IA—95%
  - Stage IB—80%
  - Stage IIA—63%
  - Stage IIB—58%
  - Stage III—30%
  - Stage IVA—16%

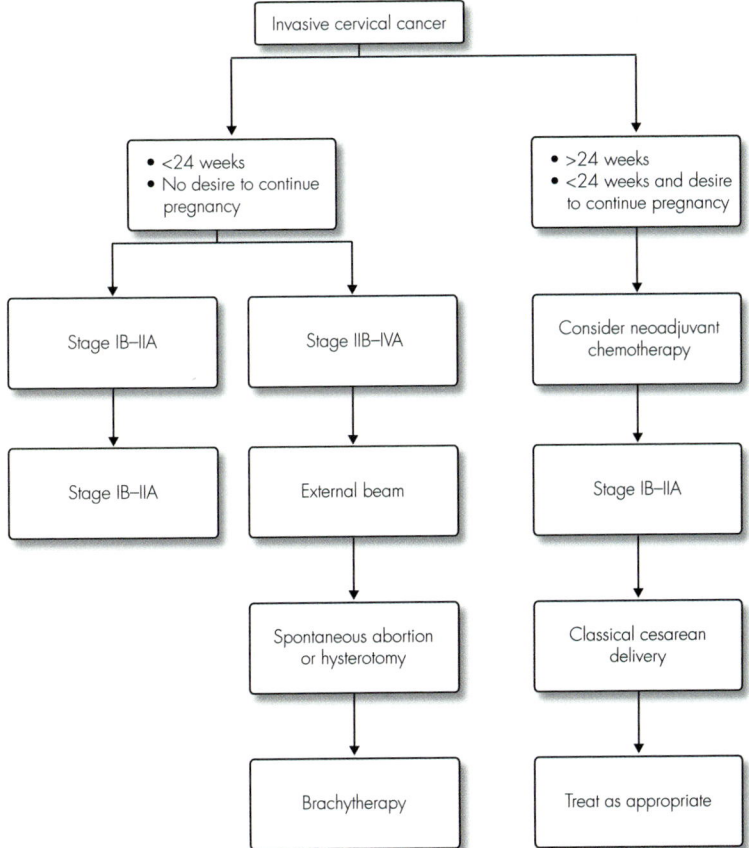

Figure 11.21. Management of cervical cancer in pregnancy
Source: Reproduced with permission from Berek JS, Hacker NF, eds. *Practical Gynecologic Oncology*. 4th Ed. Philadelphia (PA): Lippincott Williams & Wilkins; 2005.

ADNEXAL MASSES

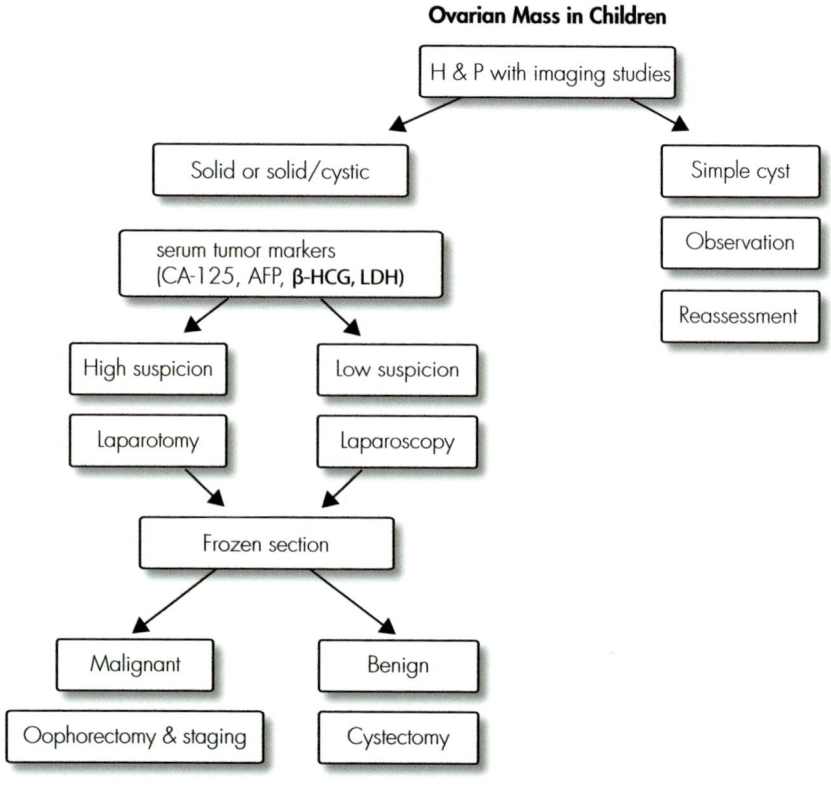

Figure 11.22. Evaluation of an adnexal mass in a pediatric patient

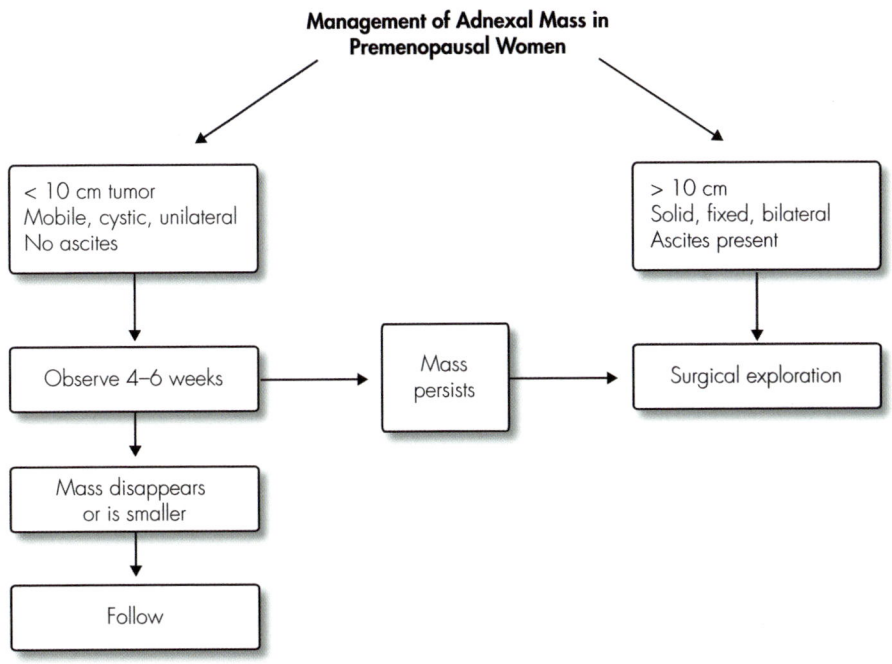

Figure 11.23. Management of an adnexal mass in a premenopausal patient

GYN-ONCOLOGY — Adnexal Masses

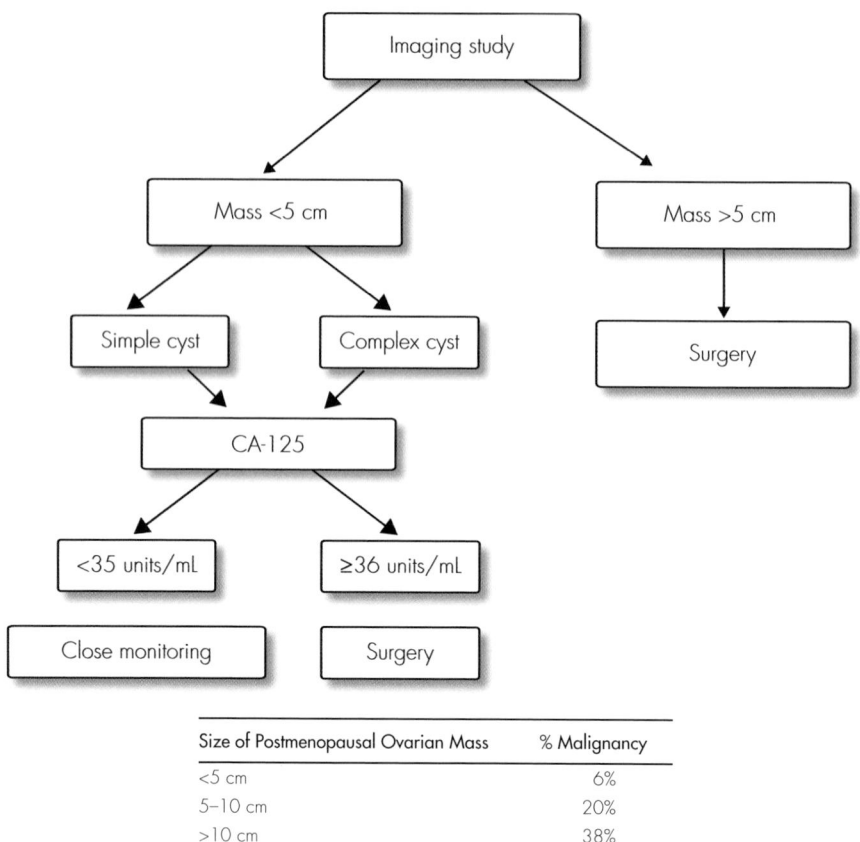

Figure 11.24. Management of an adnexal mass in postmenopausal patient

EPITHELIAL OVARIAN CANCER

Definition/Background
- Second most common gynecologic malignancy
- Most common cause of death from gynecologic malignancy
- Ovarian cancer patients usually die secondary to bowel obstruction
- No reliable screening test available
- Median age of diagnosis 60–64 years

Risk Factors
- Family history—strongest known risk factor; found in about 10–15% of women with ovarian cancer
- Hereditary nonpolyposis colorectal cancer/Lynch syndrome II (3–14% risk of ovarian cancer)
- *BRCA1*—absolute risk of developing ovarian cancer over a lifetime is 35–45%
- *BRCA2*—absolute risk of developing ovarian cancer over a lifetime is 15–25%

Protective Factors
- Multiparity
- Oral contraceptive use
- Prior breastfeeding (lactational amenorrhea and anovulation)

Symptoms/Signs
- Abdominal discomfort, upper abdominal fullness, early satiety, fatigue, urinary frequency, dyspnea
- Pelvic mass, bilateral irregularity, solid or fixed mass, ascites or nodular cul-de-sac

Histopathology
- Epithelial (59%)
- Serous cystadenocarcinoma (46%)
  - Bilateral presentation with psammoma bodies
- Mucinous (36%)
- Undifferentiated (15%)
- Endometrioid (8%)
- Clear cell (3%)
- Hobnail appearance on pathology
  - Clear cell cancers may be associated with worse prognosis
- Brenner's (2%)
- Squamous (<1%)

Pretreatment Evaluation
- Complete history and physical examination including pelvic and rectovaginal examination, CT scan, ultrasound.
- Obtain tumor markers that can include the following:
  - CA-125—Refer to gyn-oncologist: CA-125 >200 U/mL in premenopausal women, CA-125 >35 U/mL in postmenopausal women, ascites, or family history of breast or ovarian cancer in a first-degree relative (ACOG Committee opinion 2002).

- HE4—Approved by FDA in 2008 for monitoring for recurrent or progressive disease in patients with EOC. Also used as a component of the ROMA (Risk of Ovarian Malignancy Algorithm).
- CEA—Elevated in mucinous tumors and may also be elevated in cancers of the breast, pancreas, thyroid, and lung.
- OVA-1—Approved by the FDA in 2009 to further assess the likelihood of malignancy in women who are planning to have surgery for an adnexal mass. OVA-1 incorporates 5 proteins (CA125 and beta 2 microglobulin are up-regulated; transferrin, transthyretin, and apolipoprotein A1 are down-regulated).

Five-Year Survival
- Stage IA-IC = 90–83%
- Stage IIA-IIC = 86–71%
- Stage IIIA-C = 47%–32%
- Stage IV = 19%

Epithelial Ovarian Cancer — GYN-ONCOLOGY

Table 11.12. Ovarian, fallopian tube, peritoneal cancer staging and treatment

Stage		Treatment^
Stage I	Tumor confined to ovaries or fallopian tubes	
IA	Tumor limited to one ovary (capsule intact) or one fallopian tube; no surface involvement; negative ascites or washings	Observation for grade 1 tumors. For grade 2, consider observation vs. adjuvant taxane/carboplatin
IB	Tumor limited to both ovaries (capsules intact) or both fallopian tubes; no surface involvement; negative ascites or washings	Observation for grade 1 tumors. Adjuvant taxane/carboplatin for 3 vs. 6 cycles
IC	Tumor limited to one or both ovaries or fallopian tubes with any of the following:	Adjuvant taxane/carboplatin for 3–6 cycles
IC1	Surgical spill	Adjuvant taxane/carboplatin for 3 vs. 6 cycles
IC2	Capsule ruptured before surgery or tumor on ovarian or fallopian tube surface	Adjuvant taxane/carboplatin for 3 vs. 6 cycles
IC3	Malignant cells in the ascites or peritoneal washings	Adjuvant taxane/carboplatin for 3 vs. 6 cycles
Stage II	Tumor involves one or both ovaries or fallopian tubes with pelvic extension (below pelvic brim) or peritoneal cancer	
IIA	Extension and/or implants on uterus and/or tube(s) and/or ovaries	Adjuvant taxane/carboplatin for 3 vs. 6 cycles
IIB	Extension to other pelvic intraperitoneal tissues	Adjuvant taxane/carboplatin for 6 cycles
Stage III	Tumor involves one or both ovaries or fallopian tubes, or peritoneal cancer, with cytologically or histologically confirmed spread to the peritoneum outside the pelvis and/or metastasis to the retroperitoneal lymph nodes	Can consider neoadjuvant chemotherapy + interval debulking + adjuvant chemotherapy vs. primary debulking surgery + adjuvant chemotherapy*
IIIA	Positive retroperitoneal nodes and/or microscopic metastasis beyond pelvis	
IIIA1	Positive retroperitoneal lymph nodes only (cytologically or histologically proven)	
IIIA1(i)	Metastasis up to 10 mm in greatest dimension	
IIIA1(ii)	Metastasis more than 10 mm in greatest dimension	
IIIA2	Microscopic (above the brim) peritoneal involvement, with or without positive retroperitoneal lymph nodes	
IIIB	Macroscopic peritoneal metastasis beyond pelvis up to 2 cm in greatest dimension with or without positive retroperitoneal lymph nodes	
IIIC	Macroscopic peritoneal metastasis beyond pelvis more than 2 cm in greatest dimension (includes extension of tumor to capsule of liver and spleen without parenchymal involvement of either organ) with or without positive retroperitoneal lymph nodes	

(continued)

GYN-ONCOLOGY — Epithelial Ovarian Cancer

Stage		Treatment^
Stage IV	Distant metastases excluding peritoneal metastases	Can consider neoadjuvant chemotherapy + interval debulking + adjuvant chemotherapy vs. primary debulking surgery + adjuvant chemotherapy*
IVA	Pleural effusion with positive cytology	
IVB	Parenchymal metastases and metastases to extra-abdominal organs (including inguinal lymph nodes and lymph nodes outside the abdominal cavity)	

^Treatment includes surgical resection for all patients, which includes bilateral salpingo-oophorectomy, hysterectomy, omentectomy, pelvic and para-aortic lymphadenectomy, tumor debulking, possible uterolysis, possible bowel resection. Adjuvant treatment includes chemotherapy as outlined in the table.

*Intraperitoneal chemotherapy with platinum and taxane should be considered as a first-line treatment option for women with stage III ovarian, fallopian tube, peritoneal cancer after optimal cytoreductive surgery (NCI Clinical Alert in January 2006 strongly encouraged the use of IP chemotherapy in this subset of patients)

**Bevacizumab and olaparib are FDA approved for use in the relapsed setting.

Source: Prat J; FIGO Committee on Gynecologic Oncology. Staging classification for cancer of the ovary, fallopian tube, and peritoneum. *Int J Gynaecol Obstet.* 2014 Jan;124(1):1-5.

Treatment of Ovarian Cancer

- Targeted therapies such as bevacizumab and PARP inhibitors have been FDA approved.
- Bevacizumab IV + chemotherapy (either topotecan, liposomal doxorubicin, and paclitaxel) has been FDA approved in treatment of recurrent, platinum-resistant ovarian cancer.
  - Bevacizumab is an antibody against VEGF-A (ligand for VEGF receptor).
  - Any patient treated with bevacizumab should be considered at risk for new or worsening hypertension, proteinuria, thrombotic events, bleeding, altered wound healing, and gastrointestinal perforation.
  - Hypertension is the most common side effect, and management should be initiated when BP >140/90 mm Hg. Multiple antihypertensive drugs are being used to treat antiangiogenic therapy-induced hypertension, including calcium channel blockers (CCB), ACE inhibitors (ACEi), ARBs, beta-blockers, and diuretics. No clinical evidence favors one antihypertensive agent over another. In general, CCB (such as amlodipine) and ACEi are generally effective in treating antiangiogenic therapy-induced hypertension. ACEi are a good choice for treatment of antiangiogenic therapy-induced hypertension in the setting of proteinuria.
  - For proteinuria, refer to nephrologist if proteinuria is >1 g/24hrs and/or is accompanied by acute kidney injury.
- PARP 1 and PARP2 inhibitor–PO (olaparib) has been FDA approved in the treatment of recurrent ovarian cancer of patients with deleterious germline *BRCA* mutation who have been treated with three or more prior lines of chemotherapy.
  - Side effects include fatigue, thrombocytopenia, dyspepsia, altered taste, stomatitis, anemia, nausea, vomiting, diarrhea.

OVARIAN GERM CELL TUMORS
Fast Facts
- Derived from primordial germ cells.
- Germ cell tumors account for 20–25% of ovarian neoplasms but only 5% of malignant ovarian neoplasms.
- Tumors grow rapidly, but most present with stage IA disease.
- Presents in 10–30-year-olds (median age 22)—represents 70% of ovarian tumors in this age group.
- Malignant ovarian germ cell tumors occur more often in Asians/African Americans than Caucasians (3:1).

Signs and Symptoms
- Abdominal pain and mass—both symptoms seen in 85% of patients
- Precocious puberty (if estrogen-secreting tumor)
- Symptoms similar to pregnancy (from human chorionic gonadotropin [hCG] production)
- Tumors tend to be large—16 cm

Tumor Types
- Benign: Mature cystic teratoma (dermoid cyst)
- Malignant:
    - Immature teratomas are the only malignant ovarian germ cell tumors that are histologically graded.
        - <1% of all teratomas
    - Bilateral ovarian disease is most common in dysgerminomas.

Table 11.13. Types of malignant germ cell tumors

Type	%
Immature teratomas	35.6
Dysgerminomas	32.8
Endodermal sinus	14.5
Mixed germ cell tumors	5.3
Embryonal	4.1
Mature teratomas with malignant degeneration	2.9
Teratocarcinoma	2.6
Choriocarcinoma	2.1

Source: Adapted from Smith HO, Berwick M, Verschraegen CF, Wiggins C, Lansing L, Muller CY, Qualls CR. Incidence and survival rates for female malignant germ cell tumors. *Obstet Gynecol.* 2006 May;107(5):1075-85.

Dysgerminoma
- Derived from germ cells and exquisitely radiosensitive
- Tumor rarely produces hCG and ± pregnancy test in non–sexually active patient
    - Pathology shows lymphocytic infiltration

- Treatment: unilateral salpingo-oophorectomy (USO) with close inspection of other ovary (15% bilateral)
  - Adjuvant chemotherapy for all except stage I dysgerminoma and well-differentiated stage I immature teratoma Adjuvant chemotherapy (bleomycin, etoposide, cis-platin [BEP] x3) for all except stage I dysgerminoma
- Recurrence: treated with chemotherapy with good success

Endodermal Sinus Tumor
- Median age at diagnosis is 19 years
- Secretes alpha-fetoprotein
- Pathology: invaginated papillary structure with central blood vessel called "Schiller-Duvall Body"
- Treatment: surgery (USO) and chemotherapy (bleomycin, etoposide, cisplatin [BEP] x3; 95% curative)
- Prognosis: very poor, if no chemotherapy, 85% recur

Embryonal Carcinoma
- Derived from primordial germ cells
- Very rare; occurs during childhood
- Presents with precocious puberty or mass
- Secretes AFP and hCG
- Treatment: Surgery and chemotherapy (bleomycin, etoposide, cis-platin [BEP] x3)
- Prognosis: poor

Choriocarcinoma
- Gestational = characteristics similar to uterine choriocarcinoma
- Non-gestational = resistant to chemotherapy
- Secretes hCG
- Pathology: Arias stella reaction, increased aromatism, increased pleomorphism, increased mitotic activity

Gonadoblastoma
- Associated with abnormal karyotype (gonadal dysgenesis associated with presence of Y chromosome)
- Symptoms: primary amenorrhea, virilization, or genital developmental problems
- Dysgerminoma often coexists forming a mixed germ cell tumor
- Therapy: bilateral salpingo-oophorectomy
- Prognosis: good

Immature Teratoma
- Malignant corollary of cystic teratoma with three germ cell layers
- Pathology: immature embryonic elements with neural elements
- Rare, almost never bilateral, occurs in first 2 decades of life
- Prognosis: poor, but depends on grade (level of neural elements) and presence of immature implants

Ovarian Germ Cell Tumors — GYN-ONCOLOGY

Table 11.14. Tumor markers in germ cell cancer

Histology	Tumor Marker		
	AFP	hCG	LDH
Dysgerminoma	rare	rare	+
Endodermal sinus tumor (yolk sac)	++	−	+
Immature teratoma	±	−	±
Mixed germ cell tumor	±	±	±
Choriocarcinoma	−	++	±
Embryonal cancer	±	+	±
Polyembryoma	±	+	−

AFP, alpha-fetoprotein; hCG, human chorionic gonadotropin; LDH, lactate dehydrogenase.

SEX CORD-STROMAL CELL OVARIAN TUMORS

Background
- Account for 5–8% of all primary ovarian neoplasms
- Most produce steroid hormones
- Fibromas are the most common sex cord stromal tumor

Tumor Types
Granulosa-Stromal Cell Tumors
- Most common stromal tumor.
- Symptoms: hormone disturbances, precocious puberty secondary to tumor secreting estrogen.
- Pathology: Call-Exner bodies (eosinophilic substrate with few degenerated nuclei), coffee bean nuclei, microfollicular pattern, granulosa and thecal cells.
- Usually low grade and frequently associated with endometrial hyperplasia or adenocarcinoma (consider endometrial biopsy (EMB) in patient with diagnosis of granulosa cell tumor). EMB will detect endometrial hyperplasia in 25–50% of women with granulosa cell tumors and 5–10% of women with carcinoma.
- Treatment: if young, USO; if menopausal, total abdominal hysterectomy/bilateral salpingo-oophorectomy.
- Recurrence or > stage II: treat with chemotherapy or XRT.
- Prognosis = long-term survival is good (75–90%).

Sertoli-Stromal Cell Tumors
- Testosterone-producing tumors
- Symptoms: virilization
- Treatment: fertility-sparing surgery for local disease
- Prognosis: good if low grade
- Gynandroblastoma
  - Display both granulosa and Leydig cell types and tumor characteristics
- Sex cord tumor with annular tubules
- Mostly benign
- Pathology: reinke crystals (crystalized testosterone)
  - Steroid (lipid) cell tumor

Table 11.15. Tumor markers in sex cord-stromal cell tumors

	Inhibin	Testosterone	Androstenedione
Thecoma-fibroma	−	−	−
Granulosa cell	+	−	−
Gonadoblastoma	±	±	±
Sertoli-Leydig	±	+	+

VULVAR INTRAEPITHELIAL NEOPLASIA (VIN)
Background
- Premalignant condition of the vulva and refers to squamous lesions
- No routine screening
- Historically, VIN categorized as three grades: VIN 1, 2, and 3. There is no evidence that VIN1 is a cancer precursor requiring treatment; now referred to as condyloma acuminatum.
- New terminology instituted in 2012 by the Lower Anogenital Squamous Terminology (LAST) project used to describe HPV-associated squamous lesions of the anogenital tract.

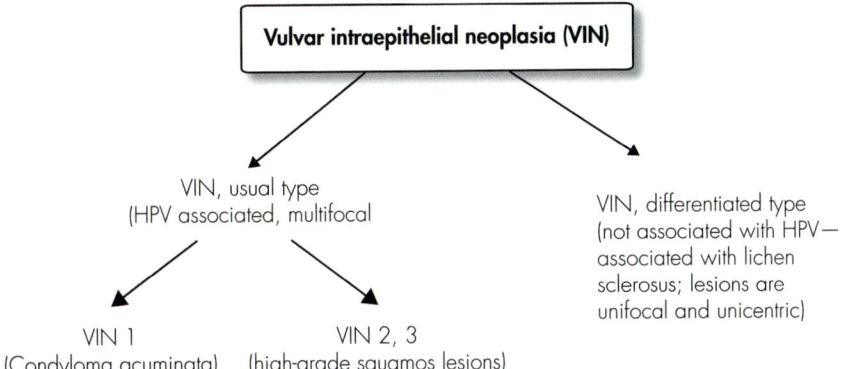

Figure 11.25. Vulvar intraepithelial neoplasia

Risk Factors for Invasive Disease
- HPV, immunodeficiency (i.e. HIV), cigarette smoking, age ≥45 years, lichen sclerosus

Diagnosis and Treatment
- Biopsy any vulvar lesion not known to be benign/nonneoplastic.
- Surgical treatment—wide local excision with gross 1 cm margins. Goals of treatment of VIN are to prevent development of vulvar squamous carcinoma and relieve symptoms while preserving normal anatomy.
- For women in whom malignancy is not suspected or has been excluded, laser ablation for those who are young or excision near the introitus can cause dyspareunia. For recurrent lesions, 250 mg of 5% imiquimod can be applied as a thin layer overnight without a cover twice a week for 16 weeks. In case of severe side effects, application could be reduced to twice a week. Lesion size reduced by more than 25% at 20 weeks in 81% of those treated (van Seters 2008). Can be used to avoid multiple excisional procedures. Use topical 5-FU rarely—mostly due to significant burning.

VULVAR CANCER

Background
- Fourth most common gynecologic malignancy (after uterine, ovarian, cervical).
- Comprises 5% of malignancies of female genital tract.
- Incidence of vulvar intraepithelial lesion has increased, but incidence of vulvar cancer has remained stable.

Risk Factors
- Postmenopausal female
- Cigarette smoking
- Vulvar dystrophy (e.g., lichen sclerosis)
- Vulvar intraepithelial lesion
- Cervical intraepithelial lesion
- HPV
- Immunodeficiency syndromes
- Prior history of cervical cancer
- European ancestry

Symptoms
- Vulvar pruritus is most common complaint among symptomatic women
- Vulvar bleeding or discharge
- Dysuria
- Dysuria or enlarged lymph nodes are less frequently encountered and signs of more advanced disease.

Clinical Manifestations
- Unifocal vulvar plaque, ulcer, mass (fleshy, nodular, or warty) on labia majora

Diagnosis
- Biopsy gross lesions to determine diagnosis and depth of stromal invasion.
- Take biopsy from center of lesion and include dermis or connective tissue to help assess depth.
- If no gross lesion visible but clinical suspicion is high, colposcopic vulvar examination with 5% acetic acid is indicated. Use copious amounts with prolonged contact with keratinized vulvar squamous epithelium.

Tumor Types
- Squamous cell—90% of all vulvar malignancies with two subtypes.
- Keratinizing, differentiated, or simple type is more common. Occurs in older women. Not related to HPV.
- Classic, warty, or Bowenoid type predominantly associated with HPV 16, 18, 33.
- Occurs in younger women.
- Melanoma is second most common—5% of all vulvar malignancies. Usually pigmented but amelanotic lesions can also occur.
- Basal cell carcinoma—2% of all vulvar malignancies.
  - Appearance of "rodent" ulcer with rolled edges and central ulceration.
  - Can also be pigmented and pearly.

Vulvar Cancer GYN-ONCOLOGY

- Sarcoma—1% of all vulvar malignancies.
- Extramammary Paget's disease—1% of all vulvar malignancies.

Workup
- Complete physical exam including inguinal, supraclavicular, and axillary nodes
- Colposcopy of cervix, vagina, and vulva

Table 11.16. Vulvar cancer staging and treatment

Stage		Treatment
Stage IA	Tumor confined to vulva or perineum, ≤ 2 cm in greatest dimension, negative nodes, stromal invasion ≤ 1 mm	Deep radical excision
Stage IB	Tumor confined to vulva or perineum, >2 cm in greatest dimension, negative nodes OR stromal invasion >1 mm	Treatment same for IB as II: If lateral lesion—radical local excision or deep radical excision with ipsilateral groin dissection or radical hemivulvectomy with en bloc ipsilateral inguinal femoral lymphadenectomy
Stage II	Tumor confined to the vulva and/or perineum, >2 cm in greatest dimension, negative nodes (lower/distal 1/3 urethra, lower/distal 1/3 vagina, anal involvement)	Treatment same for IB as II: If midline lesion—Vulvectomy with en bloc bilateral groin dissection or bilateral groin dissection with radical vulvectomy (triple incision technique)
Stage III	Tumor of any size with adjacent spread with or without extension to adjacent perineal structures (lower/distal 1/3 urethra, lower/distal 1/3 vagina, anal involvement) with positive inguinofemoral lymph nodes	Radical resection pre- or postirradiation. Rarely exenterative surgery
Stage IIIAi	One lymph node metastasis, ≥5 mm	
Stage IIIAii	One to two lymph node metastases, <5 mm	
Stage IIIBi	Two or more lymph node metastases, ≥5 mm	
Stage IIIBii	Three or more lymph node metastases, <5 mm	
Stage IIIC	Lymph node metastasis with extracapsular spread	
Stage IVA	Tumor of any size with extension to any of the following: upper/proximal 2/3 of urethra; upper/proximal 2/3 vagina, bladder mucosa, or rectal mucosa; or fixed to pelvic bone. Fixed or ulcerated regional lymph node metastasis.	
Stage IVB	Any distant metastases including pelvic lymph nodes	

Source: Reproduced with permission from Pecorelli S. Revised FIGO staging for carcinoma of the vulva, cervix, and endometrium. *Int J Gynaecol Obstet.* 2009;105(2):103-104. Copyright © 2009 International Federation of Gynecology and Obstetrics.

Table 11.17. Vaginal cancer staging

Primary Tumor (T)		
TX	–	Primary tumor cannot be assessed
T0	–	No evidence of primary tumor
Tis	–	Carcinoma in situ
T1	I	Tumor confined to vagina
T2	II	Tumor invades paravaginal tissue but not to pelvic wall
T3	III	Tumor extends to pelvic wall
T4*	IVA	Tumor invades bladder and/or bowel mucosa and/or extends beyond the true pelvis (bullous edema is not sufficient to classify a tumor as T4)
	IVB	Distant metastasis

Note: If the bladder mucosa is not involved, the tumor is stage III.

Source: Reproduced with permission from FIGO Committee on Gynecologic Oncology: Current FIGO staging for cancer of the vagina, fallopian tube, ovary, and gestational trophoblastic neoplasia. *Int J Gynaecol Obstet.* 2009;105(1):3-4. Copyright © 2009 International Federation of Gynecology and Obstetrics.

GESTATIONAL TROPHOBLASTIC DISEASE (GTD) AND GESTATIONAL TROPHOBLASTIC NEOPLASIA (GTN)

Fast Facts
- GTD comprises placental conditions: hydatidiform moles, placental site nodule, and exaggerated placental site.
- GTN comprises tumors with potential for invasion and metastases: choriocarcinoma, placental site trophoblastic tumor (PSTT), and epithelioid trophoblastic tumor.

Signs and Symptoms
- First trimester bleeding
- Size/date discrepancy
- Sudden increase in uterine size
- Passage of vesicles
- Hyperemesis gravidarum
- Early preeclampsia
- Thyrotoxicosis
- β-hCG greater than expected

Table 11.18. Features of partial and complete hydatidiform moles

Feature	Partial Mole	Complete Mole
Karyotype	Most commonly 69,XXX or 69,XXY	Most commonly 46,XX or 46,XY
Pathology		
Fetus	Often present	Absent
Amnion, fetal red blood cells	Usually present	Absent
Villous edema	Variable; focal	Diffuse
Trophoblastic proliferation	Focal, slight to moderate	Diffuses slight to severe
Clinical presentation		
Diagnosis	Missed abortion	Molar gestation
Uterine size	Small for gestational age	50% larger for gestational age
Theca lutein cysts	Rare	15–25%
Medical complications	Rare	Less than 25%
Postmolar malignant sequelae	<5%	6–32%

Source: Modified from Soper JT, Lewis JL Jr., Hammond CB. Gestational troboblastic disease. In: Hoskins WJ, Perez CA, Young RC, eds. *Principals and Practice of Gynecologic Oncology*, 2nd Ed. Philadelphia (PA): Lippincott-Raven; 1997.

Table 11.19. Diagnosis and evaluation of GTN

Diagnosis of GTN
After molar evacuation: 4 values or more of plateaued hCG (±10%) over at least 3 weeks: days 1, 7, 14, and 21
After molar evacuation: a rise of hCG of 10% or greater for 3 values or more over at least 2 weeks: days 1, 7, and 14
After molar evacuation: persistence of hCG beyond 6 months
The histologic diagnosis of choriocarcinoma, invasive mole, or PSTT
Metastatic disease without established primary site with elevated hCG; pregnancy has been excluded

Evaluation of GTN
Complete physical and pelvic examination; baseline hematologic, renal, and hepatic functions
Baseline quantitative hCG level
Chest radiograph or CT scan of chest
Brain MRI or CT scan
CT or MRI scan of abdomen and pelvis

CT, computed tomography; hCG, human chorionic gonadotropin; MRI, magnetic resonance imaging; PSTT, placental site trophoblastic tumor.

Source: Reproduced with permission from Ko, EM and Soper, JT. Gestational trophoblastic disease. In: DiSaia PJ, Creasman WT, Mannel RS, McMeekin DS, Mutch DG, eds. *Clinical Gynecologic Oncology, 8th Ed.* Philadelphia (PA): Elsevier; 2012.

Table 11.20. Management of hydatidiform mole

Evacuation: suction D&E (or hysterectomy in selected patients)
Postevacuation quantitative hCG level and chest radiograph
Monitor quantitative hCG levels every 1–2 weeks until normal value or criteria for GTN
Examination every 2–4 weeks while hCG elevated
Confirm normal hCG level, then monitor hCG levels every 1–2 months for 6–12 months
Initiate chemotherapy for GTN using indications: 1. Plateaued or rising hCG values 2. Histologic diagnosis of choriocarcinoma, invasive mole, or placental site trophoblastic tumor 3. Persistent hCG >6 months after evacuation 4. Metastatic disease

D&E, suction dilation and evacuation; GTN, gestational trophoblastic neoplasia; hCG, human chorionic gonadotropin.

Source: Reproduced with permission from Ko, EM and Soper, JT. Gestational trophoblastic disease. In: DiSaia PJ, Creasman WT, Mannel RS, McMeekin DS, Mutch DG, eds. *Clinical Gynecologic Oncology, 8th Ed.* Philadelphia (PA): Elsevier; 2012.

Table 11.21. Management of low-risk nonmetastatic or low-risk metastatic GTN

Initiate single-agent methotrexate or dactinomycin regimen
Consider hysterectomy if fertility not desired
Monitor hematologic, renal, and hepatic indices before each cycle of chemotherapy
Monitor serum hCG levels weekly during therapy
Change to alternative single-agent if resistance or severe toxicity to first agent
If resistance to alternative agent:
1. Repeat metastatic evaluation
2. Consider hysterectomy if no extrauterine metastases
3. Multiagent therapy (MAC or EMA/CO, see text)
Remission: three consecutive weekly hCG values in the normal range
1 or 2 cycles of maintenance/consolidation chemotherapy

EMA/CO, etoposide, methotrexate, actinomycin-D, cyclophosphamide and vincristine; MAC, methotrexate, actinomycin-D, and cyclophosphamide.

Source: Reproduced with permission from Ko, EM and Soper, JT. Gestational trophoblastic disease. In: DiSaia PJ, Creasman WT, Mannel RS, McMeekin DS, Mutch DG, eds. *Clinical Gynecologic Oncology, 8th Ed.* Philadelphia (PA): Elsevier; 2012.

Table 11.22. WHO prognostic scoring for GTN

Prognostic Factors	Score			
	0	1	2	4
Age (yr)	<40	≤40	—	—
Antecedent pregnancy	Mole	Abortion	Term	—
Interval mo from index pregnancy	<4	4–<7	7–<13	≥13
Pretreatment human chorionic gonadotropin (IU/L)	$<10^3$	10^3–$<10^4$	10^4–$<10^5$	$≥10^6$
Largest tumor (cm) (including uterus)	3–5	≥5	—	—
Site of metastases	Lung	Spleen, kidney	GI tract	Brain, liver
Number of metastases	—	1–4	5–8	>8
Previous failed chemotherapy	—	—	Single drug	2 or more drugs

Total score is obtained by adding the individual scores for each prognostic factor. 0–4 = low risk, 5–6 = intermediate risk, >7 = high risk

Format for reporting to International Federation of Gynecology and Obstetrics (FIGO) Annual.

Source: Reproduced with permission from Berek JS, Hacker NF, eds. *Practical Gynecologic Oncology, 4th Ed.* Philadelphia: Lippincott Williams & Wilkins; 2005.

GYN-ONCOLOGY — GTD and GTN

Table 11.23. Anatomic FIGO staging system for GTN

Stage	Criteria
I	Disease confined to the uterus
II	Disease outside of uterus but is limited to the genital structures
III	Disease extends to the lungs with or without known genital tract involvement
IV	All other metastatic sites

FIGO, International Federation of Gynecology and Obstetrics; GTN, gestational trophoblastic neoplasia.

Source: Reproduced with permission from FIGO Committee on Gynecologic Oncology. Current FIGO staging for cancer of the vagina, fallopian tube, ovary, and gestational trophoblastic neoplasia. Int J Gynaecol Obstet. 2009 Apr. 105(1):3-4. Copyright © 2009 International Federation of Gynecology and Obstetrics.

Table 11.24. Management of high-risk GTN

Evaluate for high-risk metastases: Brain, liver, kidney
Stabilize medical status of patient
Multiagent therapy with EMA/CO or MAC • Aggressive recycling may require cytokine support
Management of brain metastases (see text): • Consider early neurosurgical intervention if isolated brain lesion • Consider stereotactic or whole brain irradiation if multiple brain lesions
Management of liver metastases (see text): • Consider selective angiographic embolization or irradiation
Monitor hCG weekly during therapy
At least three cycles of maintenance chemotherapy after hCG values normalize

Source: Reproduced with permission from Ko, EM and Soper, JT. Gestational trophoblastic disease. In: DiSaia PJ, Creasman WT, Mannel RS, McMeekin DS, Mutch DG, eds. Clinical Gynecologic Oncology, 8th Ed. Philadelphia (PA): Elsevier; 2012.

Table 11.25. Surveillance during and after therapy of GTN

Monitor serum quantitative hCG levels every week during chemotherapy: 1. Response: >10% decline in hCG during one cycle 2. Plateau: ±10% change in hCG during one cycle 3. Resistance: >10% rise in hCG during one cycle or plateau for two cycles of chemotherapy
• Evaluate for new metastases • Consider alternative chemotherapy • Consider extirpation of drug-resistant sites of disease
Remission: Three consecutive normal weekly hCG values
1. Maintenance chemotherapy
Surveillance of remission: 1. hCG values every 2 weeks × 3 months 2. hCG values every month to complete 1 year of follow-up 3. hCG values every 6–12 months indefinitely; at least 3–5 years

Source: Reproduced with permission from Ko, EM and Soper, JT. Gestational trophoblastic disease. In: DiSaia PJ, Creasman WT, Mannel RS, McMeekin DS, Mutch DG, eds. Clinical Gynecologic Oncology, 8th Ed. Philadelphia (PA): Elsevier; 2012.

DENNIS SIEGLER'S* TOP TEN WAYS** TO SURVIVE GYN-ONCOLOGY

(Pre-80-Hour Work Week)***

10. Do not become angry.
9. DO NOT BECOME ANGRY.
8. DO NOT BECOME ANGRY.
7. If angry, do not become frustrated.
6. If angry and frustrated, remember there is always another GOG form to complete.⁺
5. Remember that actual OR time = requested OR time × 2.
4. Chemotherapy admissions only seem to multiply like rabbits.
3. If all else fails, examine the patient.
2. PM rounds should be completed before AM rounds begin. And the number-one way to survive gyn-onc:
1. Remember, it could be worse; you could be in internal medicine.

*Former Stanford Chief Resident 1993.
**With apologies to David Letterman.
***Younger physicians may not get the joke . . . too bad.
****Chemotherapy admissions are now rare since most chemotherapy regimens are given as outpatients.
*****GOG forms are no longer filled out by residents—all are electronic.
⁺Yes, I know that these are now done electronically.

NCCN GUIDELINES® FOR MANAGEMENT OF COMMON PROBLEMS IN GYN-ONCOLOGY PATIENTS
Pain Control

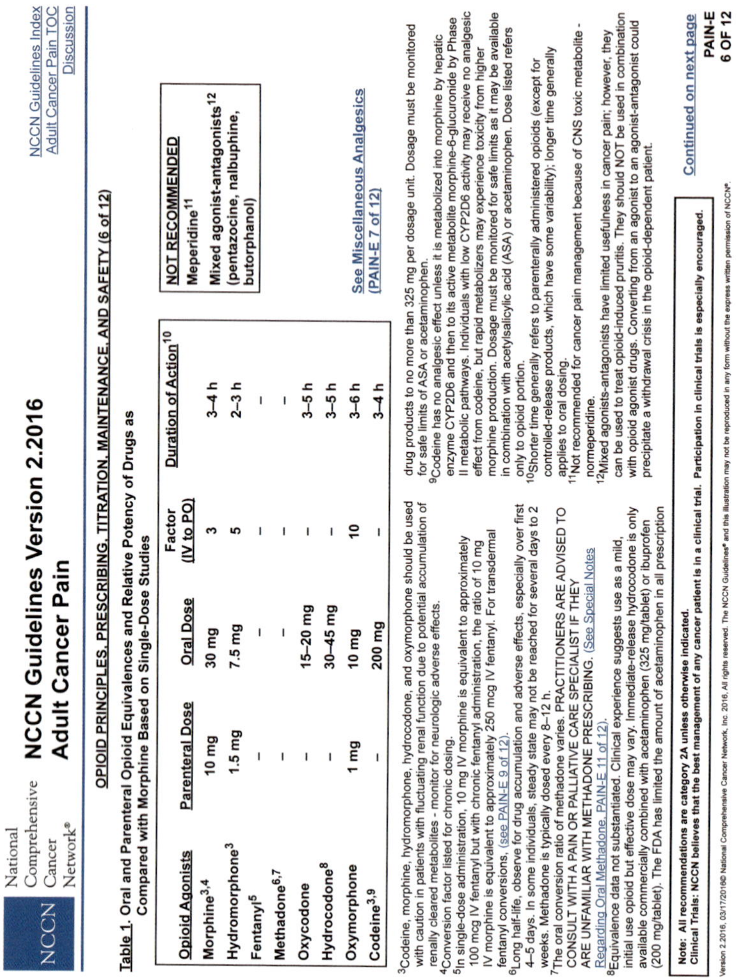

NCCN Guidelines Index
Adult Cancer Pain TOC
Discussion

NCCN Guidelines Version 2.2016
Adult Cancer Pain

OPIOID PRINCIPLES, PRESCRIBING, TITRATION, MAINTENANCE, AND SAFETY (6 of 12)

Table 1. Oral and Parenteral Opioid Equivalences and Relative Potency of Drugs as Compared with Morphine Based on Single-Dose Studies

Opioid Agonists	Parenteral Dose	Oral Dose	Factor (IV to PO)	Duration of Action[10]
Morphine[3,4]	10 mg	30 mg	3	3-4 h
Hydromorphone[3]	1.5 mg	7.5 mg	5	2-3 h
Fentanyl[5]	—	—	—	—
Methadone[6,7]	—	—	—	—
Oxycodone	—	15-20 mg	—	3-5 h
Hydrocodone[8]	—	30-45 mg	—	3-5 h
Oxymorphone	1 mg	10 mg	10	3-6 h
Codeine[3,9]	—	200 mg	—	3-4 h

NOT RECOMMENDED
Meperidine[11]
Mixed agonist-antagonists[12] (pentazocine, nalbuphine, butorphanol)

See Miscellaneous Analgesics (PAIN-E 7 of 12)

[3] Codeine, morphine, hydromorphone, hydrocodone, and oxymorphone should be used with caution in patients with fluctuating renal function due to potential accumulation of renally cleared metabolites - monitor for neurologic adverse effects.
[4] Conversion factor listed for chronic dosing.
[5] In single-dose administration, 10 mg IV morphine is equivalent to approximately 100 mcg IV fentanyl but with chronic fentanyl administration, the ratio of 10 mg IV morphine is equivalent to approximately 250 mcg IV fentanyl. For transdermal fentanyl conversions, (see PAIN-E 9 of 12).
[6] Long half-life, observe for drug accumulation and adverse effects, especially over first 4-5 days. In some individuals, steady state may not be reached for several days to 2 weeks. Methadone is typically dosed every 8-12 h.
[7] The oral conversion ratio of methadone varies. PRACTITIONERS ARE ADVISED TO CONSULT WITH A PAIN OR PALLIATIVE CARE SPECIALIST IF THEY ARE UNFAMILIAR WITH METHADONE PRESCRIBING. (See Special Notes Regarding Oral Methadone, PAIN-E 11 of 12).
[8] Equivalence data not substantiated. Clinical experience suggests use as a mild, initial use opioid but effective dose may vary. Immediate-release hydrocodone is only available commercially combined with acetaminophen (325 mg/tablet) or ibuprofen (200 mg/tablet). The FDA has limited the amount of acetaminophen in all prescription drug products to no more than 325 mg per dosage unit. Dosage must be monitored for safe limits of ASA or acetaminophen.
[9] Codeine has no analgesic effect unless it is metabolized into morphine by hepatic enzyme CYP2D6 and then to its active metabolite morphine-6-glucuronide by Phase II metabolic pathways. Individuals with low CYP2D6 activity may receive no analgesic effect from codeine, but rapid metabolizers may experience toxicity from higher morphine production. Dosage must be monitored for safe limits as it may be available in combination with acetylsalicylic acid (ASA) or acetaminophen. Dose listed refers only to opioid portion.
[10] Shorter time generally refers to parenterally administered opioids (except for controlled-release products, which have some variability); longer time generally applies to oral dosing.
[11] Not recommended for cancer pain management because of CNS toxic metabolite - normeperidine.
[12] Mixed agonists-antagonists have limited usefulness in cancer pain; however, they can be used to treat opioid-induced pruritis. They should NOT be used in combination with opioid agonist drugs. Converting from an agonist to an agonist-antagonist could precipitate a withdrawal crisis in the opioid-dependent patient.

Note: All recommendations are category 2A unless otherwise indicated.
Clinical Trials: NCCN believes that the best management of any cancer patient is in a clinical trial. Participation in clinical trials is especially encouraged.

Continued on next page
PAIN-E
6 OF 12

Figure 11.26. Adult cancer pain
Reproduced with permission from the NCCN Clinical Practice Guidelines in Oncology (NCCN Guidelines®) for Adult Cancer Pain V.2.2016. © 2016 National Comprehensive Cancer Network, Inc. All rights reserved. The NCCN Guidelines® and illustrations herein may not be reproduced in any form for any purpose without the express written permission of the NCCN. To view the most recent and complete version of the NCCN Guidelines, go online to NCCN.org. NATIONAL COMPREHENSIVE CANCER NETWORK®, NCCN®, NCCN GUIDELINES®, and all other NCCN Content are trademarks owned by the National Comprehensive Cancer Network, Inc.

Antiemesis

NCCN Guidelines Version 2.2016
Antiemesis

NCCN Guidelines Index
Antiemesis Table of Contents
Discussion

PRINCIPLES OF EMESIS CONTROL FOR THE CANCER PATIENT

- Prevention of nausea/vomiting is the goal.
  ▶ The risk of nausea/vomiting for persons receiving chemotherapy of high and moderate emetic risk lasts for at least 3 days for high and 2 days for moderate after the last dose of chemotherapy. Patients need to be protected throughout the full period of risk.
- Oral and intravenous 5-HT3 antagonists have equivalent efficacy when used at the appropriate doses.
- Consider the toxicity of the specific antiemetic(s).
- Choice of antiemetic(s) used should be based on the emetic risk of the therapy, prior experience with antiemetics, and patient factors.
- There are other potential causes of emesis in cancer patients.
  These may include:
  ▶ Partial or complete bowel obstruction
  ▶ Vestibular dysfunction
  ▶ Brain metastases
  ▶ Electrolyte imbalance: hypercalcemia, hyperglycemia, or hyponatremia
  ▶ Uremia
  ▶ Concomitant drug treatments, including opioids
  ▶ Gastroparesis: tumor or chemotherapy (eg, vincristine) induced or other causes (eg, diabetes)
  ▶ Malignant ascites
  ▶ Psychophysiologic:
    ◊ Anxiety
    ◊ Anticipatory nausea/vomiting
- For use of antiemetics for nausea/vomiting that are not related to radiation and/or chemotherapy, see NCCN Guidelines for Palliative Care.
- For multi-drug regimens, select antiemetic therapy based on the drug with the highest emetic risk. See Emetogenic Potential of Intravenous Antineoplastic Agents (AE-2).
- Consider using an H2 blocker or proton pump inhibitor to prevent dyspepsia, which can mimic nausea.
- Lifestyle measures may help to alleviate nausea/vomiting, such as eating small frequent meals, choosing healthful foods, controlling the amount of food consumed, and eating food at room temperature. A dietary consult may also be useful. See NCI's "Eating Hints: Before, During, and After Cancer Treatment." (http://www.cancer.gov/cancertopics/coping/eatinghints/page2#4)

Note: All recommendations are category 2A unless otherwise indicated.
Clinical Trials: NCCN believes that the best management of any cancer patient is in a clinical trial. Participation in clinical trials is especially encouraged.

AE-1

Figure 11.27. Principles of emesis control
Reproduced with permission from the NCCN Clinical Practice Guidelines in Oncology (NCCN Guidelines®) for Antiemesis V.2.2016. © 2016 National Comprehensive Cancer Network, Inc. All rights reserved. The NCCN Guidelines® and illustrations herein may not be reproduced in any form for any purpose without the express written permission of the NCCN. To view the most recent and complete version of the NCCN Guidelines, go online to NCCN.org. NATIONAL COMPREHENSIVE CANCER NETWORK®, NCCN®, NCCN GUIDELINES®, and all other NCCN Content are trademarks owned by the National Comprehensive Cancer Network, Inc.

GYN-ONCOLOGY — NCCN Clinical Practice Guidelines In Oncology (NCCN Guidelines®)

NCCN Guidelines Version 2.2016
Antiemesis

NCCN Guidelines Index
Antiemesis Table of Contents
Discussion

EMETOGENIC POTENTIAL OF INTRAVENOUS ANTINEOPLASTIC AGENTS[a]

High emetic risk (>90% frequency of emesis)[b,c]	Moderate emetic risk (30%–90% frequency of emesis)[b,c]		
• AC combination defined as either doxorubicin or epirubicin with cyclophosphamide • Carmustine >250 mg/m² • Cisplatin • Cyclophosphamide >1,500 mg/m² • Dacarbazine • Doxorubicin ≥60 mg/m² • Epirubicin >90 mg/m² • Ifosfamide ≥2 g/m² per dose • Mechlorethamine • Streptozocin	• Aldesleukin >12–15 million IU/m² • Amifostine >300 mg/m² • Arsenic trioxide • Azacitidine • Bendamustine • Busulfan • Carboplatin[d] • Carmustine[d] ≤250 mg/m²	• Clofarabine • Cyclophosphamide ≤1500 mg/m² • Cytarabine >200 mg/m² • Dactinomycin[d] • Daunorubicin[d] • Dinutuximab • Doxorubicin[d] <60 mg/m² • Epirubicin[d] ≤90 mg/m² • Idarubicin	• Ifosfamide[d] <2 g/m² per dose • Interferon alfa ≥10 million IU/m² • Irinotecan[d] • Melphalan • Methotrexate[d] ≥250 mg/m² • Oxaliplatin • Temozolomide • Trabectedin

Low Emetic Risk (See AE-3)
Minimal Emetic Risk (See AE-3)
Oral Chemotherapy (See AE-4)

Adapted with permission from:
Hesketh PJ, et al. Proposal for classifying the acute emetogenicity of cancer chemotherapy. J Clin Oncol 1997;15:103–109
Grunberg SM, Warr D, Gralla RJ, et al. Evaluation of new antiemetic agents and definition of antineoplastic agent emetogenicity–state of the art. Support Care Cancer. 2010;19:S43-47.

[a] Potential drug interactions between antineoplastic agents/antiemetic therapies and various other drugs should always be considered.
[b] Proportion of patients who experience emesis in the absence of effective antiemetic prophylaxis.
[c] Continuous infusion may make an agent less emetogenic.
[d] These agents may be highly emetogenic in certain patients.

Note: All recommendations are category 2A unless otherwise indicated.
Clinical Trials: NCCN believes that the best management of any cancer patient is in a clinical trial. Participation in clinical trials is especially encouraged.

Figure 11.28. Emetogenic potential of high- and moderate-risk IV antineoplastic agents
Reproduced with permission from the NCCN Clinical Practice Guidelines in Oncology (NCCN Guidelines®) for Antiemesis V.2.2016. © 2016 National Comprehensive Cancer Network, Inc. All rights reserved. The NCCN Guidelines® and illustrations herein may not be reproduced in any form for any purpose without the express written permission of the NCCN. To view the most recent and complete version of the NCCN Guidelines, go online to NCCN.org. NATIONAL COMPREHENSIVE CANCER NETWORK®, NCCN®, NCCN GUIDELINES®, and all other NCCN Content are trademarks owned by the National Comprehensive Cancer Network, Inc.

Figure 11.29. Emetogenic potential of low- and minimal-risk IV antineoplastic agents
Reproduced with permission from the NCCN Clinical Practice Guidelines in Oncology (NCCN Guidelines®) for Antiemesis V.2.2016. © 2016 National Comprehensive Cancer Network, Inc. All rights reserved. The NCCN Guidelines® and illustrations herein may not be reproduced in any form for any purpose without the express written permission of the NCCN. To view the most recent and complete version of the NCCN Guidelines, go online to NCCN.org. NATIONAL COMPREHENSIVE CANCER NETWORK®, NCCN®, NCCN GUIDELINES®, and all other NCCN Content are trademarks owned by the National Comprehensive Cancer Network, Inc.

GYN-ONCOLOGY — NCCN Clinical Practice Guidelines In Oncology (NCCN Guidelines®)

NCCN Guidelines Index
Antiemesis Table of Contents
Discussion

NCCN Guidelines Version 2.2016
Antiemesis

EMETOGENIC POTENTIAL OF ORAL ANTINEOPLASTIC AGENTS[a]

LEVEL	AGENT			
Moderate to high emetic risk	• Altretamine • Busulfan (≥4 mg/d) • Ceritinib • Crizotinib • Cyclophosphamide (≥100 mg/m²/d)	• Estramustine • Etoposide • Lenvatinib • Lomustine (single day) • Mitotane	• Olaparib • Panobinostat • Procarbazine • Temozolomide (>75 mg/m²/d) • Trifluridine/tipiracil	
Minimal to low emetic risk	• Afatinib • Alectinib • Axitinib • Bexarotene • Bosutinib • Busulfan (<4 mg/d) • Cabozantinib • Capecitabine • Chlorambucil • Cobimetinib • Cyclophosphamide (<100 mg/m²/d) • Dasatinib • Dabrafenib • Erlotinib • Everolimus • Fludarabine	• Gefitinib • Hydroxyurea • Ibrutinib • Idelalisib • Imatinib • Ixazomib • Lapatinib • Lenalidomide • Melphalan • Mercaptopurine • Methotrexate • Nilotinib • Osimertinib • Palbociclib • Pazopanib • Pomalidomide • Ponatinib	• Regorafenib • Ruxolitinib • Sonidegib • Sorafenib • Sunitinib • Temozolomide (≤75 mg/m²/d)[e] • Thalidomide • Thioguanine • Topotecan • Trametinib • Tretinoin • Vandetanib • Vemurafenib • Vismodegib • Vorinostat	

High Emetic Risk (See AE-2)
Moderate Emetic Risk (See AE-2)
Low Emetic Risk (See AE-3)
Minimal Emetic Risk (See AE-3)

Adapted with permission from:
Hesketh PJ, et al. Proposal for classifying the acute emetogenicity of cancer chemotherapy. J Clin Oncol 1997;15:103-109.
Grunberg SM, Warr D, Gralla RJ, et al. Evaluation of new antiemetic agents and definition of antineoplastic agent emetogenicity-state of the art. Support Care Cancer. 2010;19:S43-47.

[a] Potential drug interactions between antineoplastic agents/antiemetic therapies and various other drugs should always be considered.
[e] Temozolomide ≤75 mg/m²/d should be considered moderately emetogenic with concurrent radiotherapy.

Note: All recommendations are category 2A unless otherwise indicated.
Clinical Trials: NCCN believes that the best management of any cancer patient is in a clinical trial. Participation in clinical trials is especially encouraged.

Figure 11.30. Emetogenic potential of oral antineoplastic agents
Reproduced with permission from the NCCN Clinical Practice Guidelines in Oncology (NCCN Guidelines®) for Antiemesis V.2.2016. © 2016 National Comprehensive Cancer Network, Inc. All rights reserved. The NCCN Guidelines® and illustrations herein may not be reproduced in any form for any purpose without the express written permission of the NCCN. To view the most recent and complete version of the NCCN Guidelines, go online to NCCN.org. NATIONAL COMPREHENSIVE CANCER NETWORK®, NCCN®, NCCN GUIDELINES®, and all other NCCN Content are trademarks owned by the National Comprehensive Cancer Network, Inc.

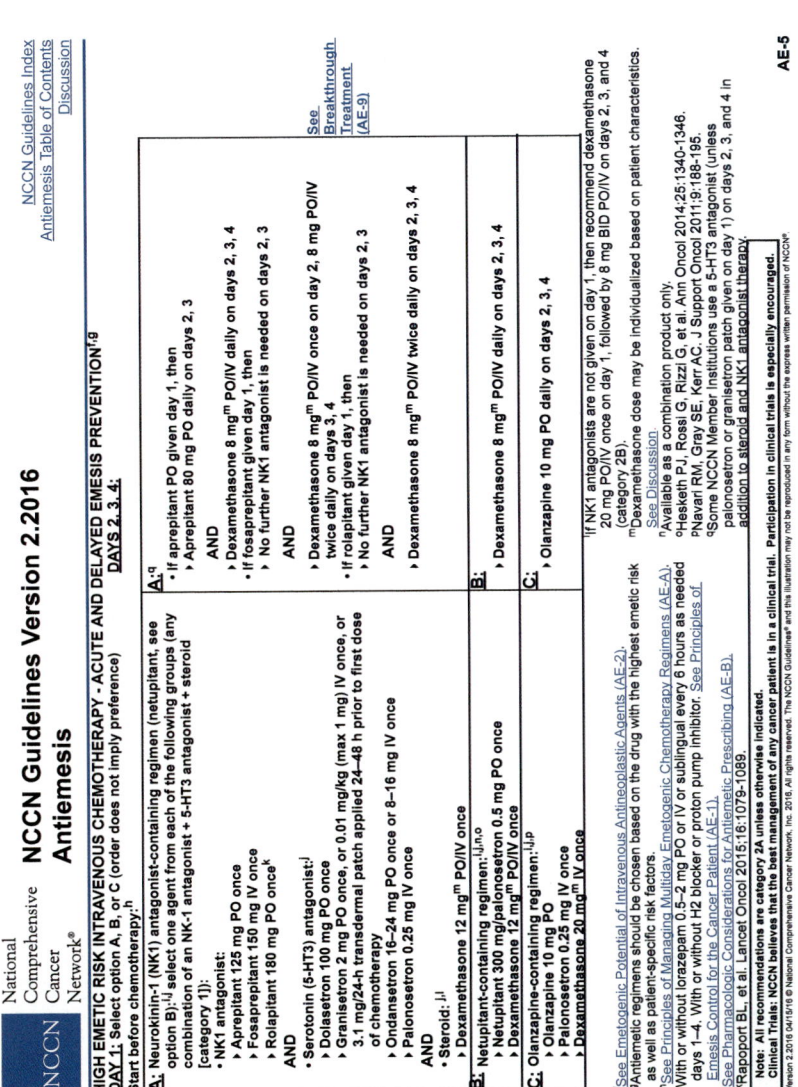

Figure 11.31. Acute and delayed emesis prevention of high emetic risk IV chemotherapy
Reproduced with permission from the NCCN Clinical Practice Guidelines in Oncology (NCCN Guidelines®) for Antiemesis V.2.2016. © 2016 National Comprehensive Cancer Network, Inc. All rights reserved. The NCCN Guidelines® and illustrations herein may not be reproduced in any form for any purpose without the express written permission of the NCCN. To view the most recent and complete version of the NCCN Guidelines, go online to NCCN.org. NATIONAL COMPREHENSIVE CANCER NETWORK®, NCCN®, NCCN GUIDELINES®, and all other NCCN Content are trademarks owned by the National Comprehensive Cancer Network, Inc.

GYN-ONCOLOGY
NCCN Clinical Practice Guidelines In Oncology (NCCN Guidelines®)

NCCN Guidelines Version 2.2016
Antiemesis

NCCN Guidelines Index
Antiemesis Table of Contents
Discussion

MODERATE EMETIC RISK INTRAVENOUS CHEMOTHERAPY - ACUTE AND DELAYED EMESIS PREVENTION[f,g]

DAY 1: Select option A, B, or C (order does not imply preference)
Start before chemotherapy:[h]

A:
Serotonin (5-HT3) antagonist + steroid (category 1) ± NK1 antagonist[i,j]
(netupitant, see option B)
- Dolasetron 100 mg PO once
- Granisetron 2 mg PO once, or 0.01 mg/kg (max 1 mg) IV once, or 3.1 mg/24-h transdermal patch applied 24–48 h prior to first dose of chemotherapy
- Ondansetron 16–24 mg PO once or 8–16 mg IV once
- Palonosetron 0.25 mg IV once (preferred)

AND
- Steroid[j]
  - Dexamethasone 12 mg[m] PO/IV once

WITH/WITHOUT
- NK1 antagonist:[j,r]
  - Aprepitant 125 mg PO once
  - Fosaprepitant 150 mg IV once
  - Rolapitant 180 mg PO once[s]

B:
Netupitant-containing regimen:[i,j,n]
- Netupitant 300 mg/palonosetron 0.5 mg PO once[r]
- Dexamethasone 12 mg[m] PO/IV once

C:
Olanzapine-containing regimen:[i,j,p]
- Olanzapine 10 mg PO
- Palonosetron 0.25 mg IV once
- Dexamethasone 20 mg[m] IV once

DAYS 2 and 3:

A:
If no NK1 antagonist given on day 1:
- Serotonin (5-HT3) antagonist monotherapy:[j,t] (Select one):
  - Dolasetron 100 mg PO daily on days 2, 3
  - Granisetron 1–2 mg PO daily or 1 mg PO BID or 0.01 mg/kg (maximum 1 mg) IV daily on days 2, 3
  - Ondansetron 8 mg PO BID or 16 mg PO daily or 8–16 mg IV daily on days 2, 3

OR
- Steroid monotherapy[j]:
  - Dexamethasone 8 mg[m] PO/IV daily on days 2, 3

If NK1 antagonist given on day 1:
- If aprepitant given day 1, then
  - Aprepitant 80 mg PO daily on days 2, 3, ± dexamethasone 8 mg PO/IV daily on days 2, 3
- If fosaprepitant given day 1, then
  - No further NK1 antagonist is needed on days 2, 3
  - ± dexamethasone on days 2, 3
- If rolapitant given day 1, then
  - No further NK1 antagonist is needed on days 2, 3
  - ± dexamethasone on days 2, 3

B:
- ± Dexamethasone 8 mg[m] PO/IV daily on days 2, 3

C:
- Olanzapine 10 mg PO daily days 2, 3

See Breakthrough Treatment (AE-9)

See Emetogenic Potential of Intravenous Antineoplastic Agents (AE-2).
[g]Antiemetic regimens should be chosen based on the drug with the highest emetic risk as well as patient-specific risk factors.
[h]See Principles of Managing Multiday Emetogenic Chemotherapy Regimens (AE-A).
[i]With or without lorazepam 0.5–2 mg PO or IV or sublingual every 6 hours as needed days 1–4. With or without H2 blocker or proton pump inhibitor See Principles of Emesis Control for the Cancer Patient (AE-1).
[j]See Pharmacologic Considerations for Antiemetic Prescribing (AE-B).

Note: All recommendations are category 2A unless otherwise indicated.
Clinical Trials: NCCN believes that the best management of any cancer patient is in a clinical trial. Participation in clinical trials is especially encouraged.

[m]Dexamethasone dose may be individualized based on patient characteristics. See Discussion
[n]Available as a combination product only.
[p]Navari RM, Gray SE, Kerr AC. J Support Oncol 2011;9:188-195.
[r]As per high emetic risk prevention, an NK1 antagonist should be added (to dexamethasone and a 5-HT3 antagonist regimen) for select patients with additional risk factors or treatment failing therapy with a steroid + 5-HT3 antagonist alone (See AE-5).
[s]Schwartzberg LS, et al. Lancet Oncol 2015;16:1071–1078.
[t]No further therapy required if palonosetron or granisetron patch given on day 1.

AE-6

Figure 11.32. Acute and delayed emesis prevention of moderate emetic risk IV chemotherapy
Reproduced with permission from the NCCN Clinical Practice Guidelines in Oncology (NCCN Guidelines®) for Antiemesis V.2.2016. © 2016 National Comprehensive Cancer Network, Inc. All rights reserved. The NCCN Guidelines® and illustrations herein may not be reproduced in any form for any purpose without the express written permission of the NCCN. To view the most recent and complete version of the NCCN Guidelines, go online to NCCN.org. NATIONAL COMPREHENSIVE CANCER NETWORK®, NCCN®, NCCN GUIDELINES®, and all other NCCN Content are trademarks owned by the National Comprehensive Cancer Network, Inc.

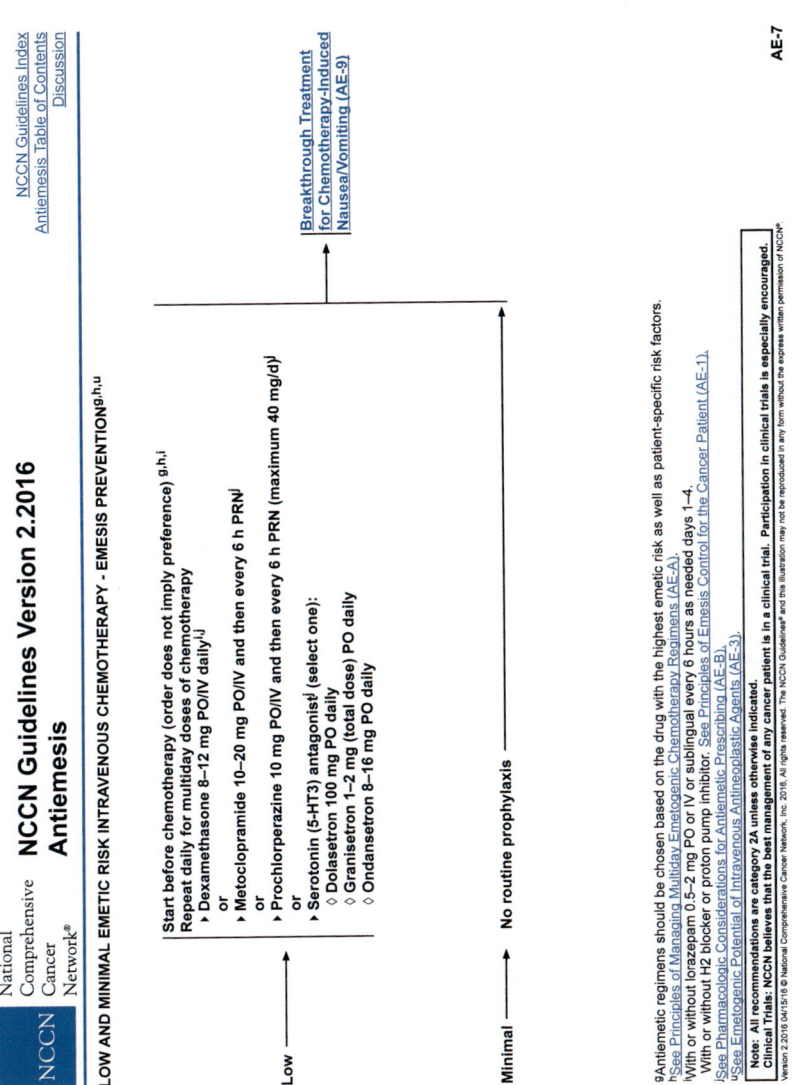

Figure 11.33. Emesis prevention of low- and minimal-risk IV chemotherapy
Reproduced with permission from the NCCN Clinical Practice Guidelines in Oncology (NCCN Guidelines®) for Antiemesis V.2.2016. © 2016 National Comprehensive Cancer Network, Inc. All rights reserved. The NCCN Guidelines® and illustrations herein may not be reproduced in any form for any purpose without the express written permission of the NCCN. To view the most recent and complete version of the NCCN Guidelines, go online to NCCN.org. NATIONAL COMPREHENSIVE CANCER NETWORK®, NCCN®, NCCN GUIDELINES®, and all other NCCN Content are trademarks owned by the National Comprehensive Cancer Network, Inc.

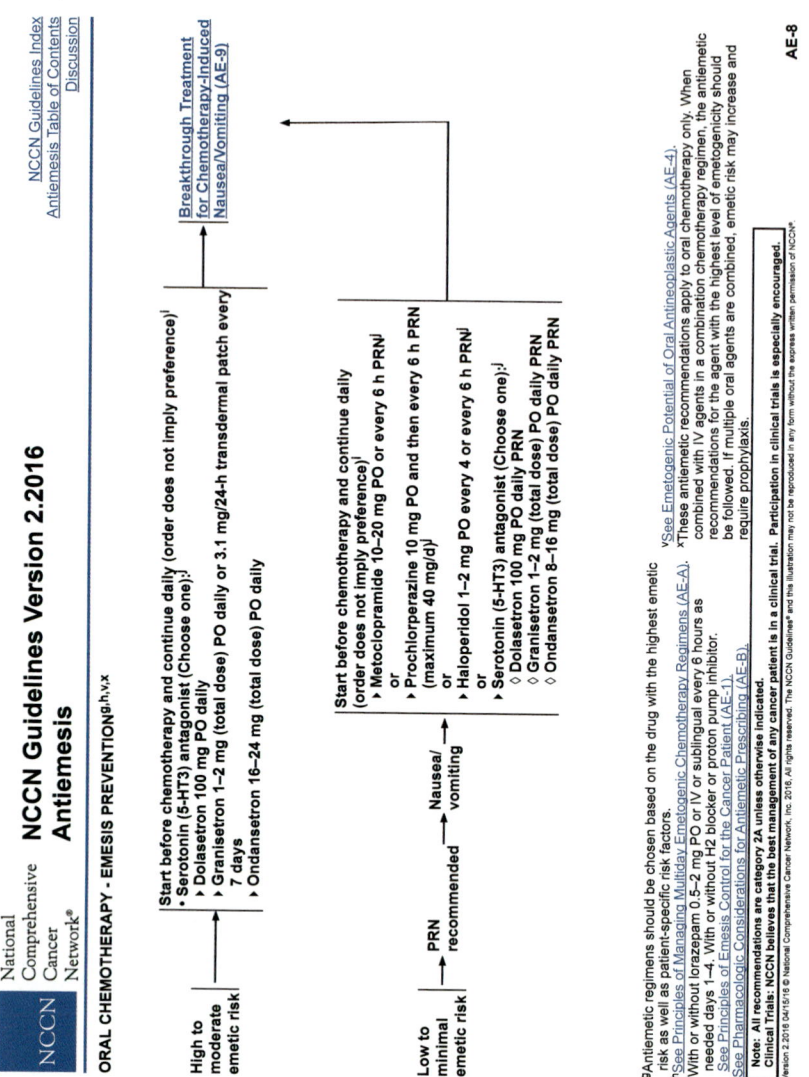

Figure 11.34. Emesis prevention of oral chemotherapy

Reproduced with permission from the NCCN Clinical Practice Guidelines in Oncology (NCCN Guidelines®) for Antiemesis V.2.2016. © 2016 National Comprehensive Cancer Network, Inc. All rights reserved. The NCCN Guidelines® and illustrations herein may not be reproduced in any form for any purpose without the express written permission of the NCCN. To view the most recent and complete version of the NCCN Guidelines, go online to NCCN.org. NATIONAL COMPREHENSIVE CANCER NETWORK®, NCCN®, NCCN GUIDELINES®, and all other NCCN Content are trademarks owned by the National Comprehensive Cancer Network, Inc.

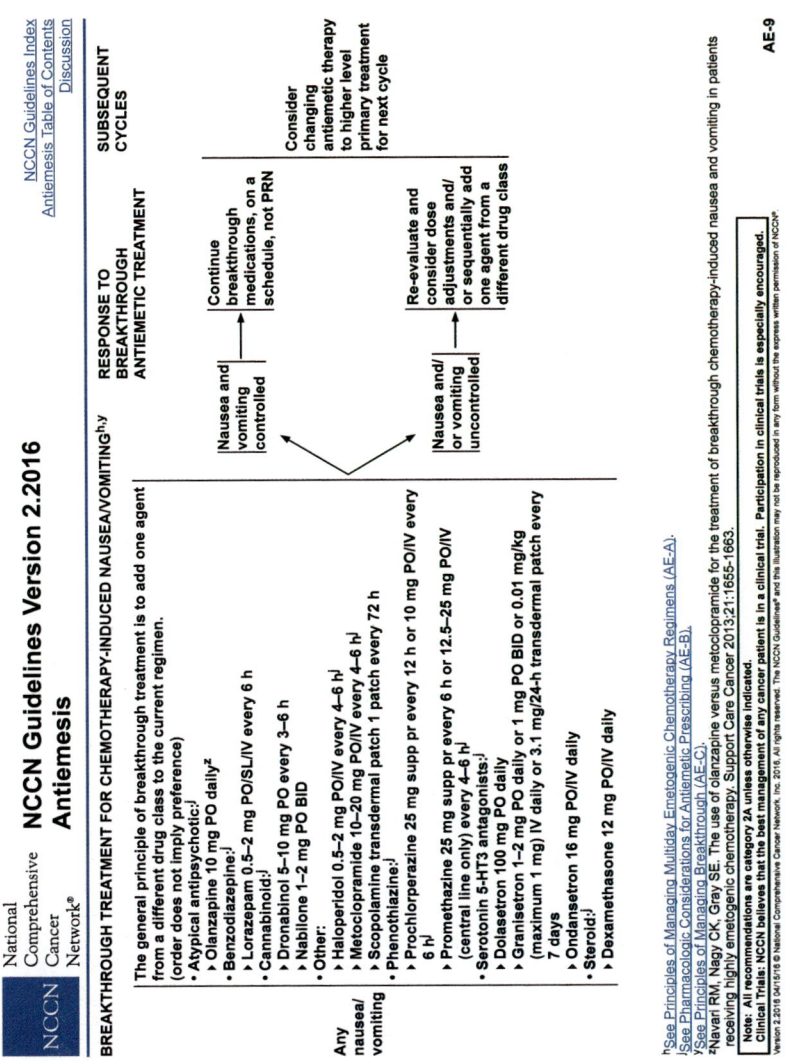

Figure 11.35. Breakthrough treatment for chemotherapy-induced nausea/vomiting
Reproduced with permission from the NCCN Clinical Practice Guidelines in Oncology (NCCN Guidelines®) for Antiemesis V.2.2016. © 2016 National Comprehensive Cancer Network, Inc. All rights reserved. The NCCN Guidelines® and illustrations herein may not be reproduced in any form for any purpose without the express written permission of the NCCN. To view the most recent and complete version of the NCCN Guidelines, go online to NCCN.org. NATIONAL COMPREHENSIVE CANCER NETWORK®, NCCN®, NCCN GUIDELINES®, and all other NCCN Content are trademarks owned by the National Comprehensive Cancer Network, Inc.

Neutropenic Fever Management

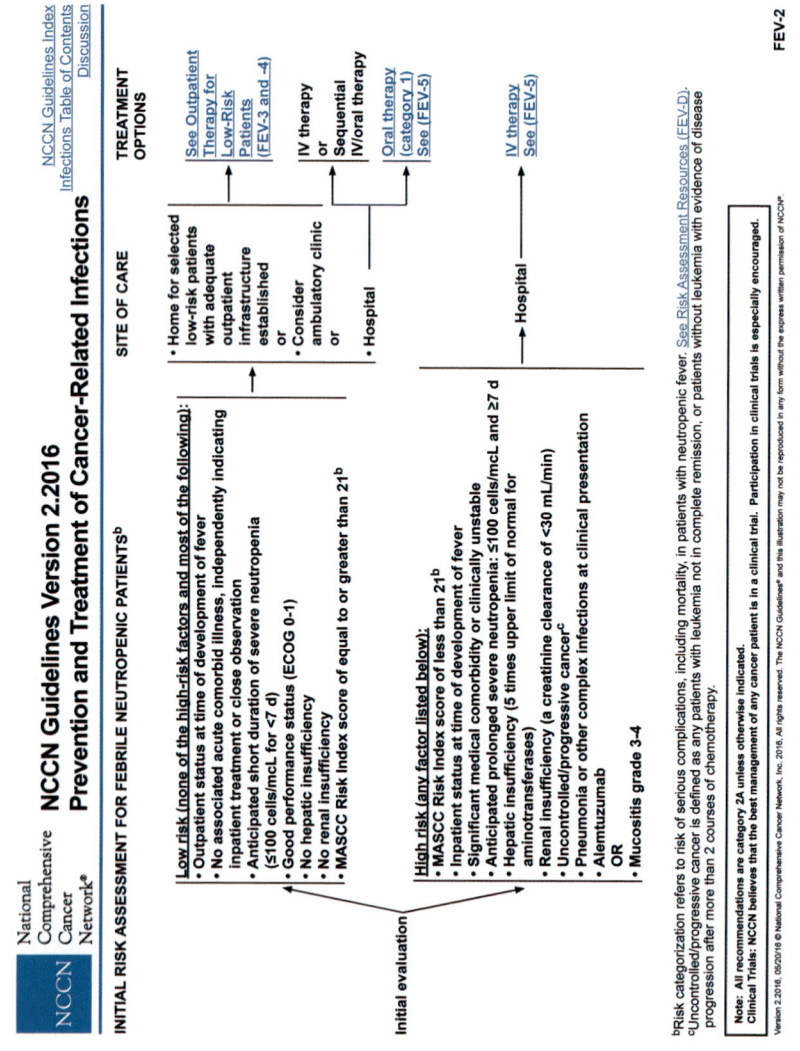

Figure 11.36. Risk assessment for febrile neutropenic patients
Reproduced with permission from the NCCN Clinical Practice Guidelines in Oncology (NCCN Guidelines®) for the Prevention and Treatment of Cancer-Related Infections V.2.2016. © 2016 National Comprehensive Cancer Network, Inc. All rights reserved. The NCCN Guidelines® and illustrations herein may not be reproduced in any form for any purpose without the express written permission of the NCCN. To view the most recent and complete version of the NCCN Guidelines, go online to NCCN.org. NATIONAL COMPREHENSIVE CANCER NETWORK®, NCCN®, NCCN GUIDELINES®, and all other NCCN Content are trademarks owned by the National Comprehensive Cancer Network, Inc.

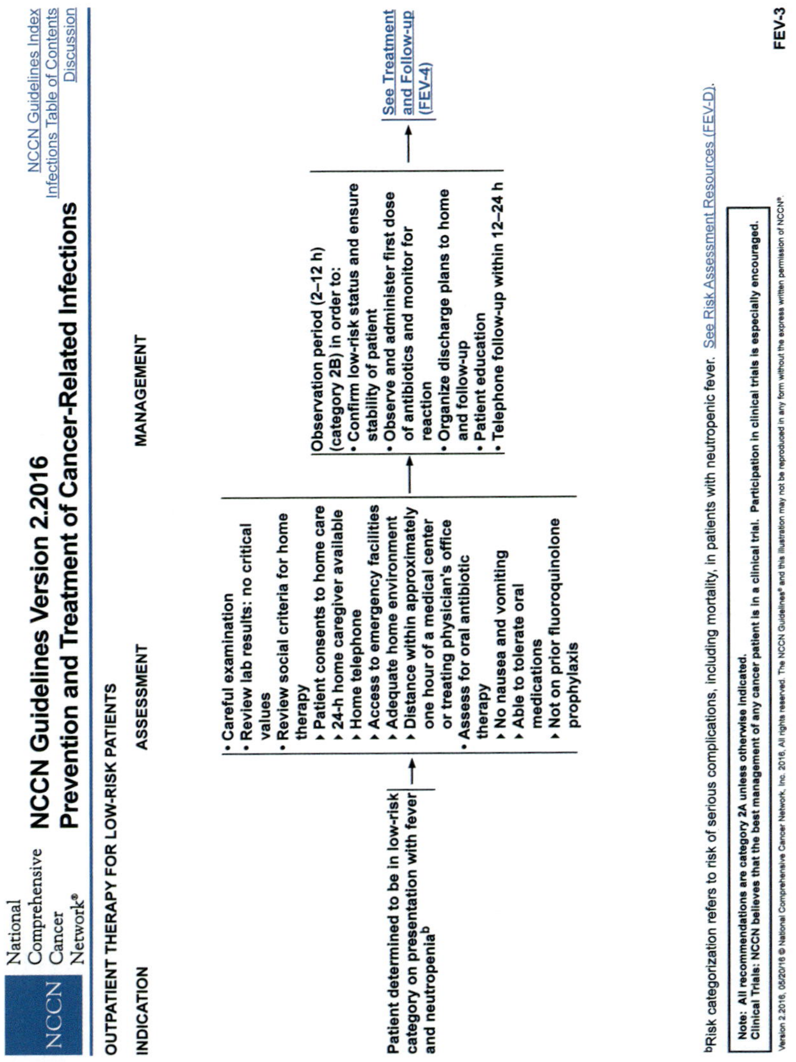

NCCN Clinical Practice Guidelines In Oncology (NCCN Guidelines®) — GYN-ONCOLOGY

NCCN Guidelines Version 2.2016
Prevention and Treatment of Cancer-Related Infections

OUTPATIENT THERAPY FOR LOW-RISK PATIENTS

INDICATION	ASSESSMENT	MANAGEMENT

Patient determined to be in low-risk category on presentation with fever and neutropenia[b]	• Careful examination
	• Review lab results: no critical values
	• Review social criteria for home therapy
	  ▸ Patient consents to home care
	  ▸ 24-h home caregiver available
	  ▸ Home telephone
	  ▸ Access to emergency facilities
	  ▸ Adequate home environment
	  ▸ Distance within approximately one hour of a medical center or treating physician's office
	• Assess for oral antibiotic therapy
	  ▸ No nausea and vomiting
	  ▸ Able to tolerate oral medications
	  ▸ Not on prior fluoroquinolone prophylaxis
		• Observation period (2–12 h) (category 2B) in order to:
		  ▸ Confirm low-risk status and ensure stability of patient
		  ▸ Observe and administer first dose of antibiotics and monitor for reaction
		  ▸ Organize discharge plans to home and follow-up
		  ▸ Patient education
		  ▸ Telephone follow-up within 12–24 h → See Treatment and Follow-up (FEV-4)

[b]Risk categorization refers to risk of serious complications, including mortality, in patients with neutropenic fever. See Risk Assessment Resources (FEV-D).

Note: All recommendations are category 2A unless otherwise indicated.
Clinical Trials: NCCN believes that the best management of any cancer patient is in a clinical trial. Participation in clinical trials is especially encouraged.

Figure 11.37. Criteria for low-risk outpatient therapy
Reproduced with permission from the NCCN Clinical Practice Guidelines in Oncology (NCCN Guidelines®) for the Prevention and Treatment of Cancer-Related Infections V.2.2016. © 2016 National Comprehensive Cancer Network, Inc. All rights reserved. The NCCN Guidelines® and illustrations herein may not be reproduced in any form for any purpose without the express written permission of the NCCN. To view the most recent and complete version of the NCCN Guidelines, go online to NCCN.org. NATIONAL COMPREHENSIVE CANCER NETWORK®, NCCN®, NCCN GUIDELINES®, and all other NCCN Content are trademarks owned by the National Comprehensive Cancer Network, Inc.

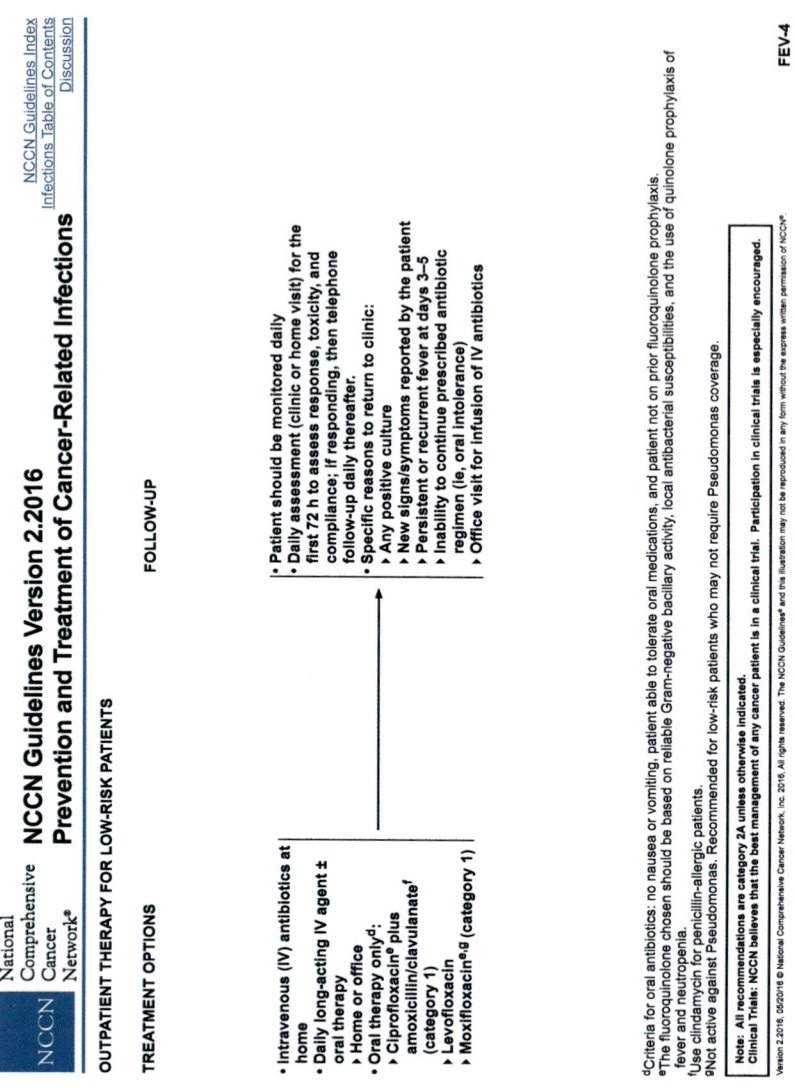

Figure 11.38. Low-risk outpatient therapy options
Reproduced with permission from the NCCN Clinical Practice Guidelines in Oncology (NCCN Guidelines®) for the Prevention and Treatment of Cancer-Related Infections V.2.2016. © 2016 National Comprehensive Cancer Network, Inc. All rights reserved. The NCCN Guidelines® and illustrations herein may not be reproduced in any form for any purpose without the express written permission of the NCCN. To view the most recent and complete version of the NCCN Guidelines, go online to NCCN.org. NATIONAL COMPREHENSIVE CANCER NETWORK®, NCCN®, NCCN GUIDELINES®, and all other NCCN Content are trademarks owned by the National Comprehensive Cancer Network, Inc.

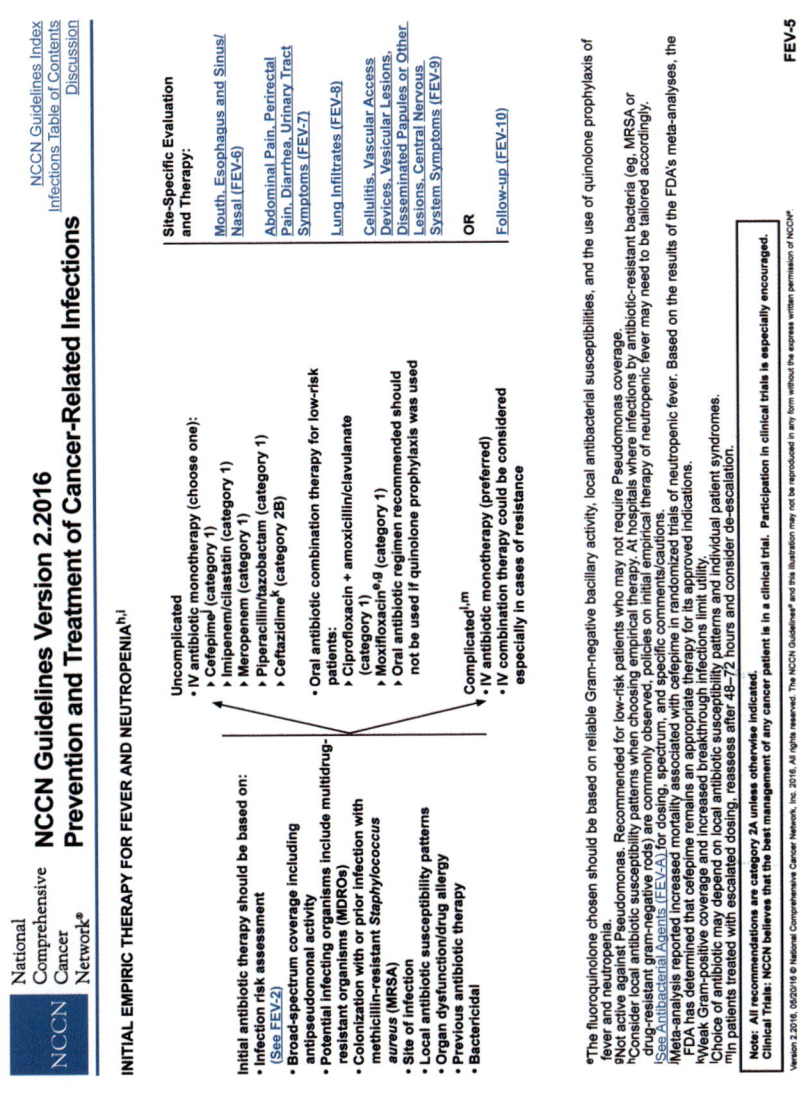

Figure 11.39. Initial empiric therapy for fever and neutropenia
Reproduced with permission from the NCCN Clinical Practice Guidelines in Oncology (NCCN Guidelines®) for the Prevention and Treatment of Cancer-Related Infections V.2.2016. © 2016 National Comprehensive Cancer Network, Inc. All rights reserved. The NCCN Guidelines® and illustrations herein may not be reproduced in any form for any purpose without the express written permission of the NCCN. To view the most recent and complete version of the NCCN Guidelines, go online to NCCN.org. NATIONAL COMPREHENSIVE CANCER NETWORK®, NCCN®, NCCN GUIDELINES®, and all other NCCN Content are trademarks owned by the National Comprehensive Cancer Network, Inc.

GYN-ONCOLOGY — NCCN Clinical Practice Guidelines In Oncology (NCCN Guidelines®)

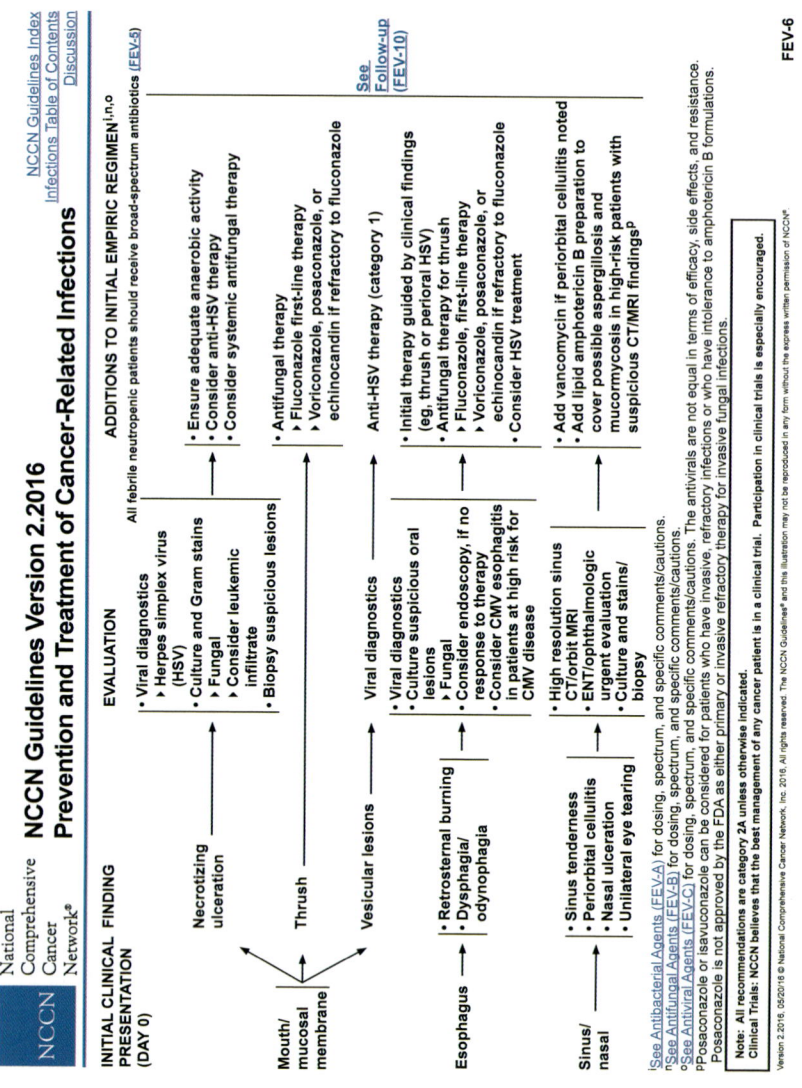

Figure 11.40. Prevention and treatment of cancer-related infections

Reproduced with permission from the NCCN Clinical Practice Guidelines in Oncology (NCCN Guidelines®) for the Prevention and Treatment of Cancer-Related Infections V.2.2016. © 2016 National Comprehensive Cancer Network, Inc. All rights reserved. The NCCN Guidelines® and illustrations herein may not be reproduced in any form for any purpose without the express written permission of the NCCN. To view the most recent and complete version of the NCCN Guidelines, go online to NCCN.org. NATIONAL COMPREHENSIVE CANCER NETWORK®, NCCN®, NCCN GUIDELINES®, and all other NCCN Content are trademarks owned by the National Comprehensive Cancer Network, Inc.

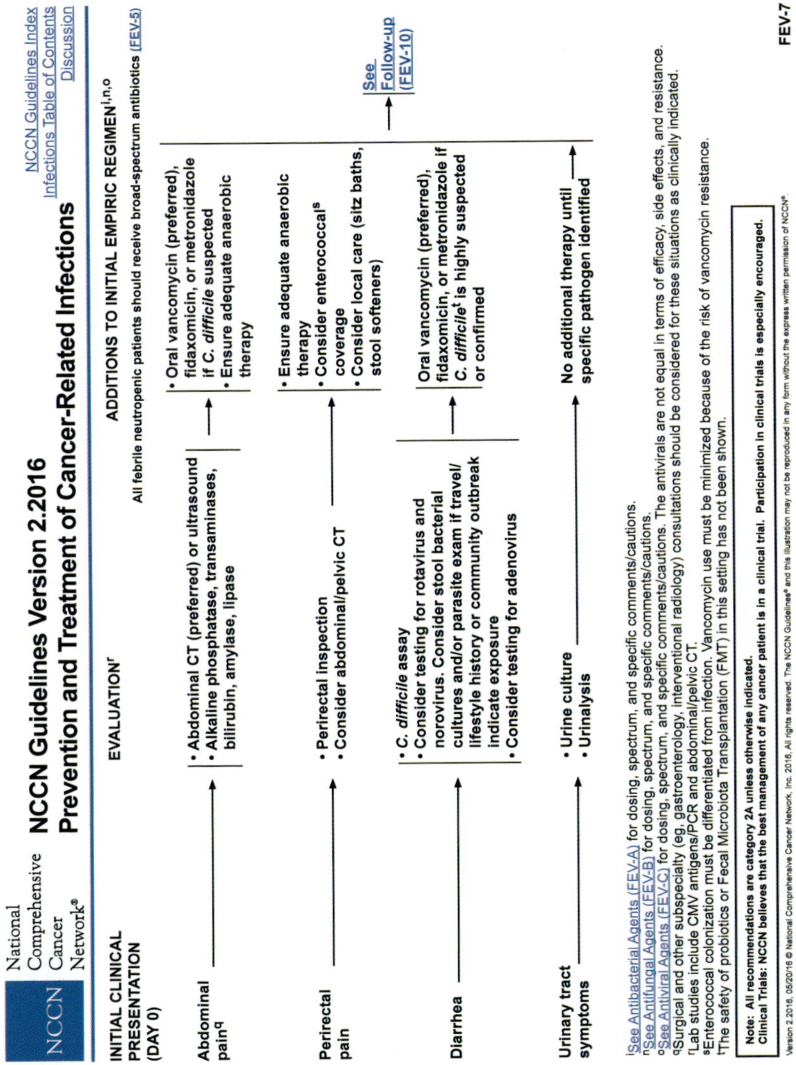

NCCN National Comprehensive Cancer Network®

NCCN Guidelines Version 2.2016
Prevention and Treatment of Cancer-Related Infections

NCCN Guidelines Index
Infections Table of Contents
Discussion

INITIAL CLINICAL PRESENTATION (DAY 0)	EVALUATION[r]	ADDITIONS TO INITIAL EMPIRIC REGIMEN[l,n,o] All febrile neutropenic patients should receive broad-spectrum antibiotics (FEV-5)	
Abdominal pain[q] →	• Abdominal CT (preferred) or ultrasound • Alkaline phosphatase, transaminases, bilirubin, amylase, lipase →	• Oral vancomycin (preferred), fidaxomicin, or metronidazole if *C. difficile* suspected • Ensure adequate anaerobic therapy	→ See Follow-up (FEV-10)
Perirectal pain →	• Perirectal inspection • Consider abdominal/pelvic CT →	• Ensure adequate anaerobic therapy • Consider enterococcal[s] coverage • Consider local care (sitz baths, stool softeners)	
Diarrhea →	• *C. difficile* assay • Consider testing for rotavirus and norovirus. Consider stool bacterial cultures and/or parasite exam if travel/lifestyle history or community outbreak indicate exposure • Consider testing for adenovirus →	Oral vancomycin (preferred), fidaxomicin, or metronidazole if *C. difficile*[t] is highly suspected or confirmed	
Urinary tract symptoms →	• Urine culture • Urinalysis →	No additional therapy until specific pathogen identified →	

[l] See Antibacterial Agents (FEV-A) for dosing, spectrum, and specific comments/cautions.
[n] See Antifungal Agents (FEV-B) for dosing, spectrum, and specific comments/cautions.
[o] See Antiviral Agents (FEV-C) for dosing, spectrum, and specific comments/cautions. The antivirals are not equal in terms of efficacy, side effects, and resistance.
[q] Surgical and other subspecialty (eg, gastroenterology, interventional radiology) consultations should be considered for these situations as clinically indicated.
[r] Lab studies include CMV antigens/PCR and abdominal/pelvic CT.
[s] Enterococcal colonization must be differentiated from infection. Vancomycin use must be minimized because of the risk of vancomycin resistance.
[t] The safety of probiotics or Fecal Microbiota Transplantation (FMT) in this setting has not been shown.

Note: All recommendations are category 2A unless otherwise indicated.
Clinical Trials: NCCN believes that the best management of any cancer patient is in a clinical trial. Participation in clinical trials is especially encouraged.

FEV-7

Figure 11.41. Prevention and treatment of cancer-related infections

Reproduced with permission from the NCCN Clinical Practice Guidelines in Oncology (NCCN Guidelines®) for the Prevention and Treatment of Cancer-Related Infections V.2.2016. © 2016 National Comprehensive Cancer Network, Inc. All rights reserved. The NCCN Guidelines® and illustrations herein may not be reproduced in any form for any purpose without the express written permission of the NCCN. To view the most recent and complete version of the NCCN Guidelines, go online to NCCN.org. NATIONAL COMPREHENSIVE CANCER NETWORK®, NCCN®, NCCN GUIDELINES®, and all other NCCN Content are trademarks owned by the National Comprehensive Cancer Network, Inc.

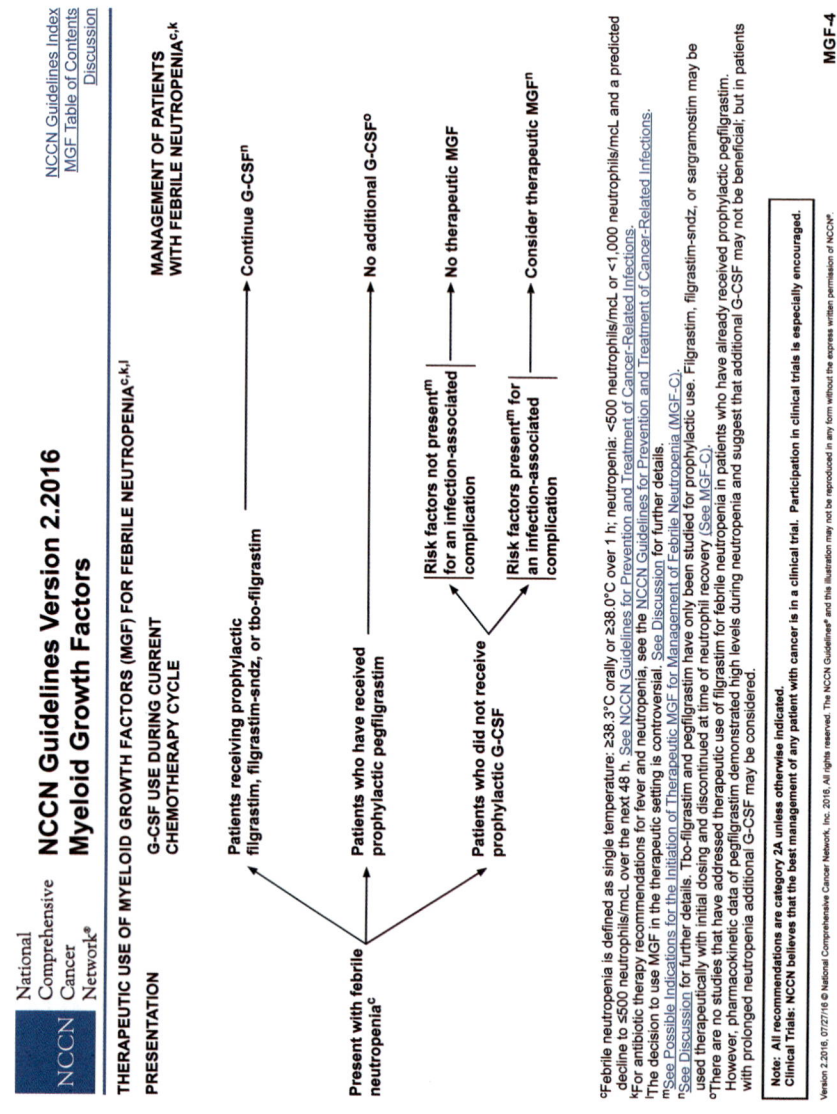

Figure 11.42. Use of myeloid growth factors for febrile neutropenia
Reproduced with permission from the NCCN Clinical Practice Guidelines in Oncology (NCCN Guidelines®) for Myeloid Growth Factors V.2.2016. © 2016 National Comprehensive Cancer Network, Inc. All rights reserved. The NCCN Guidelines® and illustrations herein may not be reproduced in any form for any purpose without the express written permission of the NCCN. To view the most recent and complete version of the NCCN Guidelines, go online to NCCN.org. NATIONAL COMPREHENSIVE CANCER NETWORK®, NCCN®, NCCN GUIDELINES®, and all other NCCN Content are trademarks owned by the National Comprehensive Cancer Network, Inc.

OTHER COMMON CLINICAL PROBLEMS IN THE GYN-ONCOLOGY PATIENT
Ileus versus Small Bowel Obstruction

Table 11.30. Comparison of SBO with ileus

Sign or Symptom	Ileus	Small Bowel Obstruction
Abdominal distension	May be present	May be present
Bowel sounds	Usually quiet or absent	May be high-pitched, may be absent
Obstipation	May be present	May be present
Pain	Mild and diffuse	Moderate to severe, colicky
Peritoneal signs	Absent	May be present
Radiography	Dilated loops of bowel, paucity of colonic gas	Dilated loops of bowel, differential air-fluid levels, paucity of colonic gas
Vomiting	May be present	May be present, may be bilious or feculent

- **Laboratory:** CBC, CMP (including magnesium). Hypokalemia worsens ileus, and magnesium depletion can lead to hypokalemia. Uremia can lead to ileus.
- **Radiography:** Plain abdominal films. Supine and upright plain films. For ileus, may show dilated loops of bowel but should demonstrate air in the colon and rectum without a transition zone. If diagnosis unclear, obtain a CT scan.
- **Management:** Supportive care: remove any inciting factors (opioids should be used sparingly and supplemented with NSAIDS or other nonopioid pain relievers), IV fluids to maintain normovolemia, electrolytes, bowel rest with sips of clear fluids at most, bowel decompression for those with moderate to severe or continuous vomiting (nasogastric tube can be placed), serial abdominal exam with repeat imaging studies if conservative measures do not improve the patient's condition in 48 to 72 hours.

Chemotherapy Extravasation Injury

Table 11.31. Treatment of chemotherapy extravasation injury

Class/Specific Agent	Local Antidote	Specific Procedure
Alkylating agents		
Cisplatin, mechlorethamine	1/3 or 1/6 M sodium thiosulfate	Mix 4–8 mL 10% sodium thiosulfate U.S.P. with 6 mL of sterile water for injection, U.S.P. for a 1/3 or 1/6 M solution. Inject 2 mL into site for each mg of mechlorethamine or 100 mg of cisplatin extravasated.
Mitomycin-C	Dimethylsulfoxide (DMSO) 50–99% (w/v)	Apply 1.5 mL to the site every 6 hr for 14 days. Allow to air-dry, do not cover.
DNA intercalators		
Doxorubicin, daunorubicin, amsacrine	Cold compresses	Apply immediately for 30–60 mins, then alternate on/off every 15 mins for 1 day.
	Dimethylsulfoxide (DMSO) 50–99% (w/v)	Apply 1.5 mL to the site every 6 hr for 14 days. Allow to air-dry, do not cover.
Vinca alkaloids		
Vinblastine, vincristine	Warm compresses, then hyaluronidase	Apply immediately for 30–60 mins, then alternate on/off every 15 mins for 1 day. Inject 150 U hyaluronidase (Wydase, others) into site.
Epipodophyllotoxins		
Etoposide, teniposide	Warm compresses, then hyaluronidase	Apply immediately for 30–60 mins, then alternate on/off every 15 mins for 1 day. Inject 150 U hyaluronidase (Wydase, others) into site.

Source: Dorr RT. Pharmacologic management of vesicant chemotherapy extravasations. In: Dorr RT, Von Hoff DD, ed. Cancer Chemotherapy Handbook, 2nd Ed. Norwalk, CT: Appleton & Lange; 1994. Reproduced with the permission of the McGraw-Hill Education.

HELPFUL TABLES

Table 11.32. Body fluid composition

	Na+	Cl–	K+	HCO_3^-	Daily production (mL)
Gastric juices	60–100	100	10	0	1,500–2,000
Duodenum	130	90	5	0–10	300–2000
Bile	145	100	5	15–35	100–800
Pancreatic juices	140	75	5	70–115	100–800
Ileum	140	100	5	15–30	2,000–3,000

Table 11.33. Steroids

		Relative Potency			Starting Doses (mg)	
Generic Name	Trade Name	Glucocorticoid and anti-inflammatory	Mineralocorticoid	Equivalent Doses (mg)	Moderate Illness	Severe Illness
Short-acting						
Hydrocortisone (cortisol)	Cortef	1	1	20	80–160	
	Solu-Cortef					
Cortisone		0.8	0.8	25	100–200	
Prednisone	Deltasone	4	0.8	5	20–40	60–100
	Meticorten					
Prednisolone	Delta-Cortef	4	0.8	5	20–40	60–100
	Meticortelone					
Methylprednisolone	Medrol	5	0.5	4	16–32	48–80
	Solu-Medrol					
Intermediate-acting						
Triamcinolone	Aristocort	5	0	4	16–32	48–80
Paramethasone	Kenacort	10	0	2	8–16	24–40
Long-acting						
Dexamethasone	Decadron	25	0	0.75	3–6	9–15
Betamethasone	Celestone	25	0	0.6	2.4–4.8	7.2–12

Source: Klearman M, Pereira M. Arthritis and rheumatologic diseases. In: Dunagan WC, Ridner ML, eds. *Manual of Medical Therapeutics*, 27th Ed. Boston: Little, Brown; 1992. Reproduced with the permission of the publisher.

INVASIVE CARDIAC MONITORING
Fast Facts
- Swan-Ganz catheter allows accurate measurement of hemodynamic parameters in acutely ill patient.
- Introduced into clinical practice in 1970.

Indications
- Sepsis with refractory hypotension or oliguria
- Unexplained or refractory pulmonary edema, heart failure, or oliguria
- Severe PIH with pulmonary edema or oliguria
- Intraoperative or intrapartum cardiovascular decompensation
- Massive blood loss and volume loss or replacement
- Adult respiratory distress syndrome (ARDS)
- Shock of undefined etiology
- Some chronic conditions, particularly associated with labor or surgery
  - NYHA Class III or IV cardiac disease (structural or physiologic)
  - Peripartum or perioperative coronary artery disease (ischemia, infarction)

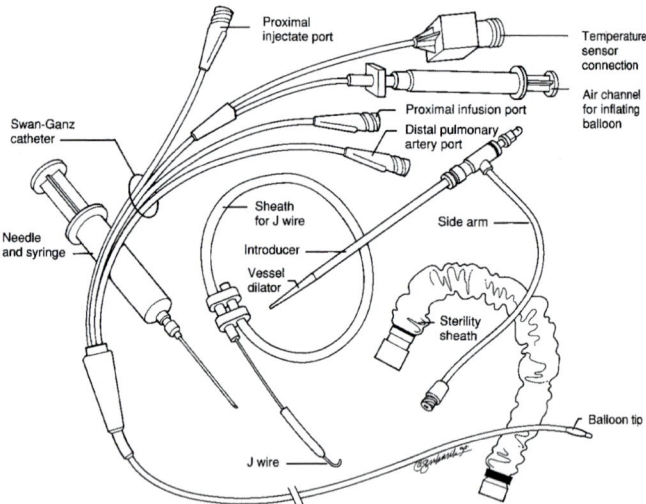

Figure 11.43. Triple lumen catheter
Distal port (upper left): Located in pulmonary artery. Attached to pressure transducer to provide continuous pulmonary artery pressure tracings and allow pulmonary capillary wedge pressure determination. Can also withdraw mixed venous blood from pulmonary artery. *Proximal port (center right):* Located in superior vena cava. Can be used in infused fluids and also used in cardiac output measurements. *Thermistor:* A temperature sensor used in determination of cardiac output.

Source: Mabie WC. Critical care obstetrics. In: Gabbe SG, Niebyl JR, Simpson JL, eds. *Obstetrics: Normal and Problem Pregnancies, 2nd Ed.* New York: Churchill Livingstone; 1991. Reproduced with the permission of the publisher.

Hemodynamic Measurements

Wedge Pressure
A measurement of left ventricular preload. The pulmonary artery wedge pressure is obtained with a balloon-tipped catheter advanced into a branch of the pulmonary artery until the vessel is occluded, forming a free communication through the pulmonary capillaries and veins to the left atrium. A true wedge position is in the lung zone where both pulmonary artery and pulmonary venous pressures exceed alveolar pressure.

Preload
Initial stretch of the myocardial fiber at end diastole. Clinically, the right and left ventricular end-diastolic pressures are assessed by the central venous pressure and wedge pressure respectively.

Afterload
Wall tension of the ventricle during ejection. Best reflected by systolic blood pressure.

Contractility
The force of myocardial contractility when preload and afterload are held constant.

Table 11.34. Hemodynamic therapy

	Decreased	Increased
Preload		
	Crystalloid	**Diuretics**
	Colloid	Furosemide
	Blood	Ethacrynic acid
		Mannitol
		Venodilators
		Furosemide
		Nitroglycerin
		Morphine
Afterload		
	Volume	**Arterial dilators**
	Inotropic support	Hydralazine
	Vasopressors	Diazoxide
	Norepinephrine	**Venous dilators**
	Phenylephrine	Nitroglycerin
	Metaraminol	**Mixed arteriovenous dilators**
		Nitroprusside
		Trimethaphan
Contractility		
	Dopamine	
	Dobutamine	
	Epinephrine	
	Calcium	
	Digitalis	

Source: Gomella LG, Braen GR, Olding MJ. Critical care. In: *Clinician's Pocket Reference: The Scut Monkey's Handbook*, 7th Ed. Norwalk, CT: Appleton & Lange; 1993. Reproduced with the permission of the publisher.

GYN-ONCOLOGY

Table 11.35. Derivation of hemodynamic parameters

Mean arterial pressure	MAP	mm Hg	$\dfrac{\text{systolic pressure} + 2 (\text{diastolic pressure})}{3}$
Stroke volume	SV	mL/beat	CO/HR
Stroke index	SI	mL/beat/m²	SV/BSA
Cardiac index	CI	L/min/m²	CO/BSA
Pulmonary vascular resistance	PVR	dynes × sec × cm⁻⁵	$\dfrac{\text{MPAP}-\text{PCWP}}{\text{CO}} \times 80$
Systemic vascular Resistance	SVR	dynes × sec × cm⁻⁵	$\dfrac{\text{MAP}-\text{CVP}}{\text{CO}} \times 80$

BSA, body surface area; CI, cardiac index; HR, hemodynamic response; MAP, mean arterial pressure; MPAP, mean pulmonary artery pressure; PCWP, capillary wedge pressure; PVR, pulmonary vascular resistance; SI, stroke index; SV, stroke volume; SVR, systemic vascular resistance.

Table 11.36. Normal hemodynamic values

		Trimester of Pregnancy		
Parameter	Nonpregnant	First	Second	Third
Heart beat (beats/min)	60–100	81	84	84
Central venous pressure (mm Hg)	5–10			
Pulmonary capillary wedge pressure (mm Hg)	6–12			
Mean arterial pressure (mm Hg)	90–110	82	84	86
Cardiac output (L/min)	4.3–6.0	6.2	6.3	6.4
Stroke volume (mL/beat)	57–71	76	75	76
Systemic vascular resistance (dynes × sec × cm⁻⁵)	900–1,400	1,087	1,093	1,119
Pulmonary vascular resistance (dynes × sec × cm⁻⁵)	<250			

Source: Adapted from Clark SL, Cotton DB, Lee W, et al. Central hemodynamic assessment of normal term pregnancy. *Am J Obstet Gynecol.* 1989;161(6 Pt 1):1439-42; and Rosenthal MH. Intrapartum intensive care management of the cardiac patient. *Clin Obstet Gynecol.* 1981;24(3):789-94.

Table 11.37. SHOCK: hemodynamic profiles

Physiologic Variable	Preload (CVP)	Pump Function (Cardiac Output/Index)	Afterload (SVR)	Tissue Perfusion (Capillary Refill Time)	Tissue Perfusion (Mixed Venous O₂ Sat)
Hypovolemic	Decreased	Decreased	Increased	Increased	Low
Cardiogenic	Increased	Decreased	Increased	Increased	Low
Distributive (septic and SIRS)	Decreased	Increased	Decreased	Decreased	High
Obstructive	Increased	Decreased	Increased	Increased	Low

Early Goal-Directed Therapy Tarets in ICU
- Administration of IVF within the first 6 hours of presentation using physiologic targets to guide fluid management
- Mean arterial pressure (MAP) ≥65 mm Hg (MAP = [(2 × diastolic) + systolic]/3)
- Urine output ≥0.5 mL/kg/hour
- Static or dynamic predictors of fluid responsiveness, eg. CVP 8–12 mm Hg
- Central venous (SV) oxyhemoglobin saturation ($ScvO_2$) ≥70%

COAGULATION CASCADE

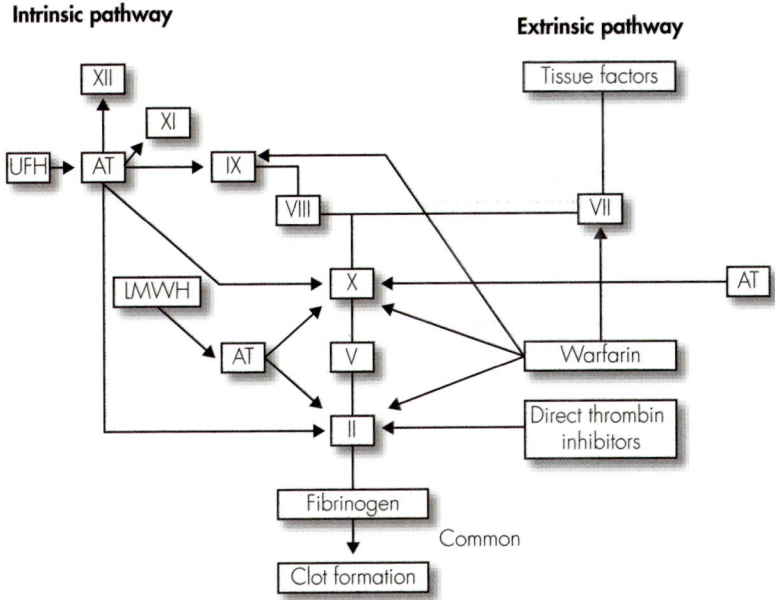

Figure 11.44. Effects of anticoagulants on the coagulation cascade
AT, antithrombin; LMWH, low-molecular-weight heparin; UFH, unfractionated heparin.
Source: Reproduced with permission from Haines ST. Update on the prevention of venous thromboembolism. *Am J Health-Syst Pharm.* 2004;7:S5–S11. © 2004, American Society of Health-System Pharmacists, Inc. All rights reserved.

THROMBOEMBOLIC PHENOMENA
Fast Facts
- First 5 to 10 days following diagnosis is most important time to begin treatment.
- For patients with proximal DVT, the greatest risk of embolization is during the first 3 months of anticoagulant therapy and in particular during the first few days following the diagnosis.
- Therapy should continue for 3–6 months in patients with cancer and VTE.
- Check baseline PT/INR/PTTT prior to initiation of anticoagulation.

Treatment Options
- Low-molecular-weight heparin (LMWH) (e.g., enoxaparin)—preferred for patients with active cancer.
- Factor Xa inhibitor (SQ)—Fondaparinux-acceptable alternative to LMWH for nonpregnant patients but insufficient evidence in patients with malignancy.
- UFH (IV)—preferred agent for patients with severe renal failure but associated with higher rates of recurrent thrombosis and major bleeding.
- Oral factor Xa inhibitors (e.g., rivaroxaban) and oral direct thrombin inhibitors (dabigatran)—acceptable alternative to LMWH for patients with normal renal function who wish to avoid daily injections and risk of bleeding with an irreversible agent.

Dosing
- LMWH
  - Enoxaparin 1 mg/kg SC every 12 hours or 1.5 mg/kg once daily.
- Dalteparin 200 units/kg once daily for the first 30 days, followed by 150 units/kg for maintenance.
- LMWH is as effective and safe as UFH and is clearly superior because therapeutic dosing is more rapidly and dependably achieved.
- Factor Xa and direct thrombin inhibitors
  - Fondaparinux 5 mg SC qd (<50kg), 7.5 mg SC qd (50–100 kg), and 10 mg SC qd (>100 kg)
  - Rivaroxaban 15 mg PO twice daily (for the first 3 weeks)
  - Apixaban 10 mg PO twice daily (for the first 7 days)
  - Edoxaban 60 mg PO once daily (and 30 mg once daily in patients with a creatinine 30 to 50 mL/minute or a body weight below 60 kg)
  - Dabigatran 150 mg PO twice daily

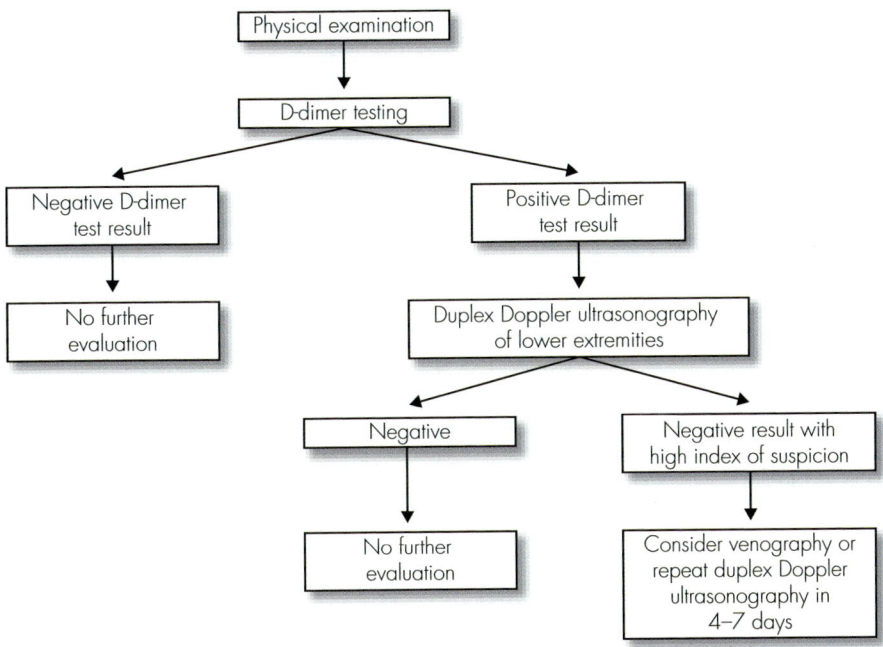

Figure 11.45. Diagnostic algorithm for deep vein thrombosis

If the duplex Doppler ultrasonography results are positive, begin anticoagulation therapy with low-molecular-weight heparin or unfractionated heparin. If contraindications for anticoagulation exist, consider placement of an inferior vena caval filter.

Source: Reproduced with permission from Krivak TC, Zorn KK. Venous thromboembolism in obstetrics and gynecology. *Obstet Gynecol.* 2007;109(3):761-77. Copyright © 2007 The American College of Obstetricians and Gynecologists.

GYN-ONCOLOGY — Thromboembolic Phenomena

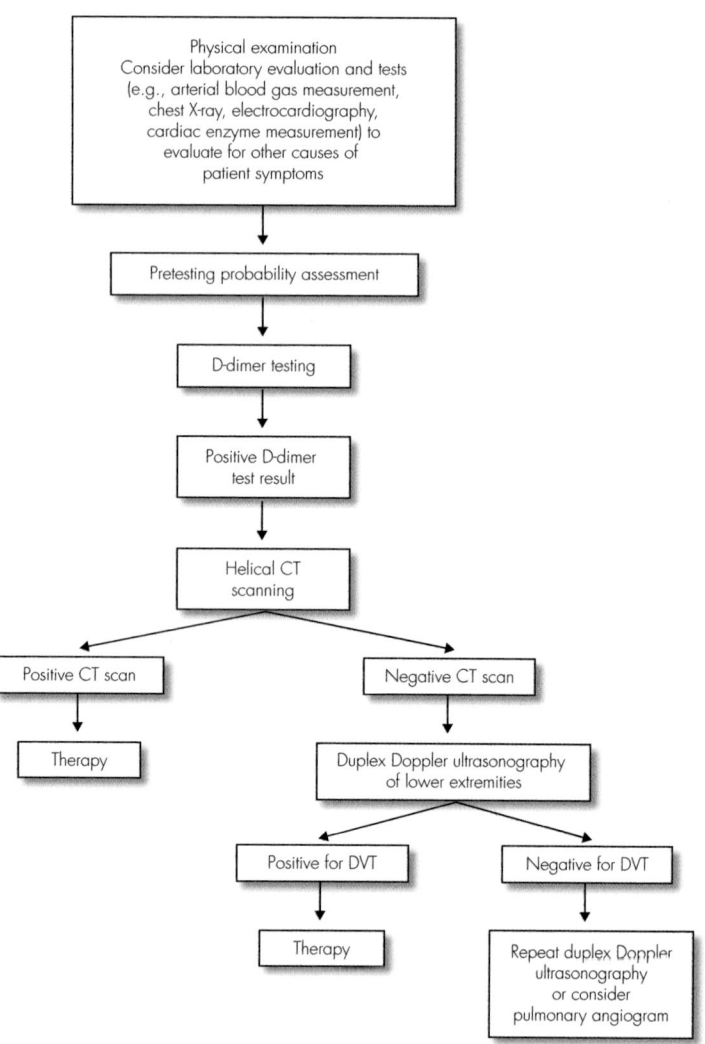

Figure 11.46. Diagnostic algorithm for pulmonary embolism
Therapy may consist of unfractionated heparin or low-molecular-weight heparin, as well as supportive care (supplemental oxygen). If the patient is unstable, thrombolytic therapy may be considered. If contraindication for coagulation exists, consider placement of inferior vena caval filter. If the D-dimer test result is negative and pretest probability is low, duplex Doppler ultrasonography of lower extremities would be considered. Withhold anticoagulation therapy if both test results are negative.
Source: Reproduced with permission from Krivak TC, Zorn KK. Venous thromboembolism in obstetrics and gynecology. *Obstet Gynecol.* 2007;109(3):761-77. Copyright © 2007 The American College of Obstetricians and Gynecologists.

Thromboembolic Phenomena — GYN-ONCOLOGY

Table 11.38. Stanford hospital guide for preventing venous thromboembolism

Low Risk (<5% Risk of DVT)

- Patient <40 yr old **and**
- Minor surgery **and**
- No additional risk factors

- No specific prophylaxis; early mobilization

Moderate Risk (10–20% Risk of DVT)

- Age 40–60 years old with no additional risk factors **or**
- Minor surgery in patients with additional risk factors

- UFH 5000 units SC q8hrs **or**
- LMWH (enoxaparin) 40 mg SC qday

Add GCS or IPC

High Risk (20–40% Risk of DVT)

- Surgery in patients >60 years old **or**
- Age 40–60 with additional risk factors

- UFH 5000 units SC q8hrs **or**
- LMWH (enoxaparin) 30 mg SC bid

Add GCS or IPC if possible

Highest Risk (40–80% Risk of DVT)

- Surgery in patient with multiple risk factors **or**
- Hip or knee arthroplasty **or**
- Hip fracture surgery **or**
- Major trauma **or**
- Spinal cord injury

- LMWH (enoxaparin) 30 mg SC bid **or**
- Fondiparinux 2.5 mg SC qday **or**
- Warfarin started day of surgery, target INR 2–3
- Add GCS or IPC if possible
- Consider extended (4 wk) out of hospital prophylaxis at discharge

DVT, deep vein thrombosis; GCS, graduated compression stockings; INR, international normalized ratio; IPC, intermittent pneumatic compression; LMWH, low-molecular-weight heparin; UFH, unfractionated heparin.

GYN-ONCOLOGY — Thromboembolic Phenomena

Table 11.39. Venous thromboembolism prophylaxis—Inova Fairfax Hospital

The presence of one (1) high-risk factor or two (2) or more other risk factors is an indication for VTE prophylaxis.

VTE High-risk Factors
Trauma (abdomen, pelvis, hip, and leg)
Major surgery (especially abdomen, pelvis, hip, and leg)
Prior history of VTE (DVT or PE)
Malignancy

Other VTE Risk Factors
Age >40 yr
Intensive care unit admission
Chronic lung disease
Respiratory failure
Pneumonia
Inflammatory disorders
Central line/venous catheter
Known thrombophilia
Active collagen vascular disorder
Serious infection
Prolonged immobility (>24 hr)
Varicose veins
Nephrotic syndrome
Sickle cell disease
Pregnancy or estrogen use
Obesity
Congestive heart failure

Anticoagulant Prophylaxis Exclusion Criteria
Active bleeding
Uncontrolled hypertension
Coagulopathy
Current anticoagulant treatment
Recent intraocular or intracranial surgery
Presence or history of heparin induced thrombocytopenia (HIT)
Significant renal insufficiency
Epidural anesthesia or spinal tap within 24 hr
Hypersensitivity to unfractionated heparin or low-molecular-weight heparin

Standard Venous Thromboembolism Prophylaxis Options
Intermittent sequential pneumatic compression device (SCD)
Heparin 5000 units SC q8hrs
Lovenox 40 mg SC daily
(Lovenox 30 mg subcutaneously daily for creatinine clearance <30 mL/min)

Table 11.40. Overview of traditional and newer antithrombotic agents.*

Agent	Route of Administration	Mechanism of Action	Recommended Interval between Last Dose and Procedure
Anticoagulant agents			
Warfarin (Coumadin, Bristol-Myers Squibb)	Oral	Inhibition of vitamin K–dependent factors II, VII, IX, and X for γ-carboxylation; and proteins C and S	1–8 days, depending on INR and patient characteristics; INR decreases to ≤1.5 in approximately 93% of patients within 5 days[48]
Unfractionated heparin	Intravenous or subcutaneous	Antithrombin activation (inhibition of factors IIa, IXa, Xa, XIa, and XIIa)	Intravenous, 2–6 hr, depending on dose; subcutaneous, 12–24 hr, depending on dose
Low-molecular-weight heparins (enoxaparin [Lovenox, Sanofi Aventis] and dalteparin [Fragmin, Eisai])	Subcutaneous	Antithrombin activation (inhibition of factor Xa and, to a lesser extent, factor IIa)	24 hr
Fondaparinux (Arixtra, GlaxoSmithKline)	Subcutaneous	Antithrombin activation (factor Xa inhibitor)	36–48 hr
Dabigatran (Pradaxa, Boehringer Ingelheim)	Oral	Direct thrombin inhibitor	1 or 2 days with creatinine clearance rate of ≥50 ml/min; 3–5 days with creatinine clearance rate of <50 ml/min
Rivaroxaban (Xarelto, Bayer HealthCare)	Oral	Direct factor Xa inhibitor	≥1 day when renal function is normal; 2 days with creatinine clearance rate of 60–90 ml/min; 3 days with creatinine clearance rate of 30–59 ml/min; and 4 days with creatinine clearance rate of 15–29 ml/min[52]
Apixaban (Eliquis, Bristol-Myers Squibb)	Oral	Direct factor Xa inhibitor	1 or 2 days with creatinine clearance rate of >60 ml/min; 3 days with creatinine clearance rate of 50–59 ml/min; and 5 days with creatinine clearance rate of <30–49 ml/min
Desirudin (Iprivask, Canyon Pharmaceuticals)	Subcutaneous	Direct thrombin inhibitor	2 hr
Antiplatelet agents			
Aspirin	Oral	Cyclooxygenase inhibitor (irreversible effect)	7–10 days
Aspirin and dipyridamole (Aggrenox, Boehringer Ingelheim)	Oral	Phosphodiesterase inhibitor	7–10 days
Cilostazol (Pletal, Otsuka Pharmaceutical)	Oral	Phosphodiesterase inhibitor	2 days
Thienopyridine agents (clopidogrel [Plavix, Sanofi Aventis], ticlopidine [Ticlid, Roche], prasugrel [Effient, Eli Lilly], and ticagrelor [Brilinta, AstraZeneca])	Oral	ADP receptor antagonist	5 days (clopidogrel and ticagrelor), 7 days (prasugrel), or 10–14 days (ticlopidine)

*ADP denotes adenosine diphosphate, aPTT activated partial thromboplastin time, FDA Food and Drug Administration, INR international normalized ratio, and PCC prothrombin complex concentrate.

†PCCs are either 3-factor or 4-factor concentrates. Nonactivated 4-factor PCCs contain factors II, VII, IX, and X and proteins C and S, and nonactivated 3-factor PCCs contain factors II, IX, and X and only small amounts of factor VII. For details, see the Supplementary Appendix.

‡Factor VIII inhibitor bypass activity provides both factor II (prothrombin) and factor Xa for rapid and sustained thrombin generation. For details, see the Supplementary Appendix.

Source: Baron TH, Kamath PS, McBane RD. Management of antithrombotic therapy in patients undergoing invasive procedures. *N Engl J Med.* 2013 May 30;368(22):2113-24.

SEPSIS SYNDROME

Definition
- Clinical syndrome of systemic toxicity (sepsis) related to infection, which often leads to cardiovascular collapse.

Fast Facts
- 70–80% are the result of gram-negative bacteria.
- 70,000–300,000 cases annually.
- 30–50% of episodes associated with septic shock.
- Mortality rate approaches 50%.

Diagnosis
Each of the Following Four:
- Clinical evidence to support a presumptive diagnosis of gram-negative infection and evidence of deleterious systemic effects.
- Core temperature T >38.3° C (101° F) or unexplained hypothermia <35.6° C.
- Tachycardia (>90 bpm) in absence of β-blockade and tachypnea (respiratory rate >20 or requiring mechanical ventilation).
- Hypotension (systolic blood pressure ≤90 mm Hg or drop in systolic blood pressure ≥40 mm Hg) in presence of adequate volume status and no antihypertensive agents.

Evidence of Systemic Toxicity or Poor End-Organ Perfusion Defined by at Least Two of the Following:
- Unexplained metabolic acidosis (pH <7.3, a base deficit of >5, or increased plasma lactate).
- Arterial hypoxia (PO_2 ≤75 mm Hg or PO_2/FiO_2 ratio <250) in patient without overt pulmonary disease.
- Acute renal failure (urinary output <30 cc/hour) for 1 hour despite acute volume loading and evidence of adequate intravascular volume.
- Recent (within 24 hours) unexplained coagulation abnormalities (increased prothrombin time/partial thromboplastin time) or unexplained platelet depression (<100,000 or decrease of 50% from baseline).
- Mental status changes.
- Elevated cardiac index (>4 L/min/m²) with low SVR (<800 dynes × sec × cm^{-5}).

Management
1. History and physical exam
2. Volume replacement
3. Blood/urine/sputum cultures
4. O_2, labs, X-rays (chest X-ray, kidney-ureter-bladder radiography, etc.)
5. Broad-spectrum antibiotics
6. Consider transfer to intensive care unit for pressor support

ABDOMINAL DEHISCENCE
Predisposing Factors
- Inadequate closure
- Previous radiation
- Infection (cellulitis must be examined)
- Poor nutrition (albumin <3.0 g/dL)

Signs and Symptoms
- Sudden wound discomfort or none at all
- Sensation of disruption by patient
- Appearance of copious, persistent serosanguineous wound drainage
- Prolonged paralytic ileus

    These signs represent dehiscence until proven otherwise.

Management
- Semi-Fowler's position
- Cover bowels/wound with sterile, wet gauze pads
- Place nasogastric tube to decompress bowel
- Initiate broad spectrum antibiotic coverage
- Plan for surgical closure if operative candidate

HEMORRHAGE

"Hypovolemia is a problem" (Teng, 1991).

Unsatisfactory Hemostasis

Signs and Symptoms
- Can be revealed or concealed
- Tachycardia, ectopy, chest pain
- Cold extremities
- Confusion secondary to hypoxia
- Abdominal distention
- Hemoperitoneum

Early recognition is crucial.

Management
- Medical stabilization
- Surgical re-exploration

Coagulopathy

Signs and Symptoms
- Unexplained bleeding from wound, IV sites, etc.
- Red top tube fails to clot
- Microangiopathic changes revealed on disseminated intravascular coagulation panel

Management
- Correction of underlying cause
- Sepsis, fetal demise, tissue necrosis, replacement of blood products

Table 11.41. Blood products

Component	Contents	Volume	Indication
Packed red blood cells	Red cells with most plasma removed	1 unit = 250–300 cc	Acute or chronic blood loss 1 unit raises Hct by 3%
Platelets	Platelets only	1 pack = 50 cc 1 pack raises platelets by 6 K; 6-pack is from 6 donors blood	Platelets <20 K in non-bleeding patient Platelets <50 K in bleeding patient
Fresh frozen-plasma (FFP)	Fibrinogen, Factor II, VII, IX, X, XI, XII, XIII and heat labile V and VII,	1 unit = 150–250 cc units 11 g albumin 500 mg fibrinogen 0.7–1.0 units clotting factor	DIC, transfusion >10 Liver disease, IgG deficiency 1 unit raises fibrinogen by 10 mg/dL
Cryoprecipitated antihemophilic factor (Cryo)	Factors VIII, XIII, von Willebrand's, fibrinogen	1 unit = 10 cc 250 mg fibrinogen 80 units factor VIII	Hemophilia A, von Willebrand's disease, fibrinogen deficiency

ACID/BASE DISTURBANCES
Interpretation of Arterial Blood Gases
- *Rule I:* A change in PCO_2 down or up of 10 mm Hg is associated with an increase or decrease of pH of 0.08 units.
- *Rule II:* A pH change of 0.15 is equivalent to a base change of 10 mEq/L.
- *Rule III:* The dose of bicarbonate (in mEq) required to fully correct a metabolic acidosis is:

$$\frac{\text{Base deficit (mEqL)} \times \text{patient weight (kg)}}{4}$$

- *Rule IV:* If the alveolar ventilation increases, PCO_2 will decrease, if alveolar ventilation decreases, PCO_2 will increase.

Source: Gomella LG, Braen GR, Olding MJ. Blood gases and acid base disorders. In: *Clinician's Pocket Reference: The Scut Monkey's Handbook*, 7th Ed. Norwalk, CT: Appleton & Lange; 1993. Reproduced with the permission of the publisher.

Table 11.42. Differential diagnosis of acid/base disturbances

	Ph	HCO_3	PCO_2
Metabolic acidosis	↓	↓↓	↓
Metabolic alkalosis	↑	↑↑	↑
Respiratory acidosis	↓	↑	↑↑
Respiratory alkalosis	↑	↓	↓↓

Metabolic Acidosis

Anion gap
- **P** araldehyde
- **L** actate
- **U** remia
- **M** ethanol
- **S** alicylates
- **E** thylene glycol
- **E** thanol
- **D** iabetic ketoacidosis

Non-anion gap
- **D** iarrhea, dilution
- **U** reteral conduit
- **R** enal tubular acidosis
- **H** yperal
- **A** cetazolamide, acid administration
- **M** ultiple myeloma

(As in Durham, NC, home of the **Duke Blue Devils!**)

Metabolic Alkalosis

Chloride responsive
(urinary chloride <10mEq/L)
- Gastrointestinal losses (emesis, nasogastric)
- Diuretics
- Chronic hypercapnea
- Cystic fibrosis

Chloride resistant
(urinary chloride >10 mEq/L)
- Cushing syndrome
- Conn's syndrome
- Exogenous steroids
- Barter's syndrome

Figure 11.47. Metabolic acidosis and alkalosis

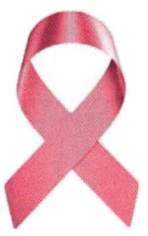

CHAPTER 12

Breast Cancer

FAST FACTS

- Breast cancer accounts for 27% of all new cases of cancer diagnosed in women.
- A woman's lifetime risk of developing breast cancer is 12.08%, or 1 in 8.
- Tumors detected at an early stage that are small and confined to the breast are more likely to be successfully treated, with a 98% 5-year survival for localized disease.
- Ten percent of cases of ovarian cancer and 3–5% of cases of breast cancer are due to germline mutations in *BRCA1* and *BRCA2*.
- More than 1,200 different mutations have been reported for *BRCA1*, and more than 1,300 different mutations have been reported for *BRCA2*.
- An estimated 1 in 300 to 1 in 800 individuals carry a mutation in *BRCA1* or *BRCA2*.
- An estimated 1 in 40 Ashkenazi Jews carries one of three founder mutations in *BRCA1* or *BRCA2*.
- For a woman with a *BRCA1* mutation, the risk of ovarian cancer is 39–46%.
- For a woman with a *BRCA2* mutation, the risk of ovarian cancer is 12–20%.
- The estimated lifetime risk of breast cancer with a *BRCA1* or *BRCA2* mutation is 65–74%.
- For women with breast cancer, the 10-year actuarial risk of developing subsequent ovarian cancer is 12.7% for *BRCA1* mutation carriers and 6.8% for *BRCA2* mutation carriers.

   Source: Data from ACOG Practice Bulletin No. 122: Breast cancer screening. *Obstet Gynecol*. 2011 Aug;118(2 Pt 1):372-82; ACOG Practice Bulletin No. 103: Hereditary breast and ovarian cancer syndrome. *Obstet Gynecol*. 2009 Apr;113(4):957-66.

Table 12.1. Risk and protective factors for developing breast cancer

	Risk Group		
	Low risk	High risk	Relative risk
Risk factors			
Deleterious *BRCA1/BRCA2* genes	Negative	Positive	3.0 to 7.0
Mother or sister with breast cancer	No	Yes	2.6
Age	30 to 34	70 to 74	18.0
Age at menarche	>14	<12	1.5
Age at first birth	<20	>30	1.9 to 3.5
Age at menopause	<45	>55	2.0
Use of contraceptive pills	Never	Past/current use	1.07 to 1.2
HRT (estrogen + progestin)	Never	Current	1.2
Alcohol	None	2 to 5 drinks/day	1.4
Breast density on mammography (percents)	0	≥75	1.8 to 6.0
Bone density	Lowest quartile	Highest quartile	2.7 to 3.5
History of a benign breast biopsy	No	Yes	1.7
History of atypical hyperplasia on biopsy	No	Yes	3.7
Protective factors			
Breast feeding (months)	≥16	0	0.73
Parity	≥5	0	0.71
Recreational exercise	Yes	No	0.70
Postmenopause body mass index (kg/m^2)	<22.9	>30.7	0.63
Oophorectomy before age 35 years	Yes	No	0.3
Aspirin	≥Once/week for ≥6 months	Nonusers	0.79

HRT: hormone replacement therapy.

Source: Adapted from Clemons M, Goss P. Estrogen and the risk of breast cancer. *N Engl J Med.* 2001 Jan 25;344(4):276-85. Review. Erratum in: *N Engl J Med.* 2001 Jun 7;344(23):1804.

Table 12.2. Breast cancer screening for average-risk patient: breast self-exam (BSE) and clinical breast exam (CBE)

American Cancer Society (ACS)	U.S. Preventive Services Task Force (USPSTF)	American College of Obstetricians and Gynecologists (ACOG)
Breast self-examination		
It is acceptable for women to choose not to do breast self-examination (BSE) or to do BSE regularly (monthly) or irregularly. Beginning in their early 20s, women should be told about the benefits and limitations of BSE. Whether a woman ever performs BSE, the importance of prompt reporting of any new breast symptoms to a health professional should be emphasized. Women who choose to do BSE should receive instruction and have their technique reviewed on the occasion of a periodic health examination.	No requirement for clinicians to teach women how to perform BSE (grade D recommendation).	Breast self-awareness should be encouraged and can include BSE; women should report any changes in their breasts to their health care providers.
Clinical breast examination		
The ACS does not recommend clinical breast examination (CBE) for breast cancer screening in average-risk women at any age. This new recommendation should not be interpreted to discount the potential value of CBE in low- and medium-resource settings where mammography screening may not be feasible. Clinical breast examination also may have a role in some groups of women at very high risk.	Insufficient current evidence to assess the additional benefits and harms of CBE beyond screening mammography in women 40 years or older.	For women aged 20–39 years, CBEs are recommended every 1–3 years. For women aged 40 years and older, CBE should be performed annually.

Table 12.3. Breast cancer screening for average-risk patients: mammography

American Cancer Society (ACS)	U.S. Preventive Services Task Force (USPSTF)	American College of Obstetricians and Gynecologists (ACOG)
Screening mammography age 40–49		
Women should have the opportunity to begin annual screening at 40–44 years of age (qualified recommendation) Women should begin regular screening mammography at age 45 years (strong recommendation) Women aged 45–54 years should be screened annually (qualified recommendation)	No requirement for routine screening mammography in women aged 40 to 49 years (grade C recommendation); the decision to start regular, biennial screening mammography before the age of 50 years should be an individual one and take into account patient context, including the patient's values regarding specific benefits and harms. Women who place a higher value on the potential benefit than the potential harms may choose to begin biennial screening between the ages of 40 and 49 years (grade C recommendation)	Women should be educated on the predictive value of screening mammography and the potential for false-positive results and false-negative results; women should be informed of the potential for additional imaging or biopsies that may be recommended based on screening results. Women aged 40 years and older should be offered screening mammography annually Biennial screening may be a more appropriate or acceptable strategy to some women, and ACOG recommends the screening strategy should therefore be determined based on the patient's individual risk and values
Screening mammography age >50		
Women aged 45–54 years should be screened annually (qualified recommendation) Women 55 years and older should transition to biennial screening or have the opportunity to continue screening annually (qualified recommendation)	Biennial screening mammography for women between the ages of 50 and 74 years (grade B recommendation) Insufficient current evidence to assess the additional benefits and harms of screening mammography in women 75 years or older	As above

Table 12.4. Breast cancer screening for average-risk patients: MRI as an adjuvant screening tool

American Cancer Society (ACS)	U.S. Preventive Services Task Force (USPSTF)	American College of Obstetricians and Gynecologists (ACOG)
Breast MRI screening as an adjunct to mammography		
The ACS recommends annual MRI screening, based on evidence from nonrandomized screening trials and observational studies, in women with the following risk factors: • BRCA mutation • First-degree relative of BRCA carrier, but untested • Lifetime risk ~20– 25% or greater, as defined by BRCAPRO or other models that are largely dependent on family history The ACS recommends annual MRI screening, based on expert consensus opinion that considers evidence of lifetime risk for breast cancer, in women with the following risk factors: • Radiation to chest between age 10 and 30 years • Li-Fraumeni syndrome and first-degree relatives • Cowden and Bannayan-Riley-Ruvalcaba syndromes and first-degree relatives with those syndromes The ACS found insufficient evidence to recommend for or against MRI screening in women with the following risk factors: • Lifetime risk 15– 20%, as defined by BRCAPRO or other models that are largely dependent on family history • Lobular carcinoma in situ (LCIS) or atypical lobular hyperplasia (ALH) • Atypical ductal hyperplasia (ADH) • Heterogeneously or extremely dense breast on mammography • Personal history of breast cancer, including ductal carcinoma in situ (DCIS) The ACS recommends against MRI screening (based on expert consensus opinion) in women at <15% lifetime risk. Finally, the ACS advises that screening decisions should be made on a case-by-case basis, as there may be particular factors to support MRI. Payment should not be a barrier.	Insufficient current evidence to assess the additional benefits and harms of either digital mammography or MRI instead of film mammography as a screening modality for breast cancer	Breast MRI is not recommended for screening women at average risk of developing breast cancer Women who are estimated to have a lifetime risk of breast cancer of 20% or greater, based on risk models that rely largely on family history (such as BRCAPRO, BODACEA, or Claus), but who are either untested or test negative for BRCA gene mutations can be offered enhanced screening For women who test positive for BRCA1 and BRCA2 mutations, enhanced screening should be recommended and risk reduction methods discussed

Table 12.5. Breast cancer screening recommendations: *BRCA* testing

American Cancer Society (ACS)	U.S. Preventive Services Task Force (USPSTF)	American College of Obstetricians and Gynecologists (ACOG)
BRCA screening		
Two decision models have been developed to estimate the likelihood that a *BRCA* mutation is present, BRCAPRO and the Breast and Ovarian Analysis of Disease Incidence and Carrier Estimation Algorithm (BOADICEA); the BOADICEA model also provides estimates of breast cancer risk. Genetic testing for a *BRCA1* or *BRCA2* mutation is generally offered to adult members of families with a known *BRCA* mutation, or to women with at least a 10% likelihood of carrying such a mutation, based on either validated family history criteria or one of the above-mentioned models.	The USPSTF recommends that primary care providers screen women who have family members with breast, ovarian, tubal, or peritoneal cancer with one of several screening tools designed to identify a family history that may be associated with an increased risk for potentially harmful mutations in breast cancer susceptibility genes (*BRCA1* or *BRCA2*). Family history factors associated with increased likelihood of potentially harmful *BRCA* mutations include breast cancer diagnosis before age 50 years, bilateral breast cancer, presence of breast and ovarian cancer, presence of breast cancer in one or more male family members, multiple cases of breast cancer in the family, one or more family members with two primary types of *BRCA*-related cancer, and Ashkenazi Jewish ethnicity. Women with positive screening results should receive genetic counseling and, if indicated after counseling, *BRCA* testing (grade B recommendation). The USPSTF recommends against routine genetic counseling or *BRCA* testing for women whose family history is not associated with an increased risk for potentially harmful mutations in the *BRCA1* or *BRCA2* genes (grade D recommendation).	Patients with greater than an approximate 20–25% chance of having an inherited predisposition to breast cancer and ovarian cancer and for whom genetic risk assessment is recommended: Women with a personal history of both breast cancer and ovarian cancer* Women with ovarian cancer* and a close relative† with ovarian cancer or premenopausal breast cancer or both Women with ovarian cancer* who are of Ashkenazi Jewish ancestry Women with breast cancer at age 50 years or younger and a close relative† with ovarian cancer* or male breast cancer at any age Women of Ashkenazi Jewish ancestry in whom breast cancer was diagnosed at age 40 years or younger Women with a close relative† with a known *BRCA1* or *BRCA2* mutation Patients with greater than an approximate 5–10% chance of having an inherited predisposition to breast cancer and ovarian cancer and for whom genetic risk assessment may be helpful: Women with breast cancer at age 40 years or younger Women with ovarian cancer, primary peritoneal cancer, or fallopian tube cancer of high grade, serous histology at any age Women with bilateral breast cancer (particularly if the first case of breast cancer was diagnosed at age 50 years or younger) Women with breast cancer at age 50 years or younger and a close relative† with breast cancer at age 50 years or younger Women of Ashkenazi Jewish ancestry with breast cancer at age 50 years or younger Women with breast cancer at any age and two or more close relatives† with breast cancer at any age (particularly if at least one case of breast cancer was diagnosed at age 50 years or younger) Unaffected women with a close relative† that meets one of the previous criteria

*Cancer of the peritoneum and fallopian tubes should be considered a part of the spectrum of the hereditary breast and ovarian cancer syndrome.

†Close relative is defined as a first-degree relative (mother, sister, daughter) or second-degree relative (grandmother, granddaughter, aunt, etc.).

Sources for Tables 12.2-12.5: Oeffinger KC, Fontham ETH, Etzioni R, et al. Breast cancer screening for women at average risk: 2015 guideline update from the American Cancer Society. *JAMA*. 2015 Oct 20:314.

(continued)

Saslow D, Boetes C, Burke W, Harms S, Leach MO, Lehman CD, et al. American Cancer Society guidelines for breast screening with MRI as an adjunct to mammography. *CA Cancer J Clin.* 2007 Mar-Apr;57(2):75-89.

US Preventive Services Task Force. Screening for breast cancer: U.S. Preventive Services Task Force recommendation statement. *Ann Intern Med.* 2009 Nov 7;151(10):716-26. Erratum in: *Ann Intern Med.* 2010 May 18;152(10):688. *Ann Intern Med.* 2010 Feb 2;152(3):199-200.

Siu AL; U.S. Preventive Services Task Force. Screening for breast cancer: U.S. Preventive Services Task Force recommendation statement. *Ann Intern Med.* 2016 Feb16;164(4):279-96.

American College of Obstetricians and Gynecologists; ACOG Committee on Society of Gynecologic Oncologists. ACOG Practice Bulletin No. 122: Breast cancer screening. *Obstet Gynecol.* 2011 Aug;118(2 Pt 1):372-82.

American College of Obstetricians and Gynecologists; ACOG Committee on Society of Gynecologic Oncologists. ACOG Practice Bulletin No. 103: Hereditary breast and ovarian cancer syndrome. *Obstet Gynecol.* 2009 Apr;113(4):957-66.

Moyer VA. Risk assessment, genetic counseling, and genetic testing for *BRCA*-related cancer in women: U.S. Preventive Services Task Force recommendation statement. *Ann Intern Med.* 2014 Feb 18;160(4):271-81.

BRCA SCREENING TOOLS

Table 12.6. Ontario family history assessment tool

Risk Factor	Points
Breast and Ovarian Cancer	
Mother	10
Sibling	7
Second-/third-degree relative	5
Breast Cancer Relative	
Parent	4
Sibling	3
Second-/third-degree relative	2
Male relative (add to above)	2
Breast Cancer Characteristics	
Onset at age 20–29 yr	6
Onset at age 30–39 yr	4
Onset at age 40–49 yr	2
Premenopausal/perimenopausal	2
Bilateral/multifocal	3
Ovarian Cancer Relative	
Mother	7
Sibling	4
Second-/third-degree relative	3
Age at Ovarian Cancer Onset	
<40 yr	6
40–60 yr	4
>60 yr	2
Age at Prostate Cancer Onset	
<50 yr	1
Age at Colon Cancer Onset	
<50 yr	1
Family Total	
Referral[†]	≥10

[†]Referral with a score of ≥10 corresponds to doubling of lifetime risk for breast cancer (22%).

Source: Reproduced with permission from Gilpin CA, Carson N, Hunter AG. A preliminary validation of a family history assessment form to select women at risk for breast or ovarian cancer for referral to a genetics center. *Clin Genet.* 2000 Oct;58(4):299-308. © John Wiley & Sons A/S.

BRCA Screening Tools

BREAST CANCER

Table 12.7. Manchester scoring system

Cancer, Age at Diagnosis	BRCA1	BRCA2
FBC, <30	6	5
FBC, 30–39	4	4
FBC, 40–49	3	3
FBC, 50–59	2	2
FBC, <59	1	1
MBC, <60	5 (if BRCA2 already tested)	8
MBC, >59	5 (if BRCA2 already tested)	5
Ovarian cancer, <60	8	5 (if BRCA1 already tested)
Ovarian cancer, >59	5	5 (if BRCA1 already tested)
Pancreatic cancer	0	1
Prostate cancer, <60	0	2
Prostate cancer, >59	0	1

FBC, female breast cancer (each breast cancer in bilateral disease is counted separately and DCIS is included); MBC, male breast cancer. Scores should be summed counting each cancer in a direct lineage, for example: proband breast cancer aged 29 years (BRCA1: 6; BRCA2: 5); mother breast cancer at aged 61 years (BRCA1: 1; BRCA2: 1, discounted as not the highest score in direct lineage); father MBC at 54 years of age (BRCA1: 5 only if BRCA2 negative; BRCA2: 8); paternal aunt breast cancer bilateral at age 43 and 52 years (BRCA1: 5; BRCA2: 5); total score: BRCA2: 18; BRCA1: 16 only after BRCA2 testing.

Source: Reproduced with permission from Evans DG, Eccles DM, Rahman N, et al. A new scoring system for the chances of identifying a BRCA1/2 mutation outperforms existing models including BRCAPRO. *J Med Genet.* 2004 Jun;41(6):474-80. Copyright © 2004 BMJ Publishing Group Ltd.

Table 12.8. Family history screen-7

#	Question	Positive Answers	ICC (PCU/GCRA)
1	Did any of your first-degree relatives have breast *or* ovarian cancer?	348 (19.4%)	0.87
2	Did any of your relatives have bilateral breast cancer?	84 (4.7%)	0.56
3	Did any man in your family have breast cancer?	2 (0.1%)	0.33
4	Did any woman in your family have breast *and* ovarian cancer?	5 (0.3%)	0.08
5	Did any woman in your family have breast cancer before the age of 50 years?	537 (29.9%)	0.79
6	Do you have two or more relatives with breast *and/or* ovarian cancer?	221 (12.2%)	0.58
7	Do you have two or more relatives with breast *and/or* bowel cancer?	251 (14.0%)	0.53

A cut point of at least one positive question determines referral for genetic evaluation by a trained specialist.

Source: Reproduced from Ashton-Prolla P, Giacomazzi J, Schmidt AV, et al. Development and validation of a simple questionnaire for the identification of hereditary breast cancer in primary care. *BMC Cancer.* 2009 Aug 14;9:283.

Table 12.9. Pedigree assessment tool

Diagnosis	Points assigned
Breast cancer at age 50 or higher[y]	3
Breast cancer prior to age 50[y]	4
Ovarian cancer at any age[ʃ]	5
Male breast cancer at any age	8
Ashkenazi Jewish heritage	4

[*]The pedigree assessment tool (PAT) score is calculated by adding the points assigned to every family member with a breast or ovarian cancer diagnosis, including second- and third-degree relatives. A separate score is calculated for both the maternal and paternal lineage and the higher of the 2 scores is assigned to the participant. For example, a woman with the following family history would have a maternal PAT score of 7 and a paternal PAT score of 12: sister diagnosed with breast cancer at age 43 (4 points), maternal aunt diagnosed with breast cancer at age 72 (3 points), paternal aunt diagnosed with ovarian cancer at age 62 (5 points), and paternal grandmother with breast cancer at age 59 (3 points). In this example, the sister is counted in both the maternal and paternal PAT score since she belongs to both genetic lineages. Likewise, a participant herself, and any of her siblings, children, grandchildren, and nieces/nephews affected with breast or ovarian cancer are included in both the maternal and paternal point total.

[y]A woman with bilateral breast cancer is assigned the sum of the 2 individual scores corresponding to her age at the time of each diagnosis. For example, a woman diagnosed with breast cancer initially at age 47 who develops a contralateral breast cancer at age 60 is assigned 7 points (4 þ 3).

[ʃ]A woman with both breast and ovarian cancer is assigned the sum of the appropriate breast cancer score (3 or 4 points depending on age at breast cancer diagnosis) plus 5 points for the ovarian cancer.

Source: Reproduced with permission from Hoskins KF, Zwaagstra A, Ranz M. Validation of a tool for identifying women at high risk for hereditary breast cancer in population-based screening. *Cancer.* 2006 Oct 15;107(8):1769-76. Copyright © 2006 American Cancer Society.

BRCA Screening Tools **BREAST CANCER**

Table 12.10. Referral scoring tool

History of **BREAST** *or* **OVARIAN** cancer in the family?
NO: (stop)
YES: (complete checklist)

	Breast Cancer at Or Before Age 50	Ovarian Cancer at Any Age
Yourself		
Mother		
Sister		
Daughter		
Mother's side		
Grandmother		
Aunt		
Father's side		
Grandmother		
Aunt		
Two (2) or more cases of breast cancer *(after age 50)* **on the same side of the family**		
Male breast cancer at *any age* **in any relative**		
Jewish ancestry		

ASSESSMENT: (**Positive Screen** = Two [2] or more checks in above table.)
POSITIVE SCREEN: _____ **NEGATIVE SCREEN:** _____

Source: Reproduced with permission from Macmillan Publishers Ltd:, Bellcross CA, Lemke AA, Pape LS, Tess AL, Meisner LT. Evaluation of a breast/ovarian cancer genetics referral screening tool in a mammography population. *Genet Med.* 2009 Nov;11(11):783-89. Copyright © 2009.

APPENDIX A
Lab Values

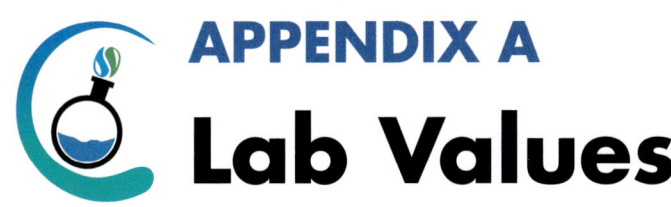

STANFORD UNIVERSITY MEDICAL CENTER LABORATORY

Hematology
Hct	35–47%
Hgb	11.7–15.7 g/dL
Plt	150–400 K/uL
WBC	4.0–11.0 K/uL
Poly	42.7–73.3%
Bands	0.0–11.0%
Mono	2.0–11.0%
Lymph	12.5–40.0%
Eos	0.0–7.5%
Baso	0.0–2.0%
RBC	3.8–5.2 MIL/uL
MCV	82–98 fl
MCH	27–34 pg
MCHC	32–36 g/dL
RDW	11.5–14.6%

Coagulation
PT-seconds	10.5–13.1 sec
PT-INR	0.89–1.11 INR
Coumadin range	
Low intensity	2.0–3.0 INR
High intensity	3.0–5.0 INR
APTT	23–33 sec
Thrombin Time	13–17 sec
Fibrinogen	160–350 mg/dL
FSP	0–10 mcg/mL
D-Dimer	0–200

Drug Levels
Carbamazepine	8–12 mcg/mL
Digoxin	0.5–2.0 mcg/mL
Lithium	0.6–1.2 mEq/L
Phenobarb	10–40 mcg/mL
Phenytoin	10–20 mcg/mL
Pro cainamide	4–8 mcg/mL
Quinidine	2.5–5.0 mcg/mL
Theophylline	5–20 mcg/mL
Vancomycin	
Peak	20–30 mcg/mL
Trough	5–10 mcg/mL
Gentamicin	
Peak	6–8 ng/mL
Trough	<2 ng/mL

Chemistry
Sodium	135–148 mEq/L
Potassium	3.5–5.3 mEq/L
Chloride	95–105 mEq/L
CO_2	24–31 mEq/L
Anion Gap	8–16 mEq/L
Osm (serum)	285–310 mOsm/kg
Glucose	70–110 mg/dl
BUN	5–25 mg/dL
Creatinine	0.5–1.4 mg/dL
Calcium	1.12–1.32 mmol/L
Phosphorus	2.5–4.5 mg/dL
Magnesium	1.5–2.0 mEq/L
Uric Acid	2.5–7.5 mg/dL
Total Protein	6.3–8.2 g/dL
Albumin	3.9–5.0 g/dL
Bilirubin, Total	0.2–1.3 mg/dL
Bilirubin, Direct	0.0–0.4 mg/dL
Alk Phos	38–126 IU/L
AST (SOOT)	8–39 IU/L
ALT (SGPT)	9–52 IU/L
Gamma GT	8–78 IU/L
Cholesterol	
Low Risk	<200 mg/dL
Moderate Risk	200–239 mg/dL
High Risk	>239 mg/dL
Triglyceride	35–135 mg/dL
Amylase	30–110 IU/L
Ammonia	9–33 mcmol/L
Ferritin	
Female 18–50 yr old	6–81 ng/mL
Female >50 yr old	14–186 ng/mL
Male	30–284 ng/mL
TIBC	240–450%
Transferrin	230–430 mg/dL
Haptoglobin	50–320 mg/dL

Source: Courtesy of Sussman H, MD, Lab Director, Stanford Health Services.

ENDOCRINE LAB VALUES

	Conventional Units	Conversion Factor	SI Units
Adrenocorticotropin hormone (ACTH)			
6:00 AM	10–80 pg/mL	0.2202	2.2–17.6 pmol/L
6:00 PM	<50 pg/mL	0.2202	<11 pmol/L
Androstenedione	60–300 ng/dL	0.0349	2.1–10.5 nmol/L
Cortisol			
8:00 AM	5–25 mcg/dL	27.9	140–700 nmol/L
4:00 PM	3–12 mcg/dL	27.9	80–330 nmol/L
10:00 PM	<50% of AM value	27.9	<50% of AM value
Dehydroepiandrosterone sulfate	80–350 mcg/dL	0.0027	2.2–9.5 mcmol/L
11-Deoxycortisol	0.05–0.25 mcg/dL	28.86	1.5–7.3 nmol/L
11-Deoxycorticosterone	2–10 ng/dL	30.3	60–300 pmol/L
Estradiol	20–400 pg/mL	3.67	70–1500 pmol/L
Estrone	30–200 pg/mL	3.7	110–740 pmol/L
FSH, reproductive years	5–30 mIU/mL	1.0	5–30 IU/L
Glucose, fasting	70–100 mg/dL	0.0556	4.0–6.0 mmol/L
Growth hormone	<10 ng/mL	1.0	<10 mcg/L
17-Hydroxyprogesterone	100–300 ng/dL	0.03	3–9 nmol/L
Insulin, fasting	5–25 mcU/mL	7.175	35–180 pmol/L
Insulin-like growth factor-I	0.3–2.2 U/mL	1000	300–2200 U/L
LH, reproductive years	5–20 mIU/mL	1.0	5–20 IU/L
Progesterone			
Follicular phase	<3 ng/mL	3.18	<9.5 nmol/L
Secretory phase	5–30 ng/mL	3.18	16–95 nmol/L
Prolactin	1–20 ng/mL	44.4	44.4–888 pmol/L
Testosterone, total	20–80 ng/dL	0.0347	0.7–2.8 nmol/L
Testosterone, free	100–200 pg/dL	0.0347	35–700 pmol/L
Thyroid stimulating hormone (TSH)	0.35–6.7 mcU/mL	1.0	3.5–6.7 mU/L
Thyroxine, free T4	0.8–2.3 ng/dL	1.29	10–30 nmol/L
Triiodothyronine, T3, total	80–220 ng/dL	0.0154	1.2–3.4 nmol/L
Triiodothyronine, T3, free	0.13–0.55 ng/dL	15.4	2.0–8.5 pmol/L
Triiodothyronine, reverse	8–35 ng/dL	15.4	120–540 pmol/L

Source: Speroff L, Glass RH, Kase NG. Clinical Assays. In: *Clinical Gynecologic Endocrinology and Infertility*, 5th Ed. Baltimore: Williams & Wilkins; 1994. Reproduced with the permission of the publisher.

ENGLISH/METRIC WEIGHT CONVERSION

								Ounces								
	0	1	2	3	4	5	6	7	8	9	10	11	12	13	14	15
Pounds																
0	0	28	57	85	113	142	170	198	227	255	283	312	341	369	397	425
1	454	482	510	539	567	595	624	652	680	709	737	765	794	822	850	879
2	907	936	964	992	1021	1049	1077	1106	1134	1162	1191	1219	1247	1276	1304	1332
3	1361	1389	1417	1446	1474	1503	1531	1559	1588	1616	1644	1673	1701	1729	1758	1786
4	1814	1843	1871	1899	1928	1956	1984	2013	2041	2070	2098	2126	2155	2183	2211	2240
5	2268	2296	2325	2353	2381	2410	2438	2466	2495	2523	2551	2580	2608	2637	2665	1786
6	2722	2750	2778	2807	2835	2863	2892	2920	2948	2977	3005	3033	3062	3090	3118	3147
7	3175	3203	3232	3250	3289	3317	3345	3374	3402	3430	3459	3487	3515	3544	3572	3600
8	3629	3657	3685	3714	3742	3770	3799	3827	3856	3884	3912	3941	3969	3997	4026	4054
9	4082	4111	4139	4167	4196	4224	4252	4281	4309	4337	4366	4394	4423	4451	4479	4508
10	4536	4564	4593	4621	4649	4678	4706	4734	4763	4791	4819	4848	4876	4904	4933	4961
11	4990	5018	5046	5075	5103	5131	5160	5188	5216	5245	5273	5301	5330	5358	5386	5415
12	5443	5471	5500	5528	5557	5585	5613	5542	5670	5698	5727	5755	5783	5812	5840	5868
13	5897	5925	5953	5982	6010	6038	6067	6095	6123	6152	6180	6209	6237	6265	6294	6322
14	6350	6379	6407	6435	6464	6492	6520	6549	6577	6605	6634	6662	6690	6719	6747	6775

All converted English weights are in grams.

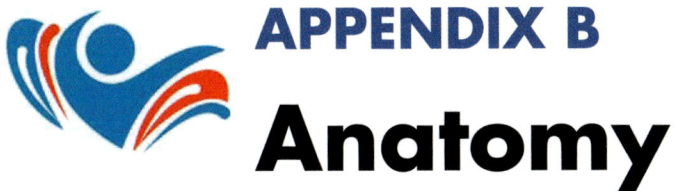

APPENDIX B
Anatomy

LOCATION OF THE URETER

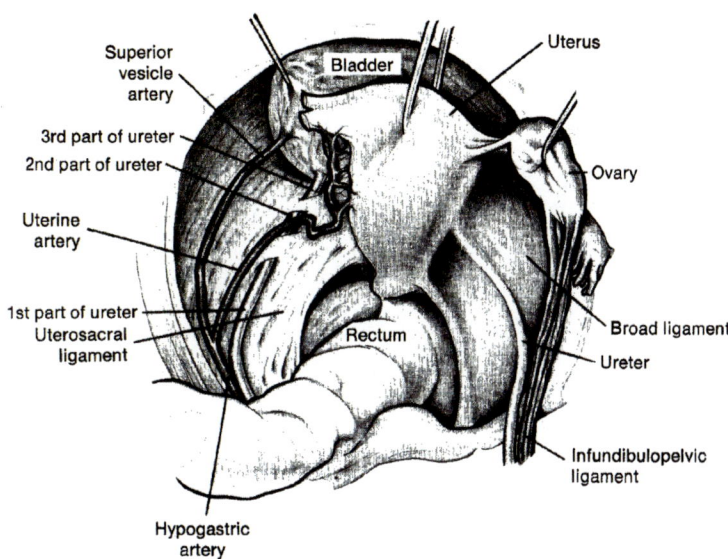

Source: Tewari KS and Monk BJ. Invasive cervical cancer. In *Clinical Gynecologic Oncology, 8th Ed.* DiSaia PJ and Creasman WT eds. Copyright 2012. Elsevier. Phladelphia. Reproduced with permission of the publisher.

FETAL CIRCULATION

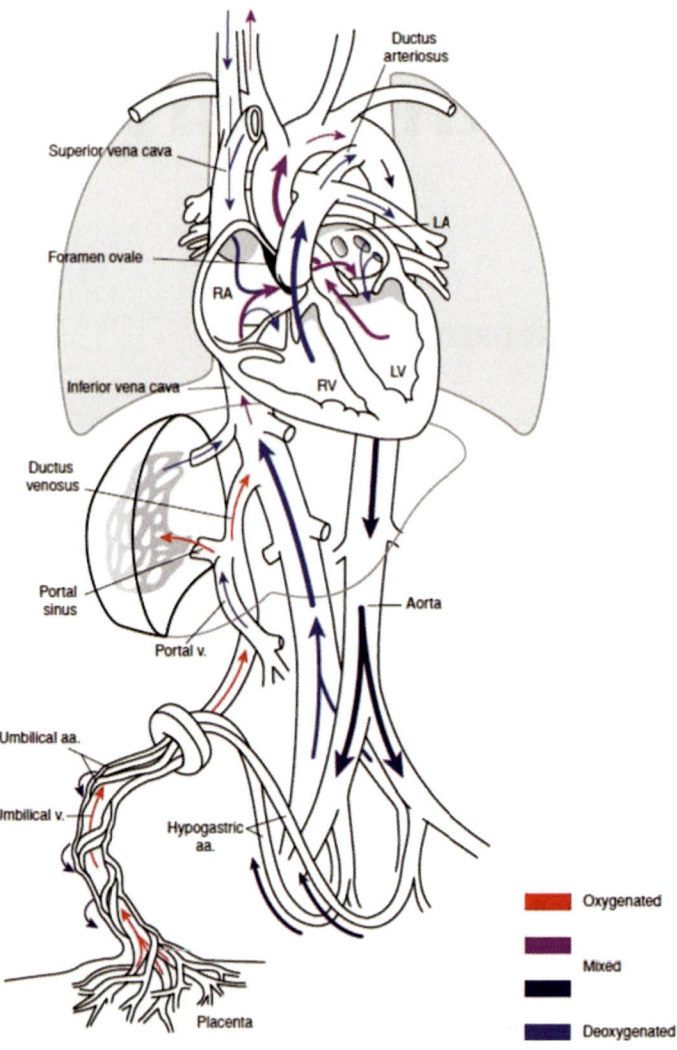

Source: Reproduced with permission from Embryogenesis and Fetal Morphological Developments in *William's Obstetrics*, *24th Ed.* Cunningham FG, Levano KJ, Bloom SL et al eds. New York. Copyright © 2014 McGraw Hill Education.

PELVIC BLOOD SUPPLY

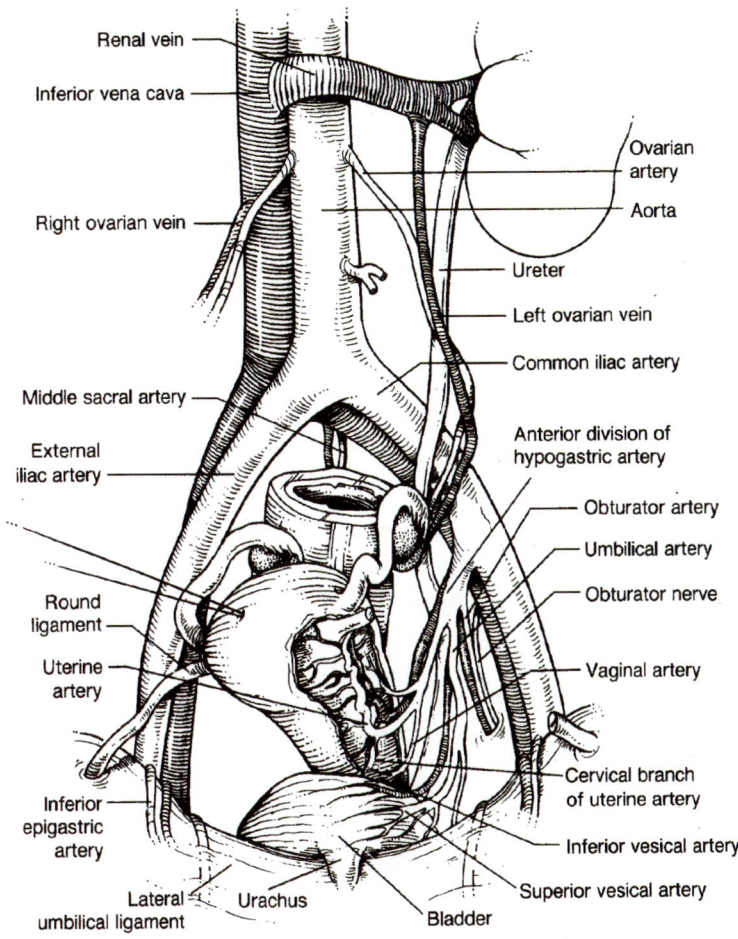

Source: DiSaia PJ. Clinical anatomy of the female pelvis. In: Scott JR, DiSaia PJ, Hammond CB, Spellacy WN, eds. *Danforth's Obstetrics and Gynecology*, 7th Ed. Philadelphia: Lippincott; 1994. Reproduced with the permission of the publisher.

ANATOMY

BONY PELVIS

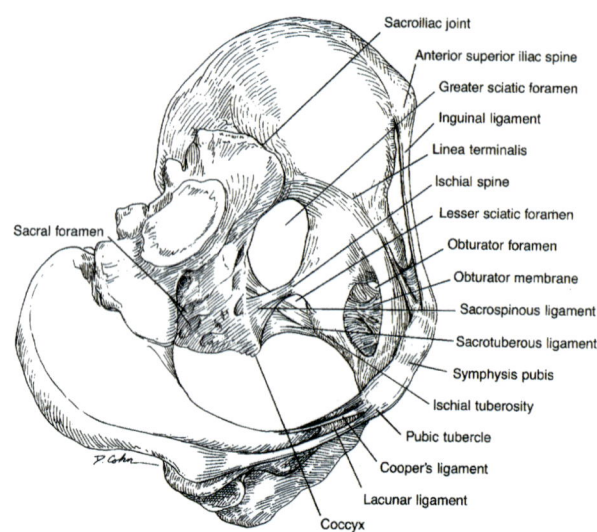

LUMBAR/SACRAL NERVE PLEXUSES

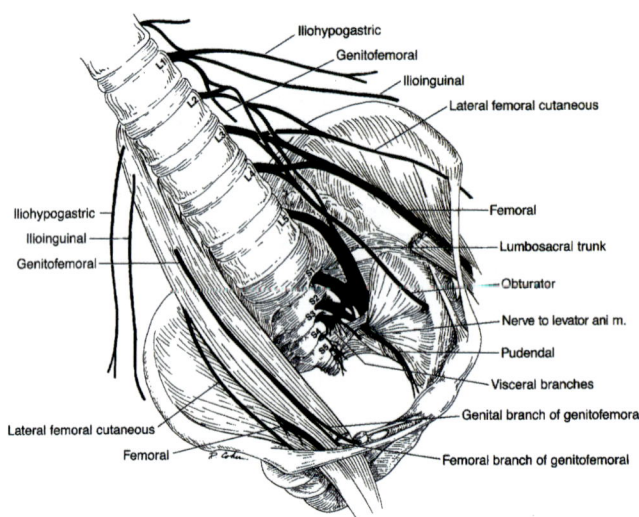

Source: Burnett LS. Anatomy. In: Jones HW, Wentz AC, Burnett LS, eds. *Novak's Textbook of Gynecology*, 11th Ed. Baltimore: Williams & Wilkins; 1988. Reproduced with the permission of the publisher.

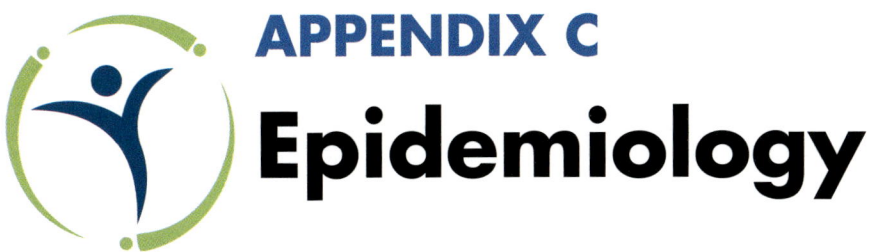

APPENDIX C
Epidemiology

DEFINITION
- The study of health and health problems in populations

Alternative Definitions
- Medical student: The worst-taught class in medical school
- Resident: A very scary field in medicine filled with math
- David Grimes' mother: A dermatology subspecialty

Epidemiologic Study Designs
- Descriptive Studies
- Analytic Studies
- Cohort Studies
- Case-Control Studies
- Experimental Studies
- Randomized Clinical Trials

Basic Terms

Prevalence $\quad \dfrac{\text{\# of people who have a disease at one point in time}}{\text{\# of persons at risk at the point}}$

Incidence $\quad \dfrac{\text{\# of new cases of disease over a period of time}}{\text{\# of persons at risk during that period}}$

Sensitivity   The proportion of subjects with the disease who have a positive test (a/a+c)
Specificity   The proportion of subjects without the disease who have a negative test (d/b+d)
Predictive value
- Positive—likelihood a positive test indicates disease (a/a+b)
- Negative—likelihood a negative test indicates lack of disease (d/d+c)

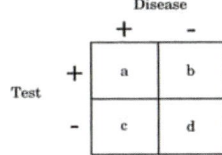

EPIDEMIOLOGY

DESCRIPTIVE STUDIES

Advantages
- Data are relatively easy to obtain.
- Cost of obtaining data is relatively low.
- Ethical problems are minimal since the researcher does not decide which health services are to be received.

Disadvantages
- No comparison group.
- Cause and effect relationships are suggested only.

Study Design

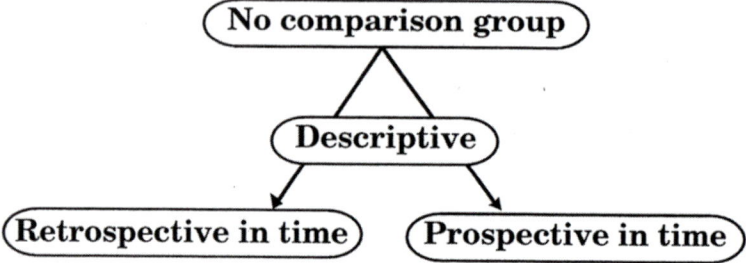

Analysis
- Tables
- Histogram
- Line graphs
- Scatter diagrams
- Other graphic representation

ANALYTIC STUDIES

Essential Features
There are at least 2 study groups:
- A group of subjects with the outcome or exposure of interest and a group of individuals without the health problem or exposure of interest.
- Association between exposure and outcome can be examined.
- Study subtypes named according to the determination of the study groups.

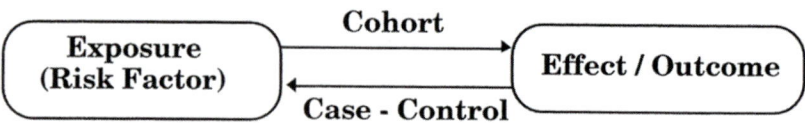

COHORT STUDIES

Advantages
- Avoids having to withhold treatment from those who wish to receive it
- Uses prospective data collection allowing standardization of eligibility criteria, the maneuver and outcome assessment
- Uses concurrent control group; cointervention less likely to influence results since it should affect both groups
- Uses prospective data collection
- Can match for potential confounders during sample selection

Disadvantages
- Impossible to ensure known confounding variables are equally distributed between groups
- Impossible to ensure that some factor unidentified by the investigator is not responsible both for exposure to the maneuver and good outcomes
- Difficult to achieve blindness to intervention with resulting bias likely (i.e., increased attention to experimental group)
- Difficult to obtain concurrent controls if therapy is in vogue
- Expensive in time, money, and subjects to do well

Study Design

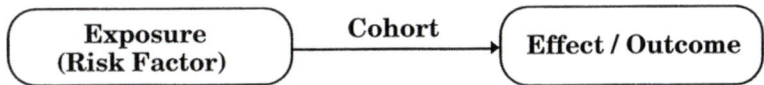

- At least two groups of subjects are studied.
- Entry into these groups is not randomized.
- Both groups of subjects are followed for a period of time to determine the frequency of the outcome in each group.
- The risk of developing the outcome for those exposed and those not exposed will be compared to see if there is a difference.
- To determine whether an association exists between an exposure (risk factor) and a future outcome (health problem).

Analysis

	Outcome		
	Yes	No	
Exposure Yes	a	b	N_1
Exposure No	c	d	N_0

$$\text{Relative Risk} = \frac{a/N_1}{c/N_0}$$

$$\text{Attributable Risk} = a/N_1 - c/N_0$$

CASE CONTROL STUDIES

Advantages
- Useful for health problems that occur infrequently
- Useful for studying health problems with long latent interval
- Less time-consuming and less expensive than cohort studies because of the convenient sampling strategy and relatively short study period

Disadvantages
- Selection bias—cases and controls are selected from two separate populations.
  - Difficult to ensure that they are comparable with respect to extraneous risk factors and other sources of distortion.
- Information bias—exposure data is collected from records or by recall after disease occurrence.
  - Records may be incomplete and recall of past events is subject to human error and selective recall.
- Inappropriate for determining incidence rates.
- Inappropriate for determining the other possible health effects of an exposure.

Study Design
- Two groups of subjects studied: one group that experiences the outcome (cases) and the other that does not (controls).
- Entry into these two groups not influenced by the investigator and therefore cannot be randomized.

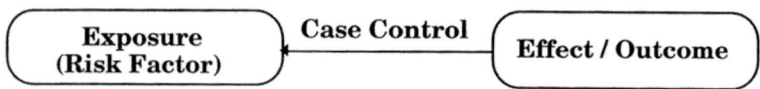

- Cases are identified during a given period of time.
- The exposure of the two groups to specific risk factors in the past is investigated.
- The likelihood that the cases were exposed to specific risk factors is then compared to the likelihood that controls were exposed to the same risk factors to see if there is a significant difference.

		Outcome	
		Yes	No
Exposure	Yes	a	b
	No	c	d

$$\text{Odds Ratio} = \frac{a/b}{c/d} = \frac{ad}{bc}$$

Analysis
- Proportion that cases and controls represent in the population is unknown.
- Estimate of the relative risk can be obtained by cross-product ratio.
- Odds ratio approximates relative risk if incidence of outcome is <5%.

RANDOMIZED CLINICAL TRIALS
Advantages
- Controls selection bias effectively
- Balances potential confounding variables
- Allows standardization of eligibility criteria, exposures, and outcome assessments
- Statistically efficient because equal numbers of exposed and unexposed can be studied
- Statistically efficient because statistical power is not lost when confounding is controlled for in the analysis
- Theoretically attractive since many statistical methods are based on random assignment
- Concurrent comparison groups

Disadvantages
- Design and implementation of an RCT may be complex.
- Extrapolation to the general population may be limited by careful selection criteria employed to conduct RCT.
- Open to ethical challenges: can exposure be ethically withheld from one group.

Study Design

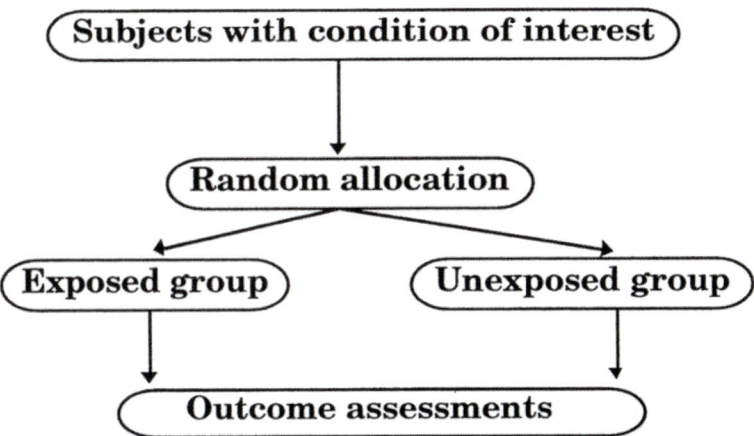

- Two groups of subjects are studied, those exposed to each of two treatments.
- Subjects are randomly assigned to one of the two treatment groups.
- Subjects are analyzed as part of the group to which they were randomized even if they fail to complete therapy (not intuitively obvious).

Analysis

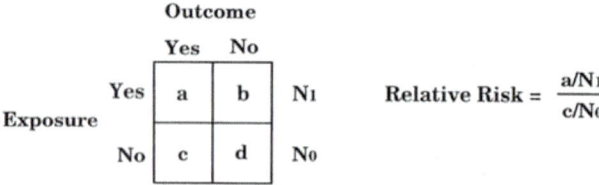

- Essentially same analysis as for cohort study with determination of RR.

STUDY SIZE AND POWER ANALYSIS
Type I Error (Alpha Error)
Probability of a study showing a statistically significant difference when no real difference exists (null hypothesis true). A *p*-value of 0.05 indicates a 5% probability of obtaining a difference when there is none.

Type II Error (Beta Error)
False-negative result is the probability of failing to show a statistically significant difference when a true difference exists.

Power
The probability of a study detecting a statistically significant difference when a real difference exists. Complement to Type II error as Power = 1 − beta.

BIAS
Selection Bias
The persons in one study group are different on some factor other than presence or absence of disease (case control) or exposure (cohort) that was not measured and therefore cannot be controlled for in the analysis.

Ascertainment Bias
The information regarding outcome in a cohort study or history of exposure in a case control study has not been obtained in an equal fashion for both subjects and controls.

Confounding
The two comparison groups differ in some characteristic, which is self-associated with both the outcome and exposure being studied but not directly involved in the causal pathway.

Random Bias
The two comparison groups differ because of chance. Confidence intervals can be computed for the RR estimate thus allowing testing of the null hypothesis.

Special thanks to David Grimes, Ken Schulz, and the Berlex Foundation

APPENDIX D
Operative Reports

CESAREAN SECTION

Preoperative Diagnosis:
1. 42-week intrauterine pregnancy
2. Failed induction
3. Inability of the fetus to tolerate labor

Postoperative Diagnosis: Same
Procedure: Primary Low Transverse Cesarean Section via Pfannenstiel
Surgeon:
Assistant:
Anesthesia: Epidural
Complications: None
EBL: 800 cc
Fluids: 1500 cc LR
Urine Output: 300 cc clear urine at end of the procedure

Indications: 20 years old G1P0 at 42 weeks, induced for postdates, late decels with oxytocin, maximum dilation 2 cm.

Findings: Male infant in cephalic presentation. Thick meconium with none below the cords, pediatrics present at delivery, Apgars 6/8, weight 2980 g. Normal uterus, tubes, and ovaries.

Procedures: The patient was taken to the operating room where epidural anesthesia was found to be adequate. She was then prepared and draped in the normal sterile fashion in the dorsal supine position with a leftward tilt. A Pfannenstiel skin incision was then made with the scalpel and carried through to the underlying layer of fascia with the bovie. The fascia was incised in the midline and the incision extended laterally with the Mayo scissors. The superior aspect of the fascial incision was then grasped with the Kocher clamps, elevated, and the underlying rectus muscles dissected off bluntly. Attention was then turned to the inferior aspect of this incision, which, in a similar fashion, was grasped, tented up with the Kocher clamps, and the rectus muscle dissected off bluntly. The rectus muscles were then separated in the midline, and the peritoneum identified, tented up, and entered sharply with the Metzenbaum scissors. The peritoneal incision was then extended superiorly and inferiorly with good visualization of the bladder. The bladder blade was then inserted and the vesicouterine peritoneum identified, grasped with the pick-ups, and entered sharply with the Metzenbaum scissors. This incision was then extended laterally and the bladder flap created digitally.

The bladder blade was then reinserted and the lower uterine segment incised in a transverse fashion with the scalpel. The uterine incision was then extended laterally with the bandage scissors. The bladder blade was removed and the infant's head delivered atraumatically. The nose and mouth were suctioned with the DeLee suction trap, and the cord clamped and cut. The infant was handed off to the waiting pediatricians. Cord gases were sent.

The placenta was then removed manually; the uterus exteriorized, and cleared of all clots and debris. The uterine incision was repaired with 1-0 chromic in a running, locked fashion. A second layer of the same suture was used to obtain excellent hemostasis. The bladder flap was repaired with 3-0 Vicryl in a running stitch and uterus returned to the abdomen. The gutters were cleared of all clots, and the peritoneum closed with 3-0 Vicryl. The fascia was reapproximated with 0 Vicryl in a running fashion. The skin was closed with staples.

The patient tolerated the procedure well. Sponge, lap, and needle counts were correct times two. Two grams of Cefotetan was given at cord clamp. The patient was taken to the recovery room in stable condition.

TUBAL LIGATION

Preoperative Diagnosis: Multiparity, desires permanent sterilization
Postoperative Diagnosis: Same
Procedure: Postpartum tubal ligation, Pomeroy method
Surgeon:
Assistant:
Anesthesia: Epidural
Complications: None
EBL: <20 cc
Fluids: 500 cc LR

Indications: 35 years old G5P4014 s/p NSVD who desires permanent sterilization. Risk/benefits of procedure discussed with patient including risk of failure of 3–5/1000 with increased risk of ectopic gestation if pregnancy occurs.

Findings: Normal uterus, tubes, and ovaries.

Procedure: The patient was taken to the operating room where her epidural was found to be adequate. A small transverse, infraumbilical skin incision was then made with the scalpel. The incision was carried down through the underlying fascia until the peritoneum was identified and entered. The peritoneum was noted to be free of any adhesions and the incision was then extended with the Metzenbaum scissors.

The patient's left fallopian tube was then identified, brought to the incision, and grasped with a Babcock clamp. The tube was then followed out to the fimbria. The Babcock clamp was then used to grasp the tube approximately 4 cm from the cornual region. A 3-cm segment of tube was then ligated with a free tie of plain gut, and excised. Good hemostasis was noted and the tube was returned to the abdomen. The right fallopian tube was then ligated, and a 3-cm segment excised in a similar fashion. Excellent hemostasis was noted, and the tube returned to the abdomen.

The peritoneum and fascia were then closed in a single layer using 3-0 Vicryl. The skin was closed in a subcuticular fashion using 3-0 Vicryl on Keith needle.

The patient tolerated the procedure well. Sponge, lap, and needle counts were correct times two. The patient was taken to the recovery room in stable condition.

Pathology: Segments of right and left fallopian tubes.

DILATION & CURETTAGE

Preoperative Diagnosis: 8-week intrauterine pregnancy with incomplete abortion
Postoperative Diagnosis: Same
Procedure: Suction dilation & curettage
Surgeon:
Assistant:
Anesthesia: Paracervical block, IV Fentanyl
Complications: None
EBL: 50 cc

Findings: 8-week–sized anteverted uterus, moderate amounts of products of conception

Procedure: The patient was taken to the Special Procedure Room in the Gynecologic Clinic after a deformed gestational sac had been noted on transvaginal ultrasound. A sterile speculum was placed in the patient's vagina and the cervix noted to be 1 cm dilated with products of conception present at the cervical os. The cervix and vagina were then swabbed with Betadine and 2 cc of Xylocaine was injected into the anterior lip of the cervix. The single tooth tenaculum was then applied to this location and 5 cc of Xylocaine was then injected at 4 o'clock and 7 o'clock to produce a paracervical block.

The uterus was then gently sounded to 9 cm, and an 8 mm suction curette advanced gently to the uterine fundus. The suction device was then activated and the curette rotated to clear the uterus of the products of conception. A sharp curettage was then performed until a gritty texture was noted. The suction curette was then reintroduced to clear the uterus of all remaining products of conception. There was minimal bleeding noted and the tenaculum removed with good hemostasis noted.

The patient tolerated the procedure well. The patient was taken to the recovery area in stable condition.

Pathology: Products of conception.

LAPAROSCOPIC TUBAL LIGATION

Preoperative Diagnosis: Multiparity, desires permanent sterilization
Postoperative Diagnosis: Multiparity, desires permanent sterilization
Procedure: Laparoscopic tubal ligation with Falope rings
Surgeon:
Assistant:
Anesthesia: General endotracheal
Complications: None
EBL: 25 cc
Fluids: 1500 cc LR
Urine Output: 100 cc clear urine at end of the procedure

Findings: Normal uterus, tubes, and ovaries

Technique: The patient was taken to the operating room where general anesthesia was obtained without difficulty. The patient was then examined under anesthesia and found to have a small anteverted uterus with normal adnexa. She was then placed in the dorsal lithotomy position and prepared and draped in the sterile fashion. A bivalve speculum was then placed in the patient's vagina and the anterior lip of the cervix grasped with the single toothed tenaculum. A HUMI uterine manipulator was then advanced into the uterus to provide a means to manipulate the uterus. The speculum was removed from the vagina.

Attention was then turned to the patient's abdomen where a 10 mm skin incision was made in the umbilical fold. The veres needle was carefully introduced into the peritoneal cavity at a 45 degree angle while tenting the abdominal wall. Intraperitoneal placement was confirmed by use of a water-filled syringe and drop in intraabdominal pressure with insufflation of CO_2 gas. The trocar and sleeve were then advanced without difficulty into the abdomen where intraabdominal placement was confirmed by the laparoscope. Pneumoperitoneum was obtained with 4 liters of CO_2 gas and the 10 mm trocar and sleeve were then advanced without difficulty into the abdomen where intraabdominal placement was confirmed by the laparoscope. A second skin incision was made 2 cm above the symphysis pubis in the midline. The second trocar and sleeve were then advanced under direct visualization.

A survey of the patient's pelvis and abdomen revealed entirely normal anatomy. The Falope ring applicator was then advanced through the second trocar sleeve and the patient's left fallopian tube was identified and followed out to the fimbriated end. The ring was applied in the mid-isthmic area with a good knuckle of tube noted and good blanching at the site of application. There was no bleeding in the mesosalpinx. The Falope ring applicator was then reloaded and the patient's right tube manipulated in a similar fashion with easy application of the Falope ring.

The instruments were then removed from the patient's abdomen, and the incision was repaired with 3-0 Vicryl. The HUMI was then removed from the vagina with no bleeding noted from the cervix. The patient tolerated the procedure well. Sponge, lap, and needle counts were correct times two. The patient was taken to the recovery room in stable condition.

TOTAL ABDOMINAL HYSTERECTOMY

Preoperative Diagnosis: 1. Hypermenorrhea and Polymenorrhea unresponsive to medical therapy
Postoperative Diagnosis: 1. Hypermenorrhea and Polymenorrhea unresponsive to medical therapy
Procedure: Total abdominal hysterectomy and bilateral salpingo-oophorectomy
Surgeon:
Assistant:
Anesthesia: General endotracheal
Complications: None
EBL: 150 cc
Fluids: 1000 cc LR
Urine Output: 200 cc clear urine at end of procedure

Findings: EUA: diffusely enlarged uterus. Operative finding: 8 × 7 cm uterus with normal tubes and ovaries bilaterally. On opening the uterus a 2 × 2 cm pedunculated myoma was noted. Frozen section revealed benign tissue. All specimens sent to pathology.

Procedure: The risks, benefits, indications, and alternatives of the procedure were reviewed with the patient and informed consent was obtained. The patient was taken to the operating room with IV running and Foley catheter in place.

The patient was placed in the supine position, given general anesthesia, prepared, and draped in the usual sterile fashion. A Pfannenstiel incision was made approximately 2 cm above the symphysis pubis and extended sharply to the rectus fascia. The fascia was then incised bilaterally with the curved Mayo scissors, and the muscles of the anterior abdominal wall were separated in the midline by sharp and blunt dissection.

The peritoneum was grasped between two pick-ups, elevated, and entered sharply with the scalpel. The pelvis was examined with the finding noted above. An O'Connor-O'Sullivan retractor was placed into the incision and the bowel packed away with moist laparotomy sponges. Two Pean clamps were placed on the cornua and used for retraction. The round ligaments on both sides were clamped, transected, and suture ligated with #0 Vicryl. The anterior leaf of the broad ligament was incised along the bladder reflection to the midline from both sides. The bladder was then gently dissected off the lower uterine segment and the cervix with a sponge stick.

The infundibulopelvic ligaments on both sides were then doubly clamped, transected, and suture ligated with #0 Vicryl. Hemostasis was visualized. The uterine arteries were skeletonized bilaterally, clamped with Heaney clamps, transected, and suture ligated with #0 Vicryl. Again, hemostasis was assured. The uterosacral ligaments were clamped on both sides, transected, and suture ligated in a similar fashion.

The cervix and uterus were amputated with the cautery. The vaginal cuff angles were closed with figure-of-eight stitches of #0 Vicryl and were transfixed to the ipsilateral cardinal and uterosacral ligaments. The remainder of the vaginal cuff was closed with a series of interrupted #0 Vicryl figure-of-eight sutures. Hemostasis was assured.

The pelvis was irrigated copiously with warmed normal saline. All laparotomy sponges and instruments were removed from the abdomen. The fascia was closed with running #0 Vicryl, and hemostasis was assured. The skin was closed with staples. Sponge, lap, needle, and instrument counts were correct times two. The patient was taken to the PACU, awake and in stable condition.

VAGINAL HYSTERECTOMY

Preoperative Diagnosis: Uterine prolapse
Postoperative Diagnosis: Uterine prolapse
Procedure: Total vaginal hysterectomy
Surgeon:
Assistant:
Anesthesia: General endotracheal
Complications: None
EBL: 100 cc
Urine Output: 200 cc clear urine at end of procedure
Fluids: 500 cc LR

Findings: EUA: small anteverted uterus with irregular contour. Operative findings: Small 7 × 6 cm irregularly shaped uterus, normal tubes, ovaries not well visualized.

Procedure: The risks, benefits, indications, and alternatives of the procedure were reviewed with the patient and informed consent was obtained. The patient was taken to the operating room with IV running and Foley catheter in place. The patient was placed in dorsolithotomy position, prepared, and draped in the usual sterile fashion.

A weighted speculum was placed into the vagina, and the cervix was grasped with a toothed tenaculum. The cervix was then injected circumferentially with 1% Xylocaine with 1:200,000 epinephrine. The cervix was then circumferentially incised with the scalpel and the bladder dissected off the pubovesical cervical fascia anteriorly with a sponge stick and the Metzenbaum scissors. The anterior cul-de-sac was entered sharply. The same procedure was performed posteriorly and the posterior cul-de-sac entered sharply without difficulty.

At this point, a Heaney clamp was placed over the uterosacral ligaments on either side. These were then transected, and suture ligated with #0 Vicryl. Hemostasis was assured. The cardinal ligaments were then clamped on both sides, transected, and suture ligated in similar fashion.

The uterine arteries and the broad ligament were then serially clamped with Heaney clamps, transected, and suture ligated on both sides. Excellent hemostasis was visualized. Both cornua were clamped with Heaney clamps, transected, and the uterus delivered. These pedicles were then suture ligated with excellent hemostasis.

The peritoneum was closed with purse-string suture of #0 Vicryl. The vaginal cuff angles were closed with figure-of-eight stitches of #0 Vicryl on both sides and transfixed to the ipsilateral cardinal and uterosacral ligaments. The remainder of the vaginal cuff was closed with figure-of-eight stitches of #0 Vicryl in interrupted fashion.

A Penrose drain was placed into the vaginal cuff between suture ligatures. All instruments were then removed from the vagina, and the patient taken out of dorsolithotomy position and awakened from general anesthesia. The patient was taken to the PACU in stable condition. Sponge, lap, needle, and instrument count was correct times two.

APPENDIX E
Spanish Primer

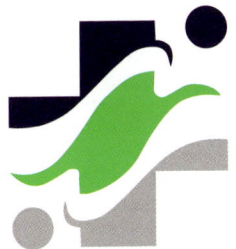

NUMBERS

one	uno (una)	sixteen	dieciséis
two	dos	seventeen	diecisiete
three	tres	eighteen	dieciocho
four	cuatro	nineteen	diecinueve
five	cinco	twenty	veinte
six	seis	thirty	trienta
seven	siete	forty	cuarenta
eight	ocho	fifty	cincuenta
nine	nueve	sixty	sesenta
ten	diez	seventy	setenta
eleven	once	eighty	ochenta
twelve	doce	ninety	noventa
thirteen	trece	hundred	cien
fourteen	catorce	thousand	mil
fifteen	quince		

YEARS

1930	mil novecientos treinta
1943	mil novecientos cuarenta y tres
1960	mil novecientos sesenta
1970	mil novecientos setenta
1974	mil novecientos setenta y cuatro

DAYS OF THE WEEK

Monday	lunes
Tuesday	martes
Wednesday	miércoles
Thursday	jueves
Friday	viernes
Saturday	sábado
Sunday	domingo

TIMES

morning	la mañana
afternoon	la tarde
evening	la tarde
night	la noche
today	hoy
tomorrow	mañana
last night	anoche
yesterday	ayer
day before yesterday	anteayer

MONTHS

January	enero
February	febrero
March	marzo
April	abril
May	mayo
June	junio
July	julio
August	agosto
September	septiembre
October	octubre
November	noviembre
December	diciembre

INTRODUCTIONS

Good morning
Buenos días

How do you feel?
Cómo se siente? Cómo esta?

My name is _____
Me llamo _____

Please
Por favor

OBSTETRIC AND GYNECOLOGIC HISTORY

At what age did you begin to menstruate?
A qué edad empezó su menstruación?

What was the first day of your last period? (menstruation, period)
Cuándo fue el primer día de su última regla? (menstruación, período)

When did you have your last period?
Cuándo fue su última regla?

Did you have a normal period?
Tuvo una regla normal? (Fue esta regla normal?)

Pregnancy
Embarazo, encinta, "gorda"

How many pregnancies have you had?
Cuántos embarazos ha tenido usted?

How many children have you had?
Cuántos niños ha tenido usted?

Are they all living?
Estan vivos todos?

What was the cause of death? At what age?
Cuál fue la causa de la muerte? A qué edad?

Have you had any problems with past pregnancies?
Ha tenido algunos problemas con sus embarazos pasados?

Bleeding? Hypertension? Toxemia?
Sangrando (hemorragia)? Alta presión de la sangre? Toxemia?

Have you had any problems with past deliveries?
Ha tenido problemas con sus partos pasados?

What was the duration of your longest (shortest) labor?
Cuántas horas duró su parto más largo (más corto)?

What was the date of your last pregnancy?
Cuál fue la fecha de su último embarazo?

What was the weight of your largest (smallest) baby at birth?
Cuánto pesó el bebé más grande (más pequeño) al nacer?

Were all your pregnancies term?
Fueron de tiempo (de nueve meses) sus otros niños?

Were there any problems with the children after birth?
Después de nacer, tuvo algún o algunos problemas con los niños?

Have you ever had a miscarriage? Was it the first, second? What date?
Ha tenido un malparto, aborto? Fue el primero, el segundo? Qué fecha?

Have you ever had a stillborn?
Ha tenido un niño que ha nacido muerto?

Have you ever had a cesarean section? What date?
Ha tenido usted una operación cesárea? Qué fecha?

PAST MEDICAL AND SURGICAL HISTORY

Have you had any operations? For what? When? In which hospital?
Ha tenido algunas operaciones? Para qué? Cuándo? En cuál hospital?

Have you had any major illnesses?
Ha tenido algunas enfermedades graves?

Have you had any accidents, fractures?
Ha tenido algunos accidentes, fracturas?

Have you ever had a blood transfusion?
Ha tenido una transfusión (infusión) de sangre?

SPANISH PRIMER

Have you been taking any medications?
Qué medicinas ha estado tomando?

Are you allergic to medicines or foods?
Es usted alérgica a medicinas o comidas?

Do you smoke? How many packs in a day (week)? Cigarettes
Fuma usted? Cuántos paquetes en un día (una semana)? Cigarillos

FAMILY HISTORY

Have you or anyone in your family had:
Usted o alguien en su familia ha tenido:

asthma	asma
cancer	cáncer
convulsions	convulsiones
diabetes	diabetes
epilepsy	epilepsia
gonorrhea	gonorrea
syphilis	sífilis
hay fever	fiebre del heno
heart disease	mala (enfermedad) del corazón
hepatitis (liver)	hepatitis (hígado)
hypertension	alta presión de la sangre
influenza	influenza, gripe
jaundice (yellow skin)	ictericia (la piel amarilla)
measles	sarampión
chickenpox	viruela
pneumonia	pulmonía, neumonía
rheumatic fever	fiebre reumática
scarlet fever	fiebre escarlatina
stroke	hemoragia cerebral
thyroid	tiroides
tuberculosis	tuberculosis
tumor	tumor
infections of the bladder, kidney	infecciones de la vejiga, de los riñones
infections of the chest, lungs	infecciones del pecho o de los pulmones

ANATOMY

head	cabeza	**heart**	corazón
eyes	ojos	**lungs (lung)**	pulmones (pulmón)
ears	oídos	**abdomen**	abdomen (vientre)
nose	nariz	**liver**	hígado
mouth	boca	**intestines**	intestinos
tongue	lengua	**appendix**	apéndice
teeth	dientes	**rectum**	recto
neck	cuello	**bladder**	vejiga
arm	brazo	**vagina**	vagina
shoulder	hombro	**cervix**	cervis
hand	la mano	**uterus**	útero (matriz)
fingers	dedos	**fallopian tubes**	las trompas, los tubos
axilla	axila	**ovaries**	ovarios
chest	pecho	**cyst**	quiste
breasts	pecho (seno)		

PRESENT PREGNANCY

Why did you come to the hospital (clinic)?
Porqué ha venido al hospital (a la clínica)?

Have you been coming to the clinics?
Ha venido a las clínicas?

How many times?
Cuántas veces?

When was the last time you came to the clinic? What date?
Cuándo fue la última vez que vinó a la clinica? Qué fecha?

In what month of your pregnancy did you start prenatal care?
En qué mes de su embarazo vio al doctor para empezar el cuidado de maternidad?

Have you had any problems with this pregnancy?
Ha tenido algunos problemas con este embarazo?

What is your due date?
Para cuándo supone será la fecha del nacimiento de su bebé?

Have you had any bleeding?
Ha sangrado?

Have you had any infections? Of what?
Ha tenido algunas infecciones? De qué?

Have you had any hypertension?
Ha tenido alta presión de la sangre?

Have you had any swelling of the hand, face, legs?
Se le han hinchado las manos, el rostro (la cara), las piernas?

How much weight have you gained? How much do you weigh? Your normal weight?
Cuánto peso ha ganado? Cuánto pesa? Su peso normalmente?

Have you had spots in front of your eyes?
Ha tenido manchas enfrente de los ojos?

Have you had (severe) headaches? How many times in a week?
Ha tenido dolores (fuertes) de la cabeza? Cuántas veces en una semana?

Have you had difficulty breathing? Lying down? After working?
Ha tenido dificultad para respirar? Al acostarse? Después de trabajar?

Do you tire easily?
Se cansa facilmente?

Have you had heart palpitations?
Ha tenido problemas del corazón?

Have you had diarrhea? Constipation?
Ha tenido diarrea? Estreñimiento?

Have you been vomiting?
Ha estado vomitando?

Have you had dysuria?
Ha tenido dolores al orinar?

LABOR AND DELIVERY

Are you going to have a baby?
Va a tener un niño?

Are you in pain?
Tiene dolor?

What time did your pains begin?
Cuándo empezaron los dolores (las contracciones)?

What time did they become regular?
A qué hora fueron (empezaron) regulares (los dolores)?

How often were they once they became regular?
Con qué frecuencia cuando empezaron regulares?

How often are your pains?
Cada cuándo le dan los dolores?

How long do they last?
Cuánto duran?

Have you had bleeding?
Ha sangrado?

Was it pinkish or bright red?
Fue de color rosado o rojo claro?

How much? A cupful? A tablespoonful? A teaspoonful?
Cuánta sangre? Una taza? Una cucharada? Una cucharadita?

Did your membranes rupture? Has your bag of waters broken?
Se le revento la bolsa de agua? (Se le) ha roto la bolsa de agua?

What time did it break?
A qué hora se le revento?

How much water did you lose? Down the legs?
Cuánta agua perdió? Se le bajó por las piernas?

Have you felt the baby move today?
Ha sentido mover el niño?

Your cervix is not dilated.
Su cuello no está dilatado.

Your cervix is dilated to 5 centimeters.
Su cuello tiene cinco centímetros.

You are in labor. Your membranes have ruptured.
Está en trabajo de parto. Sus membranas están rojas.

The heartrate of the baby is normal.
El corazón del niño está normal.

INSTRUCTIONS

Take off your clothes.
Quitese la ropa.

Take off your panties.
Quitese su ropa interior.

I am going to examine you.
Voy a examinarle.

Bend your knees.
Doble las rodillas.

Open your legs.
Abra las piernas.

Put your feet together.
Junte los pies.

Relax your body.
Descanse (relaje) el cuerpo.

Lie down on your back.
Acuestese en su espalda. (Acuestese boca arriba.)

SPANISH PRIMER — Instructions

Lie down on your right (left) side.
Acuestese del lado derecho (izquierdo).

Move down on the table.
Bajese.

Move.
Muevase.

You are going to stay in the hospital.
Se va a quedar en el hospital.

You may go home.
Se puede ir a casa.

You are in early labor.
Está en la primera parte del parto.

Stay at the hospital and walk for two hours.
Quedese aquí en el hospital y ande por dos horas.

Don't push.
No puje.

Breathe through your mouth.
Respire por la boca.

Push with your pains.
Puje con sus dolores.

Do you understand?
Entiende?

Congratulations. You have a baby boy (girl)!
Felicitaciones. Es un niño (una niña)!

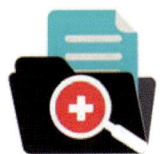

References

Aagaard-Tillery KM, Malone FD, Nyberg DA, et al. Role of second-trimester genetic sonography after Down syndrome screening. *Obstet Gynecol.* 2009 Dec;114(6):1189-96.

Abdalla H, Thum MY. Repeated testing of basal FSH levels has no predictive value for IVF outcome in women with elevated basal FSH. *Hum Reprod.* 2006 Jan;21(1):171-74.

Abdel Gadir A, Mowafi RS, Alnaser HM, et al. Ovarian electrocautery versus human menopausal gonadotrophins and pure follicle stimulating hormone therapy in the treatment of patients with polycystic ovarian disease. *Clin Endocrinol (Oxf).* 1990 Nov;33(5):585-92.

Abdul-Kadir R, McLintock C, Ducloy AS, et al. Evaluation and management of postpartum hemorrhage: consensus from an international expert panel. *Transfusion.* 2014 Jul;54(7):1756-68.

Abenhaim HA, Azoulay L, Kramer MS, et al. Incidence and risk factors of amniotic fluid embolisms: a population-based study on 3 million births in the United States. *Am J Obstet Gynecol.* 2008 Jul;199(1):49.e1-8.

Acker DB, Sachs BP, Friedman EA. Risk factors for shoulder dystocia. *Obstet Gynecol.* 1985 Dec;66(6):762-68.

American College of Obstetricians and Gynecologists. Practice Bulletin No. 40, November 2002: Shoulder dystocia. *Int J Gynaecol Obstet.* 2003 Jan;80(1):87-92.

American College of Obstetricians and Gynecologists. Committee Opinion No. 345: vulvodynia. *Obstet Gynecol.* 2006;108(4):1049-52.

American College of Obstetricians and Gynecologists. Practice Bulletin No. 88: Invasive prenatal testing for aneuploidy. *Obstet Gynecol.* 2007 Dec;110(6):1459-67.

American College of Obstetricians and Gynecologists. Practice Bulletin No. 91: Treatment of urinary tract infections in nonpregnant women. *Obstet Gynecol.* 2008 Mar;111(3):785-94.

American College of Obstetricians and Gynecologists. Practice Bulletin No. 92: Use of psychiatric medications during pregnancy and lactation. *Obstet Gynecol.* 2008;111(4).

American College of Obstetricians and Gynecologists. Practice Bulletin No. 95: Anemia in pregnancy. *Obstet Gynecol.* 2008 Jul;112(1):201-207.

American College of Obstetricians and Gynecologists. Practice Bulletin No. 96: Alternatives to hysterectomy in the management of leiomyomas. *Obstet Gynecol.* 2008 Aug;112(2 Pt 1):387-400.

American College of Obstetricians and Gynecologists. Practice Bulletin No. 102: Management of stillbirth. *Obstet Gynecol.* 2009;113(3):748-61.

American College of Obstetricians and Gynecologists. Practice Bulletin No. 103: Hereditary breast and ovarian cancer syndrome. *Obstet Gynecol.* 2009 Apr;113(4):957-66.

American College of Obstetricians and Gynecologists. Practice Bulletin No. 104: Antibiotic prophylaxis for gynecologic procedures. *Obstet Gynecol.* 2009 May;113(5):1180-9.

American College of Obstetricians and Gynecologists. Practice Bulletin No. 105: Bariatric surgery and pregnancy. *Obstet Gynecol.* 2009 Jun;113(6):1405-13.

REFERENCES

American College of Obstetricians and Gynecologists. Practice Bulletin No. 107: Induction of labor. *Obstet Gynecol.* 2009 Aug;114(2 Pt 1):386-97.

American College of Obstetricians and Gynecologists. Practice Bulletin No. 108: Polycystic ovary syndrome. *Obstet Gynecol.* 2009 Oct;114(4):936-49.

American College of Obstetricians and Gynecologists. Committee Opinion No. 455: Magnesium sulfate before anticipated preterm birth for neuroprotection. *Obstet Gynecol.* 2010 Mar;115(3):669-71.

American College of Obstetricians and Gynecologists. Practice Bulletin No. 115: Vaginal birth after previous cesarean delivery. *Obstet Gynecol.* 2010 Aug;116(2 Pt 1):450-63.

American College of Obstetricians and Gynecologists. Practice Bulletin No. 116: Management of intrapartum fetal heart rate tracings. *Obstet Gynecol.* 2010 Nov;116(5):1232-40.

American College of Obstetricians and Gynecologists. Committee Opinion No. 485: Prevention of early-onset group B streptococcal disease in newborns. *Obstet Gynecol.* 2011 Apr;117(4):1019-27.

American College of Obstetricians and Gynecologists. Technology Assessment No. 7: Hysteroscopy. *Obstet Gynecol.* 2011 Jun;117(6):1486-91.

American College of Obstetricians and Gynecologists. Practice Bulletin No. 122: Breast cancer screening. *Obstet Gynecol.* 2011 Aug;118(2 Pt 1):372-82.

American College of Obstetricians and Gynecologists. Practice Bulletin No. 124: Inherited thrombophilias in pregnancy. *Obstet Gynecol.* 2011 Sep;118(3):730-40.

American College of Obstetricians and Gynecologists. Committee Opinion No. 505: Understanding and using the U.S. Medical Eligibility Criteria For Contraceptive Use, 2010. *Obstet Gynecol.* 2011 Sep;118(3):754-60.

American College of Obstetricians and Gynecologists. *Guidelines for Perinatal Care, 7th Ed.* Washington, DC: American College of Obstetricians and Gynecologists; 2012.

American College of Obstetricians and Gynecologists. Practice Bulletin No. 127: Management of preterm labor. *Obstet Gynecol.* 2012 Jun;119(6):1308-17.

American College of Obstetricians and Gynecologists. Practice Bulletin No. 128: Diagnosis of abnormal uterine bleeding in reproductive-aged women. *Obstet Gynecol.* 2012 Jul;120(1):197-206.

American College of Obstetricians and Gynecologists. Practice Bulletin No. 129: Osteoporosis. *Obstet Gynecol.* 2012 Sep;120(3):718-34.

American College of Obstetricians and Gynecologists. Practice Bulletin No. 131: Screening for cervical cancer. *Obstet Gynecol.* 2012 Nov;120(5):1222-38.

American College of Obstetricians and Gynecologists. Practice Bulletin No. 132: Antiphospholipid syndrome. *Obstet Gynecol.* 2012 Dec;120(6):1514-21.

American College of Obstetricians and Gynecologists. Committee Opinion No. 557: Management of acute abnormal uterine bleeding in nonpregnant reproductive-aged women. *Obstet Gynecol.* 2013 Apr;121(4):891-96.

American College of Obstetricians and Gynecologists. Practice Bulletin No. 133: Benefits and risks of sterilization. *Obstet Gynecol.* 2013;121(2 Pt 1):392-404.

American College of Obstetricians and Gynecologists. Committee Opinion No. 560: Medically indicated late-preterm and early-term deliveries. *Obstet Gynecol.* 2013 Apr;121(4):908-910.

American College of Obstetricians and Gynecologists. Committee Opinion No. 561: Nonmedically indicated early-term deliveries. *Obstet Gynecol.* 2013 Apr;121(4):911-15.

American College of Obstetricians and Gynecologists. Practice Bulletin No. 134: Fetal growth restriction. *Obstet Gynecol.* 2013 May;121(5):1122-33.

REFERENCES

American College of Obstetricians and Gynecologists. Practice Bulletin No. 138: Inherited thrombophilias in pregnancy. *Obstet Gynecol.* 2013 Sep;122(3):706-717.

American College of Obstetricians and Gynecologists. Practice Bulletin No. 139: Premature rupture of membranes. *Obstet Gynecol.* 2013 Oct;122(4):918-30.

American College of Obstetricians and Gynecologists. Hypertension in pregnancy. Report of the American College of Obstetricians and Gynecologists' Task Force on Hypertension in Pregnancy. *Obstet Gynecol.* 2013 Nov;122(5):1122-31.

American College of Obstetricians and Gynecologists. Practice Bulletin No. 141: Management of menopausal symptoms. *Obstet Gynecol.* 2014 Jan;123(1):202-216.

American College of Obstetricians and Gynecologists. Practice Bulletin No. 142: Cerclage for the management of cervical insufficiency. *Obstet Gynecol.* 2014 Feb;123(2 Pt 1):372-79.

American College of Obstetricians and Gynecologists. Practice Bulletin No. 143: Medical management of first-trimester abortion. *Obstet Gynecol.* 2014 Mar;123(3):676-92.

American College of Obstetricians and Gynecologists. Practice Bulletin No. 144: Multifetal gestations: twin, triplet, and higher-order multifetal pregnancies. *Obstet Gynecol.* 2014 May;123(5):1118-32.

American College of Obstetricians and Gynecologists. Practice Bulletin No. 145: Antepartum fetal surveillance. *Obstet Gynecol.* 2014 Jul;124(1):182-92.

American College of Obstetricians and Gynecologists. Committee Opinion No. 609: Colorectal cancer screening strategies. *Obstet Gynecol.* 2014 Oct;124(4):849-55.

American College of Obstetricians and Gynecologists. Committee Opinion No. 611: Method for estimating due date. *Obstet Gynecol.* 2014 Oct;124(4):863-66.

American College of Obstetricians and Gynecologists. Practice Bulletin No. 148: Thyroid disease in pregnancy. *Obstet Gynecol.* 2015 Apr;125(4):996-1005.

American College of Obstetricians and Gynecologists. Practice Bulletin No. 151: Cytomegalovirus, parvovirus B19, varicella zoster, and toxoplasmosis in pregnancy. *Obstet Gynecol.* 2015 Jun;125(6):1510-25.

American College of Obstetricians and Gynecologists. Practice Bulletin No. 152: Emergency contraception. *Obstet Gynecol.* 2015 Sep;126(3):e1-11.

American College of Obstetricians and Gynecologists. Practice Bulletin No. 153: Nausea and vomiting of pregnancy. *Obstet Gynecol.* 2015 Sep;126(3):e12-24.

American College of Obstetricians and Gynecologists. Periviable birth. *Am J Obstet Gynecol.* 2015 Nov;213(5):604-614.

American College of Obstetricians and Gynecologists. Practice Bulletin No. 154: Operative vaginal delivery. *Obstet Gynecol.* 2015 Nov;126(5):e56-65.

American College of Obstetricians and Gynecologists. Committee Opinion No. 623: Emergent therapy for acute-onset, severe hypertension during pregnancy and the postpartum period. *Obstet Gynecol.* 2015 Feb;125(2):521-25.

American College of Obstetricians and Gynecologists. Practice Bulletin No. 160: Premature rupture of membranes. *Obstet Gynecol.* 2016 Jan;127(1):e39-51.

American College of Obstetricians and Gynecologists. Committee Opinion No. 656: Guidelines for diagnostic imaging during pregnancy and lactation. *Obstet Gynecol.* 2016 Feb;127(2):e75-80.

American College of Obstetricians and Gynecologists. Practice Bulletin No. 163: Screening for fetal aneuploidy. *Obstet Gynecol.* 2016 May;127(5):e123-37.

Adam Z, Poulin F, Papp Z. Increased risk of neural tube defects after recurrent pregnancy losses. *Am J Med Genet.* 1995 Feb 13;55(4):512.

REFERENCES

Adamson GD, Pasta DJ. Endometriosis fertility index: the new, validated endometriosis staging system. *Fertil Steril.* 2010 Oct;94(5):1609-15.

Alberman E. The epidemiology of repeated abortion. In: Beard R, Sharp F, eds. *Early Pregnancy Loss: Mechanisms and Treatment.* New York: Springer-Verlag; 1988.

Alvarez C, Marti-Bonmati L, Novella-Maestre E, et al. Dopamine agonist cabergoline reduces hemoconcentration and ascites in hyperstimulated women undergoing assisted reproduction. *J Clin Endocrinol Metab.* 2007 Aug;92(8):2931-7.

Amer SA, Li TC, Ledger WL. Ovulation induction using laparoscopic ovarian drilling in women with polycystic ovarian syndrome: predictors of success. *Hum Reprod.* 2004 Aug;19(8):1719-24.

American Association of Gynecologic Laparoscopists: Advancing Minimally Invasive Gynecology W. AAGL practice report: practice guidelines for the diagnosis and management of submucous leiomyomas. *J Minim Invasive Gynecol.* 2012 Mar-Apr;19(2):152-71.

American College of Obstetricians and Gynecologists, Society for Maternal-Fetal Medicine. Safe prevention of the primary cesarean delivery. *Am J Obstet Gynecol.* 2014 Mar;210(3):179-93.

American Diabetes Association. Standards of medical care in diabetes—2008. *Diabetes Care.* 2008 Jan;31 Suppl 1:S12-54.

American Diabetes Association. Classification and diagnosis of diabetes. *Diabetes Care.* 2015 Jan;38 Suppl:S8-S16.

American Society for Reproductive Medicine. Revised American Society for Reproductive Medicine classification of endometriosis: 1996. *Fertil Steril.* 1997 May;67(5):817-21.

American Society for Reproductive Medicine. Hormonal contraception: recent advances and controversies. *Fertil Steril.* 2008 Nov;90(5 Suppl):S103-113.

American Society for Reproductive Medicine. Multiple gestation associated with infertility therapy: an American Society for Reproductive Medicine Practice Committee opinion. *Fertil Steril.* 2012 Apr;97(4):825-34.

American Society for Reproductive Medicine. Evaluation and treatment of recurrent pregnancy loss: a committee opinion. *Fertil Steril.* 2012 Nov;98(5):1103-11.

American Society for Reproductive Medicine. Criteria for number of embryos to transfer: a committee opinion. *Fertil Steril.* 2013 Jan;99(1):44-6.

American Society for Reproductive Medicine. Medical treatment of ectopic pregnancy: a committee opinion. *Fertil Steril.* 2013 Sep;100(3):638-44.

American Society for Reproductive Medicine. Recommendations for practices utilizing gestational carriers: a committee opinion. *Fertil Steril.* 2015 Jan;103(1):e1-8.

American Society for Reproductive Medicine. Subclinical hypothyroidism in the infertile female population: a guideline. *Fertil Steril.* 2015 Sep;104(3):545-53.

Andermann E, Scriver CR, Wolfe LS, et al. Genetic variants of Tay-Sachs disease: Tay-Sachs disease and Sandhoff's disease in French Canadians, juvenile Tay-Sachs disease in Lebanese Canadians, and a Tay-Sachs screening program in the French-Canadian population. *Prog Clin Biol Res.* 1977;18:161-88.

Anderson GM, Kieser DC, Steyn FJ, et al. Hypothalamic prolactin receptor messenger ribonucleic acid levels, prolactin signaling, and hyperprolactinemic inhibition of pulsatile luteinizing hormone secretion are dependent on estradiol. *Endocrinology.* 2008 Apr;149(4):1562-70.

Anderson JE, Jorenby DE, Scott WJ, et al. Treating tobacco use and dependence: an evidence-based clinical practice guideline for tobacco cessation. *Chest.* 2002 Mar;121(3):932-41.

Anderson JM, Etches D. Prevention and management of postpartum hemorrhage. *Am Fam Physician.* 2007 Mar 15;75(6):875-82.

REFERENCES

Ashton-Prolla P, Giacomazzi J, Schmidt AV, et al. Development and validation of a simple questionnaire for the identification of hereditary breast cancer in primary care. *BMC Cancer.* 2009;9:283.

Ayvaliotis B, Bronson R, Rosenfeld D, et al. Conception rates in couples where autoimmunity to sperm is detected. *Fertil Steril.* 1985 May;43(5):739-42.

B-Lynch C. The B-Lynch suture for control of massive postpartum hemorrhage. *Cont Ob/Gyn.* 1998(Aug):93-8.

Badawy A, Shokeir T, Allam AF, et al. Pregnancy outcome after ovulation induction with aromatase inhibitors or clomiphene citrate in unexplained infertility. *Acta Obstet Gynecol Scand.* 2009;88(2):187-91.

Baerwald AR, Olatunbosun OA, Pierson RA. Effects of oral contraceptives administered at defined stages of ovarian follicular development. *Fertil Steril.* 2006 Jul;86(1):27-35.

Baghdadi LR, Abu Hashim H, Amer SA, et al. Impact of obesity on reproductive outcomes after ovarian ablative therapy in PCOS: a collaborative meta-analysis. *Reprod Biomed Online.* 2012 Sep;25(3):227-41.

Baird DD, Dunson DB, Hill MC, et al. High cumulative incidence of uterine leiomyoma in black and white women: ultrasound evidence. *Am J Obstet Gynecol.* 2003 Jan;188(1):100-107.

Bajaj K, Gross S. Carrier screening: past, present, and future. *J Clin Med.* 2014;3(3):1033-42.

Bajekal N, Li TC. Fibroids, infertility and pregnancy wastage. *Hum Reprod Update.* 2000 Nov-Dec;6(6):614-20.

Balci A, Sollie-Szarynska KM, van der Bijl AG, et al. Prospective validation and assessment of cardiovascular and offspring risk models for pregnant women with congenital heart disease. *Heart.* 2014 Sep;100(17):1373-81.

Barakat R. Current management of early-stage endometrial cancer. *OBG Management.* 2003;15(1):32.

Barbieri R. Have you made best use of the Bakri balloon in PPH? *OBG Management.* 2011;23(7):6-9.

Bardenheier B, Prevots DR, Khetsuriani N, et al. Tetanus surveillance—United States, 1995-1997. MMWR CDC surveillance summaries: *MMWR.* 1998 Jul 3;47(2):1-13.

Barnhart K, Hummel AC, Sammel MD, et al. Use of "2-dose" regimen of methotrexate to treat Ectopic pregnancy. *Fertil Steril.* 2007 Feb;87(2):250-56.

Barnhart K, van Mello NM, Bourne T, et al. Pregnancy of unknown location: a consensus statement of nomenclature, definitions, and outcome. *Fertil Steril.* 2011 Mar 1;95(3):857-66.

Barnhart KT, Schreiber CA. Return to fertility following discontinuation of oral contraceptives. *Fertil Steril.* 2009 Mar;91(3):659-63.

Baron TH, Kamath PS, McBane RD. Management of antithrombotic therapy in patients undergoing invasive procedures. *N Engl J Med.* 2013 May 30;368(22):2113-24.

Barrett JF, Hannah ME, Hutton EK, et al. A randomized trial of planned cesarean or vaginal delivery for twin pregnancy. *N Engl J Med.* 2013 Oct 3;369(14):1295-1305

Barton JR, Sibai BM. Prediction and prevention of recurrent preeclampsia. *Obstet Gynecol.* 2008 Aug;112(2 Pt 1):359-72.

Bayrak A, Saadat P, Mor E, et al. Pituitary imaging is indicated for the evaluation of hyperprolactinemia. *Fertil Steril.* 2005 Jul;84(1):181-85.

Bayram N, van Wely M, Kaaijk EM, et al. Using an electrocautery strategy or recombinant follicle stimulating hormone to induce ovulation in polycystic ovary syndrome: randomised controlled trial. *BMJ.* 2004 Jan 24;328(7433):192.

REFERENCES

Becker RH, Vonk R, Mende BC, et al. The relevance of placental location at 20-23 gestational weeks for prediction of placenta previa at delivery: evaluation of 8650 cases. *Ultrasound Obstet Gynecol.* 2001 Jun;17(6):496-501.

Beckmann C, Ling F, Herbert W. *Obstetrics and Gynecology. 3rd ed.* Baltimore: Williams & Wilkins; 1998.

Bedaiwy M, Liu J. Long-term management of endometriosis: medical therapy and treatment of infertility. *SRM.* 2010(Aug):10-14.

Bednarek PH, Creinin MD, Reeves MF, et al. Immediate versus delayed IUD insertion after uterine aspiration. *N Engl J Med.* 2011 Jun 9;364(23):2208-17.

Belfort M. Critical care in OB: part 4 navigating a thyroid storm. *Cont Ob/Gyn.* 2006;51(10):38-47.

Bellcross CA, Lemke AA, Pape LS, et al. Evaluation of a breast/ovarian cancer genetics referral screening tool in a mammography population. *Genet Med.* 2009 Nov;11(11):783-89.

Bellini C, Hennekam RC, Bonioli E. A diagnostic flow chart for non-immune hydrops fetalis. *Am J Med Genet.* 2009 May;149A(5):852-53.

Benedetti TJ, Gabbe SG. Shoulder dystocia: a complication of fetal macrosomia and prolonged second stage of labor with midpelvic delivery. *Obstet Gynecol.* 1978 Nov;52(5):526-29.

Berek J, Hacker N. *Practical Gynecologic Oncology, 4th Ed.* Philadelphia: Lippincott Williams & Wilkins; 2005.

Berghella V, Baxter J, Pereira L. Cerclage: should we be doing them? *Cont Ob/Gyn.* 2005(Dec):34-41.

Berghella V, Kuhlman K, Weiner S, et al. Cervical funneling: sonographic criteria predictive of preterm delivery. *Ultrasound Obstet Gynecol.* 1997 Sep;10(3):161-66.

Berghella V, Roman A, Daskalakis C, et al. Gestational age at cervical length measurement and incidence of preterm birth. *Obstet Gynecol.* 2007 Aug;110(2 Pt 1):311-17.

Bianchi DW, Platt LD, Goldberg JD, et al. Genome-wide fetal aneuploidy detection by maternal plasma DNA sequencing. *Obstet Gynecol.* 2012 May;119(5):890-901.

Bishop EH. Pelvic scoring for elective induction. *Obstet Gynecol.* 1964 Aug;24:266-68.

Bissonnette F, Lapensee L, Bouzayen R. Outpatient laparoscopic tubal anastomosis and subsequent fertility. *Fertil Steril.* 1999 Sep;72(3):549-52.

Blazar AS, Lambert-Messerlian G, Hackett R, et al. Use of in-cycle antimullerian hormone levels to predict cycle outcome. *Am J Obstet Gynecol.* 2011 Sep;205(3):223.e1-5.

Blumenfeld Z, Avivi I, Linn S, et al. Prevention of irreversible chemotherapy-induced ovarian damage in young women with lymphoma by a gonadotrophin-releasing hormone agonist in parallel to chemotherapy. *Hum Reprod.* 1996 Aug;11(8):1620-6.

Blumenthal PD, Edelman A. Hormonal contraception. *Obstet Gynecol.* 2008 Sep;112(3):670-84.

Bosdou JK, Venetis CA, Kolibianakis EM, et al. The use of androgens or androgen-modulating agents in poor responders undergoing in vitro fertilization: a systematic review and meta-analysis. *Hum Reprod Update.* 2012 Mar-Apr;18(2):127-45.

Branch DW, Gibson M, Silver RM. Clinical practice: recurrent miscarriage. *N Engl J Med.* 2010 Oct 28;363(18):1740-7.

Branch W. Report of the Obstetric APS Task Force: 13th International Congress on Antiphospholipid Antibodies, 13th April 2010. *Lupus.* 2011 Feb;20(2):158-64.

Branda KJ, Tomczak J, Natowicz MR. Heterozygosity for Tay-Sachs and Sandhoff diseases in non-Jewish Americans with ancestry from Ireland, Great Britain, or Italy. *Genet Test.* 2004 8(2):174-80.

Braunstein GD. False-positive serum human chorionic gonadotropin results: causes, characteristics, and recognition. *Am J Obstet Gynecol.* 2002;187(1):217-24.

REFERENCES

Bray GA. Definition, measurement, and classification of the syndromes of obesity. *Int J Obesity.* 1978;2(2):99-112.

Breitkopf DM, Frederickson RA, Snyder RR. Detection of benign endometrial masses by endometrial stripe measurement in premenopausal women. *Obstet Gynecol.* 2004 Jul;104(1):120-25.

Brigham SA, Conlon C, Farquharson RG. A longitudinal study of pregnancy outcome following idiopathic recurrent miscarriage. *Hum Reprod.* 1999 Nov;14(11):2868-71.

Brinton LA, Trabert B, Shalev V, et al. In vitro fertilization and risk of breast and gynecologic cancers: a retrospective cohort study within the Israeli Maccabi Healthcare Services. *Fertil Steril.* 2013 Apr;99(5):1189-96.

Brown HL. Trauma in pregnancy. *Obstet Gynecol.* 2009 Jul;114(1):147-60.

Burch HB, Wartofsky L. Life-threatening thyrotoxicosis: thyroid storm. *Endocrinol Metab Clin North Am.* 1993 Jun;22(2):263-77.

Burger M, Weber-Rossler T, Willmann M. Measurement of the pregnant cervix by transvaginal sonography: an interobserver study and new standards to improve the interobserver variability. *Ultrasound Obstet Gynecol.* 1997 Mar;9(3):188-93.

Burrow GN, Wortzman G, Rewcastle NB, et al. Microadenomas of the pituitary and abnormal sellar tomograms in an unselected autopsy series. *N Engl J Med.* 1981 Jan 15;304(3):156-58.

Buster J, Barnhart K. Ectopic pregnancy: a 5-step plan for medical management. *OBG Management.* 2004:74-86.

Buttram VC, Jr. Müllerian anomalies and their management. *Fertil Steril.* 1983 Aug;40(2):159-63.

Buttram VC, Jr., Reiter RC. Uterine leiomyomata: etiology, symptomatology, and management. *Fertil Steril.* 1981 Oct;36(4):433-45.

Buyalos RP, Ghosh K, Daneshmand ST. Infertile women of advanced reproductive age: variability of day 3 FSH and E2 levels. *J Reprod Med.* 1998 Dec;43(12):1023-6.

Callen P. *Ultrasonography in Obstetrics and Gynecology.* San Francisco: WB Saunders; 2000.

Camus E, Poncelet C, Goffinet F, et al. Pregnancy rates after in-vitro fertilization in cases of tubal infertility with and without hydrosalpinx: a meta-analysis of published comparative studies. *Hum Reprod.* 1999 May;14(5):1243-9.

Carraro P. Guidelines for the laboratory investigation of inherited thrombophilias: recommendations for the first level clinical laboratories. European Communities Confederation of Clinical Chemistry and Laboratory Medicine, Working Group on Guidelines for Investigation of Disease. *Clin Chem Lab Med.* 2003;41:382-91.

Collaborative Group on Hormonal Factors in Breast Cancer. Breast cancer and hormonal contraceptives: collaborative reanalysis of individual data on 53,297 women with breast cancer and 100,239 women without breast cancer from 54 epidemiological studies. *Lancet.* 1996 Jun 22;347(9017):1713-27.

Carey E, Findley A. Caring for patients with chronic pelvic pain. *Cont Ob/Gyn.* January 2015.

Carlson KJ, Miller BA, Fowler FJ, Jr. The Maine Women's Health Study: II. Outcomes of nonsurgical management of leiomyomas, abnormal bleeding, and chronic pelvic pain. *Obstet Gynecol.* 1994 Apr;83(4):566-72.

Carmichael SL, Shaw GM. Maternal corticosteroid use and risk of selected congenital anomalies. *Am J Med Genet.* 1999 Sep 17;86(3):242-44.

Carmina E, Rosato F, Janni A, et al. Extensive clinical experience: relative prevalence of different androgen excess disorders in 950 women referred because of clinical hyperandrogenism. *J Clin Endocrinol Metab.* 2006 Jan;91(1):2-6.

REFERENCES

Carr BR, Breslau NA, Givens C, et al. Oral contraceptive pills, gonadotropin-releasing hormone agonists, or use in combination for treatment of hirsutism: a clinical research center study. *J Clin Endocrinol Metab.* 1995 Apr;80(4):1169-78.

Carson SA, Buster JE. Ectopic pregnancy. *N Engl J Med.* 1993 Oct 14;329(16):1174-81.

Casey BM, Leveno KJ. Thyroid disease in pregnancy. *Obstet Gynecol.* 2006 Nov;108(5):1283-92.

Catarci T, Fiacco F, Bozzao L, et al. Empty sella and headache. *Headache.* 1994 Nov-Dec;34(10): 583-86.

Caughey AB, Hopkins LM, Norton ME. Chorionic villus sampling compared with amniocentesis and the difference in the rate of pregnancy loss. *Obstet Gynecol.* 2006 Sep;108(3 Pt 1):612-16.

Centers for Disease Control. U.S. medical eligibility criteria for contraceptive use, 2010. *MMWR.* 2010 Jun 18;59(Rr-4):1-86.

Centers for Disease Control. Testing for HCV infection: an update of guidance for clinicians and laboratorians. *MMWR.* 2013 May 10;62(18):362-65.

Centers for Disease Control. U.S. selected practice recommendations for contraceptive use, 2013: adapted from the World Health Organization selected practice recommendations for contraceptive use, 2nd edition. *MMWR.* 2013 Jun 21;62(Rr-05):1-60.

Centers for Disease Control. Sexually transmitted diseases treatment guidelines, 2015. *MMWR.* 2015;64(3):1-137.

Chandra A, Copen CE, Stephen EH. Infertility and impaired fecundity in the United States, 1982-2010: data from the National Survey of Family Growth. *National Health Statistics Reports.* 2013 Aug 14(67):1-18.

Chang MY, Chiang CH, Hsieh TT, et al. Use of the antral follicle count to predict the outcome of assisted reproductive technologies. *Fertil Steril.* 1998 Mar;69(3):505-510.

Check W, Hoskins W. Conservative management of endometrial hyperplasia: new strategies and experimental options. *OBG Management.* 2003(Sept):15-26.

Chen C. Pregnancy after human oocyte cryopreservation. *Lancet.* 1986 Apr 19;1(8486):884-86.

Chen K. UTI in pregnancy: 6 questions to guide therapy. *OBG Management.* 2004(Nov):36-53.

Chen MM, Coakley FV, Kaimal A, et al. Guidelines for computed tomography and magnetic resonance imaging use during pregnancy and lactation. *Obstet Gynecol.* 2008 Aug;112(2 Pt 1):333-40.

Cheschier N. ACOG Practice Bulletin No. 44: Neural tube defects (Replaces committee opinion number 252, March 2001). *Int J Gynaecol Obstet.* 2003 Oct;83(1):123-33.

Chou R. Nonpharmacologic therapies for acute and chronic low back pain: a review of the evidence for an American Pain Society/American. *Ann Intern Med.* 2007;147.

Chou R, Qaseem A, Owens DK, et al. Diagnostic imaging for low back pain: advice for high-value health care from the American College of Physicians. *Ann Intern Med.* 2011 Feb 1;154(3):181-89.

Chou R, Qaseem A, Snow V, et al. Diagnosis and treatment of low back pain: a joint clinical practice guideline from the American College of Physicians and the American Pain Society. *Ann Intern Med.* 2007 Oct 2;147(7):478-91.

Chow AW, Benninger MS, Brook I, et al. IDSA clinical practice guideline for acute bacterial rhinosinusitis in children and adults. *Clin Infect Dis.* 2012 Apr;54(8):e72-e112.

Christiansen OB, Pedersen B, Rosgaard A, et al. A randomized, double-blind, placebo-controlled trial of intravenous immunoglobulin in the prevention of recurrent miscarriage: evidence for a therapeutic effect in women with secondary recurrent miscarriage. *Hum Reprod.* 2002 Mar;17(3):809-816.

Christiansen OB, Steffensen R, Nielsen HS, et al. Multifactorial etiology of recurrent miscarriage and its scientific and clinical implications. *Gynecol Obstet Invest.* 2008;66(4):257-67.

REFERENCES

Christopher D, Robinson BK, Peaceman AM. An evidence-based approach to determining route of delivery for twin gestations. *Rev Obstet Gynecol.* 2011;4(3-4):109-116.

Ciccarelli E, Camanni F. Diagnosis and drug therapy of prolactinoma. *Drugs.* 1996 Jun;51(6): 954-65.

Ciotta L, Cianci A, Calogero AE, et al. Clinical and endocrine effects of finasteride, a 5 alpha-reductase inhibitor, in women with idiopathic hirsutism. *Fertil Steril.* 1995 Aug;64(2):299-306.

Clark EA, Silver RM. Long-term maternal morbidity associated with repeat cesarean delivery. *Am J Obstet Gynecol.* 2011 Dec;205(6 Suppl):S2-10.

Clark SL, Cotton DB, Lee W, et al. Central hemodynamic assessment of normal term pregnancy. *Am J Obstet Gynecol.* 1989 Dec;161(6 Pt 1):1439-42.

Clarke GN, Elliott PJ, Smaila C. Detection of sperm antibodies in semen using the immunobead test: a survey of 813 consecutive patients. *Am J Reprod Immunol Microbiol.* 1985 Mar;7(3):118-23.

Clemons M, Goss P. Estrogen and the risk of breast cancer. *N Engl J Med.* 2001 Jan 25;344(4):276-85.

Cobo A, Meseguer M, Remohi J, et al. Use of cryo-banked oocytes in an ovum donation programme: a prospective, randomized, controlled, clinical trial. *Hum Reprod.* 2010 Sep;25(9):2239-46.

Cocksedge KA, Li TC, Saravelos SH, et al. A reappraisal of the role of polycystic ovary syndrome in recurrent miscarriage. *Reprod Biomed Online.* 2008 Jul;17(1):151-60.

Colao A, Di Somma C, Loche S, et al. Prolactinomas in adolescents: persistent bone loss after 2 years of prolactin normalization. *Clin Endocrinol (Oxf).* 2000 Mar;52(3):319-27.

Condous G, Kirk E, Lu C, et al. Diagnostic accuracy of varying discriminatory zones for the prediction of ectopic pregnancy in women with a pregnancy of unknown location *Ultrasound Obstet Gynecol.* 2005 Dec;26(7):770-75.

Coomarasamy A, Williams H, Truchanowicz E, et al. A randomized trial of progesterone in women with recurrent miscarriages. *N Engl J Med.* 2015 Nov 26;373(22):2141-8.

Cooper TG, Noonan E, von Eckardstein S, et al. World Health Organization reference values for human semen characteristics. *Hum Reprod Update.* 2010 May-Jun;16(3):231-45.

Copel JA, Bahtiyar MO. A practical approach to fetal growth restriction. *Obstet Gynecol.* 2014 May;123(5):1057-69.

Copperman AB, Wells V, Luna M, et al. Presence of hydrosalpinx correlated to endometrial inflammatory response in vivo. *Fertil Steril.* 2006 Oct;86(4):972-76.

Corfman RS. Indications for hysteroscopy. *Obstet Gynecol Clin North Am.* 1988 Mar;15(1):41-9.

Coric M, Barisic D, Pavicic D, et al. Electrocoagulation versus suture after laparoscopic stripping of ovarian endometriomas assessed by antral follicle count: preliminary results of randomized clinical trial. *Arch Gynecol Obstet.* 2011 Feb;283(2):373-78.

Cosman F, de Beur SJ, LeBoff MS, et al. Clinician's guide to prevention and treatment of osteoporosis. *Osteoporos Int.* 2014 Oct;25(10):2359-81.

Couchman G, Hammond C. Physiology of reproduction. In: Scott J, DiSaia P, Hammond C, et al., editors. *Danforth's Obstetrics and Gynecology, 7th Ed.,* 7th Ed. Philadelphia: Lippincott; 1994.

Coustan D. Delivery: timing, mode, and management. In: Reece E, Coustan D, Gabbe S, editors. *Diabetes in Women: Adolescence, Pregnancy, and Menopause, 3rd Ed.* Philadelphia: Lippincott Williams & Wilkins; 2004.

Coutifaris C, Myers ER, Guzick DS, et al. Histological dating of timed endometrial biopsy tissue is not related to fertility status. *Fertil Steril.* 2004 Nov;82(5):1264-72.

Craig LB, Ke RW, Kutteh WH. Increased prevalence of insulin resistance in women with a history of recurrent pregnancy loss. *Fertil Steril.* 2002 Sep;78(3):487-90.

REFERENCES

Creasman WT, Morrow CP, Bundy BN, et al. Surgical pathologic spread patterns of endometrial cancer: a gynecologic oncology group study. *Cancer.* 1987 Oct 15;60(8 Suppl):2035-41.

Creinin MD, Fox MC, Teal S, et al. A randomized comparison of misoprostol 6 to 8 hours versus 24 hours after mifepristone for abortion. *Obstet Gynecol.* 2004 May; 103(5 Pt 1):851-59.

Creinin MD, Vittinghoff E, Schaff E, et al. Medical abortion with oral methotrexate and vaginal misoprostol. *Obstet Gynecol.* 1997 Oct;90(4 Pt 1):611-16.

Crosignani PG. Current treatment issues in female hyperprolactinaemia. *Eur J Obstet Gynecol Reprod Biol.* 2006 Apr 1;125(2):152-64.

Cuckle H, Benn P, Wright D. Down syndrome screening in the first and/or second trimester: model predicted performance using meta-analysis parameters. *Semin Perinatol.* 2005 Aug;29(4):252-57.

Cuckle HS, Wald NJ, Thompson SG. Estimating a woman's risk of having a pregnancy associated with Down's syndrome using her age and serum alpha-fetoprotein level. *Br J Obstet Gynecol.* 1987 May;94(5):387-402.

Curtis KM, Chrisman CE, Peterson HB. Contraception for women in selected circumstances. *Obstet Gynecol.* 2002 Jun;99(6):1100-12.

Cutts FT. Human papillomavirus and HPV vaccines: a review. *Bull World Health Organ.* 2007;85(09):719-26.

D'Ercole M, Della Pepa GM, Carrozza C, et al. Two diagnostic pitfalls mimicking a prolactin-secreting microadenoma. *J Clin Endocrinol Metab.* 2010 Dec;95(12):5171.

Dabirashrafi H, Bahadori M, Mohammad K, et al. Septate uterus: new idea on the histologic features of the septum in this abnormal uterus. *Am J Obstet Gynecol.* 1995 Jan;172(1 Pt 1):105-107.

Dahdouh EM, Balayla J, Garcia-Velasco JA. Impact of blastocyst biopsy and comprehensive chromosome screening technology on preimplantation genetic screening: a systematic review of randomized controlled trials. *Reprod Biomed Online.* 2015 Mar;30(3):281-89.

Dahlke JD, Mendez-Figueroa H, Rouse DJ, et al. Evidence-based surgery for cesarean delivery: an updated systematic review. *Am J Obstet Gynecol.* 2013 Oct;209(4):294-306.

Daly DC, Walters CA, Soto-Albors CE, et al. A randomized study of dexamethasone in ovulation induction with clomiphene citrate. *Fertil Steril.* 1984 Jun;41(6):844-48.

Daniell JF, Miller W. Polycystic ovaries treated by laparoscopic laser vaporization. *Fertil Steril.* 1989 Feb;51(2):232-36.

Dashe JS, Casey BM, Wells CE, et al. Thyroid-stimulating hormone in singleton and twin pregnancy: importance of gestational age-specific reference ranges. *Obstet Gynecol.* 2005 Oct;106(4):753-57.

Davies MJ, Moore VM, Willson KJ, et al. Reproductive technologies and the risk of birth defects. *N Engl J Med.* 2012 May 10;366(19):1803-13.

Davis A, Godwin A, Lippman J, et al. Triphasic norgestimate-ethinyl estradiol for treating dysfunctional uterine bleeding. *Obstet Gynecol.* 2000 Dec;96(6):913-20.

Davis AR, Kroll R, Soltes B, et al. Occurrence of menses or pregnancy after cessation of a continuous oral contraceptive. *Fertil Steril.* 2008 May;89(5):1059-63.

Davis OK, Berkeley AS, Naus GJ, et al. The incidence of luteal phase defect in normal, fertile women, determined by serial endometrial biopsies. *Fertil Steril.* 1989 Apr;51(4):582-86.

De Groot L, Abalovich M, Alexander EK, et al. Management of thyroid dysfunction during pregnancy and postpartum: an Endocrine Society clinical practice guideline. *J Clin Endocrinol Metab.* 2012 Aug;97(8):2543-65.

De Souza E, Halliday J, Chan A, et al. Recurrence risks for trisomies 13, 18, and 21. *Am J Med Genet.* 2009 Dec;149A(12):2716-22.

REFERENCES

de Villiers TJ, Gass ML, Haines CJ, et al. Global consensus statement on menopausal hormone therapy. *Climacteric*. 2013 Apr;16(2):203-204.

de Vries BB, van den Ouweland AM, Mohkamsing S, et al. Screening and diagnosis for the fragile X syndrome among the mentally retarded: an epidemiological and psychological survey: collaborative Fragile X study group. *Am J Hum Genet*. 1997 Sep;61(3):660-67.

Deaton JL, Honore GM, Huffman CS, et al. Early transvaginal ultrasound following an accurately dated pregnancy: the importance of finding a yolk sac or fetal heart motion. *Hum Reprod*. 1997 Dec;12(12):2820-3.

Dekkers OM, Pereira AM, Romijn JA. Treatment and follow-up of clinically nonfunctioning pituitary macroadenomas. *J Clin Endocrinol Metab*. 2008 Oct;93(10):3717-26.

Del Mastro L, Boni L, Michelotti A, et al. Effect of the gonadotropin-releasing hormone analogue triptorelin on the occurrence of chemotherapy-induced early menopause in premenopausal women with breast cancer: a randomized trial. *JAMA*. 2011 Jul 20;306(3):269-76.

DeLeo FR, Otto M, Kreiswirth BN, et al. Community-associated meticillin-resistant *Staphylococcus aureus*. *Lancet*. 2010;375(9725):1557-68.

Delmas PD. Markers of bone turnover for monitoring treatment of osteoporosis with antiresorptive drugs. *Osteoporos Int*. 2000;11 Suppl 6:S66-76.

Deneux-Tharaux C, Carmona E, Bouvier-Colle MH, et al. Postpartum maternal mortality and cesarean delivery. *Obstet Gynecol*. 2006 Sep;108(3 Pt 1):541-48.

Diamond MP, Legro RS, Coutifaris C, et al. Letrozole, gonadotropin, or clomiphene for unexplained infertility. *N Engl J Med*. 2015 Sep 24;373(13):1230-40.

Dickinson JE, Eriksen NL, Meyer BA, et al. The effect of preterm birth on umbilical cord blood gases. *Obstet Gynecol*. 1992 Apr;79(4):575-78.

Djahanbakhch O, McNeilly AS, Warner PM, et al. Changes in plasma levels of prolactin, in relation to those of FSH, oestradiol, androstenedione and progesterone around the preovulatory surge of LH in women. *Clinical endocrinol*. 1984 Apr;20(4):463-72.

Dolmans MM, Luyckx V, Donnez J, et al. Risk of transferring malignant cells with transplanted frozen-thawed ovarian tissue. *Fertil Steril*. 2013 May;99(6):1514-22.

Donnez J, Dolmans MM, Pellicer A, et al. Restoration of ovarian activity and pregnancy after transplantation of cryopreserved ovarian tissue: a review of 60 cases of reimplantation. *Fertil Steril*. 2013 May;99(6):1503-13.

Donnez J, Donnez O, Dolmans MM. With the advent of selective progesterone receptor modulators, what is the place of myoma surgery in current practice? *Fertil Steril*. 2014 Sep;102(3):640-48.

Dorr R. Pharmacologic management of vesicant chemotherapy extravasations. In: Dorr R, Von Hoff D, editors. *Cancer Chemotherapy Handbook, 2nd Ed*. Norwalk, CT: Appleton & Lange; 1994.

Doubilet PM, Benson CB, Bourne T, et al. Diagnostic criteria for nonviable pregnancy early in the first trimester. *N Engl J Med*. 2013 Oct 10;369(15):1443-51.

Druzin ML. Atraumatic delivery in cases of malpresentation of the very low birth weight fetus at cesarean section: the splint technique. *Am J Obstet Gynecol*. 1986.

Duffy JM, Ahmad G, Mohiyiddeen L, et al. Growth hormone for in vitro fertilization. *Cochrane Database Syst Rev*. 2010(1):CD000099.

Dugoff L, Society for Maternal-Fetal Medicine. First- and second-trimester maternal serum markers for aneuploidy and adverse obstetric outcomes. *Obstet Gynecol*. 2010 May;115(5):1052-61.

Duhl AJ, Paidas MJ, Ural SH, et al. Antithrombotic therapy and pregnancy: consensus report and recommendations for prevention and treatment of venous thromboembolism and adverse pregnancy outcomes. *Am J Obstet Gynecol*. 2007 Nov;197(5):457 e1-21.

REFERENCES

Dunaif A, Xia J, Book CB, et al. Excessive insulin receptor serine phosphorylation in cultured fibroblasts and in skeletal muscle. A potential mechanism for insulin resistance in the polycystic ovary syndrome. *J Clin Invest.* 1995 Aug;96(2):801-810.

Dunlop AL, Gardiner PM, Shellhaas CS, et al. The clinical content of preconception care: the use of medications and supplements among women of reproductive age. *Am J Obstet Gynecol.* 2008 Dec;199(6 Suppl 2):S367-72.

Dykes AC, Walker ID, McMahon AD, et al. A study of Protein S antigen levels in 3788 healthy volunteers: influence of age, sex and hormone use, and estimate for prevalence of deficiency state. *Br J Haematol.* 2001;113:636-41.

Eckert LO. Clinical practice: acute vulvovaginitis. *N Engl J Med.* 2006 Sep 21;355(12):1244-52.

Eddleman KA, Malone FD, Sullivan L, et al. Pregnancy loss rates after midtrimester amniocentesis. *Obstet Gynecol.* 2006 Nov;108(5):1067-72.

Edmonds DK, Lindsay KS, Miller JF, et al. Early embryonic mortality in women. *Fertil Steril.* 1982 Oct;38(4):447-53.

Edwards JG, Feldman G, Goldberg J, et al. Expanded carrier screening in reproductive medicine-points to consider: a joint statement of the American College of Medical Genetics and Genomics, American College of Obstetricians and Gynecologists, National Society of Genetic Counselors, Perinatal Quality Foundation, and Society for Maternal-Fetal Medicine. *Obstet Gynecol.* 2015 Mar;125(3):653-62.

Einarson A, Maltepe C, Boskovic R, et al. Treatment of nausea and vomiting in pregnancy: an updated algorithm. *Can Fam Physician.* 2007 Dec;53(12):2109-11.

El-Refaey H, Rajasekar D, Abdalla M, et al. Induction of abortion with mifepristone (RU 486) and oral or vaginal misoprostol. *N Engl J Med.* 1995 Apr 13;332(15):983-87.

Elias KA, Weiner RI. Direct arterial vascularization of estrogen-induced prolactin-secreting anterior pituitary tumors. *Proc Natl Acad Sci USA.* 1984 Jul;81(14):4549-53.

Elnashar A, Abdelmageed E, Fayed M, et al. Clomiphene citrate and dexamethazone in treatment of clomiphene citrate-resistant polycystic ovary syndrome: a prospective placebo-controlled study. *Hum Reprod.* 2006 Jul;21(7):1805-8.

Elting MW, Korsen TJ, Rekers-Mombarg LT, et al. Women with polycystic ovary syndrome gain regular menstrual cycles when ageing. *Hum Reprod.* 2000 Jan;15(1):24-8.

Empson M, Lassere M, Craig JC, et al. Recurrent pregnancy loss with antiphospholipid antibody: a systematic review of therapeutic trials. *Obstet Gynecol.* 2002 Jan;99(1):135-44.

Ergaz Z, Ornoy A. Parvovirus B19 in pregnancy. *Reproductive Toxicology.* 2006 May;21(4):421-35.

Evans DG, Eccles DM, Rahman N, et al. A new scoring system for the chances of identifying a BRCA1/2 mutation outperforms existing models including BRCAPRO. *J Med Genet.* 2004 Jun;41(6):474-80.

Falcone T, Parker WH. Surgical management of leiomyomas for fertility or uterine preservation. *Obstet Gynecol.* 2013 Apr;121(4):856-68.

Farhi J, Ashkenazi J, Feldberg D, et al. Effect of uterine leiomyomata on the results of in-vitro fertilization treatment. *Hum Reprod.* 1995 Oct;10(10):2576-8.

Farley TM, Meirik O, Collins J. Cardiovascular disease and combined oral contraceptives: reviewing the evidence and balancing the risks. *Hum Reprod Update.* 1999 Nov-Dec;5(6):721-35.

Farquhar CM, Lethaby A, Sowter M, et al. An evaluation of risk factors for endometrial hyperplasia in premenopausal women with abnormal menstrual bleeding. *Am J Obstet Gynecol.* 1999 Sep;181(3):525-29.

Feigenbaum SL, Downey DE, Wilson CB, et al. Transsphenoidal pituitary resection for preoperative diagnosis of prolactin-secreting pituitary adenoma in women: long term follow-up. *J Clin Endocrinol Metab.* 1996 May;81(5):1711-9.

REFERENCES

Felemban A, Tan SL, Tulandi T. Laparoscopic treatment of polycystic ovaries with insulated needle cautery: a reappraisal. *Fertil Steril.* 2000 Feb;73(2):266-69.

Fernandez E, La Vecchia C, Balducci A, et al. Oral contraceptives and colorectal cancer risk: a meta-analysis. *Br J Cancer.* 2001 Mar 2;84(5):722-27.

Fernandez H, Capmas P, Lucot JP, et al. Fertility after ectopic pregnancy: the DEMETER randomized trial. *Hum Reprod.* 2013 May;28(5):1247-53.

Fernandez-Carvajal I, Lopez Posadas B, Pan R, et al. Expansion of an *FMR1* grey-zone allele to a full mutation in two generations. *J Mol Diagn.* 2009 Jul;11(4):306-310.

Ferreira M, Bos-Mikich A, Hoher M, et al. Dichorionic twins and monochorionic triplets after the transfer of two blastocysts. *J Assist Reprod Genet.* 2010 Sep; 27(9-10):545-48.

FIGO. Current FIGO staging for cancer of the vagina, fallopian tube, ovary, and gestational trophoblastic neoplasia. *Int J Gynaecol Obstet.* 2009 Apr;105(1):3-4.

Forman EJ, Upham KM, Cheng M, et al. Comprehensive chromosome screening alters traditional morphology-based embryo selection: a prospective study of 100 consecutive cycles of planned fresh euploid blastocyst transfer. *Fertil Steril.* 2013 Sep;100(3):718-24.

Fourman LT, Fazeli PK. Neuroendocrine causes of amenorrhea—an update. *J Clin Endocrinol Metab.* 2015 Mar;100(3):812-24.

Franco RF, Reitsma PH. Genetic risk factors of venous thrombosis. *Hum Genet.* 2001;109: 369-84.

Francois K. Managing uterine atony and hemorrhagic shock. *Cont Ob/Gyn.* 2006(Feb):52-9.

Franssen MT, Musters AM, van der Veen F, et al. Reproductive outcome after PGD in couples with recurrent miscarriage carrying a structural chromosome abnormality: a systematic review. *Hum Reprod Update.* 2011 Jul-Aug;17(4):467-75.

Fraser IS, Critchley HO, Munro MG, et al. A process designed to lead to international agreement on terminologies and definitions used to describe abnormalities of menstrual bleeding. *Fertil Steril.* 2007 Mar;87(3):466-76.

Fraser WD, Hofmeyr J, Lede R, et al. Amnioinfusion for the prevention of the meconium aspiration syndrome. *N Engl J Med.* 2005 Sep 1;353(9):909-917.

Frattarelli JL, Lauria-Costab DF, Miller BT, et al. Basal antral follicle number and mean ovarian diameter predict cycle cancellation and ovarian responsiveness in assisted reproductive technology cycles. *Fertil Steril.* 2000 Sep;74(3):512-17.

Frattarelli JL, Levi AJ, Miller BT, et al. A prospective assessment of the predictive value of basal antral follicles in in vitro fertilization cycles. *Fertil Steril.* 2003 Aug;80(2):350-55.

Freedman RR, Roehrs TA. Lack of sleep disturbance from menopausal hot flashes. *Fertil Steril.* 2004 Jul;82(1):138-44.

Freeman EW, Sammel MD, Lin H, et al. Duration of menopausal hot flushes and associated risk factors. *Obstet Gynecol.* 2011 May;117(5):1095-1104

Freeman JS. Insulin analog therapy: improving the match with physiologic insulin secretion. *J Am Osteopath Assoc.* 2009 Jan;109(1):26-36.

Fretts RC. Etiology and prevention of stillbirth. *Am J Obstet Gynecol.* 2005 Dec;193(6):1923-35. Copyright © 2005 Elsevier.

Friederich PW, Sanson BJ, Simioni P, et al. Frequency of pregnancy-related venous thromboembolism in anticoagulant factor-deficient women: implications for prophylaxis [published errata appear in *Ann Intern Med* 1997;127:1138; *Ann Intern Med* 1997;126:835]. *Ann Intern Med.* 1996;125:955-60.

Friedman AM, Ananth CV, Prendergast E, et al. Evaluation of third-degree and fourth-degree laceration rates as quality indicators. *Obstet Gynecol.* 2015 Apr;125(4):927-37.

REFERENCES

Fritz B, Hallermann C, Olert J, et al. Cytogenetic analyses of culture failures by comparative genomic hybridisation (CGH):Re-evaluation of chromosome aberration rates in early spontaneous abortions. *Eur J Hum Genet.* 2001 Jul;9(7):539-47.

Fritz M, Speroff L. Normal and abnormal growth and pubertal development. In: *Clinical Gynecologic Endocrinology and Infertility, 8th Ed.* Philadelphia: Lippincott Williams & Wilkins; 2011.

Fritz M, Speroff L. Reproduction and the thyroid. In: *Clinical Gynecologic Endocrinology and Infertility, 8th Ed.* Philadelphia: Lippincott Williams & Wilkins; 2011.

Fruzzetti F, Bersi C, Parrini D, et al. Treatment of hirsutism: comparisons between different antiandrogens with central and peripheral effects. *Fertil Steril.* 1999 Mar;71(3):445-51.

Fujimoto VY, Clifton DK, Cohen NL, et al. Variability of serum prolactin and progesterone levels in normal women: the relevance of single hormone measurements in the clinical setting. *Obstet Gynecol.* 1990 Jul;76(1):71-8.

Gadir AA, Alnaser HM, Mowafi RS, et al. The response of patients with polycystic ovarian disease to human menopausal gonadotropin therapy after ovarian electrocautery or a luteinizing hormone-releasing hormone agonist. *Fertil Steril.* 1992 Feb;57(2):309-313.

Garber JR, Cobin RH, Gharib H, et al. Clinical practice guidelines for hypothyroidism in adults: cosponsored by the American Association of Clinical Endocrinologists and the American Thyroid Association. *Thyroid.* 2012 Dec;22(12):1200-35.

Garcia-Enguidanos A, Martinez D, Calle ME, et al. Long-term use of oral contraceptives increases the risk of miscarriage. *Fertil Steril.* 2005 Jun;83(6):1864-6.

Garcia-Velasco JA, Mahutte NG, Corona J, et al. Removal of endometriomas before in vitro fertilization does not improve fertility outcomes: a matched, case-control study. *Fertil Steril.* 2004 May;81(5):1194-7.

Gariepy A, Stanwood N. Medical management of early pregnancy failure. *Cont Ob/Gyn.* 2013(May):26-33.

Gaudet T. Complementary and alternative medicine. *Clin Update Womens Health Care.* 2011;X(4):66. American College of Obstetricians and Gynecologists. Washington, DC.

Gavin L, Moskosky S, Carter M, et al. Providing quality family planning services: recommendations of CDC and the U.S. Office of Population Affairs. *MMWR.* 2014 Apr 25;63(Rr-04):1-54.

Gerhardt A, Scharf RE, Beckmann MW, et al. Prothrombin and factor V mutations in women with a history of thrombosis during pregnancy and the puerperium. *N Engl J Med.* 2000;342:374-80.

Gibney J, Smith TP, McKenna TJ. Clinical relevance of macroprolactin. *Clinical endocrinol.* 2005 Jun;62(6):633-43.

Gillam MP, Middler S, Freed DJ, et al. The novel use of very high doses of cabergoline and a combination of testosterone and an aromatase inhibitor in the treatment of a giant prolactinoma. *J Clin Endocrinol Metab.* 2002 Oct;87(10):4447-51.

Gilliam M. Acne treatment with a low dose oral contraceptive. *Obstet Gynecol.* 2001;97(Suppl 1):S9.

Gilpin CA, Carson N, Hunter AG. A preliminary validation of a family history assessment form to select women at risk for breast or ovarian cancer for referral to a genetics center. *Clin genet.* 2000 Oct;58(4):299-308.

Gjonnaess H. Polycystic ovarian syndrome treated by ovarian electrocautery through the laparoscope. *Fertil Steril.* 1984 Jan;41(1):20-25.

Gjonnaess H. Late endocrine effects of ovarian electrocautery in women with polycystic ovary syndrome. *Fertil Steril.* 1998 Apr;69(4):697-701.

Glueck CJ, Wang P, Kobayashi S, et al. Metformin therapy throughout pregnancy reduces the development of gestational diabetes in women with polycystic ovary syndrome. *Fertil Steril.* 2002 Mar;77(3):520-25.

REFERENCES

Glujovsky D, Blake D, Farquhar C, et al. Cleavage stage versus blastocyst stage embryo transfer in assisted reproductive technology. *Cochrane Database Syst Rev.* 2012;7:Cd002118.

Gnoth C, Godehardt D, Godehardt E, et al. Time to pregnancy: results of the German prospective study and impact on the management of infertility. *Hum Reprod.* 2003 Sep;18(9):1959-66.

Gnoth C, Schuring AN, Friol K, et al. Relevance of anti-Müllerian hormone measurement in a routine IVF program. *Hum Reprod.* 2008 Jun;23(6):1359-65.

Golbus M. Chromosome aberrations and mammalian reproduction. I. In: Mastroianni L, Biggers J, editors. *Fertilization and Embryonic Development In Vitro.* New York: Plenum Press; 1981.

Goodwin AJ, Rosendaal FR, Kottke-Marchant K, et al. A review of the technical, diagnostic, and epidemiologic considerations for protein S assays. *Arch Pathol Lab Med.* 2002;126:1349-66.

Goodwin SC, Spies JB, Worthington-Kirsch R, et al. Uterine artery embolization for treatment of leiomyomata: long-term outcomes from the FIBROID Registry. *Obstet Gynecol.* 2008 Jan;111(1):22-33.

Gordon J, Speroff L. Abnormal puberty and growth problems. *Handbook for Clinical Gynecologic Endocrinology and Infertility, 6th Ed.* Philadelphia: Lippincott–Raven; 2002.

Gordts S, Campo R, Puttemans P, et al. Clinical factors determining pregnancy outcome after microsurgical tubal reanastomosis. *Fertil Steril.* 2009 Oct;92(4):1198-1202

Gosden RG, Wade JC, Fraser HM, et al. Impact of congenital or experimental hypogonadotrophism on the radiation sensitivity of the mouse ovary. *Hum Reprod.* 1997 Nov;12(11):2483-8.

Gourlay ML, Fine JP, Preisser JS, et al. Bone-density testing interval and transition to osteoporosis in older women. *N Engl J Med.* 2012 Jan 19;366(3):225-33.

Grady D. Clinical practice: management of menopausal symptoms. *N Engl J Med.* 2006 Nov 30;355(22):2338-47.

Greco E, Minasi MG, Fiorentino F. Healthy babies after intrauterine transfer of mosaic aneuploid blastocysts. *N Engl J Med.* 2015 Nov 19;373(21):2089-90.

Green J, Berrington de Gonzalez A, Sweetland S, et al. Risk factors for adenocarcinoma and squamous cell carcinoma of the cervix in women aged 20-44 years: the UK National Case-Control Study of Cervical Cancer. *Br J Cancer.* 2003 Dec 1;89(11):2078-86.

Gregory KD, Jackson S, Korst L, et al. Cesarean versus vaginal delivery: whose risks? Whose benefits? *Am J Perinatol.* 2012 Jan;29(1):7-18.

Greutmann M, Pieper PG. Pregnancy in women with congenital heart disease. *Eur Heart J.* 2015 Oct 1;36(37):2491-9.

Grimes DA, Jones LB, Lopez LM, et al. Oral contraceptives for functional ovarian cysts. *Cochrane Database Syst Rev.* 2011(9):Cd006134.

Grimes DA, Stuart GS, Levi EE. Screening women for oral contraception: can family history identify inherited thrombophilias? *Obstet Gynecol.* 2012 Oct;120(4):889-95.

Groen RS, Bae JY, Lim KJ. Fear of the unknown: ionizing radiation exposure during pregnancy. *Am J Obstet Gynecol.* 2012 Jun;206(6):456-62.

Group NHBPEPW. Report of the national high blood pressure education program working group on high blood pressure in pregnancy. *Am J Obstet Gynecol.* 2000 Jul;183(1):S1-s22.

Gupta S. Weight gain on the combined pill—is it real? *Hum Reprod Update.* 2000 Sep-Oct;6(5):427-31.

Guzick DS, Sullivan MW, Adamson GD, et al. Efficacy of treatment for unexplained infertility. *Fertil Steril.* 1998 Aug;70(2):207-213.

Guzick DS, Wing R, Smith D, et al. Endocrine consequences of weight loss in obese, hyperandrogenic, anovulatory women. *Fertil Steril.* 1994 Apr;61(4):598-604.

Haefner HK, Collins ME, Davis GD, et al. The vulvodynia guideline. *J Low Genit Tract Dis.* 2005 Jan;9(1):40-51.

REFERENCES

Hager W. Managing mastitis. *Cont Ob/Gyn.* 2004(Jan):33-47.

Haines ST. Update on the prevention of venous thromboembolism. *Am J Health Syst Pharm.* 2004 Dec 1;61(23 Suppl 7):S5-11.

Hamdy RC, Baim S, Broy SB, et al. Algorithm for the management of osteoporosis. *South Med J.* 2010 Oct;103(10):1009-15.

Hannah ME, Whyte H, Hannah WJ, et al. Maternal outcomes at 2 years after planned cesarean section versus planned vaginal birth for breech presentation at term: the international randomized Term Breech Trial. *Am J Obstet Gynecol.* 2004 Sep;191(3):917-27.

Hansen LM, Batzer FR, Gutmann JN, et al. Evaluating ovarian reserve: follicle stimulating hormone and oestradiol variability during cycle days 2-5. *Hum Reprod.* 1996 Mar;11(3):486-89.

Hare J. Gestational diabetes and the White classification. *Diabetes Care.* 1980;3:394-96.

Harwood M, Smith B. Low back pain: a primary care approach. *Clin Fam Practice.* 2005;7(2):279-303.

Haverkate F, Samama M. Familial dysfibrinogenaemia and thrombophilia. Report on a study of the SSC Subcommittee on fibrinogen. *Thromb Haemost.* 1995;73:151-61.

Hearne AE, Nagey DA. Therapeutic agents in preterm labor: tocolytic agents. *Clin Obstet Gynecol.* 2000 Dec;43(4):787-801.

Herman-Giddens ME, Slora EJ, Wasserman RC, et al. Secondary sexual characteristics and menses in young girls seen in office practice: a study from the Pediatric Research in Office Settings network. *Pediatrics.* 1997 Apr;99(4):505-512.

Hibbard JU, Ismail MA, Wang Y, et al. Failed vaginal birth after a cesarean section: how risky is it? I. Maternal morbidity. *Am J Obstet Gynecol.* 2001 Jun;184(7):1365-71; discussion 71-3.

Hill LM, DiNofrio DM, Chenevey P. Transvaginal sonographic evaluation of first-trimester placenta previa. *Ultrasound Obstet Gynecol.* 1995 May;5(5):301-303.

Hobbs L, Ort R, Dover J. Synopsis of laser assisted hair removal systems. *Skin Therapy Lett.* 2000;5(3):1-5.

Hochberg MC. Updating the American College of Rheumatology revised criteria for the classification of systemic lupus erythematosus (letter). *Arthritis Rheum.* 1997; 40:1725.

Hofbauer LC, Hamann C, Ebeling PR. Approach to the patient with secondary osteoporosis. *Eur J Endocrinol.* 2010 Jun;162(6):1009-20.

Hofle G, Gasser R, Mohsenipour I, et al. Surgery combined with dopamine agonists versus dopamine agonists alone in long-term treatment of macroprolactinoma: a retrospective study. *Exp Clin Endocrinol Diabetes.* 1998;106(3):211-16.

Hofmeyr GJ, Barrett JF, Crowther CA. Planned caesarean section for women with a twin pregnancy. *Cochrane Database Syst Rev.* 2011(12):Cd006553.

Holoch P, Wald M. Current options for preservation of fertility in the male. *Fertil Steril.* 2011 Aug;96(2):286-90.

Hook B, Kiwi R, Amini SB, et al. Neonatal morbidity after elective repeat cesarean section and trial of labor. *Pediatrics.* 1997 Sep;100(3 Pt 1):348-53.

Hook EB. Rates of chromosome abnormalities at different maternal ages. *Obstet Gynecol.* 1981 Sep;58(3):282-85.

Hornstein MD, Surrey ES, Weisberg GW, et al. Leuprolide acetate depot and hormonal add-back in endometriosis: a 12-month study. Lupron Add-Back Study Group. *Obstet Gynecol.* 1998 Jan;91(1):16-24.

Hoskins IA, Marks F, Ordorica SA, et al. Leukocyte esterase activity in amniotic fluid: normal values during pregnancy. *Am J Perinatol.* 1990 Apr;7(2):130-32.

REFERENCES

Hoskins KF, Zwaagstra A, Ranz M. Validation of a tool for identifying women at high risk for hereditary breast cancer in population-based screening. *Cancer*. 2006 Oct 15;107(8):1769-76.

Howell S, Shalet S. Gonadal damage from chemotherapy and radiotherapy. *Endocrinol Metab Clin North Am*. 1998 Dec;27(4):927-43.

Huh WK, Ault KA, Chelmow D, et al. Use of primary high-risk human papillomavirus testing for cervical cancer screening: interim clinical guidance. *Gynecol Oncol*. 2015 Feb;136(2):178-82.

Hui D, Okun N, Murphy K, et al. Combinations of maternal serum markers to predict pre-eclampsia, small for gestational age, and stillbirth: a systematic review. *J Obstet Gynaecol Can*. 2012 Feb;34(2):142-53.

Hurst BS, Hickman JM, Matthews ML, et al. Novel clomiphene "stair-step" protocol reduces time to ovulation in women with polycystic ovarian syndrome. *Am J Obstet Gynecol*. 2009 May;200(5):510.e1-4.

Iams JD. Clinical practice: prevention of preterm parturition. *N Engl J Med*. 2014 Jan 16;370(3):254-61.

Iams JD, Goldenberg RL, Mercer BM, et al. The Preterm Prediction Study: recurrence risk of spontaneous preterm birth. National Institute of Child Health and Human Development Maternal-Fetal Medicine Units Network. *Am J Obstet Gynecol*. 1998 May;178(5):1035-40.

Imudia AN, Awonuga AO, Kaimal AJ, et al. Elective cryopreservation of all embryos with subsequent cryothaw embryo transfer in patients at risk for ovarian hyperstimulation syndrome reduces the risk of adverse obstetric outcomes: a preliminary study. *Fertil Steril*. 2013 Jan;99(1):168-73.

Institute of M, National Research Council Committee to Reexamine IOMPWG. The National Academies Collection: reports funded by National Institutes of Health. In: Rasmussen KM, Yaktine AL, editors. *Weight Gain During Pregnancy: Reexamining the Guidelines*. Washington, DC: National Academies Press; 2009.

Isley M, Blumenthal P. Medical abortion: what's Old, what's new? *Cont Ob/Gyn*. 2008;April:30-38.

Jacob SE, Steele T. Corticosteroid classes: a quick reference guide including patch test substances and cross-reactivity. *J Am Acad Dermatol*. 2006 Apr;54(4):723-27.

Jacobson GF, Ramos GA, Ching JY, et al. Comparison of glyburide and insulin for the management of gestational diabetes in a large managed care organization. *Am J Obstet Gynecol*. 2005 Jul;193(1):118-24.

Jaffe R, Jauniaux E, Hustin J. Maternal circulation in the first-trimester human placenta—myth or reality? *Am J Obstet Gynecol*. 1997 Mar;176(3):695-705.

Jain T, Soules MR, Collins JA. Comparison of basal follicle-stimulating hormone versus the clomiphene citrate challenge test for ovarian reserve screening. *Fertil Steril*. 2004 Jul;82(1):180-85.

Jarvik JG, Deyo RA. Diagnostic evaluation of low back pain with emphasis on imaging. *Ann Intern Med*. 2002 Oct 1;137(7):586-97.

Jaslow CR, Carney JL, Kutteh WH. Diagnostic factors identified in 1020 women with two versus three or more recurrent pregnancy losses. *Fertil Steril*. 2010 Mar 1;93(4):1234-43.

Jasonni VM, Raffelli R, de March A, et al. Vaginal bromocriptine in hyperprolactinemic patients and puerperal women. *Acta Obstet Gynecol Scand*. 1991;70(6):493-95.

Jeng GT, Scott JR, Burmeister LF. A comparison of meta-analytic results using literature vs. individual patient data. Paternal cell immunization for recurrent miscarriage. *JAMA*. 1995 Sep 13;274(10):830-36.

Johnson J, Canning J, Kaneko T, et al. Germline stem cells and follicular renewal in the postnatal mammalian ovary. *Nature*. 2004 Mar 11;428(6979):145-50.

Johnson NP, Mak W, Sowter MC. Laparoscopic salpingectomy for women with hydrosalpinges enhances the success of IVF: a Cochrane review. *Hum Reprod*. 2002 Mar;17(3):543-48.

REFERENCES

Jonklaas J, Bianco AC, Bauer AJ, et al. Guidelines for the treatment of hypothyroidism: prepared by the american thyroid association task force on thyroid hormone replacement. *Thyroid.* 2014 Dec;24(12):1670-1751

Jordan RM, Kendall JW, Kerber CW. The primary empty sella syndrome: analysis of the clinical characteristics, radiographic features, pituitary function and cerebrospinal fluid adenohypophysial hormone concentrations. *Am J Med.* 1977 Apr;62(4):569-80.

Jovanovic L, Peterson CM. Management of the pregnant, insulin-dependent diabetic woman. *Diabetes Care.* 1980 Jan-Feb;3(1):63-8.

Kahraman K, Berker B, Atabekoglu CS, et al. Microdose gonadotropin-releasing hormone agonist flare-up protocol versus multiple dose gonadotropin-releasing hormone antagonist protocol in poor responders undergoing intracytoplasmic sperm injection-embryo transfer cycle. *Fertil Steril.* 2009 Jun;91(6):2437-44.

Kallio S, Puurunen J, Ruokonen A, et al. Antimullerian hormone levels decrease in women using combined contraception independently of administration route. *Fertil Steril.* 2013 Apr;99(5):1305-10.

Kamel HS, Darwish AM, Mohamed SA. Comparison of transvaginal ultrasonography and vaginal sonohysterography in the detection of endometrial polyps. *Acta Obstet Gynecol Scand.* 2000 Jan;79(1):60-64.

Kanis JA. Diagnosis of osteoporosis and assessment of fracture risk. *Lancet.* 2002 Jun 1;359(9321): 1929-36.

Kanis JA, Johnell O, Oden A, et al. Ten year probabilities of osteoporotic fractures according to BMD and diagnostic thresholds. *Osteoporos Int.* 2001 Dec;12(12):989-95.

Kaplowitz P. Clinical characteristics of 104 children referred for evaluation of precocious puberty. *J Clin Endocrinol Metab.* 2004 Aug;89(8):3644-50.

Katki HA, Schiffman M, Castle PE, et al. Five-year risks of CIN 3+ and cervical cancer among women with HPV testing of ASC-US Pap results. *J Low Genit Tract Dis.* 2013 Apr;17(5 Suppl 1): S36-42.

Katsuragawa H, Kanzaki H, Inoue T, et al. Monoclonal antibody against phosphatidylserine inhibits in vitro human trophoblastic hormone production and invasion. *Biol Reprod.* 1997 Jan;56(1):50-58.

Katz-Jaffe MG, Surrey ES, Minjarez DA, et al. Association of abnormal ovarian reserve parameters with a higher incidence of aneuploid blastocysts. *Obstet Gynecol.* 2013 Jan;121(1):71-7.

Kaufman RH, Adam E, Hatch EE, et al. Continued follow-up of pregnancy outcomes in diethylstilbestrol-exposed offspring. *Obstet Gynecol.* 2000 Oct;96(4):483-89.

Kaunitz AM. Injectable long-acting contraceptives. *Clin Obstet Gynecol.* 2001 Mar;44(1):73-91.

Kaunitz AM, Manson JE. Management of menopausal symptoms. *Obstet Gynecol.* 2015 Oct;126(4):859-76.

Khalaf Y, Ross C, El-Toukhy T, et al. The effect of small intramural uterine fibroids on the cumulative outcome of assisted conception. *Hum Reprod.* 2006 Oct;21(10):2640-4.

Kiddy DS, Hamilton-Fairley D, Bush A, et al. Improvement in endocrine and ovarian function during dietary treatment of obese women with polycystic ovary syndrome. *Clin Endocrinol (Oxf).* 1992 Jan;36(1):105-111.

Kim KW, Romero R, Park HS, et al. A rapid matrix metalloproteinase-8 bedside test for the detection of intraamniotic inflammation in women with preterm premature rupture of membranes. *Am J Obstet Gynecol.* 2007 Sep;197(3):292.e1-5.

Kim SS, Klemp J, Fabian C. Breast cancer and fertility preservation. *Fertil Steril.* 2011 Apr;95(5): 1535-43.

REFERENCES

Kirk E, Bottomley C, Bourne T. Diagnosing ectopic pregnancy and current concepts in the management of pregnancy of unknown location. *Hum Reprod Update*. 2014 Mar-Apr;20(2):250-61.

Kitaya K. Prevalence of chronic endometritis in recurrent miscarriages. *Fertil Steril*. 2011 Mar 1;95(3):1156-8.

Kleinhaus K, Perrin M, Friedlander Y, et al. Paternal age and spontaneous abortion. *Obstet Gynecol*. 2006 Aug;108(2):369-77.

Klinkert ER, Broekmans FJ, Looman CW, et al. A poor response in the first in vitro fertilization cycle is not necessarily related to a poor prognosis in subsequent cycles. *Fertil Steril*. 2004 May;81(5):1247-53.

Ko EM, Soper JT. Gestational trophoblastic disease. In: DiSaia P, Creasman W, Mannel R, et al., editors. *Clinical Gynecologic Oncology, 8th Ed*. Philadelphia: Elsevier; 2012.

Ko H, Yoshida EM. Acute fatty liver of pregnancy. *Can J Gastroenterol*. 2006 Jan;20(1):25-30.

Kokay IC, Petersen SL, Grattan DR. Identification of prolactin-sensitive GABA and kisspeptin neurons in regions of the rat hypothalamus involved in the control of fertility. *Endocrinology*. 2011 Feb;152(2):526-35.

Kolibianakis EM, Schultze-Mosgau A, Schroer A, et al. A lower ongoing pregnancy rate can be expected when GnRH agonist is used for triggering final oocyte maturation instead of HCG in patients undergoing IVF with GnRH antagonists. *Hum Reprod*. 2005 Oct;20(10):2887-92.

Kolte AM, van Oppenraaij RH, Quenby S, et al. Non-visualized pregnancy losses are prognostically important for unexplained recurrent miscarriage. *Hum Reprod*. 2014 May;29(5):931-37.

Krattenmacher R. Drospirenone: pharmacology and pharmacokinetics of a unique progestogen. *Contraception*. 2000 Jul;62(1):29-38.

Krivak TC, Zorn KK. Venous thromboembolism in obstetrics and gynecology. *Obstet Gynecol*. 2007 Mar;109(3):761-77.

Kundsin RB, Driscoll SG, Pelletier PA. Ureaplasma urealyticum incriminated in perinatal morbidity and mortality. *Science*. 1981 Jul 24;213(4506):474-75.

Kutteh WH. Novel strategies for the management of recurrent pregnancy loss. *Semin Reprod Med*. 2015 May;33(3):161-68.

Landon MB, Hauth JC, Leveno KJ, et al. Maternal and perinatal outcomes associated with a trial of labor after prior cesarean delivery. *N Engl J Med*. 2004 Dec 16;351(25):2581-9.

Landon MB, Spong CY, Thom E, et al. Risk of uterine rupture with a trial of labor in women with multiple and single prior cesarean delivery. *Obstet Gynecol*. 2006 Jul;108(1):12-20.

Lanigan SW. Incidence of side effects after laser hair removal. *J Am Acad Dermatol*. 2003 Nov;49(5):882-86.

Lara-Torre E, Schroeder B. Adolescent compliance and side effects with Quick Start initiation of oral contraceptive pills. *Contraception*. 2002 Aug;66(2):81-5.

Lashen H, Fear K, Sturdee DW. Obesity is associated with increased risk of first trimester and recurrent miscarriage: matched case-control study. *Hum Reprod*. 2004 Jul;19(7):1644-6.

Laufer MR, Ecker JL, Hill JA. Pregnancy outcome following ultrasound-detected fetal cardiac activity in women with a history of multiple spontaneous abortions. *J Soc Gynecol Investig*. 1994 Apr-Jun;1(2):138-42.

Laughlin SK, Baird DD, Savitz DA, et al. Prevalence of uterine leiomyomas in the first trimester of pregnancy: an ultrasound-screening study. *Obstet Gynecol*. 2009 Mar;113(3):630-35.

Lauria MR, Smith RS, Treadwell MC, et al. The use of second-trimester transvaginal sonography to predict placenta previa. *Ultrasound Obstet Gynecol*. 1996 Nov;8(5):337-40.

REFERENCES

Lavy G. Hysteroscopy as a diagnostic aid. *Obstet Gynecol Clin North Am.* 1988 Mar;15(1):61-72.

Lee TH, Liu CH, Huang CC, et al. Serum anti-Müllerian hormone and estradiol levels as predictors of ovarian hyperstimulation syndrome in assisted reproduction technology cycles. *Hum Reprod.* 2008 Jan;23(1):160-67.

Legro RS, Arslanian SA, Ehrmann DA, et al. Diagnosis and treatment of polycystic ovary syndrome: an Endocrine Society clinical practice guideline. *J Clin Endocrinol Metab.* 2013 Dec;98(12):4565-92.

Legro RS, Barnhart HX, Schlaff WD, et al. Clomiphene, metformin, or both for infertility in the polycystic ovary syndrome. *N Engl J Med.* 2007 Feb 8;356(6):551-66.

Legro RS, Brzyski RG, Diamond MP, et al. Letrozole versus clomiphene for infertility in the polycystic ovary syndrome. *N Engl J Med.* 2014 Jul 10;371(2):119-29.

Legro RS, Kunselman AR, Dodson WC, et al. Prevalence and predictors of risk for type 2 diabetes mellitus and impaired glucose tolerance in polycystic ovary syndrome: a prospective, controlled study in 254 affected women. *J Clin Endocrinol Metab.* 1999 Jan;84(1):165-69.

Lewin SN, Herzog TJ, Barrena Medel NI, et al. Comparative performance of the 2009 International Federation of Gynecology and Obstetrics' staging system for uterine corpus cancer. *Obstet Gynecol.* 2010 Nov;116(5):1141-9.

Linden JA. Clinical practice: care of the adult patient after sexual assault. *N Engl J Med.* 2011 Sep 1;365(9):834-41.

Ling F, Duff P. *Obstetrics and Gynecology: Principles and Practice.* New York: McGraw-Hill; 2001.

Lipscomb GH, Bran D, McCord ML, et al. Analysis of three hundred fifteen ectopic pregnancies treated with single-dose methotrexate. *Am J Obstet Gynecol.* 1998 Jun;178(6):1354-8.

Lipscomb GH, Givens VA, Meyer NL, et al. Previous ectopic pregnancy as a predictor of failure of systemic methotrexate therapy. *Fertil Steril.* 2004 May;81(5):1221-4.

Lipscomb GH, McCord ML, Stovall TG, et al. Predictors of success of methotrexate treatment in women with tubal ectopic pregnancies. *N Engl J Med.* 1999 Dec 23;341(26):1974-8.

Lipscomb GH, Stovall TG, Ling FW. Nonsurgical treatment of Ectopic pregnancy. *N Engl J Med.* 2000 Nov 2;343(18):1325-9.

Liston R, Sawchuck D, Young D. Fetal health surveillance: antepartum and intrapartum consensus guideline. *J Obstet Gynaecol Can.* 2007 Sep;29(9 Suppl 4):S3-56.

Liu S, Liston RM, Joseph KS, et al. Maternal mortality and severe morbidity associated with low-risk planned cesarean delivery versus planned vaginal delivery at term. *CMAJ.* 2007 Feb 13;176(4):455-60.

Lo JC, Schwitzgebel VM, Tyrrell JB, et al. Normal female infants born of mothers with classic congenital adrenal hyperplasia due to 21-hydroxylase deficiency. *J Clin Endocrinol Metab.* 1999 Mar;84(3):930-36.

Lobo RA, Shoupe D, Serafini P, et al. The effects of two doses of spironolactone on serum androgens and anagen hair in hirsute women. *Fertil Steril.* 1985 Feb;43(2):200-205.

Loder E. Triptan therapy in migraine. *N Engl J Med.* 2010 Jul 1;363(1):63-70.

Looker AC, Orwoll ES, Johnston CC, Jr., et al. Prevalence of low femoral bone density in older U.S. adults from NHANES III. *J Bone Miner Res.* 1997 Nov;12(11):1761-8.

Lucky AW, Henderson TA, Olson WH, et al. Effectiveness of norgestimate and ethinyl estradiol in treating moderate acne vulgaris. *J Am Acad Dermatol.* 1997 Nov; 37(5 Pt 1):746-54.

Luk J, Arici A. Does the ovarian reserve decrease from repeated ovulation stimulations? *Curr Opin Obstet Gynecol.* 2010 Jun;22(3):177-82.

REFERENCES

Luke B, Brown MB, Wantman E, et al. Factors associated with monozygosity in assisted reproductive technology pregnancies and the risk of recurrence using linked cycles. *Fertil Steril.* 2014 Mar;101(3):683-89.

Lurain JR. Gestational trophoblastic disease I: epidemiology, pathology, clinical presentation and diagnosis of gestational trophoblastic disease, and management of hydatidiform mole. *Am J Obstet Gynecol.* 2010 Dec;203(6):531-39.

Lydon-Rochelle M, Holt VL, Easterling TR, et al. Risk of uterine rupture during labor among women with a prior cesarean delivery. *N Engl J Med.* 2001 Jul 5;345(1):3-8.

Mabie W. Critical care obstetrics. In: Gabbe S, Niebyl J, Simpson J, editors. *Obstetrics: Normal and Problem Pregnancies*, 2nd Ed. New York: Churchill Livingstone; 1991.

Macones GA, Hankins GD, Spong CY, et al. The 2008 National Institute of Child Health and Human Development workshop report on electronic fetal monitoring: update on definitions, interpretation, and research guidelines. *Obstet Gynecol.* 2008 Sep;112(3):661-66.

Macones GA, Peipert J, Nelson DB, et al. Maternal complications with vaginal birth after cesarean delivery: a multicenter study. *Am J Obstet Gynecol.* 2005 Nov;193(5):1656-62.

Maheshwari A, Bhattacharya S. Elective frozen replacement cycles for all: ready for prime time? *Hum Reprod.* 2013 Jan;28(1):6-9.

Main EK, Goffman D, Scavone BM, et al. National Partnership for Maternal Safety. *Obstet Gynecol.* 2015;126(1):155-62.

Malone FD, Ball RH, Nyberg DA, et al. First-trimester septated cystic hygroma: prevalence, natural history, and pediatric outcome. *Obstet Gynecol.* 2005 Aug;106(2):288-94.

Manning FA. Dynamic ultrasound-based fetal assessment: the fetal biophysical profile score. *Clin Obstet Gynecol.* 1995 Mar;38(1):26-44.

Manning FA. Fetal biophysical profile. *Obstet Gynecol Clin North Am.* 1999 Dec;26(4):557-77.

March CM. Asherman's syndrome. *Semin Reprod Med.* 2011 Mar;29(2):83-94.

Marchbanks PA, McDonald JA, Wilson HG, et al. Oral contraceptives and the risk of breast cancer. *N Engl J Med.* 2002 Jun 27;346(26):2025-32.

Marks DR, Rapoport AM. Practical evaluation and diagnosis of headache. *Semin Neurol.* 17(4):307-312.

Massad LS, Einstein MH, Huh WK, et al. 2012 updated consensus guidelines for the management of abnormal cervical cancer screening tests and cancer precursors. *J Low Genit Tract Dis.* 2013 Apr;17(5 Suppl 1):S1-S27.

Matuszek B, Zakoscielna K, Baszak-Radomanska E, et al. Universal screening as a recommendation for thyroid tests in pregnant women. *Ann Agric Environ Med.* 2011;18(2):375-79.

Mayo K, Melamed N, Vandenberghe H, et al. The impact of adoption of the international association of diabetes in pregnancy study group criteria for the screening and diagnosis of gestational diabetes. *Am J Obstet Gynecol.* 2015 Feb;212(2):224 e1-9.

McCann MF, Potter LS. Progestin-only oral contraception: a comprehensive review. *Contraception.* 1994 Dec;50(6 Suppl 1):S1-195.

McDonough P. Puberty. In: *Precis, Reproductive Endocrinology: An Update in Obstetrics and Gynecology*. Washington, DC: American College of Obstetricians and Gynecologists; 1998.

McGovern PG, Legro RS, Myers ER, et al. Utility of screening for other causes of infertility in women with "known" polycystic ovary syndrome. *Fertil Steril.* 2007 Feb;87(2):442-44.

McKeigue PM, Lamm SH, Linn S, et al. Bendectin and birth defects: I. A meta-analysis of the epidemiologic studies. *Teratology.* 1994 Jul;50(1):27-37.

McLean H, Reed S, Abernathy W. *Manual for the Surveillance of Vaccine-Preventable Diseases.* Atlanta: Centers for Disease Control and Prevention; 2012.

REFERENCES

McQuivey RW. Vacuum-assisted delivery: a review. *J Matern Fetal Neonatal Med.* 2004 Sep;16(3): 171-80.

Melo M, Busso CE, Bellver J, et al. GnRH agonist versus recombinant HCG in an oocyte donation programme: a randomized, prospective, controlled, assessor-blind study. *Reprod Biomed Online.* 2009 Oct;19(4):486-92.

Meyer MC. Translating data to dialogue: how to discuss mode of delivery with your patient with twins. *Am J Obstet Gynecol.* 2006 Oct;195(4):899-906.

Meyer WR, Castelbaum AJ, Somkuti S, et al. Hydrosalpinges adversely affect markers of endometrial receptivity. *Hum Reprod.* 1997 Jul;12(7):1393-8.

Meyers C, Adam R, Dungan J, et al. Aneuploidy in twin gestations: when is maternal age advanced? *Obstet Gynecol.* 1997 Feb;89(2):248-51.

Miller DA, Miller LA. Electronic fetal heart rate monitoring: applying principles of patient safety. *Am J Obstet Gynecol.* 2012 Apr;206(4):278-83.

Miller ES, Grobman WA, Fonseca L, et al. Indomethacin and antibiotics in examination-indicated cerclage: a randomized controlled trial. *Obstet Gynecol.* 2014 Jun;123(6):1311-6.

Miller L, Hughes JP. Continuous combination oral contraceptive pills to eliminate withdrawal bleeding: a randomized trial. *Obstet Gynecol.* 2003 Apr;101(4):653-61.

Miller WL, Witchel SF. Prenatal treatment of congenital adrenal hyperplasia: risks outweigh benefits. *Am J Obstet Gynecol.* 2013 May;208(5):354-59.

Miyakis S, Lockshin MD, Atsumi T, et al. International consensus statement on an update of the classification criteria for definite antiphospholipid syndrome (APS). *J Thromb Haemost.* 2006 Feb;4(2):295-306.

Miyazaki FS, Nevarez F. Saline amnioinfusion for relief of repetitive variable decelerations: a prospective randomized study. *Am J Obstet Gynecol.* 1985 Oct 1;153(3):301-306.

Modan B, Hartge P, Hirsh-Yechezkel G, et al. Parity, oral contraceptives, and the risk of ovarian cancer among carriers and noncarriers of a *BRCA1* or *BRCA2* mutation. *N Engl J Med.* 2001 Jul 26;345(4):235-40.

Moise KJ. Fetal anemia due to non-Rhesus-D red-cell alloimmunization. *Semin Fetal Neonatal Med.* 2008 Aug;13(4):207-214.

Moise KJ, Jr., Argoti PS. Management and prevention of red cell alloimmunization in pregnancy: a systematic review. *Obstet Gynecol.* 2012 Nov;120(5):1132-9.

Molitch ME. Pregnancy and the hyperprolactinemic woman. *N Engl J Med.* 1985 May 23;312(21):1364-70.

Molitch ME, Reichlin S. Hyperprolactinemic disorders. *Disease-a-month: DM.* 1982 Jun;28(9):1-58.

Montagnana M, Trenti T, Aloe R, et al. Human chorionic gonadotropin in pregnancy diagnostics. *Clin Chim Acta.* 2011 Aug 17;412(17-18):1515-20.

Morin-Papunen L, Rantala AS, Unkila-Kallio L, et al. Metformin improves pregnancy and livebirth rates in women with polycystic ovary syndrome (PCOS): a multicenter, double-blind, placebo-controlled randomized trial. *J Clin Endocrinol Metab.* 2012 May;97(5):1492-1500

Morris JK, Wald NJ, Mutton DE, et al. Comparison of models of maternal age-specific risk for Down syndrome live births. *Prenat Diagn.* 2003 Mar;23(3):252-58.

Mosca L, Benjamin EJ, Berra K, et al. Effectiveness-based guidelines for the prevention of cardiovascular disease in women—2011 update: a guideline from the American Heart Association. *J Am Coll Cardiol.* 2011 Mar 22;57(12):1404-23.

Moses G, McGuire T. Drug interactions with complementary medicines. *Aust Prescr.* 2010;33: 177-80.

REFERENCES

Moyer VA, Force USPST. Screening for cervical cancer: U.S. Preventive Services Task Force recommendation statement. *Ann Intern Med.* 2012 Jun 19;156(12):880-91, W312.

Mulder JE. Thyroid disease in women. *Med Clin North Am.* 1998 Jan;82(1):103-125.

Munro MG, Critchley HO, Broder MS, et al. FIGO classification system (PALM-COEIN) for causes of abnormal uterine bleeding in nongravid women of reproductive age. *Int J Gynaecol Obstet.* 2011 Apr;113(1):3-13.

Munro MG, Critchley HO, Fraser IS. The FIGO systems for nomenclature and classification of causes of abnormal uterine bleeding in the reproductive years: who needs them? *Am J Obstet Gynecol.* 2012 Oct;207(4):259-65.

Mustafa SA, Brizot ML, Carvalho MH, et al. Transvaginal ultrasonography in predicting placenta previa at delivery: a longitudinal study. *Ultrasound Obstet Gynecol.* 2002 Oct;20(4):356-59.

Nageotte MP, Casal D, Senyei AE. Fetal fibronectin in patients at increased risk for premature birth. *Am J Obstet Gynecol.* 1994 Jan;170(1 Pt 1):20-25.

Narod SA, Risch H, Moslehi R, et al. Oral contraceptives and the risk of hereditary ovarian cancer. Hereditary Ovarian Cancer Clinical Study Group. *N Engl J Med.* 1998 Aug 13;339(7):424-28.

National Heart L, Blood I, National Asthma E, et al. NAEPP Expert Panel Report. Managing asthma during pregnancy: recommendations for pharmacologic treatment—2004 update. *J Allergy Clin Immunol.* 2005 Jan;115(1):34-46.

Nazac A, Gervaise A, Bouyer J, et al. Predictors of success in methotrexate treatment of women with unruptured tubal pregnancies. *Ultrasound Obstet Gynecol.* 2003 Feb;21(2):181-85.

Nelson RS, Thorson AG. Colorectal cancer screening. *Curr Oncol Rep.* 2009 Nov;11(6):482-89.

Ness RB, Grisso JA, Klapper J, et al. Risk of ovarian cancer in relation to estrogen and progestin dose and use characteristics of oral contraceptives. SHARE Study Group. Steroid Hormones and Reproductions. *Am J Epidemiol.* 2000 Aug 1;152(3):233-41.

Nestler JE. Metformin and the polycystic ovary syndrome. *J Clin Endocrinol Metab.* 2001 Mar;86(3):1430.

Neutel CI, Johansen HL. Measuring drug effectiveness by default: the case of Bendectin. *Can J Public Health.* 1995 Jan-Feb;86(1):66-70.

New MI. Extensive clinical experience: nonclassical 21-hydroxylase deficiency. *J Clin Endocrinol Metab.* 2006 Nov;91(11):4205-14.

Newfield L, Bradlow HL, Sepkovic DW, et al. Estrogen metabolism and the malignant potential of human papillomavirus immortalized keratinocytes. *Proc Soc Exp Biol Med.* 1998 Mar;217(3):322-26.

Newman RB, Goldenberg RL, Iams JD, et al. Preterm prediction study: comparison of the cervical score and Bishop score for prediction of spontaneous preterm delivery. *Obstet Gynecol.* 2008 Sep;112(3):508-515.

Newton ER. Chorioamnionitis and intraamniotic infection. *Clin Obstet Gynecol.* 1993 Dec;36(4):795-808.

Ng EH, Ajonuma LC, Lau EY, et al. Adverse effects of hydrosalpinx fluid on sperm motility and survival. *Hum Reprod.* 2000 Apr;15(4):772-77.

Ng EH, Chan CC, Tang OS, et al. Comparison of endometrial and subendometrial blood flows among patients with and without hydrosalpinx shown on scanning during in vitro fertilization treatment. *Fertil Steril.* 2006 Feb;85(2):333-38.

Nicolaides KH, Azar G, Byrne D, et al. Fetal nuchal translucency: ultrasound screening for chromosomal defects in first trimester of pregnancy. *BMJ.* 1992 Apr 4;304(6831):867-69.

REFERENCES

Niebyl JR. Clinical practice: nausea and vomiting in pregnancy. *N Engl J Med.* 2010 Oct 14;363(16):1544-50.

Nielsen J, Wohlert M. Chromosome abnormalities found among 34,910 newborn children: results from a 13-year incidence study in Arhus, Denmark. *Hum Genet.* 1991 May;87(1):81-3.

Nolin SL, Brown WT, Glicksman A, et al. Expansion of the fragile X CGG repeat in females with premutation or intermediate alleles. *American J Hum Genet.* 2003 Feb;72(2):454-64.

Nybo Andersen AM, Wohlfahrt J, Christens P, et al. Maternal age and fetal loss: population based register linkage study. *BMJ.* 2000 Jun 24;320(7251):1708-12.

O'Leary J. Stop OB hemorrhage with uterine artery ligation. *Cont Ob/Gyn Special Issue: Update on Surgery.* 1986.

Oates R. The genetics of male reproductive failure: what every clinician needs to know. *Sexual Reproduc Menop.* 2004; 2(4):213.

Oepkes D, Seaward PG, Vandenbussche FP, et al. Doppler ultrasonography versus amniocentesis to predict fetal anemia. *N Engl J Med.* 2006 Jul 13;355(2):156-64.

Ogasawara M, Aoki K, Okada S, et al. Embryonic karyotype of abortuses in relation to the number of previous miscarriages. *Fertil Steril.* 2000 Feb;73(2):300-304.

Ogilvie CM, Crouch NS, Rumsby G, et al. Congenital adrenal hyperplasia in adults: a review of medical, surgical and psychological issues. *Clinical endocrinol (Oxf).* 2006 Jan;64(1):2-11.

Ogino S, Wilson RB. Spinal muscular atrophy: molecular genetics and diagnostics. *Expert Rev Mol Diagn.* 2004 Jan;4(1):15-29.

Oktay K, Meirow D. Planning for fertility preservation before cancer treatment. *Sexual Reproduc Menop.* 2007;5(1):17-22.

Oktem O, Urman B. Understanding follicle growth in vivo. *Hum Reprod.* 2010 Dec;25(12):2944-54.

Oliveira LG, Capp SM, You WB, et al. Ondansetron compared with doxylamine and pyridoxine for treatment of nausea in pregnancy: a randomized controlled trial. *Obstet Gynecol.* 2014 Oct;124(4):735-42.

Otten JJH, Jennifer Pitzi; Meyers, Linda D. *DRI, Dietary Reference Intakes: The Essential Guide to Nutrient Requirements.* Washington, DC: National Academies Press; 2006.

Oyelese Y, Smulian JC. Placenta previa, placenta accreta, and vasa previa. *Obstet Gynecol.* 2006 Apr;107(4):927-41.

Pagotto U, Marsicano G, Fezza F, et al. Normal human pituitary gland and pituitary adenomas express cannabinoid receptor type 1 and synthesize endogenous cannabinoids: first evidence for a direct role of cannabinoids on hormone modulation at the human pituitary level. *J Clin Endocrinol Metab.* 2001 Jun;86(6):2687-96.

Paidas MJ, Ku DH, Lee MJ, et al. Protein Z, protein S levels are lower in patients with thrombophilia and subsequent pregnancy complications. *J Thromb Haemost.* 2005;3:497-501.

Palmer SN, Greenberg JA. Transcervical sterilization: a comparison of essure(r) permanent birth control system and adiana(r) permanent contraception system. *Rev Obstet Gynecol.* 2009 Spring;2(2):84-92.

Palomaki GE, Kloza EM, Lambert-Messerlian GM, et al. DNA sequencing of maternal plasma to detect Down syndrome: an international clinical validation study. *Genet Med.* 2011 Nov;13(11):913-20.

Pandey S, Maheshwari A, Bhattacharya S. Should access to fertility treatment be determined by female body mass index? *Hum Reprod.* 2010 Apr;25(4):815-20.

Park-Wyllie L, Mazzotta P, Pastuszak A, et al. Birth defects after maternal exposure to corticosteroids: prospective cohort study and meta-analysis of epidemiological studies. *Teratology.* 2000 Dec;62(6):385-92.

REFERENCES

Parsanezhad ME, Alborzi S, Motazedian S, et al. Use of dexamethasone and clomiphene citrate in the treatment of clomiphene citrate-resistant patients with polycystic ovary syndrome and normal dehydroepiandrosterone sulfate levels: a prospective, double-blind, placebo-controlled trial. *Fertil Steril.* 2002 Nov;78(5):1001-4.

Patel SJ, Reede DL, Katz DS, et al. Imaging the pregnant patient for nonobstetric conditions: algorithms and radiation dose considerations. *Radiographics.* 2007;27:1705-22.

Peaceman AM, Andrews WW, Thorp JM, et al. Fetal fibronectin as a predictor of preterm birth in patients with symptoms: a multicenter trial. *Am J Obstet Gynecol.* 1997 Jul;177(1):13-8.

Pearlstone AC, Fournet N, Gambone JC, et al. Ovulation induction in women age 40 and older: the importance of basal follicle-stimulating hormone level and chronological age. *Fertil Steril.* 1992 Oct;58(4):674-79.

Pecorelli S. Revised FIGO staging for carcinoma of the vulva, cervix, and endometrium. *Int J Gynaecol Obstet.* 2009 May;105(2):103-104.

Pellerito JS, McCarthy SM, Doyle MB, et al. Diagnosis of uterine anomalies: relative accuracy of MR imaging, endovaginal sonography, and hysterosalpingography. *Radiology.* 1992 Jun;183(3):795-800.

Pellestor F, Andreo B, Arnal F, et al. Maternal aging and chromosomal abnormalities: new data drawn from in vitro unfertilized human oocytes. *Hum Genet.* 2003 Feb;112(2):195-203.

Perlman JM, Wyllie J, Kattwinkel J, et al. Neonatal resuscitation: 2010 International Consensus on Cardiopulmonary Resuscitation and Emergency Cardiovascular Care Science with Treatment Recommendations. *Pediatrics.* 2010 Nov;126(5):e1319-44.

Petri M, Orbai AM, Alarcon GS, et al. Derivation and validation of the Systemic Lupus International Collaborating Clinics classification criteria for systemic lupus erythematosus. *Arthritis Rheum.* 2012 Aug;64(8):2677-86.

Pisarska MD, Carson SA, Buster JE. Ectopic pregnancy. *Lancet.* 1998;351(9109):1115-20.

Pitkin R. Commentary on pelvic scoring for elective induction. *Obstet Gynecol.* 2003;101(5):846.

Prat J. Staging classification for cancer of the ovary, fallopian tube, and peritoneum. *Int J Gynaecol Obstet.* 2014 Jan;124(1):1-5.

Prat J. Abridged republication of FIGO's staging classification for cancer of the ovary, fallopian tube, and peritoneum. *Cancer.* 2015 Oct 1;121(19):3452-4.

Preisler J, Kopeika J, Ismail L, et al. Defining safe criteria to diagnose miscarriage: prospective observational multicentre study. *BMJ.* 2015;351:h4579.

Price TM, Allen S, Pegram GV. Lack of effect of topical finasteride suggests an endocrine role for dihydrotestosterone. *Fertil Steril.* 2000 Aug;74(2):414-15.

Proctor JA, Haney AF. Recurrent first trimester pregnancy loss is associated with uterine septum but not with bicornuate uterus. *Fertil Steril.* 2003 Nov;80(5):1212-5.

Quintero RA, Morales WJ, Allen MH, et al. Staging of twin-twin transfusion syndrome. *J Perinatol.* 1999 Dec;19(8 Pt 1):550-55.

Raffi F, Metwally M, Amer S. The impact of excision of ovarian endometrioma on ovarian reserve: a systematic review and meta-analysis. *J Clin Endocrinol Metab.* 2012 Sep;97(9):3146-54.

Rai R, Backos M, Rushworth F, et al. Polycystic ovaries and recurrent miscarriage—a reappraisal. *Hum Reprod.* 2000 Mar;15(3):612-15.

Rai R, Cohen H, Dave M, et al. Randomised controlled trial of aspirin and aspirin plus heparin in pregnant women with recurrent miscarriage associated with phospholipid antibodies (or antiphospholipid antibodies). *BMJ.* 1997 Jan 25;314(7076):253-57.

REFERENCES

Ramakrishnan K, Scheid DC. Ectopic pregnancy: expectant management of immediate surgery? *J Fam Pract*. 2006 Jun;55(6):517-22.

Ramin SM, Gilstrap LC, 3rd, Leveno KJ, et al. Umbilical artery acid-base status in the preterm infant. *Obstet Gynecol*. 1989 Aug;74(2):256-58.

Reddy UM, Abuhamad AZ, Levine D, et al. Fetal imaging: executive summary of a joint Eunice Kennedy Shriver National Institute of Child Health and Human Development, Society for Maternal-Fetal Medicine, American Institute of Ultrasound in Medicine, American College of Obstetricians and Gynecologists, American College of Radiology, Society for Pediatric Radiology, and Society of Radiologists in Ultrasound Fetal Imaging workshop. *Obstet Gynecol*. 2014 May;123(5):1070-82.

Redmond GP, Olson WH, Lippman JS, et al. Norgestimate and ethinylestradiol in the treatment of acne vulgaris: a randomized, placebo-controlled trial. *Obstet Gynecol*. 1997 Apr;89(4):615-22.

Reeves SA, Gibbs RS, Clark SL. Magnesium for fetal neuroprotection. *Am J Obstet Gynecol*. 2011 Mar;204(3):202 e1-4.

Reimold SC, Rutherford JD. Clinical practice: valvular heart disease in pregnancy. *N Engl J Med*. 2003 Jul 3;349(1):52-9.

Reindollar RH, Byrd JR, McDonough PG. Delayed sexual development: a study of 252 patients. *Am J Obstet Gynecol*. 1981 Jun 15;140(4):371-80.

Reindollar RH, Novak M, Tho SP, et al. Adult-onset amenorrhea: a study of 262 patients. *Am J Obstet Gynecol*. 1986. Sep;155(3):531-43.

Remohi J, Gallardo E, Levy M, et al. Oocyte donation in women with recurrent pregnancy loss. *Hum Reprod*. 1996 Sep;11(9):2048-51.

Resnik R. Intrauterine growth restriction. *Obstet Gynecol*. 2002 Mar;99(3):490-96.

Rienzi L, Romano S, Albricci L, et al. Embryo development of fresh "versus" vitrified metaphase II oocytes after ICSI: a prospective randomized sibling-oocyte study. *Hum Reprod*. 2010 Jan;25(1):66-73.

Riggs JW, Blanco JD. Pathophysiology, diagnosis, and management of intraamniotic infection. *Semin Perinatol*. 1998 Aug;22(4):251-59.

Riley RJ, Johnson JW. Collecting and analyzing cord blood gases. *Clin Obstet Gynecol*. 1993 Mar;36(1):13-23.

Rizzuto I, Behrens RF, Smith LA. Risk of ovarian cancer in women treated with ovarian stimulating drugs for infertility. *Cochrane Database Syst Rev*. 2013;8:Cd008215.

Rodriguez-Pinilla E, Martinez-Frias ML. Corticosteroids during pregnancy and oral clefts: a case-control study. *Teratology*. 1998 Jul;58(1):2-5.

Rodriguez-Wallberg KA, Oktay K. Fertility preservation in women with breast cancer. *Clin Obstet Gynecol*. 2010 Dec;53(4):753-62.

Romero R, Dey SK, Fisher SJ. Preterm labor: one syndrome, many causes. *Science*. 2014 Aug 15;345(6198):760-65.

Romero R, Yoon BH, Mazor M, et al. A comparative study of the diagnostic performance of amniotic fluid glucose, white blood cell count, interleukin-6, and gram stain in the detection of microbial invasion in patients with preterm premature rupture of membranes. *Am J Obstet Gynecol*. 1993 Oct;169(4):839-51.

Roque M, Lattes K, Serra S, et al. Fresh embryo transfer versus frozen embryo transfer in in vitro fertilization cycles: a systematic review and meta-analysis. *Fertil Steril*. 2013 Jan;99(1):156-62.

REFERENCES

Rosati P, Guariglia L. Clinical significance of placenta previa detected at early routine transvaginal scan. *J Ultrasound Med*. 2000 Aug;19(8):581-85.

Rosenberger LH, Politano AD, Sawyer RG. The surgical care improvement project and prevention of post-operative infection, including surgical site infection. *Surg Infect*. 2011 Jun;12(3): 163-68.

Rosenthal MH. Intrapartum intensive care management of the cardiac patient. *Clin Obstet Gynecol*. 1981 Sep;24(3):789-807.

Rossi AC, D'Addario V. Maternal morbidity following a trial of labor after cesarean section vs. elective repeat cesarean delivery: a systematic review with metaanalysis. *Am J Obstet Gynecol*. 2008 Sep;199(3):224-31.

Royal College of Obstetricians and Gynecologists. *Clinical Guidance: Combined Hormonal Contraception*. London: Faculty of Sexual and Reproductive Healthcare; 2012.

Royal College of Obstetricians and Gynecologists. *Ectopic Pregnancy and Miscarriage: Diagnosis and Initial Management in Early Pregnancy of Ectopic Pregnancy and Miscarriage. NICE Clinical Guidelines, No. 154*. London; 2012.

Royar J, Becher H, Chang-Claude J. Low-dose oral contraceptives: protective effect on ovarian cancer risk. *Int J Cancer*. 2001 Nov 20;95(6):370-74.

Rubinek T, Hadani M, Barkai G, et al. Prolactin (PRL)-releasing peptide stimulates PRL secretion from human fetal pituitary cultures and growth hormone release from cultured pituitary adenomas. *J Clin Endocrinol Metab*. 2001 Jun;86(6):2826-30.

Rudick B, Ingles S, Chung K, et al. Characterizing the influence of vitamin D levels on IVF outcomes. *Hum Reprod*. 2012 Nov;27(11):3321-7.

Sachdev R, Kemmann E, Bohrer MK, et al. Detrimental effect of hydrosalpinx fluid on the development and blastulation of mouse embryos in vitro. *Fertil Steril*. 1997 Sep;68(3):531-33.

Sacks FM, Campos H. Dietary therapy in hypertension. *N Engl J Med*. 2010 Jun 3;362(22): 2102-12.

Sakornbut E. How to treat pregnant patients with asthma. *Cont Ob/Gyn*. 2003(Apr):26-43.

Saleh A, Morris D, Tan SL, et al. Effects of laparoscopic ovarian drilling on adrenal steroids in polycystic ovary syndrome patients with and without hyperinsulinemia. *Fertil Steril*. 2001 Mar;75(3):501-504.

Sam S, Legro RS, Essah PA, et al. Evidence for metabolic and reproductive phenotypes in mothers of women with polycystic ovary syndrome. *Proc Natl Acad Sci USA*. 2006 May 2;103(18):7030-5.

Saslow D, Solomon D, Lawson HW, et al. American Cancer Society, American Society for Colposcopy and Cervical Pathology, and American Society for Clinical Pathology screening guidelines for the prevention and early detection of cervical cancer. *CA Cancer J Clin*. 2012 May-Jun;62(3):147-72.

Saslow D, Solomon D, Lawson HW, et al. American Cancer Society, American Society for Colposcopy and Cervical Pathology, and American Society for Clinical Pathology screening guidelines for the prevention and early detection of cervical cancer. *J Low Genit Tract Dis*. 2012 Jul;16(3):175-204.

Saul RA, Tarleton JC. *FMR1*-related disorders. In: Pagon RA, Adam MP, Ardinger HH, et al., editors. *Gene Reviews*. Seattle: Seattle University of Washington; 1993.

Sayed GH, Zakherah MS, El-Nashar SA, et al. A randomized clinical trial of a levonorgestrel-releasing intrauterine system and a low-dose combined oral contraceptive for fibroid-related menorrhagia. *Int J Gynaecol Obstet*. 2011 Feb;112(2):126-30.

REFERENCES

Schaff EA, Eisinger SH, Stadalius LS, et al. Low-dose mifepristone 200 mg and vaginal misoprostol for abortion. *Contraception.* 1999 Jan;59(1):1-6.

Schaff EA, Fielding SL, Westhoff C. Randomized trial of oral versus vaginal misoprostol at one day after mifepristone for early medical abortion. *Contraception.* 2001 Aug;64(2):81-5.

Scheerer LJ, Lam F, Bartolucci L, et al. A new technique for reduction of prolapsed fetal membranes for emergency cervical cerclage. *Obstet Gynecol.* 1989 Sep;74(3 Pt 1):408-410.

Scheffer GJ, Broekmans FJ, Dorland M, et al. Antral follicle counts by transvaginal ultrasonography are related to age in women with proven natural fertility. *Fertil Steril.* 1999 Nov;72(5):845-51.

Schildkraut JM, Calingaert B, Marchbanks PA, et al. Impact of progestin and estrogen potency in oral contraceptives on ovarian cancer risk. *J Natl Cancer Inst.* 2002 Jan 2;94(1):32-8.

Schimberni M, Morgia F, Colabianchi J, et al. Natural-cycle in vitro fertilization in poor responder patients: a survey of 500 consecutive cycles. *Fertil Steril.* 2009 Oct;92(4):1297-1301

Schlechte J, Dolan K, Sherman B, et al. The natural history of untreated hyperprolactinemia: a prospective analysis. *J Clin Endocrinol Metab.* 1989 Feb;68(2):412-18.

Schlechte JA. Long-term management of prolactinomas. *J Clin Endocrinol Metab.* 2007 Aug;92(8):2861-5.

Schlesselman J, Collins J. The influence of steroids on gynecologic cancers. In: Fraser I, Jansen R, editors. *Estrogens and Progestogens in Clinical practice.* London: Churchill Livingstone; 1999.

Schreiber CP. The pathophysiology of primary headache. *Prim Care.* 2004 Jun;31(2):261-76, v-vi.

Schreinemachers DM, Cross PK, Hook EB. Rates of trisomies 21, 18, 13 and other chromosome abnormalities in about 20,000 prenatal studies compared with estimated rates in live births. *Hum Genet.* 1982;61(4):318-24.

Schwartz D, Mayaux MJ. Female fecundity as a function of age: results of artificial insemination in 2193 nulliparous women with azoospermic husbands. Federation CECOS. *N Engl J Med.* 1982 Feb 18;306(7):404-406.

Scott JR. Vaginal birth after cesarean delivery: a common-sense approach. *Obstet Gynecol.* 2011 Aug;118(2 Pt 1):342-50.

Scott RT, Jr., Elkind-Hirsch KE, Styne-Gross A, et al. The predictive value for in vitro fertility delivery rates is greatly impacted by the method used to select the threshold between normal and elevated basal follicle-stimulating hormone. *Fertil Steril.* 2008 Apr;89(4):868-78.

Scott RT, Jr., Hofmann GE, Oehninger S, et al. Intercycle variability of day 3 follicle-stimulating hormone levels and its effect on stimulation quality in in vitro fertilization. *Fertil Steril.* 1990 Aug;54(2):297-302.

Scott RT, Opsahl MS, Leonardi MR, et al. Life table analysis of pregnancy rates in a general infertility population relative to ovarian reserve and patient age. *Hum Reprod.* 1995 Jul;10(7):1706-10.

Seckl MJ, Sebire NJ, Berkowitz RS. Gestational trophoblastic disease. *Lancet.* 2010;376(9742):717-29.

Seckl MJ, Sebire NJ, Fisher RA, et al. Gestational trophoblastic disease: ESMO Clinical Practice Guidelines for diagnosis, treatment and follow-up. *Ann Oncol.* 2013 Oct;24 Suppl 6:vi39-50.

Seki K, Kato K, Shima K. Parallelism in the luteinizing hormone responses to opioid and dopamine antagonists in hyperprolactinemic women with pituitary microadenoma. *J Clin Endocrinol Metab.* 1986 Nov;63(5):1225-8.

Sergentanis TN, Diamantaras AA, Perlepe C, et al. IVF and breast cancer: a systematic review and meta-analysis. *Hum Reprod Update.* 2014 Jan-Feb;20(1):106-123.

REFERENCES

Servey J, Chang J. Over-the-counter medications in pregnancy. *Am Fam Physician.* 2014 Oct 15;90(8):548-55.

Sethi N. Pregnancy and epilepsy—managing both, in one patient. *OBG Management.* 2011;23(8):18-24.

Sharara FI, Scott RT, Jr., Seifer DB. The detection of diminished ovarian reserve in infertile women. *Am J Obstet Gynecol.* 1998 Sep;179(3 Pt 1):804-812.

Sharp HT. Assessment of new technology in the treatment of idiopathic menorrhagia and uterine leiomyomata. *Obstet Gynecol.* 2006 Oct;108(4):990-1003.

Shepard TH, Brent RL, Friedman JM, et al. Update on new developments in the study of human teratogens. *Teratology.* 2002 Apr;65(4):153-61.

Sherman S, Pletcher BA, Driscoll DA. Fragile X syndrome: diagnostic and carrier testing. *Genet Med.* 2005 Oct;7(8):584-87.

Shibuya Y, Kyono K. A successful birth of healthy monozygotic dichorionic diamniotic (DD) twins of the same gender following a single vitrified-warmed blastocyst transfer. *J Assist Reprod Genet.* 2012 Mar;29(3):255-57.

Sibai B. Preeclampsia: 3 preemptive tactics. *OBG Management.* 2005;17(2):20-32.

Sibai B. Managing an eclamptic patient. *OBG Management.* 2005;17(5):37-50.

Sibai BM. Imitators of severe preeclampsia. *Obstet Gynecol.* 2007 Apr;109(4):956-66.

Sibai BM. Evaluation and management of severe preeclampsia before 34 weeks' gestation. *Am J Obstet Gynecol.* 2011 Sep;205(3):191-98.

Sibai BM. Etiology and management of postpartum hypertension-preeclampsia. *Am J Obstet Gynecol.* 2012 Jun;206(6):470-75.

Siegel RL, Miller KD, Jemal A. Cancer statistics, 2015. *CA: a cancer journal for clinicians.* 2015 Jan-Feb;65(1):5-29.

Signore C, Freeman RK, Spong CY. Antenatal testing-a reevaluation: executive summary of a Eunice Kennedy Shriver National Institute of Child Health and Human Development workshop. *Obstet Gynecol.* 2009 Mar;113(3):687-701.

Signore C, Hemachandra A, Klebanoff M. Neonatal mortality and morbidity after elective cesarean delivery versus routine expectant management: a decision analysis. *Semin Perinatol.* 2006 Oct;30(5):288-95.

Silberstein SD, Holland S, Freitag F, et al. Evidence-based guideline update: pharmacologic treatment for episodic migraine prevention in adults: report of the Quality Standards Subcommittee of the American Academy of Neurology and the American Headache Society. *Neurology.* 2012 Apr 24;78(17):1337-45.

Silver RM, Landon MB, Rouse DJ, et al. Maternal morbidity associated with multiple repeat cesarean deliveries. *Obstet Gynecol.* 2006 Jun;107(6):1226-32.

Simpson JL, Carson SA, Chesney C, et al. Lack of association between antiphospholipid antibodies and first-trimester spontaneous abortion: prospective study of pregnancies detected within 21 days of conception. *Fertil Steril.* 1998 May;69(5):814-20.

Singh S, Best C, Dunn S, et al. Abnormal uterine bleeding in pre-menopausal women. *J Obstet Gynaecol Can.* 2013 May;35(5):473-79.

Siristatidis C, Sergentanis TN, Kanavidis P, et al. Controlled ovarian hyperstimulation for IVF: impact on ovarian, endometrial and cervical cancer—a systematic review and meta-analysis. *Hum Reprod Update.* 2013 Mar-Apr;19(2):105-123.

Siu AL, Force USPST. Screening for breast cancer: U.S. Preventive Services Task Force recommendation statement. *Ann Intern Med.* 2016 Feb 16;164(4):279-96.

REFERENCES

Smith GC, Pell JP, Cameron AD, et al. Risk of perinatal death associated with labor after previous cesarean delivery in uncomplicated term pregnancies. *JAMA.* 2002 May 22-29;287(20):2684-90.

Smith HO, Berwick M, Verschraegen CF, et al. Incidence and survival rates for female malignant germ cell tumors. *Obstet Gynecol.* 2006 May;107(5):1075-85.

Smith JS, Green J, Berrington de Gonzalez A, et al. Cervical cancer and use of hormonal contraceptives: a systematic review. *Lancet.* 2003 Apr 5;361(9364):1159-67.

Smith M, Calabro V, Chong B, et al. Population screening and cascade testing for carriers of SMA. *Eur J Hum Genet.* 2007 Jul;15(7):759-66.

Smith R. Finding the best approach to dysmenorrhea. *Cont Ob/Gyn.* 2006(Nov):54-60.

Smith RA, von Eschenbach AC, Wender R, et al. American Cancer Society guidelines for the early detection of cancer: update of early detection guidelines for prostate, colorectal, and endometrial cancers. Also: update 2001—testing for early lung cancer detection. *CA: Cancer J Clinicians.* 2001 Jan-Feb;51(1):38-75.

Smotrich DB, Widra EA, Gindoff PR, et al. Prognostic value of day 3 estradiol on in vitro fertilization outcome. *Fertil Steril.* 1995 Dec;64(6):1136-40.

Society for Maternal-Fetal Medicine, Norton ME, Chauhan SP, et al. Society for maternal-fetal medicine (SMFM) clinical guideline #7: nonimmune hydrops fetalis. *Am J Obstet Gynecol.* 2015 Feb;212(2):127-39.

Society for Maternal-Fetal Medicine. Progesterone and preterm birth prevention: translating clinical trials data into clinical practice. *Am J Obstet Gynecol.* 2012 May;206(5):376-86.

Somigliana E, Infantino M, Benedetti F, et al. The presence of ovarian endometriomas is associated with a reduced responsiveness to gonadotropins. *Fertil Steril.* 2006 Jul;86(1):192-96.

Sonmezer M, Oktay K. Fertility preservation in female patients. *Hum Reprod Update.* 2004 May-Jun;10(3):251-66.

Speiser PW, Azziz R, Baskin LS, et al. Congenital adrenal hyperplasia due to steroid 21-hydroxylase deficiency: an Endocrine Society clinical practice guideline. *J Clin Endocrinol Metab.* 2010 Sep;95(9):4133-60.

Spellacy WN, Miller S, Winegar A, et al. Macrosomia—maternal characteristics and infant complications. *Obstet Gynecol.* 1985 Aug;66(2):158-61.

Speroff L, DeCherney A. Evaluation of a new generation of oral contraceptives. The Advisory Board for the New Progestins. *Obstet Gynecol.* 1993 Jun;81(6):1034-47.

Spitz IM, Bardin CW, Benton L, et al. Early pregnancy termination with mifepristone and misoprostol in the United States. *N Engl J Med.* 1998 Apr 30;338(18):1241-7.

Spong CY, Berghella V, Wenstrom KD, et al. Preventing the first cesarean delivery: summary of a joint Eunice Kennedy Shriver National Institute of Child Health and Human Development, Society for Maternal-Fetal Medicine, and American College of Obstetricians and Gynecologists Workshop. *Obstet Gynecol.* 2012 Nov;120(5):1181-93.

Stajner T, Bobic B, Klun I, et al. Prenatal and early postnatal diagnosis of congenital toxoplasmosis in a setting with no systematic screening in pregnancy. *Medicine (Baltimore).* 2016 Mar;95(9):e2979.

Steege JF, Siedhoff MT. Chronic pelvic pain. *Obstet Gynecol.* 2014 Sep;124(3):616-29.

Stein ZA. A woman's age: childbearing and child rearing. *Am J Epidemiol.* 1985 Mar;121(3):327-42.

Steinauer J, Pritts EA, Jackson R, et al. Systematic review of mifepristone for the treatment of uterine leiomyomata. *Obstet Gynecol.* 2004 Jun;103(6):1331-6.

Steinberger E, Smith KD, Tcholakian RK, et al. Testosterone levels in female partners of infertile couples. Relationship between androgen levels in the woman, the male factor, and the incidence of pregnancy. *Am J Obstet Gynecol.* 1979 Jan 15;133(2):133-38.

REFERENCES

Stephenson MD, Awartani KA, Robinson WP. Cytogenetic analysis of miscarriages from couples with recurrent miscarriage: a case-control study. *Hum Reprod.* 2002 Feb;17(2):446-51.

Stern C, Chamley L. Antiphospholipid antibodies and coagulation defects in women with implantation failure after IVF and recurrent miscarriage. *Reprod Biomed Online.* 2006 Jul;13(1):29-37.

Stewart EA. Clinical practice: uterine fibroids. *N Engl J Med.* 2015 Apr 23;372(17):1646-55.

Stewart EA, Rabinovici J, Tempany CM, et al. Clinical outcomes of focused ultrasound surgery for the treatment of uterine fibroids. *Fertil Steril.* 2006 Jan;85(1):22-9.

Stewart FH, Harper CC, Ellertson CE, et al. Clinical breast and pelvic examination requirements for hormonal contraception: current practice vs. evidence. *JAMA.* 2001 May 2;285(17):2232-9.

Stockdale CK, Lawson HW. 2013 Vulvodynia Guideline update. *J Low Genit Tract Dis.* 2014 Apr;18(2):93-100.

Stovall TG, Ling FW. Ectopic pregnancy: diagnostic and therapeutic algorithms minimizing surgical intervention. *J Reprod Med.* 1993 Oct;38(10):807-812.

Strandell A, Lindhard A. Why does hydrosalpinx reduce fertility? The importance of hydrosalpinx fluid. *Hum Reprod.* 2002 May;17(5):1141-5.

Strandell A, Lindhard A, Eckerlund I. Cost-effectiveness analysis of salpingectomy prior to IVF, based on a randomized controlled trial. *Hum Reprod.* 2005 Dec;20(12):3284-92.

Strandell A, Lindhard A, Waldenstrom U, et al. Hydrosalpinx and IVF outcome: cumulative results after salpingectomy in a randomized controlled trial. *Hum Reprod.* 2001 Nov;16(11):2403-10.

Stuenkel CA, Davis SR, Gompel A, et al. Treatment of symptoms of the menopause: an Endocrine Society clinical practice guideline. *J Clin Endocrinol Metab.* 2015 Nov;100(11):3975-4011.

Surawicz CM, Brandt LJ, Binion DG, et al. Guidelines for diagnosis, treatment, and prevention of *Clostridium difficile* infections. *Am J Gastroenterol.* 2013 Apr;108(4):478-98; quiz 99.

Surrey ES, Voigt B, Fournet N, et al. Prolonged gonadotropin-releasing hormone agonist treatment of symptomatic endometriosis: the role of cyclic sodium etidronate and low-dose norethindrone "add-back" therapy. *Fertil Steril.* 1995 Apr;63(4):747-55.

Swanson D, Block R, Mousa SA. Omega-3 fatty acids EPA and DHA: health benefits throughout life. *Adv Nutr.* 2012 Jan;3(1):1-7.

Taipale P, Hiilesmaa V, Ylostalo P. Transvaginal ultrasonography at 18-23 weeks in predicting placenta previa at delivery. *Ultrasound Obstet Gynecol.* 1998 Dec;12(6):422-25.

Tan EM, Cohen AS, Fries JF, et al. The 1982 revised criteria for the classification of systemic lupus erythematosus. *Arthritis Rheum* 1982; 25:1271.

Tan PC, Subramaniam RN, Omar SZ. Labour and perinatal outcome in women at term with one previous lower-segment Caesarean: a review of 1000 consecutive cases. *Aust N Z J Obstet Gynaecol.* 2007 Feb;47(1):31-6.

Tanis BC, van den Bosch MA, Kemmeren JM, et al. Oral contraceptives and the risk of myocardial infarction. *N Engl J Med.* 2001 Dec 20;345(25):1787-93.

Tarani L, Lampariello S, Raguso G, et al. Pregnancy in patients with Turner's syndrome: six new cases and review of literature. *Gynecol endocrinol.* 1998 Apr;12(2):83-7.

Tartagni M, Schonauer MM, Cicinelli E, et al. Intermittent low-dose finasteride is as effective as daily administration for the treatment of hirsute women. *Fertil Steril.* 2004 Sep;82(3):752-55.

Teichmann AT, Brill K, Albring M, et al. The influence of the dose of ethinylestradiol in oral contraceptives on follicle growth. *Gynecol endocrinol.* 1995 Dec;9(4):299-305.

REFERENCES

Tewari KS, Sill MW, Long HJ 3rd, et al. Improved survival with bevacizumab in advanced cervical cancer. *N Engl J Med.* 2014 Feb 20;370(8):734-43.

Thiboutot D, Archer DF, Lemay A, et al. A randomized, controlled trial of a low-dose contraceptive containing 20 microg of ethinyl estradiol and 100 microg of levonorgestrel for acne treatment. *Fertil Steril.* 2001 Sep;76(3):461-68.

Thompson SA, Lyons TL, Makowski EL. Outcomes of twin gestations at the University of Colorado Health Sciences Center, 1973-1983. *J Reprod Med.* 1987 May;32(5):328-39.

Thorneycroft IH, Stanczyk FZ, Bradshaw KD, et al. Effect of low-dose oral contraceptives on androgenic markers and acne. *Contraception.* 1999 Nov;60(5):255-62.

Tian L, Shen H, Lu Q, et al. Insulin resistance increases the risk of spontaneous abortion after assisted reproduction technology treatment. *J Clin Endocrinol Metab.* 2007 Apr;92(4):1430-3.

Tita AT, Andrews WW. Diagnosis and management of clinical chorioamnionitis. *Clin Perinatol.* 2010 Jun;37(2):339-54.

Toner JP, Seifer DB. Why we may abandon basal follicle-stimulating hormone testing: a sea change in determining ovarian reserve using antimullerian hormone. *Fertil Steril.* 2013 Jun;99(7):1825-30.

Towner D, Castro MA, Eby-Wilkens E, et al. Effect of mode of delivery in nulliparous women on neonatal intracranial injury. *N Engl J Med.* 1999 Dec 2;341(23):1709-14.

Townsley DM. Hematologic complications of pregnancy. *Semin Hematol.* 2013 Jul;50(3):222-31.

Trent M. Pelvic inflammatory disease. *Pediatr Rev.* 2013 Apr;34(4):163-72.

Trio D, Strobelt N, Picciolo C, et al. Prognostic factors for successful expectant management of Ectopic pregnancy. *Fertil Steril.* 1995 Mar;63(3):469-72.

Trussell J. Contraceptive efficacy. I. In: Hatcher R, Trussell J, Nelson A, et al., editors. *Contraceptive Techology: Twentieth Revised Edition.* New York: Ardent Media; 2011.

Tsoumpou I, Kyrgiou M, Gelbaya TA, et al. The effect of surgical treatment for endometrioma on in vitro fertilization outcomes: a systematic review and meta-analysis. *Fertil Steril.* 2009 Jul;92(1):75-87.

Tulandi T, Al-Took S. Laparoscopic ovarian suspension before irradiation. *Fertil Steril.* 1998 Aug;70(2):381-83.

Tulandi T, Martin J, Al-Fadhli R, et al. Congenital malformations among 911 newborns conceived after infertility treatment with letrozole or clomiphene citrate. *Fertil Steril.* 2006 Jun;85(6):1761-5.

Turi A, Giannubilo SR, Bruge F, et al. Coenzyme Q10 content in follicular fluid and its relationship with oocyte fertilization and embryo grading. *Arch Gynecol Obstet.* 2012 Apr;285(4): 1173-6.

Uncu G, Kasapoglu I, Ozerkan K, et al. Prospective assessment of the impact of endometriomas and their removal on ovarian reserve and determinants of the rate of decline in ovarian reserve. *Hum Reprod.* 2013 Aug;28(8):2140-5.

Urman B, Yakin K. Does dehydroepiandrosterone have any benefit in fertility treatment? *Curr Opin Obstet Gynecol.* 2012 Jun;24(3):132-35.

Vacca A. Vacuum-assisted delivery: improving patient outcomes and protecting yourself against litigation. *OBG Management.* 2004:S1–S7.

van Bael M, Natowicz MR, Tomczak J, et al. Heterozygosity for Tay-Sachs disease in non-Jewish Americans with ancestry from Ireland or Great Britain. *J Med Genet.* 1996 Oct;33(10):829-32.

van Leeuwen FE, Klip H, Mooij TM, et al. Risk of borderline and invasive ovarian tumours after ovarian stimulation for in vitro fertilization in a large Dutch cohort. *Hum Reprod.* 2011 Dec;26(12):3456-65.

REFERENCES

van Leeuwen I, Branch DW, Scott JR. First-trimester ultrasonography findings in women with a history of recurrent pregnancy loss. *Am J Obstet Gynecol.* 1993 Jan; 168(1 Pt 1):111-14.

van Seters M, van Beurden M, ten Kate FJ, et al. Treatment of vulvar intraepithelial neoplasia with topical imiquimod. *N Engl J Med.* 2008 Apr 3;358(14):1465-73.

Vance ML. Treatment of patients with a pituitary adenoma: one clinician's experience. *Neurosurg Focus.* 2004 Apr 15;16(4):E1.

Verani JR, McGee L, Schrag SJ. Prevention of perinatal group B streptococcal disease—revised guidelines from CDC, 2010. *MMWR.* 2010 Nov 19;59(Rr-10):1-36.

Verhelst J, Abs R, Maiter D, et al. Cabergoline in the treatment of hyperprolactinemia: a study in 455 patients. *J Clin Endocrinol Metab.* 1999 Jul;84(7):2518-22.

Visser GH, de Valk HW. Is the evidence strong enough to change the diagnostic criteria for gestational diabetes now? *Am J Obstet Gynecol.* 2013 Apr;208(4):260-64.

Volker P, Grundker C, Schmidt O, et al. Expression of receptors for luteinizing hormone-releasing hormone in human ovarian and endometrial cancers: frequency, autoregulation, and correlation with direct antiproliferative activity of luteinizing hormone-releasing hormone analogues. *Am J Obstet Gynecol.* 2002 Feb;186(2):171-79.

Vollenhoven BJ, Lawrence AS, Healy DL. Uterine fibroids: a clinical review. *Br J Obstet Gynaecol.* 1990 Apr;97(4):285-98.

von Hertzen H, Honkanen H, Piaggio G, et al. WHO multinational study of three misoprostol regimens after mifepristone for early medical abortion. I: efficacy. *Br J Obstet Gynaecol.* 2003 Sep;110(9):808-818.

von Hertzen H, Huong NT, Piaggio G, et al. Misoprostol dose and route after mifepristone for early medical abortion: a randomised controlled noninferiority trial. *Br J Obstet Gynaecol.* 2010 Sep;117(10):1186-96.

Vossen CY, Preston FE, Conard J, et al. Hereditary thrombophilia and fetal loss: a prospective follow-up study. *J Thromb Haemost.* 2004;2:592-96.

Wallace WH, Kelsey TW. Human ovarian reserve from conception to the menopause. *PLoS One.* 2010;5(1):e8772.

Wallach EE, Vu KK. Myomata uteri and infertility. *Obstet Gynecol Clin North Am.* 1995 Dec;22(4):791-99.

Wang X, Chen C, Wang L, et al. Conception, early pregnancy loss, and time to clinical pregnancy: a population-based prospective study. *Fertil Steril.* 2003 Mar;79(3):577-84.

Warburton D, Fraser FC. Spontaneous abortion risks in man: data from reproductive histories collected in a medical genetics unit. *Am J Hum Genet.* 1964 Mar;16:1-25.

Weenen C, Laven JS, Von Bergh AR, et al. Anti-Müllerian hormone expression pattern in the human ovary: potential implications for initial and cyclic follicle recruitment. *Mol Hum Reprod.* 2004 Feb;10(2):77-83.

Weiderpass E, Baron JA, Adami HO, et al. Low-potency oestrogen and risk of

Weinbaum CM, Williams I, Mast EE, et al. Recommendations for identification and public health management of persons with chronic hepatitis B virus infection. *MMWR.* 2008 Sep 19;57(Rr-8):1-20.

Wendel GD, Jr., Stark BJ, Jamison RB, et al. Penicillin allergy and desensitization in serious infections during pregnancy. *N Engl J Med.* 1985 May 9;312(19):1229-32.

Westhoff C, Heartwell S, Edwards S, et al. Initiation of oral contraceptives using a quick start compared with a conventional start: a randomized controlled trial. *Obstet Gynecol.* 2007 Jun;109(6):1270-6.

REFERENCES

White PC, Speiser PW. Congenital adrenal hyperplasia due to 21-hydroxylase deficiency. *Endocrine rev.* 2000 Jun;21(3):245-91.

White YA, Woods DC, Takai Y, et al. Oocyte formation by mitotically active germ cells purified from ovaries of reproductive-age women. *Nature Med.* 2012 Mar;18(3):413-21.

Wiebe E, Dunn S, Guilbert E, et al. Comparison of abortions induced by methotrexate or mifepristone followed by misoprostol. *Obstet Gynecol.* 2002 May; 99(5 Pt 1):813-19.

Wilcox AJ, Weinberg CR, Baird DD. Timing of sexual intercourse in relation to ovulation. Effects on the probability of conception, survival of the pregnancy, and sex of the baby. *N Engl J Med.* 1995 Dec 7;333(23):1517-21.

Wild RA, Umstot ES, Andersen RN, et al. Androgen parameters and their correlation with body weight in one hundred thirty-eight women thought to have hyperandrogenism. *Am J Obstet Gynecol.* 1983 Jul 15;146(6):602-606.

Williams RS, Littell RD, Mendenhall NP. Laparoscopic oophoropexy and ovarian function in the treatment of Hodgkin disease. *Cancer.* 1999 Nov 15;86(10):2138-42.

Wirth B, Schmidt T, Hahnen E, et al. De novo rearrangements found in 2% of index patients with spinal muscular atrophy: mutational mechanisms, parental origin, mutation rate, and implications for genetic counseling. *Am J Hum Genet.* 1997 Nov;61(5):1102-11.

Witter F, Devoe L. Update on successful induction of labor. *Adv Studies Med.* 2005;5(9D):S888-S98.

Wong IL, Morris RS, Chang L, et al. A prospective randomized trial comparing finasteride to spironolactone in the treatment of hirsute women. *J Clin Endocrinol Metab.* 1995 Jan;80(1):233-38.

Workowski KA, Bolan GA. Sexually transmitted diseases treatment guidelines, 2015. *MMWR.* 2015 Jun 5;64(Rr-03):1-137.

Wright JD, Hassan K, Ananth CV, et al. Use of guideline-based antibiotic prophylaxis in women undergoing gynecologic surgery. *Obstet Gynecol.* 2013 Dec;122(6):1145-53.

Xenakis EM, Piper JM, Conway DL, et al. Induction of labor in the nineties: conquering the unfavorable cervix. *Obstet Gynecol.* 1997 Aug;90(2):235-39.

Yeomans ER, Hauth JC, Gilstrap LC, 3rd, et al. Umbilical cord pH, PCO_2, and bicarbonate following uncomplicated term vaginal deliveries. *Am J Obstet Gynecol.* 1985 Mar 15;151(6):798-800.

Yerushalmi GM, Gilboa Y, Jakobson-Setton A, et al. Vaginal mifepristone for the treatment of symptomatic uterine leiomyomata: an open-label study. *Fertil Steril.* 2014 Feb;101(2):496-500.

Young RL, Goldzieher JW, Elkind-Hirsch K. The endocrine effects of spironolactone used as an antiandrogen. *Fertil Steril.* 1987 Aug;48(2):223-28.

Youssef MA, van Wely M, Hassan MA, et al. Can dopamine agonists reduce the incidence and severity of OHSS in IVF/ICSI treatment cycles? A systematic review and meta-analysis. *Hum Reprod Update.* 2010 Sep-Oct;16(5):459-66.

Yu J, Chen Z, Ni Y, et al. *CFTR* mutations in men with congenital bilateral absence of the vas deferens (CBAVD): a systemic review and meta-analysis. *Hum Reprod.* 2012 Jan;27(1):25-35.

Yucelten D, Erenus M, Gurbuz O, et al. Recurrence rate of hirsutism after 3 different antiandrogen therapies. *J Am Acad Dermatol.* 1999 Jul;41(1):64-8.

Zhang J, Landy HJ, Branch DW, et al. Contemporary patterns of spontaneous labor with normal neonatal outcomes. *Obstet Gynecol.* 2010 Dec;116(6):1281-7.

Zotz RB, Gerhardt A, Scharf RE. Inherited thrombophilia and gestational venous thromboembolism. *Best Pract Res Clin Haematol.* 2003;16:243-59.

Illustrations

FIGURES

Figure 1.1.	Vaccines indicated for various medical conditions	9
Figure 1.2.	Body mass index (BMI) nomogram	15
Figure 1.3.	Flow diagram for CVD preventative care in women	20
Figure 1.4.	Algorithm summarizing the initiation of statin therapy	23
Figure 1.5.	Algorithm for the initiation of statin therapy in individuals without ASCVD	25
Figure 1.6.	Statin therapy: monitoring therapeutic response and adherence	27
Figure 1.7.	Algorithm for the management of high blood pressure in adults	37
Figure 1.8.	Antihyperglycemic therapy in type 2 diabetes: general recommendations	39
Figure 1.9.	Approach to starting and adjusting insulin in type 2 diabetes	40
Figure 1.10.	Typical migraine evolution over time	49
Figure 1.11.	Algorithm for the diagnostic evaluation of back pain	51
Figure 1.12.	Algorithm for the management of acute bacterial rhinosinusitis	54
Figure 2.1.	Management algorithm for prevention and treatment of nausea and vomiting of pregnancy	63
Figure 2.2.	Caldwell-Moloy classification of the female pelvis	69
Figure 2.3.	Average labor curves by parity in singleton, term pregnancies	74
Figure 2.4.	Algorithm for spontaneous labor	75
Figure 2.5.	Algorithm for induction of labor	83
Figure 2.6.	Types of forceps	88
Figure 2.7.	Proper placement of the vacuum cup	91
Figure 2.8.	Location of uterine incision in types of cesarean delivery	97
Figure 2.9.	Druzin splint maneuver	97
Figure 2.10.	Algorithm for neonatal resuscitation	103
Figure 2.11.	Clinical assessment of the trauma patient more than 20 weeks of gestation	112
Figure 2.12.	Labor and delivery observation after maternal trauma	113
Figure 2.13.	Intrauterine resuscitation measures	120
Figure 2.14.	A standardized ABCD approach to EFM management	122
Figure 2.15.	Typical setup for amnioinfusion	124
Figure 2.16.	Management of abruption	128
Figure 2.17.	Types of placenta previa	129
Figure 2.18.	Diagram demonstrating the technique for transvaginal sonography of placenta previa	131
Figure 2.19.	Management algorithm for postpartum hemorrhage	135
Figure 2.20.	Sequential interventions for managing postpartum hemorrhage	136
Figure 2.21.	Uterine artery ligation	137
Figure 2.22.	B-Lynch suture for postpartum hemorrhage	138
Figure 2.23.	Manual insertion of a Bakri balloon	139
Figure 2.24.	Reduction of uterine inversion	141
Figure 2.25.	McDonald cerclage	144
Figure 2.26.	Modified Shirodkar cerclage	145
Figure 2.27.	Transabdominal cerclage	146
Figure 2.28.	Technique to reduce prolapsed membranes before performing cerclage	147
Figure 2.29.	Pathways to preterm delivery	148
Figure 2.30.	Algorithm for the screening and treatment of pregnant women to reduce the risk of preterm birth	149

ILLUSTRATIONS — Figures

Figure 2.31.	Triage protocol for PTL symptoms	153
Figure 2.32.	Algorithm for selection of candidates and administration of magnesium sulfate for fetal neuroprotection	155
Figure 2.33.	Percentage of survival by gestational age	158
Figure 2.34.	Percentage with severe or moderate disability by gestational age among surviving newborns	158
Figure 2.35.	Presentation of twins presenting in labor or at term	163
Figure 2.36.	Algorithm for route of delivery of twin pregnancy	165
Figure 2.37.	CDA 2008 and IADPSG algorithms for diagnosis of GDM	178
Figure 2.38.	Pharmacokinetic profiles of human insulins compared with insulin analogs and endogenous insulin	181
Figure 2.39.	Management of gestational hypertension or preeclampsia without severe features	187
Figure 2.40.	Management of severe preeclampsia at less than 34 weeks gestation	188
Figure 2.41.	Recommended evaluation and management of women with postpartum hypertension	197
Figure 2.42.	Flowchart for fetal and placental evaluation following fetal demise	201
Figure 2.43.	Algorithm for the evaluation of nonimmune hydrops	205
Figure 2.44.	Evaluation of obstetric patients with a positive indirect Coombs test result	209
Figure 2.45.	Algorithm for the clinical management of the red cell alloimmunized pregnancy	211
Figure 2.46.	Algorithm for determining the results of cell-free fetal DNA testing to determine the fetal RHD status	212
Figure 2.47.	Risk assessment and prevention of VTE and adverse pregnancy outcome	224
Figure 2.48.	The pattern of changes in serum concentrations of thyroid function studies and hCG according to gestational age	230
Figure 2.49.	Gestational age-specific thyroid stimulating hormone nomogram	231
Figure 2.50.	Management of hyperthyroidism in pregnancy	233
Figure 2.51.	Management of thyroid storm	235
Figure 2.52.	Management of hypothyroidism	237
Figure 3.1.	Outcomes in autosomal recessive genetic diseases	239
Figure 3.2.	Cystic fibrosis genotype-phenotype correlation	246
Figure 3.3.	Risk of SMA is variable in patients with normal carrier screening result depending upon number of copies and gene location	250
Figure 3.4.	Summary of Alpha Thalassemia	252
Figure 3.5.	Summary of Beta Thalassemia	253
Figure 4.1.	Fetal anatomic landmarks	273
Figure 4.2.	Fetal intracranial anatomy	274
Figure 4.3.	Fetal echocardiography	276
Figure 4.4.	Endovaginal ultrasonography	277
Figure 4.5.	Basic principles of scanning	278
Figure 4.6.	Measurement of the cervical length for preterm labor risk assessment	280
Figure 5.1.	Twelve-month conception rates following discontinuation of various contraceptive methods	298
Figure 5.2.	Rates of amenorrhea for continuous vs. monthly oral contraceptives	301
Figure 5.3.	Available IUDs	317
Figure 5.4.	Algorithm for locating lost IUD strings	318
Figure 5.5.	Types of tubal ligation	320
Figure 6.1.	PALM-COEIN classification of abnormal uterine bleeding	324
Figure 6.2.	Evaluation of premenopausal abnormal bleeding	332
Figure 6.3.	Evaluation of postmenopausal abnormal bleeding	333
Figure 6.4.	Options for global endometrial ablation	335
Figure 6.5.	Locations of ectopic pregnancy	336
Figure 6.6.	Algorithm for the management of ectopic pregnancy	339
Figure 6.7.	Single-dose MTX treatment failure based on β-hCG levels	342
Figure 6.8.	Body surface nomogram	343
Figure 6.9.	Classification of ultrasound findings for a woman with a positive pregnancy test	344
Figure 6.10.	Algorithm for the management of pregnancy of unknown location (PUL)	346
Figure 6.11.	Algorithm for the evaluation of false positive beta-hCG	348
Figure 6.12.	Steps in obtaining samples for a sexual assault evidence collection kit and medical-history taking	353
Figure 6.14.	American Society for Reproductive Medicine revised classification of endometriosis	362
Figure 6.15.	Endometriosis fertility index surgery form	365

Figures

ILLUSTRATIONS

Figure	Title	Page
Figure 6.16.	Amino acid sequence of GnRH and GnRH-agonists	366
Figure 6.17.	Diagnosis and treatment algorithm for urinary incontinence	377
Figure 6.18.	Evaluation and treatment algorithm for urinary incontinence	378
Figure 6.19.	Vulvodynia treatment algorithm	380
Figure 6.20.	FIGO classification of system for leiomyomas	383
Figure 7.1.	Algorithm for screening for group B streptococcal (GBS) colonization and use of intrapartum prophylaxis for women with preterm labor (PTL)	390
Figure 7.2.	Algorithm for screening for group B streptococcal (GBS) colonization and use of intrapartum prophylaxis for women with preterm premature rupture of membranes (PPROM)	391
Figure 7.3.	Algorithm for secondary prevention of early-onset group B streptococcal (GBS) disease among newborns	392
Figure 7.4.	Recommended regimens for intrapartum antibiotic prophylaxis for prevention of early-onset group B streptococcal (GBS) disease	393
Figure 7.5.	Evaluation of the patient with mastitis	397
Figure 7.6.	Typical serologic course of acute hepatitis B	400
Figure 7.7.	Progression to chronic hepatitis B	401
Figure 7.8.	Recommended testing sequence for identifying current hepatitis C virus (HCV) infection	406
Figure 7.9.	Pulmonary tuberculosis control plan	409
Figure 7.10.	Algorithm for the management of pregnant patient exposed to rubella	423
Figure 7.11.	Algorithm for the diagnosis of congenital toxoplasmosis	426
Figure 7.12.	Updated interim guidance: testing algorithm for a pregnant woman with possible Zika virus exposure not residing in an area with active Zika virus transmission	430
Figure 7.13.	Risk factors that contribute to increased incidence of UTI in pregnancy	440
Figure 7.14.	Algorithm for the management of asymptomatic bacteriuria or acute cystitis in pregnancy	441
Figure 7.15.	Algorithm for the management of acute pyelonephritis in pregnancy	442
Figure 8.1.	Probability of conception as a function of timing of intercourse	464
Figure 8.2.	Effect of age on the cumulative pregnancy rate in a donor insemination program	465
Figure 8.3.	Threshold values for FSH in IVF	468
Figure 8.4.	Percentage of ovarian reserve related to increasing age	471
Figure 8.5.	Location of Y chromosome deletions related to azoospermia (DAZ)	476
Figure 8.6.	OCP/LTL protocol for IVF	483
Figure 8.7.	LTL protocol for IVF	484
Figure 8.8.	OCP/microdose GnRH-agonist protocol for IVF	485
Figure 8.9.	OCP/GnRH-antagonist protocol for IVF	486
Figure 8.10.	Sequence of oocyte maturation, fertilization, and embryo development	487
Figure 8.11.	Percentages of ART cycles using fresh nondonor eggs or embryos that resulted in pregnancies, live births, and singleton live births, by age of woman, 2013	489
Figure 8.12.	Algorithm for the management of ovarian hyperstimulation syndrome (OHSS)	492
Figure 8.13.	Reciprocal and Robertsonian translocations	499
Figure 8.14.	Gamete permutations in reciprocal translocation	500
Figure 8.15.	Gamete permutations in Robertsonian translocation	500
Figure 8.16.	Options for female gamete preservation	512
Figure 8.17.	Letrozole/gnRH-antagonist protocol for ART patients with estrogen-sensitive cancer	513
Figure 9.1.	The normal reproductive cycle	518
Figure 9.2.	The life history of germ cells	519
Figure 9.3.	Average age of appearance of pubertal events	521
Figure 9.4.	Tanner staging of breast and pubic hair	522
Figure 9.5.	Algorithm for the evaluation of amenorrhea	536
Figure 9.6.	Ultrasonographic appearance of the PCOS ovary	541
Figure 9.7.	Frequency of elevated androgens in women with PCOS	541
Figure 9.8.	Predictive value of elevated testosterone for presence of a virilizing ovarian or adrenal tumor	542
Figure 9.9.	Prevalence of autosomal recessive genetic disorders by ethnic group	546
Figure 9.10.	Nomogram for ACTH stimulation test	548
Figure 9.11.	Steroid hormone synthesis	550
Figure 9.12.	Steroid hormone synthesis	551
Figure 9.13.	Sources of androgen production	553
Figure 9.14.	Most commonly reported symptoms in patients with hyperprolactinemia	555
Figure 9.15.	Correlation between the pituitary size and serum PRL level (ng/mL)	557

ILLUSTRATIONS — Figures

Figure	Title	Page
Figure 9.16.	Anatomic changes resulting in empty sella syndrome	559
Figure 9.17.	Algorithm for the evaluation of thyroid dysfunction	564
Figure 10.1.	Algorithm for menopausal symptom management	573
Figure 10.2.	Ten-year probability of sustaining any osteoporotic fracture in women by age and T-score	581
Figure 10.3.	Lifetime risk of hip fractures in women aged 50 years according to bone mineral density or T-score at the hip	582
Figure 10.4.	Algorithm for the management of osteoporosis	583
Figure 11.1.	Cancer statistics 2015	591
Figure 11.2.	Progression from normal to dysplasia in the cervical epithelium	601
Figure 11.3.	Unsatisfactory cytology	605
Figure 11.4.	Cytology NILM but EC/TZ Absent/Insufficient	605
Figure 11.5.	Management of women ≥ age 30 who are cytology negative but HPV positive	606
Figure 11.6.	Management of women with atypical squamous cells of undetermined significance (ASC-US) on cytology	606
Figure 11.7.	Management of women ages 21–24 years with either atypical squamous cells of undetermined significance (ASC-US) or low-grade squamous intraepithelial lesions (LSIL)	607
Figure 11.8.	Management of women with low-grade squamous intraepithelial lesions (LSIL)	607
Figure 11.9.	Management of pregnant women with low-grade squamous intraepithelial lesions (LSIL)	608
Figure 11.10.	Management of women with atypical squamous cells: cannot exclude high-grade SIL (ASC-H)	608
Figure 11.11.	Management of women ages 21–24 yr with atypical squamous cells: cannot exclude high-grade SIL (ASC-H) and high-grade squamous intraepithelial lesion (HSIL)	609
Figure 11.12.	Management of women with high-grade squamous intraepithelial lesion (HSIL)	609
Figure 11.13.	Initial workup of women with atypical glandular cells (AGC)	610
Figure 11.14.	Subsequent management of women with atypical glandular cells (AGC)	610
Figure 11.15.	Management of women with no lesion or biopsy-confirmed cervical intraepithelial neoplasia—grade 1 (CIN1) preceded by "lesser abnormalities"	611
Figure 11.16.	Management of women with no lesion or biopsy-confirmed cervical intraepithelial neoplasia—grade 1 (CIN1) preceded by ASC-H or HSIL cytology	611
Figure 11.17.	Management of women with no lesion or biopsy-confirmed cervical intraepithelial neoplasia—grade 1 (CIN1)	612
Figure 11.18.	Management of women with biopsy-confirmed cervical intraepithelial neoplasia—grades 2 and 3 (CIN2, 3)	612
Figure 11.19.	Management of young women with biopsy-confirmed cervical intraepithelial neoplasia—grades 2 and 3 (CIN2, 3) in special circumstances	613
Figure 11.20.	Management of women diagnosed with adenocarcinoma in situ (AIS) during a diagnostic excisional procedure	613
Figure 11.21.	Management of cervical cancer in pregnancy	619
Figure 11.22.	Evaluation of an adnexal mass in a pediatric patient	620
Figure 11.23.	Management of an adnexal mass in a premenopausal patient	621
Figure 11.24.	Management of an adnexal mass in postmenopausal patient	622
Figure 11.25.	Vulvar intraepithelial neoplasia	631
Figure 11.26.	Adult cancer pain	640
Figure 11.27.	Principles of emesis control	641
Figure 11.28.	Emetogenic potential of high- and moderate-risk IV antineoplastic agents	642
Figure 11.29.	Emetogenic potential of low- and minimal-risk IV antineoplastic agents	643
Figure 11.30.	Emetogenic potential of oral antineoplastic agents	644
Figure 11.31.	Acute and delayed emesis prevention of high emetic risk IV chemotherapy	645
Figure 11.32.	Acute and delayed emesis prevention of moderate emetic risk IV chemotherapy	646
Figure 11.33.	Emesis prevention of low- and minimal-risk IV chemotherapy	647
Figure 11.34.	Emesis prevention of oral chemotherapy	648
Figure 11.35.	Breakthrough treatment for chemotherapy-induced nausea/vomiting	649
Figure 11.36.	Risk assessment for febrile neutropenic patients	650
Figure 11.37.	Criteria for low-risk outpatient therapy	651
Figure 11.38.	Low-risk outpatient therapy options	652
Figure 11.39.	Initial empiric therapy for fever and neutropenia	653
Figure 11.40.	Prevention and treatment of cancer-related infections	654
Figure 11.41.	Prevention and treatment of cancer-related infections	655
Figure 11.42.	Use of myeloid growth factors for febrile neutropenia	656

Tables

Figure 11.43.	Triple lumen catheter	660
Figure 11.44.	Effects of anticoagulants on the coagulation cascade	665
Figure 11.45.	Diagnostic algorithm for deep vein thrombosis	667
Figure 11.46.	Diagnostic algorithm for pulmonary embolism	668
Figure 11.47.	Metabolic acidosis and alkalosis	675

TABLES

Table 1.1.	Summary of screening, prevention, and counseling recommendations for adults <65 years	1
Table 1.2.	Summary of screening, prevention, and counseling recommendations for adults ≥65 years	4
Table 1.3.	Screening guidelines for the early detection of colorectal cancer and adenomas for average-risk women aged 50 years and older	6
Table 1.4.	Colorectal cancer screening options based upon risk factors	8
Table 1.5.	Recommended weekly and occasional food purchases for one person following a healthful diet containing 2100 kcal and 1500 mg of sodium	10
Table 1.6.	Directory reference intakes (DRIs): recommended dietary allowances and adequate intakes, vitamins	12
Table 1.7.	Directory reference intakes (DRIs): recommended dietary allowances and adequate intakes, elements	14
Table 1.8.	Body mass index nomogram	16
Table 1.9.	Body mass index table	18
Table 1.10.	Classification of CVD risk in women	19
Table 1.11.	High-, moderate-, and low-intensity statin therapy	22
Table 1.12.	Secondary causes of hyperlipidemia most commonly encountered in clinical practice	28
Table 1.13.	Adult dosing, side effects, and drug interactions of lipid-lowering drugs	29
Table 1.14.	Properties of statins	31
Table 1.15.	Lifestyle modification recommendations	33
Table 1.16.	Evidence-based dosing for antihypertensive drugs	34
Table 1.17.	Strategies to dose antihypertensive drugs	35
Table 1.18.	Guideline comparisons of goal BP and initial drug therapy for adults with hypertension	36
Table 1.19.	Initial evaluation of type 2 diabetes	38
Table 1.20.	Properties of available glucose-lowering agents in the U.S. and Europe that may guide individualized treatment choices in patients with type 2 diabetes	41
Table 1.21.	Agents to help smokers quit	44
Table 1.22.	Limits of drug detection in urine and blood samples according to length of time from last use	45
Table 1.23.	The TWEAK screening test for alcohol abuse	46
Table 1.24.	The CAGE screening test for alcohol abuse	46
Table 1.25.	Characteristics of migraine, cluster, and tension-type headaches	47
Table 1.26.	Available triptans and their doses	48
Table 1.27.	Classification of migraine preventive therapies (available in the United States)	50
Table 1.28.	Summary of the nonsurgical treatment options for low back pain	52
Table 1.29.	Drug interactions with complementary medicines	55
Table 1.30.	Commonly used botanicals and vitamins and their possible effects in the surgical patient	57
Table 2.1.	Routine prenatal laboratories	60
Table 2.2.	Contraindicated medications for patients receiving odansetron	62
Table 2.3.	Pharmacologic treatment of nausea and vomiting in pregnancy	64
Table 2.4.	New recommendations for total and rate of weight gain during pregnancy	66
Table 2.5.	Classifications of anemia in pregnancy	67
Table 2.6.	Classification of the bony pelvis	69
Table 2.7.	Average measurements of the female pelvis	70
Table 2.8.	Guidelines for redating gestational age based upon ultrasonography	71
Table 2.9.	Comparison of FLM laboratory testing options (all testing requires amniotic fluid)	73
Table 2.10.	Spontaneous labor progress stratified by cervical dilation and parity	74
Table 2.11.	Bishop scoring for cervical ripening	76
Table 2.12.	Attributes of commercially available prostaglandin analogues	77
Table 2.13.	Neonatal and infant mortality rates associated with late-preterm and early-term deliveries	79

Table 2.14.	Recommendations for timing of delivery when conditions complicate pregnancy at or after 34 weeks of gestation	80
Table 2.15.	Risk of shoulder dystocia (%) as a function of birthweight	84
Table 2.16.	Criteria for types of forceps delivery	86
Table 2.17.	ACOG summary recommendations for operative vaginal delivery	87
Table 2.18.	Relative risks based upon delivery method	87
Table 2.19.	Classification and use of vacuum delivery cups	89
Table 2.20.	Indications for cesarean delivery	92
Table 2.21.	Risk of adverse maternal and neonatal outcomes by mode of delivery	93
Table 2.22.	Recommendations for safe prevention of primary cesarean delivery	94
Table 2.23.	Summary of operative techniques in cesarean delivery	96
Table 2.24.	Maternal morbidity of women who had cesarean delivery without labor	98
Table 2.25.	Placenta previa and accreta by number of cesarean deliveries	99
Table 2.26.	Comparison of clinical practice guidelines for VBAC	101
Table 2.27.	Composite maternal risks from elective repeat cesarean delivery and trial of labor after previous cesarean delivery	101
Table 2.28.	Composite neonatal morbidity elective repeat cesarean delivery and trial of labor after previous cesarean delivery	102
Table 2.29.	Incidence and relative risk of uterine rupture during a second delivery among women with a prior cesarean delivery	102
Table 2.30.	Apgar score	104
Table 2.31.	Indications for antepartum fetal surveillance	105
Table 2.32.	Interpretation of contraction stress test	106
Table 2.33.	Biophysical profile	106
Table 2.34.	Management based on biophysical profile score	108
Table 2.35.	Maternal risk factors and estimated risk of stillbirth and reported strategies for antepartum fetal surveillance	109
Table 2.36.	Summary of key points from the imaging guidelines	114
Table 2.37.	Effects of gestational age and radiation dose on radiation-induced teratogenesis	115
Table 2.38.	Estimated fetal radiation absorption per procedure or event	115
Table 2.39.	Electronic fetal monitoring definitions	117
Table 2.40.	Three-tiered fetal heart rate interpretation system	119
Table 2.41.	Various intrauterine resuscitative measures for category II or category III tracings or both	121
Table 2.42.	A simplified ABCD checklist	123
Table 2.43.	Umbilical cord gas values for arterial and venous blood in term newborns	125
Table 2.44.	Umbilical cord gas values for arterial blood in preterm newborns	125
Table 2.45.	Evidence and strength of association linking major risk factors with placental abruption	126
Table 2.46.	Ultrasonographic criteria for diagnosis of placental abruption	127
Table 2.47.	Studies of second-trimester transvaginal sonography in the prediction of placenta previa at delivery	130
Table 2.48.	Maternal adaptation to blood loss	132
Table 2.49.	Blood component therapy	133
Table 2.50.	Duke University obstetric bleeding emergency transfusion algorithm	133
Table 2.51.	Uterotonic therapy	134
Table 2.52.	Current Society for Maternal-Fetal Medicine recommendations regarding use of progestogens to prevent preterm birth	150
Table 2.53.	Predicted probability of delivery before week 32 by cervical length (millimeters) and gestational age in weeks at time of measurement	151
Table 2.54.	Determining risk of preterm delivery in parous women at 24 weeks gestation	152
Table 2.55.	Predictive value of FFN testing in women with signs and symptoms of preterm labor	152
Table 2.56.	Predictive value of FFN testing in women with risk factors for preterm delivery but no symptoms	152
Table 2.57.	Common tocolytic agents	154
Table 2.58.	Inclusion criteria, treatment regimens, and outcomes of large randomized control trials of magnesium neuroprotection and cerebral palsy	156
Table 2.59.	General guidance regarding obstetric interventions for threatened and imminent periviable birth by best estimate of gestational age	157
Table 2.60.	Management of PROM based on gestational age	160

Tables

Table 2.61.	Timing of embryonic division in monozygotic twinning	162
Table 2.62.	Morbidity and mortality in multiple pregnancies	163
Table 2.63.	Staging for twin-twin transfusion syndrome	164
Table 2.64.	Number of cesarean sections needed to prevent one instance of composite morbidity and mortality	164
Table 2.65.	Risk factors associated with fetal intrauterine growth restriction	167
Table 2.66.	Evaluation and management of the IUGR fetus	167
Table 2.67.	Timing of delivery in cases of intrauterine growth restriction	168
Table 2.68.	Medical management of asthma in pregnancy	169
Table 2.69.	NAEPP asthma classification	170
Table 2.70.	Dosages of commonly used asthma medications in pregnancy	170
Table 2.71.	Drugs for treating an acute severe asthma exacerbation in pregnancy	171
Table 2.72.	Maternal cardiovascular and offspring risk scores and modified WHO classification of maternal risk	172
Table 2.73.	Recommendations for the evaluation and care of women of childbearing age with mechanical valve prostheses who are taking anticoagulants	174
Table 2.74.	Classification of valvular heart lesions according to maternal, fetal, and neonatal risk	175
Table 2.75.	Fetal effects of, maternal indications for, and risks associated with drugs used in the treatment of maternal valvular heart disease	176
Table 2.76.	Arguments in favor and against use of IADPSG threshold OGTT values for diagnosing GDM	179
Table 2.77.	Pharmacokinetic profiles of insulin analogs and human insulins	180
Table 2.78.	Anticipated insulin dosage as a function of gestational age	181
Table 2.79.	Insulin drip sliding scale for patients in labor	182
Table 2.80.	Management of DKA during pregnancy	183
Table 2.81.	White classification of diabetes	183
Table 2.82.	Diagnostic criteria for preeclampsia	184
Table 2.83.	Severe features of preeclampsia (any of these findings)	184
Table 2.84.	Risk factors for preeclampsia	185
Table 2.85.	Preconception risk factors for preeclampsia	185
Table 2.86.	Pregnancy-related risk factors for preeclampsia	186
Table 2.87.	Complication rates in women with superimposed preeclampsia vs. women without hypertension	186
Table 2.88.	Order set for severe intrapartum or postpartum hypertension initial first-line management with labetalol	189
Table 2.89.	Order set for severe intrapartum or postpartum hypertension initial first-line management with hydralazine	190
Table 2.90.	Order set for severe intrapartum or postpartum hypertension initial first-line management with oral nifedipine	191
Table 2.91.	Magnesium sulfate toxicity	191
Table 2.92.	Laboratory evaluation of preeclampsia	192
Table 2.93.	Antihypertensive agents used for urgent blood pressure control in pregnancy	192
Table 2.94.	Common oral antihypertensive agents in pregnancy	193
Table 2.95.	Signs and symptoms of eclampsia	193
Table 2.96.	Usual times of onset of eclampsia	194
Table 2.97.	Maternal complications associated with preeclampsia	194
Table 2.98.	Management of eclamptic seizure	195
Table 2.99.	Evaluation and management of women at risk for preeclampsia recurrence	196
Table 2.100.	Etiology and differential diagnosis of postpartum hypertension	198
Table 2.101.	Frequency of various signs and symptoms among imitators of preeclampsia–eclampsia	198
Table 2.102.	Frequency and severity of laboratory findings among imitators of preeclampsia–eclampsia	199
Table 2.103.	Characteristics of common liver disease in pregnancy	199
Table 2.104.	Estimate of stillbirth risk for selected maternal risk factors	202
Table 2.105.	Elements of the stillbirth evaluation	203
Table 2.106.	Etiologies of nonimmune hydrops fetalis	207
Table 2.107.	Therapy for selected etiologies of nonimmune hydrops	208
Table 2.108.	Non-Rhesus-D antibodies associated with hemolytic disease of the fetus and newborn	210
Table 2.109.	Classification criteria for systemic lupus erythematosus: clinical and immunologic criteria used in the SLICC classification system	213

ILLUSTRATIONS — Tables

Table	Title	Page
Table 2.110.	Revised classification criteria for the antiphospholipid syndrome	217
Table 2.111.	Treatment of pregnant women with APS	218
Table 2.112.	Risk of venous thromboembolism with different thrombophilias	219
Table 2.113.	How to test for thrombophilias	220
Table 2.114.	Anticoagulation regimen definitions	221
Table 2.115.	Recommended thromboprophylaxis for pregnancies complicated by inherited thrombophilias	221
Table 2.116.	Prevalence and risk of reoccurrence of adverse pregnancy outcome without thrombophilia	223
Table 2.117.	Relative risk of recurrent VTE in pregnancy	223
Table 2.118.	Characteristics of thrombocytopenia	226
Table 2.119.	Commonly used antiepileptic	227
Table 2.120.	Changes in thyroid function studies in normal pregnancy and in thyroid disease	231
Table 2.121.	Diagnostic criteria for thyroid storm	234
Table 3.1.	Ethnic-specific genetic carrier screening	242
Table 3.2.	Genetic disorders in the Ashkenazi Jewish population	243
Table 3.3.	Current ACOG and ACMG screening guidelines	244
Table 3.4.	Carrier frequency for cystic fibrosis, Fragile X, and spinal muscular atrophy	244
Table 3.5.	*CFTR* mutations in men with congenital absence of the vas deferens	245
Table 3.6.	Risk of expansion of Fragile X in next generation	247
Table 3.7.	Types of SMA	249
Table 3.8.	Incidence of chromosome abnormalities by maternal age	255
Table 3.9.	Chromosomal abnormalities at amniocentesis	256
Table 3.10.	Features of common chromosome abnormalities	257
Table 3.11.	Aneuploid risk of most common major anomalies	258
Table 3.12.	Management of ultrasonographic markers for aneuploidy	259
Table 3.13.	Characteristics, advantages, and disadvantages of common screening tests for aneuploidy	263
Table 3.14.	Adverse pregnancy outcomes associated with maternal serum markers for aneuploidy	265
Table 3.15.	Management recommendations for women with maternal serum markers for aneuploidy but without evident aneuploidy	266
Table 3.16.	Neural tube defect pathophysiology	267
Table 3.17.	Safety of common over-the-counter medications during pregnancy	268
Table 3.18.	Psychiatric medications during pregnancy and breastfeeding	270
Table 3.19.	Medications contraindicated during pregnancy	271
Table 4.1.	Guidelines for transvaginal ultrasonographic diagnosis of pregnancy failure in a woman with an intrauterine pregnancy of uncertain viability*	279
Table 4.2.	Diagnostic and management guidelines related to the possibility of a viable intrauterine pregnancy in a woman with a pregnancy of unknown location*	279
Table 5.1.	Percentage of women experiencing an unintended pregnancy during the first year of typical use and the first year of perfect use of contraception, and the percentage continuing use at the end of the first year	283
Table 5.2.	Classification of migraine	285
Table 5.3.	Reductions in cancer risks with use of specific contraceptive methods compared with nonusers	285
Table 5.4.	Medical eligibility criteria for contraceptive use	286
Table 5.5.	Pharmacologic profiles of progesterone and various progestins	293
Table 5.6.	Summary of oral contraceptives and cancer	297
Table 5.7.	Currently available oral contraceptives	302
Table 5.8.	Timing of initiation of Nexplanon	312
Table 5.9.	Options for emergency contraception	313
Table 5.10.	Oral contraceptives that can be used for emergency contraception in the United States	314
Table 5.11.	Five-year cumulative pregnancy rates and side effects leading to discontinuation of IUD	316
Table 5.12.	Some characteristics of essure and adiana	321
Table 5.13.	Pregnancy rates by sterilization methods	322
Table 6.1.	Suggested "normal" limits for menstrual parameters in the midreproductive years	323
Table 6.2.	Systemic etiologies for abnormal uterine bleeding	325
Table 6.3.	Genital tract disorders leading to abnormal uterine bleeding	325
Table 6.4.	Causes of abnormal uterine bleeding by age group	326
Table 6.5.	Clinical screening for an underlying disorder of hemostasis in the patient with excessive bleeding	328
Table 6.6.	Summary of initial evaluation of the patient with abnormal uterine bleeding	328

Tables

Table 6.7.	Medical options to treat acute abnormal uterine bleeding	330
Table 6.8.	Medical options to treat abnormal uterine bleeding	331
Table 6.9.	Outcomes of endometrial ablation	334
Table 6.10.	Contraindications to global endometrial ablation	334
Table 6.11.	Recommended preoperative checklist for global endometrial ablation	334
Table 6.12.	Useful ultrasonographic findings in the evaluation of women at risk for an ectopic pregnancy	337
Table 6.13.	Treatment outcomes for ectopic pregnancy	338
Table 6.14.	Contraindications to MTX therapy of ectopic pregnancy	340
Table 6.15.	Single-dose MTX treatment protocol for ectopic pregnancy	340
Table 6.16.	Two-dose MTX treatment protocol for ectopic pregnancy	341
Table 6.17.	Multi-dose MTX treatment protocol for ectopic pregnancy	341
Table 6.18.	Caveats for physicians and patients regarding the use of MTX	342
Table 6.19.	Predictors of failure of methotrexate treatment for ectopic pregnancy	342
Table 6.20.	Causes of false-positive serum hCG	347
Table 6.21.	Management of spontaneous abortion	349
Table 6.22.	Absolute contraindications to mifepristone/misoprostol for medical abortion	350
Table 6.23.	Comparison of common medical abortion regimens	351
Table 6.24.	Drug therapies for the prevention of sexually transmitted infections and pregnancy after sexual assault	354
Table 6.25.	Medical treatment of chronic pelvic pain	357
Table 6.26.	Strategies for treating primary dysmenorrhea	359
Table 6.27.	Progestins in the medical management of endometriosis	361
Table 6.28.	Descriptions of least function terms for Endometriosis Fertility Index scoring	364
Table 6.29.	Add-back therapy for patients treated with GnRH-agonists	367
Table 6.30.	Use of add-back therapy for patients on long-term GnRH-agonists	367
Table 6.31.	Options for evaluation of the uterus	369
Table 6.32.	Comparison of hysteroscopic distension media	370
Table 6.33.	Patient-controlled analgesia	371
Table 6.34.	Post-operative pain management	372
Table 6.35.	Common findings for the different types of urinary incontinence	373
Table 6.36.	Differential diagnosis of urinary incontinence in women	373
Table 6.37.	Common causes of transient urinary incontinence	374
Table 6.38.	DIAPPERS mnemonic for transient causes of urinary incontinence	374
Table 6.39.	Common medications used to treat urinary incontinence	375
Table 6.40.	Therapy to facilitate urine storage/bladder filling	376
Table 6.41.	Treatment options for vulvodynia	381
Table 6.42.	Complications of uterine fibroids during pregnancy	384
Table 7.1.	Procedures for collecting clinical specimens for culture of group B *Streptococcus* (GBS) at 35–37 weeks' gestation	387
Table 7.2.	Comparison of key points in the 2002 and 2010 centers for disease control and prevention guidelines for the prevention of perinatal group B streptococcal disease	388
Table 7.3.	Indications and nonindications for intrapartum antibiotic prophylaxis to prevent early-onset group B streptococcal (GBS) disease	389
Table 7.4.	Clinical diagnosis of chorioamnionitis	395
Table 7.5.	Drug regimens for the treatment of mastitis	398
Table 7.6.	Patient information: what to do if you develop mastitis	398
Table 7.7.	Overview of viral hepatitis	399
Table 7.8.	Interpretation of serologic test results* for hepatitis B	402
Table 7.9.	Interpretation of serologic test results for hepatitis B	403
Table 7.10.	Recommended doses of currently licensed formulation for hepatitis B vaccine	404
Table 7.11.	Interpretation of results of tests for hepatitis C virus (HCV) infection and further actions	405
Table 7.12.	Use of antiretroviral drugs during pregnancy	410
Table 7.13.	What to start: initial combination regimens for antiretroviral-naive pregnant women	411
Table 7.14.	HIV-infected pregnant women who have never received antiretroviral drugs (antiretroviral naive)	413
Table 7.15.	HIV-infected pregnant women who are currently receiving antiretroviral therapy	413
Table 7.16.	HIV-infected pregnant women who have previously received antiretroviral treatment or prophylaxis but are not currently receiving any antiretroviral medications	414

Table 7.17.	Monitoring of the woman and fetus during pregnancy	415
Table 7.18.	Antiretroviral drug resistance and resistance testing in pregnancy	416
Table 7.19.	Lack of viral suppression	417
Table 7.20.	Stopping antiretroviral drugs during pregnancy	417
Table 7.21.	Intrapartum antiretroviral therapy/prophylaxis	418
Table 7.22.	Transmission and mode of delivery	419
Table 7.23.	Other intrapartum management considerations	419
Table 7.24.	Postpartum management	420
Table 7.25.	Serological criteria for the determination of the *Toxoplasma gondii* infection stage in acquired toxoplasmosis	424
Table 7.26.	Criteria for the timing of *Toxoplasma gondii* infection versus conception in pregnant women and after childbirth	425
Table 7.27.	Clinical management of a pregnant woman with suspected Zika virus infection	431
Table 7.28.	Immunization during pregnancy	432
Table 7.29.	Key information regarding currently available human papillomavirus vaccines	439
Table 7.30.	Treatment regimens for uncomplicated acute bacterial cystitis	443
Table 7.31.	Diagnostic tests available for vaginitis	444
Table 7.32.	2015 CDC guidelines for treatment of vulvovaginal candidiasis	445
Table 7.33.	Diagnostic testing for STIs	446
Table 7.34.	2015 CDC guidelines for treatment of chlamydia	447
Table 7.35.	2015 CDC guidelines for treatment of gonorrhea	447
Table 7.36.	2015 CDC guidelines for treatment of bacterial vaginosis	448
Table 7.37.	2015 CDC guidelines for treatment of trichomoniasis	448
Table 7.38.	Ulcerative lesions in sexually transmitted diseases	449
Table 7.39.	2015 CDC guidelines for treatment of HSV	451
Table 7.40.	2015 CDC guidelines for treatment of syphilis	452
Table 7.41.	Classification, clinical presentation, and adverse perinatal effects of syphilis	453
Table 7.42.	Oral desensitization protocol for pregnant women with allergies to penicillin	453
Table 7.43.	2015 CDC guidelines for treatment of pelvic inflammatory disease (PID)	456
Table 7.44.	2015 CDC guidelines for external anogenital warts	457
Table 7.45.	Comparison of treatment modalities for external anogenital warts	457
Table 7.46.	Reported clearance and recurrence rates for EGW therapies	458
Table 7.47.	Recommendations for tetanus prophylaxis in routine wound management	459
Table 7.48.	Antimicrobial prophylactic regimens by procedure	460
Table 7.49.	Rates of resistance and dosing of oral agents for treatment of community acquired MRSA infections	461
Table 7.50.	Diagnostic testing for *C. difficile*	462
Table 7.51.	CDI severity scoring system and summary of recommended treatments	462
Table 8.1.	Etiology of infertility	464
Table 8.2.	Prevalence of infertility	465
Table 8.3.	Probability for natural conception by age and month of trying	466
Table 8.4.	Clinical usefulness of AMH values	470
Table 8.5.	Comparison of ovarian reserve markers FSH and AMH	470
Table 8.6.	Normal values for semen analysis	473
Table 8.7.	Hormone profiles of men with normal and abnormal spermatogenesis	474
Table 8.8.	Live birth rates in PCOS patients using clomiphene vs. letrozole	478
Table 8.9.	"Rule of 5s" and "rule of 7s" for ovulation induction	478
Table 8.10.	Use of electrocautery and/or recombinant FSH for ovulation induction in the PCOS patient	479
Table 8.11.	Live birth, multiple live birth, clinical pregnancy, multiple clinical pregnancy, and conception rates per cycle	480
Table 8.12.	Gonadotropin preparations	482
Table 8.13.	Gonadotropin-releasing hormone agonist/antagonist preparations	483
Table 8.14.	Criteria for number of embryos to transfer in IVF	488
Table 8.15.	Risk of birth defects following IVF or IVF/ICSI	490
Table 8.16.	Mechanism of adverse effect of hydrosapinx upon ART success	495
Table 8.17.	Incidence of sporadic miscarriage (SM) or recurrent miscarriage (RM) in different age groups	497
Table 8.18.	Prognostic value of transvaginal ultrasound observation of embryonic heart activity	498
Table 8.19.	Etiologies of evidence-based tests when evaluating recurrent pregnancy loss	498

Tables — ILLUSTRATIONS

Table 8.20.	Risk of an abnormal live birth in a patient with a translocation	501
Table 8.21.	Estimating the probability of a miscarried embryo/fetus with an abnormal karyotype according to the number of previous miscarriages and maternal age	502
Table 8.22.	Comparison of congenital and acquired uterine anomalies identified in women (primary vs. secondary RPL)	503
Table 8.23.	Revised classification criteria for the antiphospholipid syndrome	507
Table 8.24.	Treatment of pregnant women with APS	508
Table 8.25.	Rate of pregnancy loss in subsequent pregnancy in patients with a history of recurrent pregnancy loss	509
Table 8.26.	Prognosis for livebirth in patients with recurrent pregnancy loss	510
Table 8.27.	Fertility preservation options	515
Table 9.1.	Suggested normal limits for menstrual parameters in the midreproductive years	519
Table 9.2.	Tanner staging of breast and pubic hair	522
Table 9.3.	Relative frequency of delayed pubertal abnormalities	525
Table 9.4.	Distribution of diagnoses in 80 girls referred for precocious puberty	526
Table 9.5.	Types of benign pubertal variants	527
Table 9.6.	Clinical characteristics of forms of early pubertal development	528
Table 9.7.	Etiologies of GnRH-independent and GnRH-dependent precocious puberty	529
Table 9.8.	Central (gonadotropin-dependent) precocious puberty	530
Table 9.9.	Peripheral precocity (gonadotropin-independent precocious puberty)	531
Table 9.10.	Distribution of causes of primary amenorrhea	533
Table 9.11.	Mnemonic for primary amenorrhea differential diagnosis: XMAS	534
Table 9.12.	Mayer-Rokitansky-Kuster-Hauser syndrome (müllerian agenesis) vs. androgen insensitivity syndrome	534
Table 9.13.	Distribution of causes of secondary amenorrhea	535
Table 9.14.	Causes of intrauterine adhesions	535
Table 9.15.	Recommended diagnostic schemes for polycystic ovary syndrome by varying expert groups	537
Table 9.16.	Other diagnoses to exclude in all women before making a diagnosis of PCOS	538
Table 9.17.	Diagnoses to consider excluding in select women, depending on presentation	539
Table 9.18.	Suggested evaluation for patients with polycystic ovary syndrome	540
Table 9.19.	Accepted values for glucose tolerance testing	542
Table 9.20.	Prevalence of different androgen excess disorders in 950 women referred because of clinical hyperandrogenism organ dysfunction	543
Table 9.21.	Potential long-term consequences of polycystic ovary syndrome	543
Table 9.22.	Prevalence of nonclassic congenital adrenal hyperplasia (NCCAH) by ethnic group	547
Table 9.23.	Interpretation of Cortrosyn stimulation test in evaluation of CAH	547
Table 9.24.	Different forms of the prolactin hormone	554
Table 9.25.	Prevalence of increased prolactin with the following signs and symptoms	555
Table 9.26.	Potential causes of hyperprolactinemia	556
Table 9.27.	Dopamine agonists commonly used in the treatment of hyperprolactinemia	560
Table 9.28.	Hormonal assessment of the clinically nonfunctional pituitary mass	563
Table 9.29.	Changes in thyroid function test results in normal pregnancy and in thyroid disease	565
Table 9.30.	Comparison of the recommendations of different organizations in evaluation and treatment of hypothyroidism	566
Table 10.1.	Stages of the menopausal transition	571
Table 10.2.	Definitions of the spectrum of menopause	572
Table 10.3.	Onset and duration of hot flushes in the menopausal transition	574
Table 10.4.	Approved oral estrogen products for menopausal symptoms	575
Table 10.5.	Treatment options for menopausal vasomotor symptoms	576
Table 10.6.	Treatment options for menopausal vaginal symptoms	577
Table 10.7.	Approved transdermal estrogen products for menopausal symptoms	578
Table 10.8.	Approved vaginal estrogen products for menopausal symptoms	579
Table 10.9.	Diagnostic tests in the work-up of secondary osteoporosis	584
Table 10.10.	Government-approved drugs for postmenopausal osteoporosis	586
Table 11.1.	Pathologic classification of endometrial hyperplasia	592
Table 11.2.	Regression, persistence, and progression rates of endometrial hyperplasia	592
Table 11.3.	Risk factors for endometrial carcinoma	595
Table 11.4.	Endometrial cancer: staging and treatment	597

ILLUSTRATIONS — Tables

Table 11.5.	Frequency of nodal metastases in endometrial cancer	598
Table 11.6.	Risk factors associated with precancerous changes and cancer of the cervix	599
Table 11.7.	Common genital HPV genotypes	600
Table 11.8.	Risk of CIN2, CIN3, and cancer based on cytology and HPV status in women 30–64 years of age	602
Table 11.9.	Cervical cytology screening guideline recommendations	603
Table 11.10.	Risk of progression and rate of regression	604
Table 11.11.	Cervical cancer staging and treatment	617
Table 11.12.	Ovarian, fallopian tube, peritoneal cancer staging and treatment	625
Table 11.13.	Types of malignant germ cell tumors	627
Table 11.14.	Tumor markers in germ cell cancer	629
Table 11.15.	Tumor markers in sex cord-stromal cell tumors	630
Table 11.16.	Vulvar cancer staging and treatment	633
Table 11.17.	Vaginal cancer staging	634
Table 11.18.	Features of partial and complete hydatidiform moles	635
Table 11.19.	Diagnosis and evaluation of GTN	636
Table 11.20.	Management of hydatidiform mole	636
Table 11.21.	Management of low-risk nonmetastatic or low-risk metastatic GTN	637
Table 11.22.	WHO prognostic scoring for GTN	637
Table 11.23.	Anatomic FIGO staging system for GTN	638
Table 11.24.	Management of high-risk GTN	638
Table 11.25.	Surveillance during and after therapy of GTN	638
Table 11.30.	Comparison of SBO with ileus	657
Table 11.31.	Treatment of chemotherapy extravasation injury	658
Table 11.32.	Body fluid composition	659
Table 11.33.	Steroids	659
Table 11.34.	Hemodynamic therapy	662
Table 11.35.	Derivation of hemodynamic parameters	663
Table 11.36.	Normal hemodynamic values	663
Table 11.37.	SHOCK: hemodynamic profiles	663
Table 11.38.	Stanford hospital guide for preventing venous thromboembolism	669
Table 11.39.	Venous thromboembolism prophylaxis—Inova Fairfax Hospital	670
Table 11.40.	Overview of traditional and newer antithrombotic agents.*	671
Table 11.41.	Blood products	674
Table 11.42.	Differential diagnosis of acid/base disturbances	675
Table 12.1.	Risk and protective factors for developing breast cancer	678
Table 12.2.	Breast cancer screening for average-risk patient: breast self-exam (BSE) and clinical breast exam (CBE)	679
Table 12.3.	Breast cancer screening for average-risk patients: mammography	680
Table 12.4.	Breast cancer screening for average-risk patients: MRI as an adjuvant screening tool	681
Table 12.5.	Breast cancer screening recommendations: *BRCA* testing	682
Table 12.6.	Ontario family history assessment tool	684
Table 12.7.	Manchester scoring system	685
Table 12.8.	Family history screen-7	685
Table 12.9.	Pedigree assessment tool	686
Table 12.10.	Referral scoring tool	687

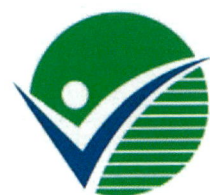

Index

A

abdominal dehiscence, 673
abdominal hysterectomy, 706
abnormal uterine bleeding, 323–334
  age-related causes, 326t
  chronic patterns, 330t
  clinical screening, 328t
  endometrial carcinoma, 594
  fibroids and, 384
  initial evaluation, 327, 328t, 333f
  laboratory testing, 327
  menstrual normal limits, 323t
  PALM-COEIN classification, 324f
  secondary evaluation, 329, 333f–333f
  systemic etiologies, 325t
  treatment, 329, 330t, 331, 331t, 332t
abortion, spontaneous
  management of, 349t, 350t, 351t
abruptio placentae. See placental abruption
acid/base disturbances, 675, 675t
acne
  oral contraceptives and, 301
acquired anemia, 67t
acromegaly
  hyperprolactinemia, 562
  PCOS diagnosis vs., 539t
acupressure/acupuncture
  nausea and vomiting in pregnancy, 61
acute sinusitis, 53, 54t
add-back therapy
  gonadotropin-releasing hormone (GnRH) analogs, 366, 367t
adenomas
  screening for older women, 6t–7t
adnexal masses, 620f, 621f, 622f
adoption
  genetics testing and, 262
adrenocorticotropic hormone (ACTH)
  congenital adrenal hyperplasia nomogram, 548f

adults
  immunization schedule for, 9f
  screening, prevention, and counseling recommendations for, 1t–3t
adverse reactions
  gonadotropin-releasing hormone (GnRH) analogs, 366
  injectable contraceptives, 308–309
  progestin-only oral contraceptives, 306
  transdermal contraceptives, 307
age
  abnormal uterine bleeding patterns and, 326t
  cervical dysplasia/cervical intraepithelial neoplasia management and, 606f, 607f
  diminished ovarian reserve and, 471–472, 471f
  infertility prevalence and, 465f
  maternal age, fetal chromosome abnormalities incidence and, 255t
  onset of puberty, 520, 521f
  recurrent pregnancy loss and, 497, 497t
alcohol abuse
  CAGE screening test, 46t
  TWEAK screening test, 46t
alpha-globin genes, 251, 252f
alpha-thalassemia, 251, 252f
alternative medicine/botanicals
  drug interactions, 55t–56t
  effects in surgical patients, 57t
amenorrhea
  evaluation algorithm, 536f
  oral contraceptives and, 300–301, 301f
  postcontraceptive risk of, 299
  primary amenorrhea, 533, 533t, 534t
  secondary, 534, 535t

American College of Obstetricians and Gynecologists (ACOG) guidelines
  cervical insufficiency, 142–143
  genetic screening, 244t
  operative vaginal delivery, 87t
  recurrent pregnancy loss, 498
  urinary tract infections in pregnancy, 443
American Society for Colposcopy and Cervical Pathology (ASCCP), 604
American Society for Reproductive Medicine (ASRM)
  endometriosis classifications, 362f–363f
  recurrent pregnancy loss definition, 498
amniocentesis
  fetal chromosome abnormalities, 256t
  genetics testing and, 262
amnioinfusion, 124, 124f, 125t
Androgen Excess-Polycystic Ovary Syndrome Society Task Force
  PCOS ultrasound criteria, 538
androgen insensitivity syndrome, 523, 534t
androgen levels
  hirsutism, 552
  hyperandrogenism organ dysfunction, 543t
  polycystic ovarian syndrome, 541f
  sources of androgen production, 552t
androgen-secreting tumor
  PCOS diagnosis vs., 539t
anemia, in pregnancy, 67t–68t
aneuploidies, 254, 258t
  gamete/embryo donation, 261
  maternal serum test and pregnancy outcomes, 265t–266t
  screening benefits and limits for, 263t–264t
  ultrasonographic markers, 259t

765

INDEX

antenatal steroids
  preterm birth risk and, 153–154
antepartum care
  HIV and pregnancy, 415t, 416t
antepartum fetal surveillance, 105–107, 105t, 106t, 108t, 109t–111t
  diagnostic imaging, 114, 114t, 115t–116t
  multiple gestation, 162–163
anthrax
  immunization during pregnancy, 436
antiandrogens
  polycystic ovarian syndrome, 544
antibiotic prophylaxis, 460t
*antibiotic typo on pg. 460, 460
anticoagulation regimen
  guidelines, 671t
  thromboembolic disorders in pregnancy, 221t
antiepileptics
  in pregnancy, 227t, 229
antihistamines
  nausea and vomiting in pregnancy, 64t
antihyperglycemic therapy
  type 2 diabetes, 39f
antihypertensive drugs
  dosing strategies, 35t
  evidence-based dosing, 34t
  guidelines for, 32–33
  in pregnancy, 192t, 193t
anti-Müllerian Hormone (AMH)
  ovarian reserve testing, 469, 470t
antineoplastic agents
  emetogenic potential, 642f, 643f
antiphospholipid syndrome (APS) in pregnancy, 217t
  management of, 218t
  recurrent pregnancy loss and, 506, 507t, 508–509
antiretroviral drugs
  intrapartum therapy in pregnancy and, 418t
  resistance in pregnancy, 416t
  stopping during pregnancy, 417t
  use during pregnancy, 410t, 411t–412t, 413t, 414t
antismoking agents, 44t–45t
antisperm antibodies
  semen analysis, 473
anti-thyroid antibody testing, 567t–568t
antral follicle count (AFC)
  ovarian reserve testing, 470–471
aortic arch scan, 276f
Apgar score, 104t

aromatase inhibitors
  ovulation induction, 477
arterial blood gases interpretation, 675, 675t
arteriosclerotic cardiovascular diseases (ASCVD)
  risk of, 21
  statin therapy for, 21, 23f–24f, 26
Ashkenazi Jewish disorders, 242, 242t, 243t
assisted reproductive technologies (ART), 482–494
  cancer risk of fertility treatments, 490
  definitions, 482
  embryo transfer, 488, 488t
  hydrosalpinx and, 495t
  oocyte retrieval, 486–487, 487f
  ovarian hyperstimulation syndrome and, 491–494, 492f
  ovarian stimulation protocols and doses, 483–486, 483f–486f
  postretrieval hormonal management, 488
asthma
  in pregnancy, 169, 169t, 170t, 171t
atypical squamous cells of undetermined significance (ASC-US)
  cervical dysplasia/intraepithelial neoplasia, 606f
autosomal recessive inheritance
  congenital adrenal hyperplasia, 546f
  gene mutations, male factor infertility, 475
  screening for, 239–240, 239f

B

bacterial vaginosis
  CDC treatment guidelines, 448t
Bakri balloon
  postpartum hemorrhage tamponade, 139, 139f
barrier contraceptives, 291
BCG vaccine
  immunization during pregnancy, 436
beta-globin genes, 252–253
beta-human chorionic gonadotropin
  false-positive test result, 347, 347t, 348f
  methotrexate for ectopic pregnancy and, 338, 342t
beta-thalassemia, 252, 253f

bevacizumab IV
  ovarian cancer, 626
biophysical profile (BPP)
  fetal assessment, 106t, 107, 108t
birth defects
  in vitro fertilization and risk of, 490, 490t
birthweight
  shoulder dystocia risk and, 84t
Bishop scoring for cervical ripening, 76t
bisphosphonates
  osteoporosis treatment, 586t
blood component therapy
  post partum hemorrhage, 133t
blood pressure
  antihypertensive agents in pregnancy and, 192t, 193t
  comparison of goal BP and drug therapy, 36t
  hypertension, 32
  management algorithm, 37t
blood products, 674t
blood samples
  drug abuse detection limits, 45t
B-Lynch suture
  postpartum hemorrhage, 138f
body fluid composition, 659t
body mass index (BMI)
  gestational diabetes, 179
  nomogram, 15f, 16t–17t
  table, 18t
body surface nomogram
  ectopic pregnancy, 343f
bone turnover biochemical markers
  osteoporosis assessment, 585
bony pelvis
  anatomy, 694f
  classification, 69t
botanicals. See alternative medicine/botanicals
brachial plexus injury
  shoulder dystocia, 85
BRCA 1/BRCA 2
  breast cancer screening, 682t, 684t
  ovarian cancer risk, 623
breakthrough bleeding
  oral contraceptives, 300
breast abscess, 397–398, 397f
breast cancer
  incidence and prevalence, 677
  oral contraceptives and, 296
  risk and protective factors, 678t
  screening guidelines, 679–687
breastfeeding
  mastitis and breast abscess, 397–398, 397f

766

INDEX

maternal varicella and, 421
oral contraceptives, 298–299
psychiatric medications during, 270t
tuberculosis and, 408
bromocriptine
 hyperprolactinemia, 560t, 561

C

cabergoline
 hyperprolactinemia, 560t, 561
CAGE screening test
 alcohol abuse, 46t
calcitonin
 osteoporosis treatment, 587t
Caldwell-Maloy pelvic classification, 69f
caloric requirements
 in pregnancy, 66
cancer. See also specific cancers
 antineoplastic agents, emetogenic potential, 642f, 643f
 break-through chemotherapy, 649f
 cancer-related infections, 654f, 655f
 chemotherapy, break-through treatment, 649f
 chemotherapy, emetogenic potential, 645f, 646f, 647f, 648f
 contraception and risk reduction of, 285t
 fertility treatment and risk of, 490
 ileus vs. small bowel obstruction, 657t
 low-risk outpatient therapy, 651f, 652f
 neutropenic fever management, 650f, 653f, 656f
 oral contraceptives and, 296–297, 297t
 pain management guidelines, 640f
 prevalence and incidence statistics, 591f
carbohydrate metabolism
 oral contraceptives, 294
cardiovascular disease
 hypercholesterolemia, 21–28
 lipid lowering drugs, 29t–30t
 women's risk of, 19t, 20f
carrier screening, 239–244
 ACOG/ACMG guidelines, 244t
 alpha-thalassemia, 251, 252f
 autosomal recessive inheritance, 239–240, 239t

cystic fibrosis, 244t
ethnic specific screening, 242, 242t
Fragile X, 244t, 248
pan ethnic/extended carrier screening, 241
spinal muscular atrophy, 244t, 249–250, 250f
catheters
 triple lumen catheter, 660, 660f
CDA 2008 algorithm
 gestational diabetes screening, 178f
CDC treatment guidelines
 external genital warts, 457t
 herpes simplex virus, 451t
 pelvic inflammatory disease, 456t
 sexually transmitted diseases, 447t–448t
 syphilis, 452t, 453t
cell-free DNA test, 264t
cerclage, cervical insufficiency, 142–143
 emergency/rescue cerclage, 146–147
 McDonald cerclage, 143, 144f
 membrane prolapse, 147f
 Shirodkar cerclage, modification, 143, 145f
 transabdominal cerclage, 143, 146f
cerebral palsy
 magnesium sulfate and reduction of, 156f
cervical cancer
 evaluation, 615–616
 follow-up, 618
 incidence and prevalence, 615
 lymphovascular space invasion/stromal invasion, 618t
 oral contraceptives and, 296
 in pregnancy, 619f
 risk factors, 615
 staging and treatment, 617t, 618–619
cervical cap (Pretif), 291
cervical dilation
 normal labor, 74t
cervical dysplasia/cervical intraepithelial neoplasia
 adenocarcinoma in situ, 613f
 ASCCP definitions, 604
 atypical glandular cells, 610f
 atypical squamous cells: cannot exclude high-grade SIL, 608f, 609f
 atypical squamous cells of undetermined significance, 606f
 cervical dysplasia screening, 601, 603t

cytology screening guidelines, 604t
 diagnosis, 602
 genital HPV genotypes, 600t
 grade 1 lesions, 611f, 612f
 grade 2 and 3 lesions, 612f, 613f
 high-grade squamous intraepithelial lesion (HSIL), 609f
 low-grade squamous intraepithelial lesions, 607f
 management, 614
 overview, 599
 pathophysiology, 600, 601f
 in pregnancy, management of, 608f, 613f, 614
 risk factors, 599t, 602t, 604t
 unsatisfactory cytology, 605f
cervical insufficiency, 142–143, 143f, 144f, 145–146, 145f, 146f
cervical ripening
 Bishop scoring for, 76t
 Cook® cervical ripening balloon, 78
cervix
 measurement criteria, 280–281, 280f
cesarean delivery, 91–99
 Druzin splint maneuver, 96, 97f
 indications, 91t
 maternal morbidity, 98t
 multiple gestation, 164, 164t
 neonatal morbidity and mortality, 102t
 operative reports, 701–702
 operative techniques, 96t
 placenta previa and accreta and, 99t
 prevention of, 94t–95t
 risks associated with, 92t
 shoulder dystocia, 84
 uterine incision, 96, 97f
chemotherapy
 break-through treatment, 649f
 emetogenic potential, 645f, 646f, 647f, 648f
 extravasation injury, 658f
chlamydia
 CDC treatment guidelines, 447t
chorioamnionitis, 394, 395f
choriocarcinoma, 627t, 628, 629t
chorionic villus sampling (CVS), 262
chromosome abnormalities
 features, 257t
 fetal assessment, 254–260, 255t, 256t, 501, 502t
 recurrent pregnancy loss and, 499, 499f–500f, 501, 501t
 testicular function impairment, 475

767

INDEX

chronic hypertension, 184
  preeclampsia and, 186, 186t
chronic sinusitis, 53
cleft deformities
  methylprednisolone and, 61
clinical pelvimetry, 69–70, 69f, 69t–70t
clomiphene (SERM)
  ovulation induction, 477, 478t
  resistance to, alternative optioncs, 478
clomiphene citrate challenge test (CCCT)
  ovarian reserve testing, 469
Clostridium difficile infection, 462t
cluster headache
  characteristics and classification, 47, 47t
coagulation cascade, 665f
coagulopathy, 674
Cochrane Library Review
  on ovarian drilling, 479
colorectal cancer
  oral contraceptives and, 297
  risk factor-based screening, 8t
  screening for older women, 6t–7t
colposcopy
  ASCCP definitions, 604
  cervical dysplasia/cervical intraepithelial neoplasia diagnosis, 602, 602t
complementary medicines
  drug interactions, 55t–56t
  effects in surgical patients, 57
complications of pregnancy
  maternal heart disease, 172t, 173
  preeclampsia, 194t, 196t
  recurrent pregnancy loss, 497–510
  thromboembolic disorders, 224f, 223t
  thrombophilias, risk of, 223t
  timing of delivery and, 80t–82t
  uterine fibroids, 384t
  venous thromboembolism risk assessment and prevention, 223t
conception probability, 463, 464f
  by age and month of trying, 466f
condoms, 283t, 291
congenital adrenal hyperplasia
  Cortrosyn stimulation test, 547t
  maternal carrier, treatment for, 548–549
  PCOS diagnosis, 538t

peripheral precocious puberty and, 532t
  prevalence, 546f, 547t
congenital anomalies
  uterus, 502, 503f
congenital heart disase
  maternal, preganancy and, 172t–173t
congenital malformations
  epilepsy in pregnancy and, 228
contingent screening test, 263t
contraception
  barrier contraceptives, 291
  cancer risk reduction and, 285t
  choices in, 283t–284t
  emergency postcoital oral contraception, 313, 313t, 314t–315t
  female sterilization, 319, 320f, 321, 321t, 322t
  injectable contraceptives, 308–309
  intrauterine device, 316, 316t, 317f, 318f
  medical eligibility criteria, 286t–290t
  migraine and, 285t
  oral contraceptives, 292–306
  transdermal contraceptives, 307
  vaginal contraceptive ring, 310
contraction stress test, 106t
Cook® cervical ripening balloon, 78
Coombs test
  isoimmunization evaluation, 209f
Copper T 380A IUD, 316, 317f
corticosteroids
  antenatal steroids, 153–154
  nausea and vomiting in pregnancy and, 61
Cortrosyn stimulation test
  congenital adrenal hyperplasia, 547t
craniopharyngioma, 524
cryopreservation
  gametes, 511–512
CTFR mutations, 245, 245t
Cushing syndrome
  hyperprolactinemia, 558
  PCOS diagnosis *vs.*, 539t
cyproterone acetate (Androcur)
  polycystic ovarian syndrome, 544
cystic fibrosis
  carrier screening, 244t
  gene mutations, male factor infertility, 475
  pathophysiology and genetics, 245–246, 245t, 246f
cytomegalovirus, 427

D

day 3 hormone testing
  ovarian reserve testing, 468–469, 468f
deep vein thrombosis, 666, 667f
delivery
  cesarean delivery, 91–99
  HIV in pregnancy and mode of, 419t
  insulin management during, 182, 182t
  intrauterine growth restriction, 168t
  multiple gestation, 164, 164t, 165f
  operative vaginal delivery, 86–91
  pregnancy complications and timing of, 80t–82t
  preterm, 151, 152t, 153–154, 153f, 154t, 155f, 156t
  risk assessment by mode of, 92t
  vaginal birth after cesarean, 100–102
de novo mutations
  spinal muscular atrophy, 249–250
Depo-Provera contraceptive, 283t
dexamethasone
  congenital adrenal hyperplasia, 548–549
dexamethasone testing
  hyperprolactinemia, 558
diabetes mellitus, 38–43
  in pregnancy, 178–183
  White classification of, 183t
diabetic ketoacidosis (DKA)
  during pregnancy, 183, 183t
diagnostic imaging
  guidelines in pregnancy, 114, 114t, 115t–116t
diaphragm contraception, 283t, 291
DIAPPERS mnemonic
  urinary incontinence treatment, 374t
diet
  gestational diabetes, 179
Dietary Approaches to Stop Hypertension (DASH) diet, 32
dilation and curettage, 704
disability
  gestational age and incidence of, 158f
dizygotic twinning, 162
donor egg IVF, 482
dopamine agonists
  hyperprolactinemia, 560t, 561

768

INDEX

dopamine antagonists
  nausea and vomiting in pregnancy, 64t
doxylamine
  nausea and vomiting in pregnancy, 61, 64t
drug abuse
  urine and blood sample detecion limits, 45t
drug interactions
  alternative medicines, 55t–56t
  antiepileptics, 229
  odansetron, contraindicated medications with, 62t
Druzin splint maneuver
  cesarean delivery, 96, 97f
dual-energy X-ray absorptiometry (DXA)
  osteoporosis diagnosis, 584t, 585
Duke University obstetric bleeding emergency transfusion algorithm, 133t
dysgerminoma, 627–628, 627t, 629t
dysmenorrhea, primary, 359t

E

early goal-directed therapy, intensive care unit, 664
echocardiography, fetal, 276f
eclampsia
  management, 195t
  onset of, 194t
  signs and symptoms, 193t
ectopic pregnancy
  body surface nomography, 343f
  diagnosis, 336, 337t
  locations, 336f
  pregnancy of unknown location (PUL) vs., 345
  therapy options for, 338, 339f, 340t, 341t, 342t, 343f
  treatment outcomes, 338t
eflornithine
  polycystic ovarian syndrome, 544
electrolysis
  polycystic ovarian syndrome, 545
elements
  DRI/RDA intake guidelines, 14t
embryo cryopreservation, 511–512
embryonal carcinoma, 627t, 628, 629t
embryo transfer
  in vitro fertilization, 488, 488t, 489f
emergency postcoital oral contraception, 313, 313t, 314t–315t

emesis control
  NCCN guidelines, 641f
empty sella syndrome, 558, 558f
endocrine function
  lab values, 690
  recurrent pregnancy loss and, 504
endodermal sinus tumor, 627t, 628, 629t
endometrial ablation, 334, 334t, 335f
endometrial cancer
  oral contraceptives and, 296
endometrial carcinoma
  bleeding patterns, 594
  follow-up protocol, 598
  histopathology, 595
  incidence and prevalence, 594
  nodal metastases frequency, 598t
  risk factors, 595t
  screening and diagnosis, 596
  staging, 597t
  treatment, 596, 597t
endometrial hyperplasia, 592–593, 592t
endometrioma
  removal, 495–496
endometriosis
  ASRM classification, 362f–363f
  fertility index, 364, 364t, 365f
  medical management of, 360, 361t
  pathophysiology, 360
endomyometritis, 396
end-organ perfusion
  sepsis syndrome, 672
endovaginal ultrasonography, 277–278, 277f
epidemiology
  analytic studies, 696
  bias in, 700
  case control studies, 698
  cohort studies, 697
  definition, 695
  descriptive studies, 696
  randomized clinical trials, 699–700
  study designs, 695
  study size and power analysis, 700
  terminology, 695
epilepsy in pregnancy, 227–229
  congenital malformations, 228
  fetal complications, 228
epithelial ovarian cancer, 623–624

Essure Adiana sterilization procedure, 321, 321t
estradiol
  menopausal therapy, 575t–580t
  osteoporosis treatment, 586t–588t
  ovarian reserve testing, 468–469
estrogen
  menopausal therapy with, 575t–580t
  in oral contraceptives, 292
  osteoporosis treatment, 586t–588t
ethnic specific genetic screening, 242, 242t
eugonadal puberty, 523
Evra patch contraceptive, 283t
extended carrier screening (ECS), 241
external genital warts, 457t, 458t
extravasation injury, chemotherapy, 658f

F

Factor V Leiden mutation
  recurrent pregnancy loss and, 505
fallopian tube cancer
  staging and treatment, 625t
family history
  breast cancer screening, 685t
fast track and standard treatment trial (FASTT)
  infertility treatment and, 480–481
fatty liver
  preeclampsia mimic and, 198t, 199t–200t
febrile morbidity, 396
female sterilization, 319, 320f, 321, 321t, 322t
fertility. See also infertility
  endometriosis fertility index, 364, 364t, 365f
  oral contraceptive use and, 298, 298f
  preservation options, 514, 515t
fertility awareness-based contraception, 283t
fetal anatomy scan, 273f–276f, 275
fetal assessment
  anatomic landmarks, 273f
  chromosome abnormalities, 254–260, 255t, 256t
  diagnostic imaging, 114, 114t, 115t–116t
  fetal anatomy scan, 273f–276f

769

INDEX

fetal assessment (*continued*)
  intracranial anatomy, 274f
  intrapartum evaluation, 117t–119t, 120f, 121f, 122f, 123t
  intrauterine fetal demise, 201f, 202t, 203t–204t
  intrauterine growth restriction, 167–168, 167t
  maternal heart disease, fetal effects, 176t–177t
  nonstress test, 105
  radiation absorption estimation, 115t–116t
fetal chromosomal abnormality, 501, 502t
fetal circulation
  anatomy, 692f
fetal echocardiography, 276f
fetal fibronectin testing (FFT)
  preterm birth prediction, 152t
fetal heart rate (FHR)
  ABCD checklist, 123t
  ABCD management approach, 122f
  EFM definitions, 117t–118t
  induction of labor and, 79
  intrauterine resuscication, 120f, 121t
  management of tracings, algorithm for, 120f
  three-tiered FHR interpretation, 119t
fetal lung maturity (FLM)
  respiratory distress syndrome, 72–73, 73t
fetal neuroprotection
  magnesium sulfate for, 155f, 156t
fibroblast culture
  nonimmune hydrops, 205t, 206
fibroids
  abnormal uterine bleeding and, 384
  infertility and, 384
  prevalence and classification, 383, 383f
  treatment, 385–386
finasteride
  polycystic ovarian syndrome, 544
flexion point
  vacuum extraction delivery, 89, 90f–91f
folate supplements
  epilepsy in pregnancy and, 229
  in pregnancy, 66
Foley catheter
  labor induction and, 78

follicle-stimulating hormone (FSH)
  ovarian reserve testing, 468, 468f, 470t
food purchase recommendations
  single adults, 10t–11t
forceps delivery, 86–91
  criteria, 86t
  types of forceps, 88f
four-chamber heart scan, 275f
fracture risk assessment tool (FRAX)
  osteoporosis, 582
Fragile X syndrome
  carrier screening, 244t, 248
  diminished ovarian reserve screening and, 471–472, 471f
  pathophysiology and genetics, 247–248
  risk of expansion, 247f
free androgen index
  recurrent pregnancy loss and, 504

G

gamete/embryo donation, 261
gamete intrafallopian transfer, 482
gamete preservation, 511–515, 512f, 513f, 515t
Gaskin maneuver
  shoulder dystocia, 85
genetics
  ACOG/ACMG guidelines, 244t
  amniocentesis, 262
  carrier screening, 239–244
  chorionic villus sampling, 263
  chromosome abnormalities in fetus, 254–260
  cystic fibrosis, 245, 245t
  gamete/embryo donation, 261
  hemoglobinopathies, 251–253
  male factor infertility, 475
  maternal serum screening, 262
  neonatal testing, 262
  neural tube defects, 267t
  pregnancy genetics testing, 261–262
  preimplantation genetic diagnosis, 261
  preimplantation genetic screening, 489–490
  psychiatric medications during pregnancy and breastfeeding, 270t
  recurrent pregnancy loss and, 499, 499f–500f, 501, 501t
  teratogenicity, 268t–269t
  testing, 261–266

genotype-phenotype correlation
  cystic fibrosis, 245–246, 246f
  Fragile X syndrome, 247–248
  spinal muscular atrophy, 249
germ cells
  life history of, 519f
  tumors, 531t, 627–628, 627t, 629t
gestational age
  assessment, 71, 71t
  percentage of survival and, 158f
  periviable birth and, 157, 157f, 157t
  preterm birth prediction and, 151t
  preterm premature rupture of membrane management and, 159–161, 160t
  preterm premature rupture of membranes and, 159–161, 160t
  radiation dose and, 115t
  thyroid function studies and, 230f
gestational diabetes
  management, 179–183, 180t, 181f, 181t, 182, 182t, 183t
  screening for, 178, 178f, 179t
gestational thrombocytopenia, 225, 226t
gestational trophoblastic disease/gestational trophoblastic neoplasia (GTD/GTN), 635, 635t, 636t, 637t, 638t
ginger extract
  nausea and vomiting in pregnancy, 65t
glucocorticoids
  congenital adrenal hyperplasia, 548–549
  contraindications in congenital adrenal hyperplasia treatment, 549
  nausea and vomiting in pregnancy, 65t
  ovulation induction, 478
glucose-lowering agents
  type 2 diabetes, 41t–43t
glucose monitoring
  gestational diabetes, 179
glucose tolerance testing
  polycystic ovarian syndrome, 542, 542t
gonadal dysgenesis, 523
gonadoblastoma, 627t, 628, 629t
gonadotoxicity
  gamete preservation and, 511, 512f

770

INDEX

gonadotropin
  ovarian hyperstimulation syndrome and, 491–494, 492f
  ovulation induction, 478, 482t
  precocious puberty and, 529, 530t
gonadotropin-releasing hormone (GnRH) analogs, 366, 366f, 367t
  fibroid treatment, 385
  gamete preservation, 514
  oral contraceptive-gonadotropin-releasing hormone agonist protocol, 483
  ovulation induction, 478, 483, 483t
gonorrhea
  CDC treatment guidelines, 447t
granulosa-stromal cell tumors, 630, 630t
Graves' disease
  in pregnancy, 232, 233f, 234t, 235t
group B *streptococcus*, 387–393
  culture protocols, 387t
  intrapartum antibiotic prophylaxis, 389t, 390f, 391f, 393f
  prevention guidelines, 388t
  screening/prophylaxis algorithm, 390f, 391f
  secondary prevention in newborns, 392f
gyn-oncology. *See* cancer; specific cancers

H

hair removal systems
  polycystic ovarian syndrome, 545
Hashimoto's disease
  in pregnancy, 236, 237f
HbBarts hydrops fetalis, 251, 252f
headache
  characteristics and classification, 47, 47t
health screening, 1t–9t
heart
  fetal anatomy scan of, 275f
heart disease
  fetal effects, maternal indications, 176f–177t
  in pregnancy, 172–177, 172t–175t
HELLP syndrome, 198t, 199t–200t, 225
hemodynamic measurements, 661, 663f
hemodynamic therapy, 663t
Hemoglobin H disease, 251, 252f
hemoglobinopathies, 251–253
hemolytic disease of fetus and newborn, 209f, 210t

hemorrhage, 674
hemorrhagic stroke
  oral contraceptives, 294
hemostasis
  abnormal uterine bleeding and, 328t
  unsatisfactory, 674
hepatitis, 198t, 199t–200t
  overview, 399t
hepatitis A
  immunization during pregnancy, 433
hepatitis B
  immunization during pregnancy, 433
  progression, 401f
  serologic course, 400f, 402t, 403t
  vaccines, 403, 404t
hepatitis C
  overview, 405, 405t, 406f
hepatotoxicity
  statin therapy, 21
hereditary nonpolyposis colorectal cancer
  ovarian cancer risk, 623
herpes simplex virus (HSV), 450–451, 451t
hirsutism, 552, 553f
homan chorionic gonadotropin (hCG)
  thyroid function studies and, 230f
hormone profiles
  male factor infertility, 474, 474t
  nonfunctional pituitary mass, 563t
  postretrieval hormonal management, ART protocols, 488
  steroid hormone biosynthesis, 550f, 551f
hot flushes, menopausal, 574–575, 574t, 575t
HPV testing
  cervical dysplasia/cervical intraepithelial neoplasia, 601–602, 602t
human chorionic gonadotropin (hCG)
  methotrexate for ectopic pregnancy and, 338, 342f
human immunodeficiency virus (HIV) infection
  antepartum care, 415t, 416t
  delivery procedures and, 419t
  intrapartum care, 418t, 419t
  lack of viral suppression, 417t
  postpartum care, 420t
  pregnancy and, 410–420
  tuberculosis in pregnancy and, 407–408, 409f

human papillomavirus (HPV)
  cervical cancer risk, 615
  cervical dysplasia/cervical intraepithelial neoplasia, 600–601, 600t
  cervical dysplasia/cervical intraepithelial neoplasia cytology, 606f
  immunization during pregnancy, 433, 439f
hydatidiform mole, 635, 635t, 636t
hydralazine
  hypertension management and, 190t
hydrops, nonimmune
  etiology, 207t
  evaluation algorithm, 205f–206f
  therapy, 208t
hydrosalpinx
  ART and, 495t
5-Hydroxytryptamine$_3$-receptor antagonists
  nausea and vomiting in pregnancy, 65t
hyperandrogenism organ dysfunction
  androgen levels, 543t
hypercholesterolemia, 21–28
hyperglycemia
  antihyperglycemic therapy, 39f
hyperlipidemia
  secondary causes, 28t
hyperprolactinemia
  etiology, 556t, 558
  pathophysiology, 554–555, 555f, 555t
  pregnancy and, 560
  prolactin secreting pituitary adenomas, 557, 557f
  treatment, 558–562, 559t, 560t
hypertension, 32–37. *See also* preeclampsia
  antihypertensive agents in pregnancy, 192t, 193t
  classification, 184–186
  hydralazine for management of, 190t
  labetalol for management of, 189t
  management algorithm, 187f–188f
  nifedipine for management of, 191t
  oral contraceptives, 294
  pharmacologic management, 32–33
  postpartum, 197f, 198t
  in pregnancy, 184–200

771

INDEX

hyperthyroidism
 in pregnancy, 232, 233f, 234t, 235t
 recurrent pregnancy loss and, 504
hypogonadal puberty, 523
hypogonadotropic hypogonadism, 524
hypothyroidism
 evaluation and treatment overview, 566t–569t
 peripheral precocious puberty and, 532t
 in pregnancy, 236, 237f
 recurrent pregnancy loss and, 504
 treatment, 569t
hypoxic-ischemic encephalopathy
 shoulder dystocia, 85
hysterectomy
 abdominal, 706
 cervical cancer, 618
 endometrial cancer, 596, 597t
 vaginal, 707
hysteroscopy
 abnormal uterine bleeding, 329
 overview, 369, 369t, 370t
 sterilization, 321, 321t

I

IADPSG algorithm, 178f, 179t
ICSI
 defined, 482
ileus
 cancer patients, 657t
immature teratoma, 627t, 628, 629t
immune hydrops, 205f
immune thrombocytopenia purpura, 225, 226t
immunization. *See also* specific diseases
 adult schedule for, 9f
 during pregnancy, 432t, 433–437, 439t
immunology
 recurrent pregnancy loss and, 506, 507t, 508–509
imperforate hymen, 523
Implanon contraceptive, 284t
implant progestin contraceptive, 311, 312t
inborn errors of metabolism
 nonimmune hydrops, 205t, 206
incontinence
 urinary incontinence, 373t, 374t, 375t, 376t, 377f–378f
induced labor, 76–83
 algorithm for, 83f

infant mortality rates
 late-term/early term deliveries, 79t
infectious disease. *See also* specific diseases
 cancer-related infections, 654f, 655f
 recurrent pregnancy loss and, 505
infertility. *See also* fertility
 advanced fertility treatments, 480–481
 assisted reproductive technologies, 482–494, 482t, 483f, 483t, 484f, 485f, 486f, 487f, 489f, 490t, 492f
 diagnostic evaluation, 466–467
 duration of, 466, 466t
 etiology of, 464t
 fibroids and, 384
 gamete preservation, 511–515, 512f, 513f, 515t
 male factor infertility, 473–476, 473t, 474t, 476f
 maternal age and, 465f
 ovarian reserve, 468–469, 468f, 470t, 471–472, 471f
 overview, 463–464, 464f
 ovulation induction treatment, 477–481, 478t, 480t
 prevalence, 465f
 recurrent pregnancy loss, 497–510, 497t, 498t, 499f, 500f, 501t, 502t, 503t, 506t–507t, 508t, 509t, 510t
 surgical treatment of, 495–496, 495t
influenza
 immunization during pregnancy, 433
inherited anemia, 67t
injectable contraceptives, 308–309
Inova Fairfax Hospital
 venous thromboembolism prophylaxis, 670t
insulin
 gestational diabetes, 180, 180t, 181f, 181t
 in labor and delivery, 182, 182t
 type 2 diabetes, administration guidelines, 40f
insulin-dependent diabetes
 pregnancy and, 183, 183t
insulin resistance
 polycystic ovarian syndrome, 542, 542t
 recurrent pregnancy loss and, 504
insulin-sensitizing drugs
 polycystic ovarian syndrome, 545

integrated screening test, 263t
intensive care unit (ICU)
 early goal-directed therapy, 664
International Federation of Gynecology and Obstetrics (FIGO)
 gestational trophoblastic disease/gestational trophoblastic neoplasia (GTD/GTN), 638t
 leiomyoma classification system, 383, 383f
intra-amniotic infection, 394, 395t
intracranial anatomy
 fetal assessment, 274f
intrapartum antibiotic prophylaxis
 group B *streptococcus*, 389t, 390f, 391f
 HIV in pregnancy and, 418t, 419t
 prevention of early-onset group B streptococcal disease, 392f
 procedures, 460t
 sexual assault patients, STD prevention, 354t
intrapartum care
 HIV in pregnancy and, 418t, 419t
intrapartum fetal evaluation
 amnioinfusion, 124, 124f, 125t
 fetal heart rate patterns, 117t–119t
intrauterine adhesions, 535t
intrauterine devices, 283t–284t, 316, 316t, 317f, 318f
 lost string location algorithm, 318f
intrauterine fetal demise, 201f. *See also* stillbirth
 isoimmunization, 209f
 nonimmune hydrops, 205f–206f, 207t, 208t
 ultrasound diagnosis, 279t
intrauterine growth restriction (IUGR), 167–168, 167t
 ultrasound diagnosis, 279t
intrauterine insemination (IUI), 480
intrauterine resuscitation, 120f, 121t
invasive cardiac monitoring, 660, 660f
in vitro fertilization (IVF)
 birth defects risk, 490, 490t
 definition, 482
 diminished ovarian reserve screening and, 471–472, 471f
 donor egg IVF, 482
 embryo transfer, 488, 488t, 489f
 endometrioma removal and, 495–496
 oral contraceptive-gonadotropin-releasing hormone agonist protocol, 483, 483f
 preimplantation genetic screening, 489–490

772

INDEX

iron supplements
  in pregnancy, 66
Irving tubal ligation, 320f
ischemic stroke
  oral contraceptives, 294
isoimmunization, 209f, 210t, 211–212

J

Japanese encephalitis
  immunization during pregnancy, 436

K

Kallmann syndrome, 524
Kroener fimbriectomy, 320f

L

labetalol
  hypertension management and, 189t
labor. *See also* delivery
  abnormal labor/induction of labor, 76–83
  cesarean delivery, 91–99
  induction algorithm, 83f
  infant mortality rates, late term/early term deliveries, 79t, 80t–83t
  insulin management during, 182, 182t
  multiple gestation and presentation, 163f
  normal labor, 74f, 74t, 75f
  operative vaginal delivery, 86–91
  pregnancy complications, 80t–83t
  preterm labor, 148–151, 148f, 152t, 153–154, 153f, 154t, 155f, 156t
  trauma in pregnancy and, 113f
  vaginal birth after cesarean, 100–102
laboratory testing
  abnormal uterine bleeding, 327
  hirsutism, 552
  infertility, 466
  lab values, 689–690
  polycystic ovarian syndrome, 540t
  preeclampsia, 192t
  prenatal visits, 60t
laparoscopic tubal ligation, 319
  operative report, 705
laparoscopy
  ectopic pregnancy, 338, 339f
  ovarian cautery/drilling, 479, 479t

overview, 368
tubal patency testing, 467
laser-assisted hair removal
  polycystic ovarian syndrome, 545
latent TB infection (LTBI), 407–408, 409f
LDL-C response
  hypercholesterolemia, 21
least function score
  endometriosis fertility index, 364, 364t, 365f
leiomyoma
  classification, 383, 383f
letrozole
  gamete preservation and, 512, 512f
  ovulation induction, 477, 478t
  resistance to, alternative options, 478
Levonorgestrel IUD, 317f
levonorgestrel-releasing intrauterine system (IUS)
  fibroid treatment, 385
Leydic cell tumor
  peripheral precocious puberty, 531t
lichen sclerosus
  vulvar dystrophies, 379
lifestyle counseling
  hypercholesterolemia, 21
  hypertension, 32–34, 33t
  polycystic ovarian syndrome, 477
lipid lowering drugs, 29t–30t
liver cancer
  oral contraceptives and, 297
liver disease in pregnancy, 198t, 199t–200t
long axis left ventricle scan, 275f
low back pain, 51–52, 51f, 52t
  diagnostic evaluation, 51f
  nonsurgical management of, 52t
lumbar/sacral nerve plexuses, 694f
luteal-gonadotropin-releasing hormone agonist protocol
  ovarian stimulation, 484, 484f
luteal phase
  deficiency, recurrent pregnancy loss and, 504
  menstrual cycle, 517, 518f
Lynch syndrome
  ovarian cancer risk, 623

M

macroadenomas
  hyperprolactinemia, 557–559
  in pregnancy, 560
macrocytic anemia, 68t

macrosomia
  shoulder dystocia risk and, 84t
Madiener tubal ligation, 320f
magnesium sulfate
  fetal neuroprotection, 155f, 156t
  toxicity, 191t
magnetic resonance imaging (MRI)
  breast cancer screening, 681t
male factor infertility, 473–476, 473t, 474t, 476f
mammography
  guidelines for, 680t
Manchester scoring system
  breast cancer screening, 685t
mastitis, 397–398, 397f
maternal age
  fetal chromosome abnormalities incidence and, 255t
maternal morbidity and mortality
  cesarean delivery, 98t
  chorioamnionitis, 394, 395t
  ectopic pregnancy, 336f
  epilepsy and, 228
  febrile morbidity and endomyometritis, 396
  maternal heart disease, 172–177
  postpartum hemorrhage, 132, 132t
  preeclampsia, 194t
  thrombocytopenia, 225, 226t
  thromboembolic disorders, 219–223
  twin gestation, 162, 163t
  vaginal birth after cesarean, 101t
  varicella and, 421
maternal serum screening (MSS), 262
  aneuploidies, pregnancy outcomes, 265t
  no evident aneuploidy, 266t
Mayer-Rokitansky-Kuster-Hauser syndrome, 523, 534t
McCune-Albright syndrome, 530, 532t
McRobert's maneuver
  shoulder dystocia, 84
mean corpuscular volume (MCV)
  anemias and, 68t
measles, mumps, rubella (MMR) vaccine
  immunization during pregnancy, 433–434
medications. *See also* specific drugs
  abnormal uterine bleeding, 330t
  contraindications during pregnancy, 271t
  psychiatric medications, 270t
  teratogenicity, 268t–269t
  urinary incontinence, 375t

773

INDEX

meningococcal vaccine
  immunization during pregnancy, 434
menopause
  abnormal uterine bleeding after, 333f
  hormone replacement therapy, 589
  hot flushes, 574–575, 574t, 575
  management algorithm, 573f
  overview, 571
  postmenopausal osteoporosis, 581–588
  spectrum definitions, 572t
  stages of, 571t
  symptom management, 575t, 576t
  transdermal estrogen for, 578t
  vaginal estrogen products, 579t–580t
  vaginal symptoms, 577t
  vasomotor symptoms, 576t
menstrual cycle
  normal bleeding parameters for, 323t, 519t
  normal reproductive cycle, 517, 518f, 519t
mentocervical diameter
  vacuum extraction delivery, 90f, 91
metabolic acidosis, 675f
metformin
  ovulation induction and, 477
  polycystic ovarian syndrome, 545
methimazole
  hyperthyroidism in pregnancy and, 232
methotrexate
  contraindications in ectopic pregnancy for, 340t
  ectopic pregnancy, 338, 339f, 340t, 341t, 343t
  limitations and failures in ectopic pregnancy of, 342f, 342t
methylprednisolone
  cleft deformities and, 61
metoclopramide
  nausea and vomiting in pregnancy and, 61
microadenomas
  hyperprolactinemia, 557–559
  in pregnancy, 560
microcytic anemia, 68t
microdose gonadotropin-releasing hormone agonist flare stimulation protocol, 484, 485f
middle cerebral artery
  Doppler evaluation, 210

mifepristone/misoprostol
  spontaneous abortion management, 350t
  uterine fibroids, 386
migraine headache
  classification, 285t
  evolution over time, 49t
  preventive treatment, 50t
  triptan therapy, 48t–49t
migraine headaches, 47–50
  characteristics and classification, 47, 47t
  preventive treatment, 50t
minerals
  DRI/RDA intake guidelines, 14t
monozygotic twinning, 162t
MRSA infections, 461t
Müllerian agenesis, 523, 534t
multiple gestation, 162–166, 162t
myeloid growth factors
  neutropenic fever management, 656f
myocardial infarction
  oral contraceptives, 294

N

NAEPP asthma classification, 170t
National Comprehensive Cancer Network (NCCN)
  break-through chemotherapy, 649f
  cancer pain management guidelines, 640f
  cancer-related infections, 654f, 655f
  emesis control, 641f
  emetogenic potential, chemotherapy, 645f, 646f, 647f, 648f
  emetogenic potential antineoplastic agents, 642f, 643f
  low-risk outpatient therapy, 651f, 652f
  neutropenic fever management, 650f, 653f, 656f
nausea, in pregnancy, 61–65
  management algorithm for, 63f
  pharmacologic treatment, 61, 63f. 64t–65t
neonatal care
  antepartum fetal surveillance, 105t
  Apgar score, 104t
  genetics testing and, 262
  group B *streptococcus* secondary prevention and, 392f
  maternal varicella and, 421
  resuscitation algorithm, 103f

neonatal morbidity and mortality
  cesarean and vaginal birth after cesarean deliveries, 102t
  epilepsy and, 228
  twin gestation, 162, 163f
neonatal resuscitation, 103f
neural tube defects
  pathophysiology, 267t
neutropenic fever management, 650f, 653f, 656f
Nexplanon, 311, 312t
nifedipine
  hypertension management and, 191t
nonimmune hydrops
  etiology, 207t
  evaluation algorithm, 205f–206f
  therapy, 208t
noninvasive prenatal testing (NIPT), 261–262
nonneoplastic epithelial disorders
  vulvar dystrophies, 379
nonpharmacological treatment
  nausea and vomiting in pregnancy, 61
non-Rhesus-D antibodies
  hemolytic disease of fetus and newborn, 209f, 210t, 211f, 212f
nonstress test
  fetal assessment, 105
normocytic anemia, 68t
nuchal translucency test, 264t
nutrition
  body mass index (BMI) nomogram, 15f, 16t–17t
  body mass index (BMI) table, 18t
  elements, DRI/RDA intake guidelines, 14t
  food purchase recommendations, single person, 10t–11t
  in pregnancy, 66
  vitamins, DRI/RDA intake guidelines, 12t–13t
NuvaRing contraceptive, 283t

O

obesity
  recurrent pregnancy loss and, 504
odansteron (zofran)
  contraindicated medications with, 61t
  nausea and vomiting in pregnancy and, 61
older adults
  screening, prevention, and counseling recommendations for, 4t–5t

774

INDEX

Ontario family history assessment tool breast cancer screening, 684t
oocyte cryopreservation, 513
oocyte retrieval protocols, 486–487, 487f
oophoropexy (ovarian transposition), 514
operative reports, 701–707
operative vaginal delivery, 86–91. *See also* forceps delivery; vacuum extraction
  ACOG summary recommendations, 87t
  risk assessment, 87t
oral contraceptive-gonadotropin-releasing hormone antagonist protocol
  ovarian stimulation, 485, 486f
oral contraceptives, 283t, 292–306
  cancer and, 296–297, 297t
  currently available compounds, 302t–305t
  emergency postcoital oral contraception, 313, 313t, 314t–315t
  management issues, 300–301, 301f
  metabolic effects, 294–295
  ovarian stimulation protocols and doses, 483–486, 483f–486f
  overview, 292
  polycystic ovarian syndrome, 544
  progestin only compounds, 306
  reproduction and, 298–299, 298f
  steroid components, 292, 293t
oral desensitization protocol
  pregnancy and penicillin allergy and, 452t, 453t
oral hypoglycemics
  in pregnancy, 181
osteoporosis, postmenopausal, 581–588
  diagnostic testing, 584t
  fracture risk assessment tool, 582
  management algorithm, 583f
  prevalence and incidence, 581, 581f, 582f
  therapeutic response assessment, 585
  treatment, 586t–588t
ovarian cancer
  epithelial, 623–624
  germ cell tumors, 627–628, 627f, 629t
  oral contraceptives and, 296
  sex cord-stromal cell tumors, 630, 630t
  staging and treatment, 625t, 626

ovarian cautery/drilling, 479, 479t
ovarian cysts
  oral contraceptives and, 301
  peripheral precocious puberty, 531t
ovarian hyperstimulation syndrome (OHSS), 491–494, 492f
ovarian insufficiency
  PCOS diagnosis *vs.*, 539t
ovarian reserve
  diminished ovarian reserve, 471–472, 471f
  tests for, 467–471
ovarian stimulation protocols and doses, 483–486, 483f–486f
ovarian tissue cryopreservation and transplantation, 513
ovulation induction
  clomiphene/letrozole resistance, 477–478, 478t
  glucocorticoids, 478
  gonadotropins for, 478
  overview, 477
  for PCOS patients, 477, 478t

P

pain management
  NCCN cancer pain management guidelines, 640f
  postoperative gynecological patients, 371, 371t, 372t
PALM-COEIN abnormal uterine bleeding classification, 324f
pan ethnic genetic screening, 241
Pap test
  cervical dysplasia/cervical intraepithelial neoplasia, 601–602
parathyroid hormone
  osteoporosis treatment, 587t
Parkland tubal ligation, 320f
PARP inhibitors
  ovarian cancer, 626
patient-controlled analgesia
  postoperative gynecological patients, 371t
pedigree assessment tool (PAT)
  breast cancer screening, 686t
pelvic inflammatory disease (PID)
  sexually transmitted disease and, 454–456, 456t
pelvic pain
  evaluation of, 355–356
  primary dysmenorrhea, 359t
  treatment, 357t–358t
pelvimetry, clinical, 69–70, 69f, 69t–70t

pelvis
  blood supply, 693f
  classification, 69t
  measurement, 70t
Perinatal Quality Foundation, 281
peritoneal cancer
  staging and treatment, 625t
periviable birth, 157, 157f, 157t
pharmacologic treatment
  nausea and vomiting in pregnancy, 61, 63f. 64t–65t
phenothiazines
  nausea and vomiting in pregnancy, 61, 64t
pitocin, 78–79
pituitary gland
  nonfunctional pituitary mass, 563t
  size and serum PRL levels, 557f
  tumors, 558
placenta accreta
  cesarean delivery, 99t
placental abruption, 126–127, 126t, 127t, 128f
placental assessment
  intrauterine fetal demise, 201f
placenta previa, 129–131
  cesarean delivery, 99t
  evaluation, 131f
  management, 130
  risk factors, 130
  types of, 129f
placentation
  multiple gestation, 162
pneumococcal vaccines
  immunization during pregnancy, 434
polio vaccine (IPV)
  immunization during pregnancy, 434
polycystic ovarian syndrome (PCOS)
  androgen elevation, 541t
  diagnostic criteria, 537t
  glucose tolerance testing, 542, 542t
  incidence and prevalence, 537
  ovulation induction and, 477, 478t
  patient evaluation, 540f
  recurrent pregnancy loss and, 504
  treatment, 543–545, 543t
  ultrasound criteria, 538, 538t, 539t, 540t, 541f
  virilizing ovarian/adrenal tumor, 542, 542f, 543t
Pomeroy tubal ligation, 320f
postoperative management
  gynecological surgery, 371, 371t, 372t

775

INDEX

postpartum care
  HIV in pregnancy and, 420t
postpartum hemorrhage, 132–139
  blood component therapy, 133t
  B-Lynch suture for, 138f
  etiology and risk factors, 132
  management algorithm, 135f–136f, 137
  maternal adaptation to blood loss, 132t
  tamponade treatment, 139f
  uterine artery ligation, 137f
  uterotonic therapy, 134t
postpartum hypertension, 197f, 198t
postpartum oral contraceptive use, 299
postpartum tubal ligation, 319
postpill amenorrhea, 299
preeclampsia. See also hypertension
  chronic hypertension and, 186, 186t
  diagnostic criteria, 184t
  features of, 184t
  imitators of, 198t, 199t–200t
  laboratory evaluation of, 192t
  management algorithm, 187f–188f
  maternal complications, 194t
  recurrence risk assessment, 196t
  risk factors, 185t, 186t
  thrombocytopenia and, 225, 226t
pregnancy
  asthma in, 169, 169t, 170t, 171t
  cervical cancer management, 619f
  complications, timing of delivery and, 80t–82t
  congenital adrenal hyperplasia in, 548–549
  contraindicated medications in, 271t
  ectopic pregnancy, 336, 336f, 337t, 338, 338t, 339f, 340t, 341t, 342t, 343t
  failed pregnancy, ultrasonography, 279t
  first trimester failure, management of, 349t, 350t, 351t
  genetics testing in, 261–262
  human immunodeficiency virus (HIV) infection during, 410–420
  immunization during, 432t, 433t–437t, 439t
  intrauterine device and risk of, 316t
  nausea and vomiting in, 61–65
  nutrition in, 66
  oral contraceptive use during, 298
  oral desensitization protocol, penicillin allergy and, 452t, 453t
  PCOS diagnosis vs., 539t
  prolactinomas in, 560
  psychiatric medications during, 270t
  recurrent pregnancy loss, 497–510
  sterilization methods and risk of, 322t
  thyroid disease screening and, 566t–569t
  trauma in, 112f–113f
  tuberculosis in, 407–408, 409f
  of unknown location (PUL), 344–345, 344f, 346f
  urinary tract infections in, 440–443, 440f, 441f, 442f, 443t
  uterine fibroid complications during, 384f
prehypertension, 32
preimplantation genetic diagnosis (PGD), 261
  in vitro fertilization, 489–490
prenatal visits
  documentation and review guidelines, 59
  routine laboratory testing, 60t
preterm birth, 148–150, 148f
  gestational age and risk of, 151t
  periviable birth, 157, 157t, 158f
  prediction, 151, 151t
  prevention algorithm, 149f
  progestogen guidelines for, 150t
  risk assessment, 152t
  screening and treatment algorithm, 149f, 150
  tocolytics for prevention of, 154t
  triage protocol for, 153t
  umbilical cord gas values for arterial blood in, 125t
preterm labor
  antenatal streroids and, 153–154
  diagnosis, 148
  fetal fibronectin testing, 152t
  intrapartum prophylaxis during, 390f
  magnesium sulfate, for neuroprotection, 155f, 156f
  overview, 148
  pathways, 148f
  predicted probability, 151, 151t
  prevention algorithm, 149f–150f
  progestogens for prevention of, 150t
  risk assessment, 152t
  tocolytics for, 154t
  triage protocol, 153f
preterm premature rupture of membranes (PPROM), 159–161, 160t
  intrapartum antibiotic prophylaxis for, 391f
primary care, 1–57
  health screening, 1t–9t
primary dysmenorrhea treatment, 359t
progesterone
  ulipristal acetate (progesterone receptor modulator), fibroid treatment, 385
progestin
  endometriosis management, 360, 361t
  implant contraceptives, 311, 312t
  in oral contraceptives, 292, 293t, 306
  polycystic ovarian syndrome, 544
progestoten
  preterm labor prevention, 150t
prolactin
  biochemistry, 554, 554t
  PCOS diagnosis, 538t
  prolactin secreting pituitary adenomas, 557, 557f
prolactinomas, 557, 557f
  in pregnancy, 560
prolapsed membranes
  reduction of, 147f
propylthiouracil (PTU)
  hyperthyroidism in pregnancy and, 232
prostaglandin analogues
  labor induction and, 77t
prothrombin G20210A mutation
  recurrent pregnancy loss and, 505
psychiatric medications
  during pregnancy and breastfeeding, 270t
puberty
  central/true precocious puberty, 529, 530t
  defined, 520
  delayed or interrupted puberty, 523–524, 525t
  onset, 520, 521f
  peripheral precocious puberty, 530, 531t–532t
  physical changes, 520
  Tanner staging, 522f, 522t
  variants and precocious puberty, 526, 526t, 527t, 528t, 529t

INDEX

pulmonary artery-ductus arteriosus scan, 276f
pulmonary embolism
 diagnostic algorithm, 668f
 incidence in pregnancy, 219, 219t

Q

quad screening test, 263t

R

radiation-induced teratogenesis, 115t
radiation therapy
 cervical cancer, 618
 fetal absorption, 115t–116t
 hyperprolactinemia, 562
radical trachelectomy
 cervical cancer, 618
RANK ligand inhibitor
 osteoporosis treatment, 587t
rape tray contents, 352
reciprocal translocations
 recurrent pregnancy loss, 499, 499f–500f, 501, 501t
recurrent pregnancy loss, 497–510
 antiphospholipid syndrome, 506, 507t, 508–509
 definitions, 498
 endocrine factors, 504
 etiology, 498t
 genetic factors, 499, 499f
 incidence and prevalence, 497, 497t
 livebirth prognosis, 510t
 microbiologic factors, 505
 treatment options, 509–510, 509t, 510t
 uterine anomalies, 502–503, 503f
recurrent sinusitis, 53
red blood cell production
 anemias and, 67t
red cell alloimmunized pregnancy, 211f
referral scoring tool
 breast cancer screening, 687t
reproductive function
 normal menstrual parameters, 519t
 normal reproductive cycle, 519f
 oral contraceptives and, 298–299, 298t
respiratory distress syndrome, 72–73, 73t
Robertsonian translocations
 recurrent pregnancy loss, 499, 499f–500f, 501, 501t

round cells
 semen analysis, 474
Royal College of Obstetrics and Gynecology (RCOG)
 recurrent pregnancy loss definition, 498
rubella, 422, 423f
 immunization during pregnancy, 433–434
Rubin's Screw Maneuver
 shoulder dystocia, 84
"Rule of 5s"
 for ovulation induction, 478t
"Rule of 7s"
 for ovulation induction, 478t

S

salpingectomy
 ectopic pregnancy, 338, 339f
Sawyer syndrome, 524
seizures
 eclampsia, 193t–195t
 epilepsy, in pregnancy, 227–228
semen analysis
 male factor infertility, 473–476, 473t
Sephardic Jewish disorders, 242–243, 242t
sepsis syndrome, 672
sequential stepwise screening test, 263t
Sertoli-stromal cell tumors, 630, 630t
serum integrated screening test, 264t
sex chromosome abnormalities, 254
sex cord-stromal cell tumors, 630, 630t
sexual assault
 follow-up care, 354
 patient evaluation, 352, 353f
 STD prophylaxis options, 354t
sexually transmitted disease (STD)
 CDC 2015 guidelines, 447t–448t
 diagnostic testing, 446t
 external genital warts, 457t, 458t
 herpes simplex virus, 450–451, 451t
 pelvic inflammatory disease and, 454–456, 456t
 sexual assault patients, prophylaxis options, 354t
 syphilis, 452t, 453t
 ulcerative lesions, 449t
Shirodkar cerclage, modification, 143, 145f
short axis of great vessels scan, 276f
shoulder dystocia, 84–85, 84t
sickle cell disease, 253

side effects
 injectable contraceptives, 308–309
 intrauterine devices, 316f
 progestin-only oral contraceptives, 306
 transdermal contraceptives, 307
Siegler, Dennis, 639
sinusitis, 53–54, 54t
small bowel obstruction
 cancer patients, 657t
smallpox vaccine (vaccinia)
 immunization during pregnancy, 436–437
smoking
 cessation therapy agents, 44t–45t
Society for Maternal-fetal Medicine
 progestogens for preterm birth prevention, 150t
sonohysterography
 abnormal uterine bleeding, 329
Spanish primer, 709–716
spermatogenesis
 male factor infertility, 474t, 475–476, 476f
sperm cryopreservation, 511
spermicide contraception, 283t, 291
spinal muscular atrophy (SMA)
 carrier screening, 244t, 249–250, 250f
 classification, 249t
 pathophysiology and genetics, 249–250
spironolactone
 polycystic ovarian syndrome, 544
sponge contraception, 283t
spontaneous abortion
 management of, 349t, 350t, 351t
 recurrent pregnancy loss, 497, 497t
spontaneous labor algorithm, 75f
sporadic miscarriage
 incidence and prevalence, 497, 497t
squamous cell hyperplasia
 atypical squamous cells: cannot exclude high-grade SIL, 608f, 609f
 atypical squamous cells of undetermined significance (ASC-US), 606f
 high-grade squamous intraepithelial lesion (HSIL), 609f
 low-grade squamous intraepithelial lesions, 607f, 608f
 vulvar dystrophies, 379
Stanford Hospital Guide
 thromboembolic prevention guidelines, 669t

777

INDEX

Stanford University Medical Center Laboratory
  lab values, 689
statin therapy
  initiation, 21–22, 23f–26f
  intensity level of treatment, 22t
  non-ASCVD patients, 25f–26f
  properties of statins, 31t
  therapeutic response and adherence, 27f
sterilization, 284t
  female, 319, 320f, 321, 321t, 322t
  pregnancy rates by methods, 322t
steroid hormones
  biosynthesis, 550f, 551f
steroids
  in oral contraceptives, 292, 293t
  table of, 659t
stillbirth
  evaluation of, 202t–204t
  intrauterine fetal demise, 201f
  risk assessment and testing guidelines, 109t–111t
superovulation treatment, 480
  ovarian hyperstimulation syndrome and, 491–494, 492f
surgical patients
  complementary medicine effects in, 57t
syphilis, 452t, 453t
systemic lupus erythematosus (SLE) in pregnancy
  classification criteria, 213t–216t
  common complaints, 216
  laboratory tests, 216
systolic/diastolic blood flow (S/D ratio)
  fetal assessment, 107

T

tamponade treatment
  postpartum hemorrhage, 139f
tension-type headache
  characteristics and classification, 47, 47t
teratogenecity
  OTC medications, 268t–269t
teratoma, immature, 627t, 628, 629t
testosterone
  virilizing adrenal or ovarian tumor, 542, 542f
tetanus, diphtheria, and pertussis/tetanus diphtheria (Tdap/Td)
  immunization during pregnancy, 434–435

tetanus prophylaxis, 459t
thrombocytopenia, 225, 226t
thromboembolic disorders
  anticoagulation regimen, 221t, 671t
  diagnosis, 220, 220t
  incidence in pregnancy, 219
  phenomena in, 666, 667f, 668f, 669f
  prevention guidelines, 669t
  recurrence prevention and risk, 223t
  risk assessment, 219t
  thromboprophylaxis, 221t–222t
  venous thromboembolism prophylaxis, 670t
thrombophilias
  incidence in pregnancy, 219, 219t
  recurrent pregnancy loss and, 505
  testing for, 219t
  thromboprophylaxis for, 221t–222t
thromboprophylaxis
  thrombophilia in pregnancy, 221t–222t
thyroid disease. *See also* hyperthyroidism; hypothyroidism
  dysfunction evaluation algorithm, 564f
  hyperthyroidism, 232, 233f, 234t, 235t
  hypothyroidism, 236, 237f
  overview, 564
  PCOS diagnosis and, 538t
  in pregancy, 230f–231f, 231t
  pregnancy and screening for, 566t–569t
  recurrent pregnancy loss and, 504
  thyroid function test, 565t
thyroid function test, 565t
  in pregnancy, 230f, 231f, 231t
thyroid hormones
  gestational age and, 230f, 231f
thyroid stimulating hormone
  gestational age and nomogram of, 231f
thyroid storm
  diagnostic criteria, 234t
  management algorithm, pregnancy, 235f
thyrotoxicosis, maternal complications from, 232
thyroxine levels
  hyperthyroidism in pregnancy and, 232
tobacco use, 44t–45t

tocolytics
  preterm birth prevention, 154t
TOLAC delivery technique, 100–102
Top Ten Ways to Survive Gyn-oncology, 639
total body radiography
  nonimmune hydrops, 205t, 206
total motile count (TMC)
  semen analysis, 473
toxoplasmosis, 424, 424f, 425t, 426f
trachelectomy, radical
  cervical cancer, 618
tranexamic acid
  uterine fibroids, 386
transabdominal cerclage, 143, 146f
transdermal contraceptives, 307
transdermal estrogen
  menopausal therapy with, 578t
transfusion
  Duke University obstetric bleeding emergency transfusion algorithm, 133t
transsphenoidal microsurgical resection
  hyperprolactinemia, 561–562
transvaginal cervical length
  ultrasound measurement, 280–281, 280f
transvaginal ultrasonography, 277–278, 277f
  abnormal uterine bleeding, 329
  embryonic heart activity, 498t
  placenta previa, 130f, 131f
trauma
  in pregnancy, 112f–113f
travel
  immunization during pregnancy for, 436
trichomoniasis
  CDC treatment guidelines, 448t
triple lumen catheter, 660, 660f
triple screening test, 263t
triptans
  migraine headaches, 48t–49t
tubal factor-hydrosalpinges, 495
tubal ligation
  laparoscopic, 319
  operative reports, 703, 705
  postpartum, 319
  reversal, 495
tubal patency testing, 466–467
tuberculosis
  in pregnancy, 407–408, 409f
Turner syndrome, 523
TWEAK screening test
  alcohol abuse, 46t

INDEX

twins
  delivery management, 164, 164t, 165–166, 165f
  labor and presentation of, 163t
  management of, 162–166, 162t
  morbidity and mortality rates, 163t, 164t
twin to twin transfusion syndrome (TTTS), 164, 164t
  nonimmune hydrops, 205f
type 1 diabetes. *See* insulin-dependent diabetes
type 2 diabetes
  antihyperglycemic therapy, 39f
  glucose-lowering agents, 41t–43t
  initial evaluation, 38t–39t
  insulin adminstration guidelines, 40f
typhoid
  immunization during pregnancy, 436

U

Uchida tubal ligation, 320f
ulcerative lesions in STI, 449t
ulipristal acetate (progesterone receptor modulator)
  fibroid treatment, 385
ultrasonography
  abnormal uterine bleeding, 329
  aneuploidy markers, 259t–260t
  ectopic pregnancy, 337t
  endovaginal, 277f
  fetal anatomy scan, 273f–276f
  placental abruption, 127t
  placenta previa, 130t
  polycystic ovarian syndrome, 538, 538t, 539t, 540f, 541f
  pregnancy failure, 279t
  pregnancy of unknown location (PUL), 344–345, 344f, 346f
  transvaginal, 277–278, 277f
  transvaginal cervical length, 280–281, 280f
umbilical artery Dopplers, 107
umbilical cord gas assessment, 125t
ureter
  anatomy, 691f
urinary incontinence, 373t, 374t, 375t, 376t, 377f–378t
urinary tract infections (UTIs)
  in pregnancy, 440–443, 440f, 441f, 442f, 443t
urine samples
  drug abuse detection limits, 45t
urine storage/bladder filling therapy, 376t

urogynecology, 373t, 374t, 375t, 376t, 377f–378t
uterine anomalies
  acquired, 503
  congenital, 502, 503f
uterine artery ligation, 137f
uterine bleeding
  abnormal, 323–334
uterine fibroids and polyps
  abnormal uterine bleeding and, 384
  infertility and, 384, 495
  prevalence and classification, 383, 383t
  treatment, 385–386
uterine incision
  cesarean delivery, 96, 97f
uterine inversion, 140, 141f
uterine rupture
  shoulder dystocia and, 85
  vaginal birth after cesarean, 101t
uterotonic therapy
  post partum hemorrhage, 134t
uterus
  hysteroscopic evaluation of, 369t

V

vaccines. *See also* specific diseases
  hepatitis B, 403, 404t
  medical indications for, 9f
  during pregnancy, 432t, 433–437, 439t
  varicella, 421
vacuum extraction, 89–91, 89t, 90f–91f
vaginal birth after cesarean (VBAC), 100–102
  clinical practice guidelines, 101t
  risk assessment, 101t
vaginal cancer, 634f
vaginal contraceptive ring, 310
vaginal delivery
  operative, 86–91
vaginal hysterectomy, 707
vaginal septum, 523
vaginitis, 444t, 445t
valvular heart disease
  maternal, pregnancy and, 174t–175t
varicella, 421
  immunization during pregnancy, 435
vas deferens congenital anomalies
  CTFR mutations, 245, 245t
venous thromboembolism (VTE)
  incidence in pregnancy, 219, 219t
  oral contraceptives, 294

prophylaxis, 670t
recurrence risk of, 223t
risk assessment and prevention, 223t
vibroacoustic stimulation (VAS)
  fetal assessment, 105
viral hepatitis. *See* hepatitis
viral suppression
  HIV in pregnancy and absence of, 417t
virilizing adrenal tumor, 542, 542f
  peripheral precocious puberty and, 532t
virilizing ovarian tumor, 542, 542f
vitamin B6
  nausea and vomiting in pregnancy, 61, 64t
vitamin K supplementation
  epilepsy in pregnancy and, 229
vitamins
  DRI/RDA intake guidelines, 12t–13t
vomiting
  emesis control in cancer therapy, 641f
  emetogenic potential, antineoplastic agents, 642f, 643f, 644f
  emetogenic potential, chemotherapy, 645f, 646f, 647f, 648f
  management algorithm for, 63f
  pharmacologic treatment, 61, 63f. 64t–65t
  in pregnancy, 61–65
vulvar cancer, 632–633, 633f
vulvar dystrophies, 379
vulvar intraepithelial neoplasia (VIN), 631, 631f
vulvodynia, 380f, 381t–382t
vulvovaginal candidiasis, 445t

W

weight gain
  oral contraceptives and, 301
  in pregnancy, 66, 66t
weight loss
  polycystic ovarian syndrome, 477, 543
WHO prognostic scoring
  gestational trophoblastic disease/gestational trophoblastic neoplasia (GTD/GTN), 637t
Wilms' tumor, 524
withdrawal contraception, 283t
women
  cardiovascular disease in, 19t, 20f
  colorectal cancer and adenoma screening for, 6t

INDEX

Wood's Screw
    shoulder dystocia, 85

X

X-linked inheritance
    Fragile X syndrome, 247
XMAS mnemonic for primary amenorrhea, 534t

Y

Y-chromosome microdeletions
    spermatogenic impairment, 475–476, 476f
yellow fever
    immunization during pregnancy, 437

Z

Zavenelli maneuver
    shoulder dystocia, 85
Zika virus, 428–429, 430f, 431t
Zoster vaccine
    immunization during pregnancy, 436
zygote intrafallopian transfer, 482